QUANTITATIVE MRI OF THE SPINAL CORD

Academic Press is an imprint of Elsevier
525 B Street, Suite 1800, San Diego, CA 92101-4495, USA
32 Jamestown Road, London NW1 7BY, UK
225 Wyman Street, Waltham, MA 02451, USA

Notices
No responsibility is assumed by the publisher for any injury and/or damage to persons or property as
a matter of products liability, negligence or otherwise, or from any use or operation of any methods,
products, instructions or ideas contained in the material herein.

Because of rapid advances in the medical sciences, in particular, independent verification of diagnoses
and drug dosages should be made.

British Library Cataloguing-in-Publication Data
A catalogue record for this book is available from the British Library

Library of Congress Cataloging-in-Publication Data
A catalog record for this book is available from the Library of Congress

ISBN: 978-0-12-396973-6

For information on all Academic Press publications
visit our website at elsevierdirect.com

Typeset by TNQ Books and Journals
www.tnq.co.in

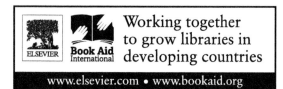

Dedication

To my parents, my sister and to Serge,
J.C.A

To my family,
C.W.K

Contents

I

QUANTITATIVE BIOMARKERS IN THE SPINAL CORD: WHAT FOR?

1.1 Rationale for Quantitative MRI of the Human Spinal Cord and Clinical Applications

KHALED ABDEL-AZIZ, OLGA CICCARELLI

1.2 Inflammatory Demyelinating Diseases

ISTVAN PIRKO, CHARLES R.G. GUTTMANN

1.3A Traumatic Spinal Cord Injury: Acute Spinal Cord Injury and Prognosis

DAVID W. CADOTTE, MICHAEL G. FEHLINGS

1.3B Traumatic Spinal Cord Injury: Chronic Spinal Cord Injury and Recovery

JOHN KRAMER, PATRICK FREUND, ARMIN CURT

II

PHYSICS OF MRI

2.1 Array Coils

JULIEN COHEN-ADAD, LAWRENCE L. WALD

2.2 B_0 Inhomogeneity and Shimming

JÜRGEN FINSTERBUSCH

Preface

According to the legend, in about 250 AD, Saint Denis, the first bishop of Paris, had his head chopped off. He then picked up his head and walked about 10 kilometers from Montmartre to his grave. There have been multiple reports of *cephalophoria* (from the greek *képhalê*, head and *phorein*, carry), which is an episode where a decapitated character gets up, picks up his head, and carries on walking. These stories suggest a great deal about the role of the spinal cord, which is not simply a relay between the brain and the peripheral system, but is also capable of generating complex functional patterns, adapting and reorganizing itself. About 1700 years later, magnetic resonance imaging (MRI) made it possible to "see" the spinal cord from outside the body, providing new elements to elucidate the enigma of *cephalophoria*.

Why this book? MRI of the spinal cord has tremendous potential for improving diagnosis/prognosis in neurodegenerative diseases and trauma as well as for developing and monitoring treatment strategies. In particular, quantitative techniques are being developed that provide a variety of imaging biomarkers sensitive to tissue integrity and neuronal function. Although most of these techniques have been validated and applied in the brain over the past 20 years, quantitative spinal cord MRI is underutilized, both in research and in the clinic, which is a direct consequence of the difficulties related to the numerous artifacts and low signal sensitivity that characterizes the spine region. Even though recent developments in a number of areas, including phased-array coils, acquisition protocols, and processing techniques, helped improving and sometimes overcoming some of the challenges, only modest efforts have been dedicated to make these developments available to the broader community of researchers and clinicians. To date, there is no consensus on how to apply these techniques to the spinal cord. As a consequence, only very few multidisciplinary centers around the world can benefit from state-of-the-art quantitative techniques of the spinal cord. Although there are several books on quantitative MRI of the brain, including the excellent book of Paul Tofts, there are none dedicated to quantitative MRI of the spinal cord. This gives the rationale for having a textbook that reviews and synthesizes recent scientific advances on quantitative techniques in the spinal cord with contributions from many leaders in this research field.

What's in the book? After presenting in section 1 the major clinical needs for quantitative markers of the spinal cord, section 2 covers the hardware and technical challenges inherent to spinal cord imaging. Section 3 then focuses on structural quantitative techniques (diffusion, magnetization transfer, relaxation, atrophy measurements), section 4 on functional and vascular characterization, while section 5 is dedicated to metabolic measurements using magnetic resonance spectroscopy.

The purpose of this book is clear: focus on the technical aspects of spinal cord MRI for an easier translation to their clinical use. Description of cutting edge research techniques as well as more established methods are included. Acquisition and analysis aspects are covered. The majority of the book contains technical details on each quantitative technique. However, it remains accessible for most researchers/clinicians familiar with MRI who wish to apply these techniques. Most existing books on spinal cord MRI focus on qualitative rather than quantitative techniques used in clinical routine, e.g., T1/T2/PD-weighted MRI. Our book essentially focuses on quantitative spinal cord MRI from a technical point of view aiding adoption by a wider community. Moreover this textbook includes "cooking recipes" (wherever applicable) at the end of each section to help researchers and clinicians implementing these methods in their practice. To summarize, this book:

- Introduces the theory behind each quantitative technique;
- Reviews their applications in the human spinal cord and describes their pros/cons;
- Proposes a simple protocol for applying each quantitative technique to the spinal cord.

How did it start? Ironically, the idea of editing a book on *Quantitative MRI of the spinal cord* first emerged during the international *Human Brain Mapping* conference, which took place in 2011 in Quebec City, Canada. During this meeting, JCA organized a symposium on *Diffusion and Functional MRI of the Spinal Cord: Methods and Clinical Application*. This symposium caught the attention of the publisher, who approached JCA with the idea of a book. CWK was one of the speakers and started discussing with JCA the need for such a book, trying to encourage him to take on this challenge. Elsevier followed up the initial discussion, contacted the editors, CWK and JCA, who joined efforts to bring together this exciting project. It is with great satisfaction and appreciation of all contributors' help that both editors, two years later, are proud of stating that they have survived the experience by completing this book!

Contributors

Khaled Abdel-Aziz Department of Brain Repair and Rehabilitation, UCL Institute of Neurology, University College London, London, UK

Daniel C. Alexander Centre for Medical Image Computing, Department of Computer Science, University College London, London, United Kingdom

Yaniv Assaf Department of Neurobiology, George S. Wise Faculty of Life Sciences, Tel Aviv University, Tel Aviv, Israel

Walter H. Backes Department of Radiology, Maastricht University Medical Center, Maastricht, The Netherlands

Roland Bammer Center for Quantitative Neuroimaging, Department of Radiology, Stanford University, Stanford, CA, USA

Robert L. Barry Vanderbilt University Institute of Imaging Science, Vanderbilt University, Nashville, TN, USA; Department of Radiology and Radiological Sciences, Vanderbilt University, Nashville, TN, USA

Jonathan C.W. Brooks Clinical Research Imaging Centre (CRiCBristol), University of Bristol, Bristol, UK

David W. Cadotte Division of Neurosurgery, Department of Surgery, University of Toronto; Krembil Neuroscience Center, Toronto Western Hospital, University Health Network, ON, Canada

Mara Cercignani Clinical Imaging Science Centre, Brighton and Sussex Medical School, University of Sussex, Falmer, East Sussex, UK

Olga Ciccarelli Department of Brain Repair and Rehabilitation, UCL Institute of Neurology, University College London, London, UK

Julien Cohen-Adad Institute of Biomedical Engineering, Polytechnique Montreal; Functional Neuroimaging Unit, CRIUGM, Université de Montréal, Montreal, QC, Canada

Armin Curt Spinal Cord Injury Center, University Hospital Balgrist, University of Zürich, Zürich, Switzerland

Enrico De Vita Lysholm Department of Neuroradiology, National Hospital for Neurology and Neurosurgery, London, UK; Academic Neuroradiological Unit, Department of Brain Repair and Rehabilitation, Institute of Neurology, University College London, London, UK

Richard D. Dortch Vanderbilt University Institute of Imaging Science, Vanderbilt University, Nashville, TN, USA; Department of Radiology and Radiological Sciences, Vanderbilt University, Nashville, TN, USA; Department of Biomedical Engineering, Vanderbilt University, Nashville, TN, USA

Benjamin M. Ellingson Department of Radiological Sciences, David Geffen School of Medicine, University of California-Los Angeles, Los Angeles, CA, USA

Michael G. Fehlings Division of Neurosurgery, Department of Surgery, University of Toronto; Krembil Neuroscience Center, Toronto Western Hospital, University Health Network, ON, Canada

Massimo Filippi Institute of Experimental Neurology, Division of Neuroscience, San Raffaele Scientific Institute, Vita-Salute San Raffaele University, Milan, Italy

Jürgen Finsterbusch Department of Systems Neuroscience, University Medical Center Hamburg-Eppendorf, Institut für Systemische Neurowissenschaften, Hamburg, Germany

Patrick Freund Spinal Cord Injury Center, University Hospital Balgrist, University of Zürich, Zürich, Switzerland

John C. Gore Vanderbilt University Institute of Imaging Science, Vanderbilt University, Nashville, TN, USA; Department of Radiology and Radiological Sciences, Vanderbilt University, Nashville, TN, USA; Department of Biomedical Engineering, Vanderbilt University, Nashville, TN, USA; Department of Physics and Astronomy, Vanderbilt University, Nashville, TN, USA

Charles R.G. Guttmann Center for Neurological Imaging, Brigham and Women's Hospital, Harvard Medical School, Boston, MA, USA

Samantha J. Holdsworth Center for Quantitative Neuroimaging, Department of Radiology, Stanford University, Stanford, CA, USA

Mark A. Horsfield Department of Cardiovascular Sciences, University of Leicester, Leicester, UK

Mina Kim Department of Diagnostic Radiology, University of Hong Kong, Hong Kong, China

John Kramer Spinal Cord Injury Center, University Hospital Balgrist, University of Zürich, Zürich, Switzerland

Cornelia Laule Radiology Department, and Pathology and Laboratory Medicine Department, University of British Columbia, Vancouver, Canada

Alex MacKay Radiology Department, and Physics and Astronomy Department, University of British Columbia, Vancouver, Canada

Robbert J. Nijenhuis Department of Radiology, University Medical Center Utrecht, Utrecht, The Netherlands

Istvan Pirko Department of Neurology, Mayo Clinic, College of Medicine, Rochester, MN, USA

Emine U. Saritas Department of Bioengineering, University of California, Berkeley, CA, USA; Department of Electrical and Electronics Engineering, Bilkent University, Ankara, Turkey

Torben Schneider Department of Neuroinflammation, UCL Institute of Neurology, University College London, London, UK

Seth A. Smith Vanderbilt University Institute of Imaging Science, Vanderbilt University, Nashville, TN, USA; Department of Radiology and Radiological Sciences, Vanderbilt University, Nashville, TN, USA; Department of Biomedical Engineering, Vanderbilt University, Nashville, TN, USA; Department of Physics and Astronomy, Vanderbilt University, Nashville, TN, USA

Bhavana S. Solanky NMR Research Unit, Department of Neuroinflammation, Institute of Neurology, University College, London, UK

Paul E. Summers Department of Biomedical, Metabolic and Neural Sciences, University of Modena and Reggio Emilia, Modena, Italy; and Department of Radiology, European Institute of Radiology, Milan, Italy

Lawrence L. Wald A.A. Martinos Center for Biomedical Imaging, Massachusetts General Hospital, Harvard Medical School, Charlestown, MA, USA; Harvard-MIT Division of Health Sciences and Technology, MIT, Cambridge, MA, USA

Claudia A.M. Wheeler-Kingshott NMR Research Unit, Department of Neuroinflammation, Queen Square MS Centre, UCL Institute of Neurology, University College London, London, UK

Acknowledgements

The editors are grateful to all the contributors for accepting the daunting task of writing a chapter, their invaluable scientific contribution, their diligence, professionalism and positive attitude throughout the whole process. The editors also thank the publishers, Mica Haley for having initiated the first contact, and April Graham and Laura Jackson for her precious support during the long path of edition.

JCA: I would like to thank CWK for being part of this creation, it was a real pleasure to work on this exciting project with her. I am indebted to all my teachers and mentors, notably Drs. Pierre Jannin, Habib Benali, Lawrence Wald, Bruce Rosen and Caterina Mainero as well as my students and former and current colleagues, Drs. Claudine Gauthier, Rick Hoge, Julien Doyon, Frédéric Lesage, Kawin Setsompop, Jonathan Polimeni, Thomas Witzel, Boris Keil, Wei Zhao, Azma Mareyam, Jennifer McNab, Himanshu Bhat, Keith Heberlein, Raphael Paquin, Christophe Grova and Pierre Bellec, for their support, helpful discussions and pleasant time spent together. I wish also to thank my parents, my sister and my close friends, for their continuous love and support. I would like to express my particular gratitude to Dr. Serge Rossignol, who indirectly initiated this book by inoculating me his passion, knowledge and rigorous scientific method for the study of spinal cord. I dedicate this book to him.

CWK: I am really grateful to JCA for involving me in the adventure of this book. I wish also to thank Glen, my husband, my children, Liam, Shane and Slade, all my group, my colleagues, students and postdocs, who sometimes have had to share my time with this book; in particular, I'd like to thank Torben and Bhavana who are also authors of two of the chapters. My gratitude goes definitely to Profs. David H Miller and Alan J Thompson who have supported me over the years and who truly taught me the importance of spinal cord involvement in disease, and Profs. Paul Tofts and Gareth J Barker who were key in my formation and my understanding of how essential it is to develop quantitative MRI techniques. But my acknowledgments can't be complete without mentioning my colleagues and dearest friends, Drs. Olga Ciccarelli and Mara Cercignani, with whom I continuously share the excitement (and struggles) of pushing MRI forward, in our joint effort of advancing medicine.

Introduction to "Quantitative MRI of the Spinal Cord"

MRI is the most versatile technique to study the central nervous system and provides a wealth of biochemical and biophysical information that supports the diagnostic processes in a variety of neurological and psychiatric diseases. Unlike CT, not only the contrast and information content in MRI can be manipulated in a seemingly endless manner to highlight anatomical features such as fiber orientation, but also the physiological parameters such as perfusion and metabolism, in a non-invasive fashion. The unprecedented opportunities to quantify brain tissue properties harbor important information to unravel disease mechanisms for researchers and provide prognostic to patients.

However, the advantage of MRI to determine quantitative tissue properties also comes at a price—the resulting information is often hard to quantify unambiguously. Difficulties to quantify MRI properties in an accurate and precise manner reflect variation in scanner performance across space and time on a given machine, but certainly across scanners with variability in software and hardware platforms. Even simple quantitative measures like brain volume and rate of atrophy are prone to difficulties in standardizing image quality and hamper implementation of quantitative MRI measures in daily practice or even in multicenter research studies.

The level of complexity increases when using MRI to study the spinal cord, an extremely relevant but rather small structure. Despite its undisputed clinical relevance to depict a host of pathological conditions, even qualitative interpretation of spinal cord MRI is endangered by additional technical caveats, such as increased susceptibility and pulsation artifacts. Any radiologist can testify that obtaining good quality routine spinal cord imaging is much more challenging than obtaining good quality brain MRI scans, and that manufacturer settings often are insufficient, certainly at 3 T. Quantitative MRI of the spine therefore is an extremely challenging endeavor, requiring not only full understanding of the quantitative MRI, but also a successful combat of specific spinal artifacts.

This book takes up the challenge to discuss quantitative MRI of the spinal cord and continues from where the seminal textbook, *Quantitative MRI of the Brain* by Paul Tofts stops. It discusses the technical and clinical issues related to quantitative MRI and provides the reader insight into the application of this versatile technique in its most challenging—yet clinically most meaningful—region. Being composed by experts around the globe who have devoted much of their time to master these advanced techniques in such an eloquent area, this volume depicts the biophysical background, technical implementation, and clinical interpretation of quantitative MRI in the spinal cord. For those frightened to apply these techniques, it even provides "cooking recipes", advising how to implement such techniques successfully and overcome the many hurdles that I have witnessed myself when trying to capitalize on the promises of MRI, which is such a delicate region, especially when trying to apply advanced pulse-sequences at high field.

With these challenges in mind, I trust the readers will appreciate the careful text of this volume edited by Julien Cohen-Adad and Claudia Wheeler-Kingshott and gain access to the theoretical and practical knowledge that will enable them to capitalize on the promises of quantitative MRI in such a challenging region.

Frederik Barkhof
Professor of Neuroradiology, Department of Radiology,
VU University Medical Centre, Amsterdam, The Netherlands.

PART I

QUANTITATIVE BIOMARKERS IN THE SPINAL CORD: WHAT FOR?

Rationale for Quantitative MRI of the Human Spinal Cord and Clinical Applications

Khaled Abdel-Aziz, Olga Ciccarelli

Department of Brain Repair and Rehabilitation, UCL Institute of Neurology, University College London, London, UK

1.1.1 INTRODUCTION

Neuroaxonal injury of the spinal cord occurs in a broad spectrum of clinically and pathologically heterogeneous neurodegenerative diseases, typically with serious clinical consequences for patients.[1–4] Typically, the clinical syndrome produced by injury to the spinal cord includes weakness or paralysis of the limbs and trunk, with sensory disturbance and dysfunction of the gastrointestinal and genitourinary sphincters. The spinal cord is therefore an important region of interest for biomedical research. However, magnetic resonance imaging (MRI) of the spinal cord is more challenging than that of the brain due to the smaller cross-sectional area of the spinal cord, motion artifacts from cerebrospinal fluid (CSF) flow with each cardiac and respiratory cycle, and susceptibility to artifacts from surrounding tissues.[5–7] Advances in neuroimaging techniques and postprocessing have allowed progress to be made in recent years, with a subsequent rise in the number of studies investigating spinal cord diseases using MRI.

WHAT IS QUANTITATIVE MRI (qMRI)?

As opposed to structural MRI (e.g., T1- or T2-weighted imaging), *quantitative MRI (qMRI)* aims at providing values that are intrinsic to the tissue properties. qMRI has the advantage of providing absolute and normative values that could be used for diagnosis, prognosis, multiple-site studies, and ultimately clinical trials.

The development of new quantitative MRI (qMRI) techniques, which are more sensitive to change in underlying tissue microstructure and metabolism, is providing insights into the pathogenesis of a growing number of neurological diseases, and is showing promise for studying potential biomarkers of disease progression.

Thoughtfully designed mechanistic MRI studies can complement histopathological studies in understanding pathophysiological processes occurring in vivo, helping to identify important mediators of disease and therefore inform rational drug design. The insights gained from recent studies into cellular and pathophysiological abnormalities in multiple sclerosis (MS) have aided our understanding of the disease and may be valuable in future therapeutic trials of neuroprotective agents.[8] It is predicted that qMRI will play an important role in drug trials, since qMRI-derived measures can be used as biomarkers of disease progression and to monitor treatment response. In addition, it is anticipated that qMRI might be used to risk stratify and characterize patients on entry into trials. A recent study showing that longitudinal changes in whole-brain and tract-specific diffusion tensor imaging (DTI) indices and the magnetization transfer ratio (MTR) can be reliably quantified, suggesting that clinical trials using these outcome measures are feasible.[9] While similar, longitudinal studies in patients with spinal cord diseases are currently lacking, this will no doubt be the focus of future work. In fact, it is essential that reliable imaging biomarkers of the spinal cord are validated to prepare us for the emergence of neuroprotective drugs.

This chapter will briefly review the qMRI techniques most commonly applied to the spinal cord, and then focus on reviewing data from qMRI studies in patients with neurodegenerative spinal cord disease, and in animal

3

models. The clinical and pathophysiological significance of the results of these studies will be discussed, and future directions of research will be proposed (studies discussed are summarized in Table 1.1.1). DTI, MR spectroscopy, and magnetization transfer imaging will also be discussed in more detail in chapters 3 and 5 of this book.

1.1.2 QUANTITATIVE MRI TECHNIQUES

MOST COMMONLY USED SPINAL CORD qMRI TECHNIQUES (MAINLY IN THE RESEARCH SETTING)

Diffusion-weighted imaging is sensitive to microstructural tissue damage, including axonal orientation and demyelination.

Magnetization transfer imaging provides information on the structural integrity of the spinal cord and is most often used to derive information regarding myelination status.

Functional MRI measures neuronal activity by detecting associated changes in blood flow.

MR spectroscopy is sensitive to metabolic changes occurring in pathology that reflect important underlying biological mechanisms.

Volumetric imaging offers the possibility of calculating atrophy measurements, which give information about axonal loss, especially when repeated over time.

1.1.2.1 Diffusion Tensor Imaging

Diffusion imaging methods in the spinal cord are extensively described in Chapter 3. The DTI model can be used to derive indices that quantitatively describe the directional diffusivity of extracellular water within white matter tracts. Data from animal studies have suggested that DTI-derived indices reflect underlying tissue structure. In particular, in animal models, such as experimental allergic encephalomyelitis (EAE), demyelination within white matter tracts leads to an increase in radial diffusivity (RD),[45] while axonal loss is expected to cause a reduction in axial diffusivity (AD)[46,47] (see Chapter 3.1). However, the situation is more complicated in human diseases, and it is likely that both demyelination and axonal loss influence both RD and AD; furthermore, changes in RD can be observed in animal models even in the absence of myelin changes.[48]

Among the best known DTI parameters is fractional anisotropy (FA), which reflects the underlying tissue microstructure, including the coherence of white matter fibers.[49–51] In addition to FA, RD, and AD, the mean diffusivity (MD) can be obtained. This parameter is very sensitive to a general change in tissue microstructure that allows water molecules to move less or more freely; for example, a reduction of the MD has been detected following acute neurological insults, but in chronic neurological disease, or where cellular necrosis leads to increased membrane permeability, a relative increase in the MD value can be seen.[52]

Therefore, despite the difficulties in extrapolating from animal studies to human studies, spinal cord DTI-derived parameters have the potential to be used as biomarkers of both myelin and axonal integrity, and they have been demonstrated to significantly change over time after an acute injury, such as an acute demyelinating lesion.[25]

FA, RD, AD, and MD can be measured within the spinal cord using regions of interest (ROIs), which can be drawn on the basis of the user's anatomical knowledge or can be measured within tracts, which are reconstructed using fiber-tracking (FT) algorithms. Probabilistic tractography algorithms allow the user to obtain an estimate of white matter connectivity within the spinal cord, which may be affected as a consequence of disease. Temporal changes in DTI metrics may become a useful method for monitoring disease progression or response to future neuroprotective agents in neurodegenerative diseases. The ability to visualize the major white matter tracts within the spinal cord also has potential clinical applications for preoperative surgical planning. Detailed imaging of the fiber tracts preoperatively can provide information regarding the integrity of tracts and allow the clinician to predict the potential benefit from surgery more accurately; slow-growing spinal tumors may efface tracts, leaving them relatively intact and making surgical resection less complicated, while more aggressive, invasive tumors are more likely to cause significant structural disruption to the tracts, which increases the risk of significant postoperative neurological deficits. Presurgical assessments of this type will empower clinicians and patients to proceed with surgery only when there is a favorable risk–benefit ratio.

Wheeler-Kingshott et al.[5] reported a uniform MD along the cervical spinal cord, but found a higher FA in the middle and lower sections of the cervical cord compared with the upper cervical cord. Regional differences in DTI metrics of the cervical cord have also been reported by Mamata et al.[53] who reported higher mean values for the apparent diffusion coefficient (ADC) and FA in the upper cervical cord (C2–C3) than in the lower level (C4–C7) in healthy volunteers. These findings suggest that regional DTI measures should be compared between patients and controls whenever possible, since averaging values of DTI measures may dilute the effect of focal pathology. For DTI studies that are discussed in this chapter, spinal level is summarized in Table 1.1.1.

TABLE 1.1.1 Summary of Clinical Imaging Studies Discussed within this Chapter

Studies	Field Strength	Disease	Region of Interest	Findings
Brex et al.[10]	1.5 T	CIS	15 mm of cord, centered at C2/3	Spinal cord area was significantly smaller in patients with abnormal brain MRI at presentation
Losseff et al.[11]	1.5 T	MS	15 mm of cord, centered at C2/3	Strong correlation between spinal cord area and EDSS. Greatest cord volume loss in patients with progressive MS
Ingle et al.[12]	1.5 T	PPMS	15 mm of cord, centered at C2/3	Correlation between spinal cord area and EDSS. Rates of cord atrophy and brain atrophy over 5 years do not correlate
Kendi et al.[13]	1.5 T	MS	C3−7	Lower NAA in patients than controls
Ciccarelli et al.[14]	1.5 T	RRMS (spinal cord relapse)	C1−3	NAA was lower in patients than controls and correlated with upper limb function; Ins concentration in patients correlated with EDSS. FA was lower in posterior columns and lateral corticospinal tracts of patients; RD correlated with disability
Blamire et al.[15]	2 T	MS	C2/3	Lower NAA in patients than controls. Spinal NAA correlated with the cerebellar subscore of the neurological assessment
Henning et al.[16]	3 T	MS	C2/3	Lower NAA and Ins and elevated Cho in a single MS patient compared to controls
Marliani et al.[17]	3 T	MS	C2/3	Lower NAA and elevated Ins and Cho in patients compared to controls
Ciccarelli et al.[7,18]	1.5 T	RRMS (spinal cord relapse)	C1−3	Lower NAA at onset of relapse, which recovers over 6 months in patients who improve clinically
Ciccarelli et al.[19]	3 T	NMO and RRMS	C1−3	Lower Ins:Cr ratios in NMO patients compared to RRMS and controls
Valsasina et al.[20]	1.5 T	MS	C1−5	Decreased FA in patients with MS. Average cord FA correlates with EDSS
Oh et al.[21,22]	3 T	MS	C3−4	FA, MD, RD, AD, and MTR are significantly different between patients and controls and correlate with sensorimotor function
Agosta et al.[23,24]	3 T	MS	C2/3	Lower FA and higher MD in patients than controls. Cord FA lower in PPMS than RRMS. FA at baseline predictive of disability on follow-up (mean 2.4 years)
Freund et al.[25]	1.5 T	RRMS (spinal cord relapse)	C1−3	RD at onset of spinal cord relapse predicts clinical recovery
Rovaris et al.[26]	1.5 T	PPMS	Cervical cord	Average MTR lower in PPMS patients than controls
Filippi et al.[27]	1.5 T	MS	Cervical cord	Patients had lower average MTR of the cervical cord than controls. Lowest MTR histogram peaks were seen in PPMS. Peak position and height of MTR histogram were predictive of locomotor disability
Rovaris et al.[28]	1.5 T	Early, nondisabling RRMS	Cervical cord	Average cord MTR and mean histogram peak height values did not differ between patients and controls

(Continued)

I. QUANTITATIVE BIOMARKERS IN THE SPINAL CORD: WHAT FOR?

TABLE 1.1.1   Summary of Clinical Imaging Studies Discussed within this Chapter—cont'd

Studies	Field Strength	Disease	Region of Interest	Findings
Rovaris et al.[29]	1.5 T	CIS	Cervical cord	Mean values of MTR histogram-derived metrics were not different between CIS patients and healthy controls
Charil et al.[30]	1.5 T	RRMS	Cervical cord	Average cervical cord MTR was correlated with a relapse rate over 18 months
Agosta et al.[23,24]	1.5 T	RRMS	Cervical cord	Spinal gray matter average MTR lower in RRMS than controls, and correlates with EDSS
Cheran et al.[31]	3 T	SCI	Whole cord	Reduction in FA, MD, and AD throughout the cervical cord, with maximal FA reduction at site of T2-weighted signal abnormality
Shanmuganathan et al.[32]	3 T	SCI	Whole cord	Reductions in whole-cord ADC, ADC, and FA at injury site compared with controls
Elliot et al.[33]	3 T	Chronic whiplash	C1–C3	Lower NAA:Cr ratios (but not Cho:Cr ratios) than healthy controls
Kachramanoglou et al.[34]	3 T	Brachial plexus reimplantation	C1–C3	Increased Ins:Cr ratios in patients compared to controls
Kara et al.[35]	3 T	CSM		Increase in ADC and decrease in FA at site of the stenosis
Holly et al.[36]	1.5 T	CSM	C1–C3	Lower NAA:Cr ratio in patients, with lactate peaks detected in nearly half of patients with T2-weighted signal abnormality
Hatem et al.[37]		Syringomyelia	C3–C7	Decreased FA. Mean FA correlates with clinical scores
Nair et al.[38]	3 T	ALS	C1–C6	FA 12% lower than controls RD 15% higher than controls No difference in MD and AD between patients and controls
Carew et al.[39,40]	3 T	ALS and presymptomatic SOD1-positive patients	C1–2	NAA:Cr and NAA:Ins ratios reduced in SOD1+ subjects and ALS compared to controls Ins:Cr reduced in SOD1+ but not ALS NAA:Cho reduced in ALS but not SOD1+ subjects
Vargas et al.[41]	1.5 T	Cohort of mixed spinal tumors		Reduction in FA. ADC increased in 3 out of 5 patients
Ducreux et al.[42]	1.5 T	Spinal astrocytoma	Cervical and thoracic cord	Reduced FA
Ozanne et al.[43]	1.5 T	Spinal AVMs	Cervical cord	Reduced FA. FA reduction associated with clinical scores
Qian et al.[44]	3 T	NMO	C1–C6	Reduced FA and increased RD and MD. Good correlation between DTI metrics and clinical scores

Abbreviations: AD: axial diffusivity; ADC: apparent diffusion coefficient; ALS: amyotrophic lateral sclerosis; AVM: arteriovenous malformation; Cho: choline containing compounds; CIS: clinically isolated syndrome; Cr: creatine + phosphocreatine; CSM: cervical spondylitic myelopathy; DTI: diffusion tensor imaging; EDSS: expanded disability severity score; FA: fractional anisotropy; Ins: myo-inositol; MD: mean diffusivity; MS: multiple sclerosis; MTR: magnetic transfer ratio; NAA: *N*-acetylaspartate; NMO: neuromyelitis optica; PPMS: primary progressive multiple sclerosis; RD: radial diffusivity; RRMS: relapsing remitting multiple sclerosis; SCI: spinal cord injury; SOD1: superoxide dismutase 1.

1.1.2.2 Proton Magnetic Resonance Spectroscopy

Proton magnetic resonance spectroscopy (MRS) (see Chapter 5) is a powerful tool that allows quantification of metabolite concentrations from human tissue in vivo. Reliable quantification of metabolites from the spinal cord using 1.5 T scanners has been limited to a few metabolites, namely N-acetylaspartate (NAA), choline (Cho), and creatine (Cr).[13,54] However, over the past decade, developments in imaging acquisition and postprocessing, together with a wider availability of high-field-strength scanners, which allow increased separation of metabolite peaks, have permitted the study of metabolites with more specific relevance to the pathogenesis of neurological diseases, such as glutamate-glutamine (Glx) and myo-inositol (Ins).[16,55,56]

NAA is synthesized by neuronal mitochondria,[57] and it is commonly used as a marker of axonal integrity and/or metabolic dysfunction in neuroimaging studies. More recently, studies modeling NAA concentrations in the spinal cord with other markers of axonal integrity, such as cross-sectional cord area, demonstrate that mathematically derived estimates of mitochondrial function can be made from spectroscopic data.[7] The development of such imaging biomarkers of mitochondrial function has wide implications for studying a large number of neurological diseases in which mitochondrial dysfunction is thought to be important. Although changes in NAA are not disease specific, they can be detected early in the disease course, making them a sensitive indicator of neuroaxonal injury when conventional imaging fails to detect any change.[58]

NAA concentrations can be expressed as absolute values, or more commonly as ratios with Cr or Cho. The Cr signal, which is a composite peak of creatine and phosphocreatine, is a better reference signal as levels are thought to be quite constant in the nervous system. In neurological disease, however, changes in the resonance intensity of both Cr and Cho have been suggested; for example, changes in Cho are thought to reflect increases in the steady-state levels of membrane phospholipids released during myelin breakdown, as is seen in active demyelinating disease.[59]

Lactate is produced as a by-product when cells within the nervous system respire under anaerobic conditions. Elevations in brain lactate have been detected using MRS in cerebral ischemia,[60] brain tumors,[61] and mitochondrial disease.[62] Although it is thought that lactate may be a relevant marker in spinal cord pathology, it is likely to be produced in much smaller concentrations, making its detection in healthy subjects difficult, if not impossible.[36]

As with DTI, it is possible that the spinal cord level is an important methodological consideration with MRS experiments. A small study by Edden et al. found a nonsignificant variation in metabolite concentrations between the upper cervical cord and the medulla.[63] Additional work is needed to evaluate whether metabolite concentrations differ between cervical, thoracic, and lumbar segments of the spinal cord.

1.1.2.3 Magnetization Transfer Imaging

Magnetization transfer imaging (see Chapter 3.4) is based on the interaction between hydrogen protons bound to macromolecules, such as those associated with lipids and lipoproteins, and the free protons normally imaged by MRI. MTR, obtained by magnetization transfer imaging, can be used as an indirect marker of demyelination and possibly axonal loss.[64,65] In patients with MS, high-resolution magnetization transfer measurements from the spinal cord have demonstrated that it is possible to assess tissue damage, including demyelination (and possibly axonal loss) of specific spinal pathways, with good accuracy.[66] However, in neurodegenerative diseases other than MS, the use of magnetization transfer imaging has largely been confined to studies of brain changes, and very few studies have focused on the spinal cord. Brain MTR has been incorporated as an exploratory endpoint to assess treatment efficacy in large multicenter trials,[67,68] and similar studies of spinal cord disease are still awaited. Relevant studies of spinal cord disease that have used MTR will be discussed in this chapter.

1.1.3 APPLICATION OF QUANTITATIVE MRI TECHNIQUES TO SPINAL CORD DISEASE

This section will give an overview of the applications of qMRI in the spinal cord, including a wide spectrum of clinical applications. Given the high number of studies of qMRI in MS and the potential relevance of qMRI in spinal cord injury, these two applications will be expanded in chapters 1.2 (demyelinating diseases) and 1.3 (trauma).

1.1.3.1 Multiple Sclerosis

MS is an inflammatory disorder of the central nervous system characterized by inflammation, demyelination, incomplete remyelination, axonal loss, and gliosis. Clinically evident signs and symptoms then develop that reflect impaired salutatory conduction at affected sites.[69] At disease onset, MS can present either with a relapsing, remitting clinical course or with progressive accumulation of neurological symptoms and disability.[70] The lifetime risk is thought to be approximately 1 in 400, making MS the commonest cause of progressive neurological disability affecting young people.[69]

MS is characterized by the recurrent formation of multifocal plaques in both white matter and gray matter. The white matter plaques are readily visible on T2-weighted and proton density (PD)-weighted MRI, and imaging of these lesions at the onset of the first clinical symptoms predicts conversion to clinically definite MS with good accuracy.[71] Imaging of white matter lesions has subsequently been incorporated into the diagnostic criteria for MS since 2001.[72–74]

The availability of good histopathological data on MS plaques and their visibility on PD and T2 imaging have made them a convenient marker of disease progression, but lesion frequency and volumes do not always explain the degree of clinical disability in patients. qMRI research has therefore tried to fill this gap to improve our understanding of the mechanisms causing disability in MS.

As the most visually evident imaging abnormality in MS, focal T2 lesions might be expected to be the predominant substrate of disability. but spinal cord lesion load does not correlate well with disability,[75] even when disability is determined by using a clinical measure such as the expanded disability severity score (EDSS), which is heavily weighted toward spinal cord functions, such as ambulation. In fact, spinal cord T2 lesions are often clinically silent. Asymptomatic spinal cord lesions have been reported in about 50% of patients with clinically isolated syndromes (CIS) and early MS.[76,77]

This clinico-radiological paradox might partly be explained by difficulties in accurately quantifying neurological dysfunction,[78] but it is more likely to be explained by the lack of sensitivity and specificity of conventional MRI techniques for detecting microscopic histopathological change. Axonal loss, which is the principal substrate for disability in MS, occurs largely independently of T2-weighted lesions.[79] New quantitative MRI techniques, which are more sensitive to change in underlying tissue microstructure and metabolism within the spinal cord, show much better correlation with disability[14,25,80] and can more accurately discriminate between patients with similar T2 lesion loads on the basis of disability.[80]

We will now review studies that used volumetric imaging, MRS, DTI, and MTR of the spinal cord in patients with MS.

1.1.3.1.1 Spinal Cord Atrophy

Spinal cord atrophy can be an early feature of MS, progresses with time, and reflects underlying axonal loss. In patients presenting with CIS suggestive of MS, evidence of cord atrophy can be seen even in the absence of spinal cord symptoms.[10] However, spinal cord volume loss is most marked in progressive forms of MS and greatest in secondary progressive MS (SPMS).[11] Interestingly, the rate of spinal cord atrophy in primary progressive MS (PPMS) does not correlate with the rate of brain atrophy, which suggests the presence of two independent disease processes causing injury to the brain and spinal cord.[12]

Spinal cord atrophy measured using MRI is reproducible and correlates strongly with disability in cross-sectional and longitudinal studies,[11,81,82] making it both a potentially useful tool for measuring disease progression and an endpoint in clinical trials of neuroprotective agents. To date, two MS clinical trials have included cord cross-sectional area as an exploratory endpoint,[83,84] and it shows promise for use in future trials, especially in progressive MS patients.

A technical consideration is that research into spinal cord atrophy in MS is moving away from the use of the whole cross-sectional area of the cord at C2–C3, as proposed by Losseff,[11] using a semiautomated edge detection method, and proposing either a new method, such as the active surface model,[85] or new combinations of acquisitions and methods.[86] In addition, gray matter and white matter volume calculation within the cord is now possible,[87] and voxel-based morphometry has been successfully applied to the spinal cord of MS patients.[88] Whether these more advanced techniques will provide additional information on patients' clinical course has to be established.

1.1.3.1.2 Spinal Cord Spectroscopy

All cross-sectional, spinal cord MRS studies in MS published to date (Table 1.1.1) have reported a reduction in NAA in patients with MS when compared to healthy controls.[13–16,55] In one study, cervical cord NAA was shown to correlate with clinical disability,[14] but most of these early exploratory studies did not report significant clinical correlations. In a previous longitudinal study, we demonstrated that following cervical cord relapse, NAA levels in the upper cervical cord are low, compared to controls, but, as patients recover from their relapse, the NAA concentration can recover. Using a model that uses cord area as a surrogate marker of axonal density, we proposed that changes in NAA were not entirely due to axonal loss but also reflected mitochondrial dysfunction, and we concluded that recovery in NAA following relapse was partially explained by recovering mitochondrial function.[18]

In a study of patients with chronic spinal cord lesions, the cervical cord Cho:Cr ratio was elevated,[17] which may reflect ongoing remyelination within plaques, although this finding has not been reproduced in other cohort studies. Unlike the brain, where elevated Cr has been reported, Cr has not been shown to change in the spinal cord.

Ins is the best available in vivo glia-specific marker.[89] Elevated Ins is seen in the brain of patients with CIS who convert to MS, suggesting that gliosis may be a process of pathogenic importance in MS.[90] In the cervical cord, Ins is marginally increased in patients with MS at the onset of a spinal cord relapse and was shown to correlate with disability in one study.[14] Another study showed a reduced Ins concentration in the spinal cord of a single MS patient.[16] We have recently proposed that Ins may be useful to distinguish MS patients from neuromyelitis optica (NMO) patients, because NMO lesions seen in a case series of patients were found to show reduced Ins compared to levels in MS patients and healthy controls, suggesting that reduced Ins may reflect the astrocytic damage that is typical of NMO lesions.[19]

1.1.3.1.3 Spinal Cord DTI

A number of research groups have developed DTI protocols for studying spinal cord injury in MS patients. Using histogram analyses, early cross-sectional studies demonstrated a reduction in cervical cord FA in MS patients and that average FA independently correlated with the degree of disability.[20] Later studies used diffusion-based tractography of the major spinal cord pathways and demonstrated that tract-specific DTI measures from the major spinal pathways correlated more specifically to system-specific and global clinical dysfunction.[14,21]

Longitudinal studies examining the relationship between DTI metrics and future clinical disability in MS have shown promise; Agosta et al. reassessed patients after a mean follow-up of 2.4 years and observed that cervical cord MD increased and FA decreased on follow-up and that FA at baseline was predictive of disability on follow-up.[23] A similar study examining patients at the onset of a cervical cord relapse found that RD was more sensitive at predicting clinical recovery at 6 months.[25] Such studies suggest that in MS patients, DTI metrics are more reflective of clinical disability than conventional imaging and are potentially of prognostic value.

1.1.3.1.4 Spinal Cord MTR

In cross-sectional studies, spinal cord MTR was much lower in patients with MS than in controls, and it was significantly lowest in patients with progressive forms of the disease.[26,27,91] Average MTR and MTR histogram height correlate with disability, with functions associated with spinal pathways, in particular, most closely associated to MTR-derived metrics.[27,92] However, it may be the case that patients with early relapsing remitting multiple sclerosis (RRMS) and CIS have normal MTR histograms.[28,29] More recently, a large study found that MTR discriminates between high and low disability levels best in patients with fewer spinal cord lesions and less accurately when there is a heavy lesion load.[22] Interestingly, only a moderate correlation has been found between average brain MTR and MTR from the cervical cord, which further supports the theory that cervical cord damage in MS occurs due to different mechanisms from those affecting the brain.[91] Tissue-specific MTR studies in patients with RRMS have demonstrated that gray matter average MTR was lower in patients than in healthy controls,[24] which is in keeping with the postmortem studies showing extensive gray matter demyelination in the spinal cords of MS patients.[93]

Longitudinal spinal cord MTR data are limited; in a small study of untreated RRMS patients, average cervical cord MTR was correlated with a relapse rate over 18 months but was not predictive of EDSS change.[30]

1.1.3.2 Neuromyelitis Optica

NMO is an inflammatory and demyelinating disease of the central nervous system, characterized by the preferential involvement of the spinal cord and optic nerve, but it is clinically and immunologically distinct from MS.[1,94] Brain MTR and DTI studies on 1.5 T systems have reported abnormalities within normal-appearing brain tissue of patients with NMO, which is suggestive of microstructural tissue damage,[95,96] although these findings have not been reproduced by others.[97] An investigation of the normal-appearing white matter of the spinal cord using 3 T DTI demonstrated significant abnormalities in DTI metrics within the spinal cord in a small cohort of 10 NMO patients.[44] Compared to healthy controls, patients had significantly reduced FA and increased MD and RD. There were strong correlations between DTI metrics and clinical scores within the NMO group, again suggesting that DTI can be a sensitive marker of tract integrity. Although one should be cautious when drawing conclusions from studies with such small numbers, the increase in RD, which is commonly seen in patients with demyelinating disease,[45] is thought to account for the decrease in FA, suggesting that demyelination, rather than axonal injury, is the major substrate of disability in this patient group.[44] As mentioned in Section 1.1.3.1.2, in a recent case series, we demonstrated that Ins may be a useful marker to distinguish NMO from MS.[19]

1.1.3.3 Acute Trauma

1.1.3.3.1 Acute Spinal Cord Injury

Traumatic spinal cord injury (SCI) is a devastating condition that primarily affects young males with an annual incidence of 15–40 cases per million.[98–100] The commonest mechanisms of primary injury in human SCI are compression, contusion, laceration, transection, and traction of the spinal cord.[101] Following the primary insult, several pathophysiological mechanisms produce secondary injury, including spinal cord edema, ischemia, free radical damage, electrolyte imbalance, excitotoxicity, inflammation, and apoptosis.[99,102] Spinal cord MRI findings on conventional T2-weighted imaging, such as hemorrhage, edema, and swelling, are commonly seen in complete motor and sensory SCI and are considered predictive of a poor neurological outcome.[103]

In a retrospective study of 20 victims of blunt force trauma with cervical spine injuries, diffusion imaging showed a significant reduction in whole-cord ADC in patients compared with healthy controls. FA values were significantly reduced at the site of injury, but no significant difference in whole-cord FA was found between patients and controls.[32] The greatest differences in whole-cord ADC and FA were seen in those patients with hemorrhagic cord contusions. In a similar series, Cheran et al. found significant reductions in MD and AD throughout all regions of the cervical cord following blunt trauma, with maximal reductions in FA at the site of injury.[31] RD was increased only in patients with non-hemorrhagic contusions. American Spinal Injury Association (ASIA) clinical motor scores correlated positively with MD, AD, and RD, and there was a negative correlation with FA (Figure 1.1.1). The data coming from both studies indicate that DTI-derived parameters are sensitive to spinal cord contusion and that MD and AD are the most sensitive markers of extent of cord injury in this group of patients. In patients with nonhemorrhagic contusions, all four DTI parameters were predictive of disability, with MD again being most significant (Figure 1.1.1). In both studies, the greatest DTI parameter changes were seen in patients with hemorrhagic contusion. The lack of correlation in this group with ASIA scores may be largely explained by the presence of large volumes of hemorrhage at the injury site, which may mean that the blood content of the extracellular space is contributing to diffusion anisotropy, which may not be truly reflective of axonal injury.

To date, studies have been limited by small cohort sizes; larger, prospective, follow-up studies are now needed to corroborate the findings to date and assess how long-term outcomes relate to changes in DTI parameters at time of injury.

1.1.3.3.2 Whiplash

Single-voxel MRS of the cervical cord in patients with chronic whiplash (>6 months post injury) shows reduced NAA:Cr ratios when compared with healthy controls, which has been interpreted as reflecting underlying neuroaxonal injury.[33] Reductions in the NAA:Cr ratio of a similar magnitude in patients when compared with controls were seen in some studies of cervical myelopathy.[36] The findings are curious; although neurological symptoms and signs are not a usual feature of whiplash injuries, a subclinical spinal injury is suggested by the findings, and it has been suggested that a persistently abnormal afferent input, following injury to peripheral structures, may be the explanation.[33]

1.1.3.3.3 Brachial Plexus Injury

Brachial plexus injuries can occur as a result of trauma to the shoulder, inflammation within the nerves making up the brachial plexus, or due to tumor invasion. In young adults, avulsion injuries, in which the nerve roots are torn from the spinal cord, are most commonly caused by motorcycle accidents. Injuries of this type are classed as "longitudinal spinal cord injuries" due to the damage that occurs to the cord.[104] The nerve roots forming the brachial plexuses are avulsed from their origin, causing variable degrees of disability in the affected limb, with a plegic, anesthetized upper limb in the most severe of cases, involving all five dorsal and ventral roots. In experimental models of lumbar root avulsion, motor neurone cell death and Wallerian degeneration are described.[105] Reimplantation of avulsed spinal ventral roots has been shown to enable significant and useful regrowth of motor axons in both experimental animal models and humans, rescuing lesioned motor neurones from death.[106]

Kachramanoglou et al.[34] carried out a ¹H-MRS study of the upper (C1–C3) spinal cord, and demonstrated that patients undergoing lower cervical root reimplantation surgery following brachial plexus avulsion showed a significantly higher Ins:Cr ratio when compared to healthy controls (Figure 1.1.2); this suggests that a reactive, gliotic process may occur above the site of the lesion, probably in response to the Wallerian degeneration of avulsed neuronal fibers, which has been demonstrated in animal models of root avulsion.[105] Interestingly, the finding of a higher Ins:Cr ratio was associated with greater disability of the arm, higher pain scores, and shorter time from injury. The authors proposed that gliotic changes might therefore normalize over time, reflecting reorganization within the cord.

Sprague-Dawley rats, who undergo root implantation following avulsion of the L5 ventral root, demonstrate differing gene expression from those that don't undergo implantation (Figure 1.1.3).[106] While cell death gene expression is similar in treated and untreated rats, genes related to neurite development and neurogenesis show a much more prominent response after reimplantation than after avulsion only. Significantly, the inflammatory response is more obvious after avulsion than after

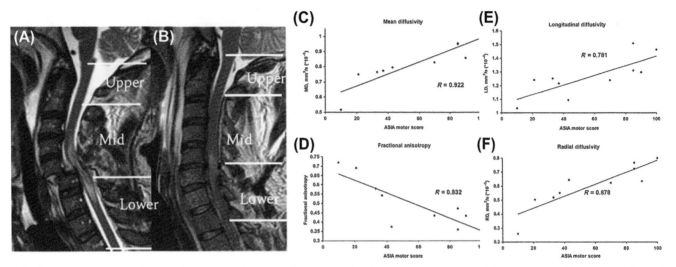

FIGURE 1.1.1 On the left, sagittal T2-weighted images demonstrate the three anatomic regions of the cervical cord (upper, middle, and lower). Hemorrhagic (A) and nonhemorrhagic (B) cord contusions are seen. On the right, scatter graphs illustrating the relationship between DTI parameters and the severity of injury measured at the injury site for the nonhemorrhagic group: (C) mean diffusivity, (D) fractional anisotropy, (E) axial diffusivity, and (F) radial diffusivity. *Source: Adapted from Ref. 31 with permission from J Neurotrauma.*

replantation, which may help explain the spectroscopy findings in humans.[34] Although the MRS study did not demonstrate lower NAA concentrations in the patient population, it may be that these changes would be detectable only in a control group of patients with chronic brachial plexus avulsion who did not undergo root reimplantation. Future studies could address these issues with a view to proposing an imaging marker for forthcoming clinical trials with stem cell transplantation in patients with brachial plexus avulsion.[107]

1.1.3.4 Chronic Spondylitic Myelopathy

Cervical spondylitic myelopathy (CSM) is a common degenerative disease that occurs most frequently in elderly patients and is characterized by intervertebral disc degeneration. As disc degeneration occurs, mechanical stresses result in osteophytic bars, which form along the ventral aspect of the spinal canal, causing narrowing of the spinal canal; this, in turn, produces myelopathic symptoms.[108,109] Conventional MRI is commonly used in clinical practice for diagnostic purposes and may show narrowing in disc spaces, ligament thickening, and narrowing of the canal, with T2 high signal change in the cord at the level of narrowing.[110] However, T2 hyperintensity is seen only in between 15% and 65% of patients,[110–113] which can sometimes lead to delays in surgical intervention.

Diffusion imaging has shown promise for detecting cord injury earlier in patients who don't exhibit hyperintense lesions on T2-weighted MRI. An increase in ADC and decrease in FA at the level of spinal canal narrowing are typically seen.[35,53,114,115] However, the use of nonstenotic segments of patients' spinal cords as controls

instead of healthy controls in some studies could have skewed the control data as mean values for the ADC and FA are higher in the upper cervical cord (C2–C3) than in the lower level (C4–C7).[35,53] However, a large body of evidence from brain DTI studies highlights the sensitivity of DTI for detecting "occult" injury, and it is likely that DTI metrics of the spinal cord reflect tissue injury in the absence of T2 changes in this patient group. Future, controlled, longitudinal studies are needed to establish whether earlier surgical intervention on the basis of DTI abnormalities improves patient outcomes. More likely, in the near term, studies could be designed to determine whether DTI can predict the outcome of conservative treatment.[35]

MR spectroscopy data from patients with CSM are limited. A single study performed using a 1.5 T system has shown significantly lower NAA:Cr ratios in patients with CSM than in healthy controls, which are suggestive of neuroaxonal loss and/or mitochondrial dysfunction.[36] A lactate peak was observed on the spectra obtained from nearly one-half of the patients with evidence of T2 hyperintensity on structural imaging, but from only one (13%) of the eight patients without a T2-weighted signal abnormality. The presence of a lactate peak suggests cellular ischemia, which is thought to play a role in the pathogenesis of CSM. A trend for lower NAA:Cr ratios in CSM patients with a positive lactate signal than in those without it was detected, but it did not reach statistical significance.[36]

1.1.3.5 Syringomyelia

Syringomyelia is characterized by the cavitation of the central spinal canal, which slowly expands, causing

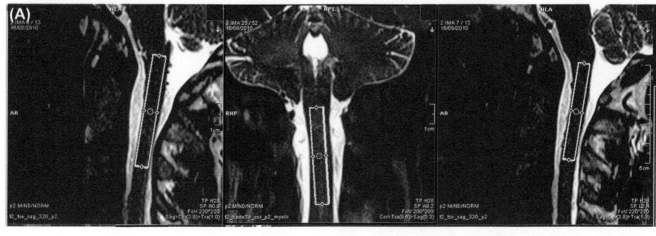

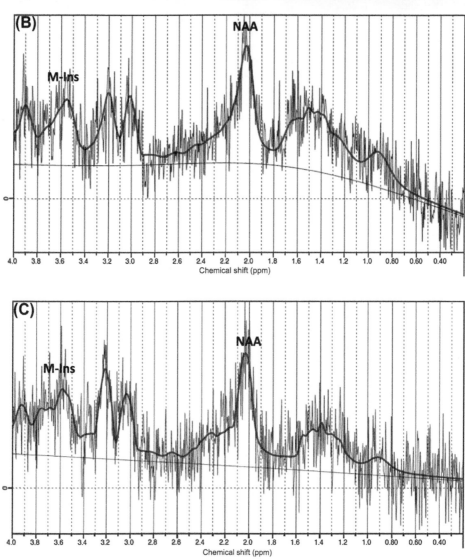

FIGURE 1.1.2 (A) T2-weighted images showing MR spectroscopic voxel placement between C1 and C3 in a patient (left and center) and a control (right). (B) Spectrum showing an increased Ins:Cr ratio in a patient following reimplantation surgery for brachial plexus avulsion injury compared to a spectrum obtained in a healthy control (C). *Source: Courtesy of Dr C Kachramanoglou, UCL Institute of Neurology.*

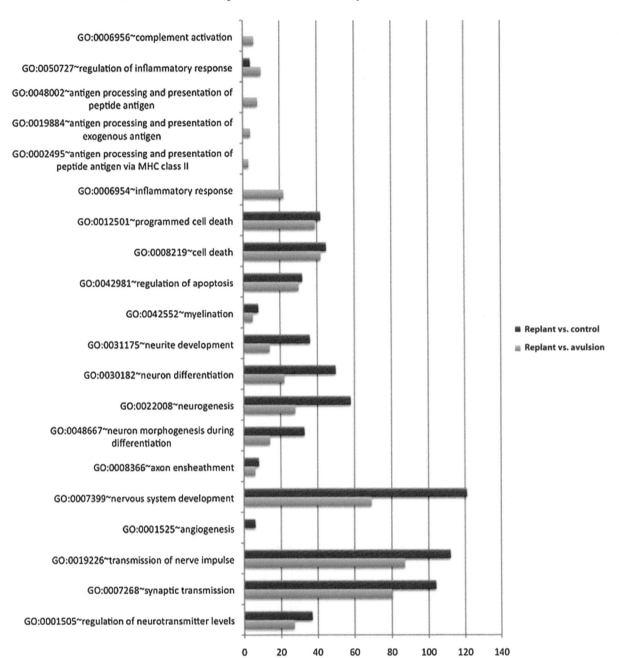

FIGURE 1.1.3 A diagram illustrating the number of significantly regulated genes in rats after root avulsion and avulsion plus reimplantation. The x-axis indicates the number of genes that have undergone significant changes in expression. Note that this number includes both up- and downregulated genes. The number of cell death genes is similar in the two groups, while genes related to neurite development and neurogenesis show a much more prominent response after reimplantation than after avulsion only. The inflammatory response is more obvious after avulsion than after reimplantation. *Source: Adapted from Ref. 106 with permission from Frontiers in Neurology.*

compression of the spinal cord parenchyma and subsequently producing neurological symptoms. Syringomyelia can affect any of the long tracts within the spinal cord, but it most commonly affects the spinothalamic tracts, and it typically produces a loss of pain and temperature sensation in a "cape distribution" over the back and shoulders. Expansion of the syrinx can produce symptoms of limb weakness, neuropathic pain, sensory loss, and bowel, bladder, and autonomic disturbance.

A small number of studies have assessed the spinal somatosensory pathways with diffusion imaging in patients with syringomyelia.[37,116,117] Hatem et al. used DTI with three-dimensional fiber tracking and demonstrated that patients with cervical syrinx and established thermatosensory impairment in the hands have lower FA in the somatosensory fibers than healthy controls[37]; in patients, the mean FA at two levels within the cervical cord (C3–C4 and C6–C7) correlated with both clinical and electrophysiological measures of sensory deficit.[37] ADC measures in the same patient group were less clinically meaningful. These findings suggest that an objective and quantitative assessment of spinal somatosensory system dysfunction is possible with DTI in syringomyelia as well as MS patients. Similar patterns of FA reductions were found by Roser et al., who in addition demonstrated that FA values normalize beyond the borders of the lesion,[117] suggesting that white matter tracts are preserved distal to the syrinx.

A recent study assessing the neuropathic pain and functional alterations of the sensory tracts within the spinal cord showed that patients with syringomyelia, with or without neuropathic pain, were indistinguishable on the basis of quantitative sensory testing alone and DTI–FT analyses; however, in patients with neuropathic pain, a greater pain intensity correlated with more abnormal MRI measures of diffusion indices.[116] In particular, higher average daily pain intensity was correlated with a lower FA and a lower number of reconstructed nerve fibers from tractography. In contrast, higher paresthesia and dysesthesia correlated with a greater number of reconstructed nerve fibers. The authors have chosen to use a single spinal level for DTI measures (C3–C4) due to physiological variations in DTI metrics at different spinal segments, which have been mentioned in this chapter. Although methodologically sound, three of the patients studied had syrinxes that did not involve this anatomical level, which may have caused some bias in the results. Allowing for this, these results do seem to suggest that the degree of damage within the spinal white matter, and not gray matter alone, is relevant to both the type and intensity of pain experienced by patients with syringomyelia.

1.1.3.6 Amyotrophic Lateral Sclerosis

Amyotrophic lateral sclerosis (ALS) is a neurodegenerative disease that leads to degeneration of the upper and lower motor neurones in the ventral horn of the spinal cord. Patients ultimately develop a combination of both upper and lower motor neurone signs with a progressive loss of bulbar and limb function. The vast majority ($\sim$95%) of cases occur sporadically, with an incidence in Europe of 2–3 cases per 100,000 individuals in the general population, and an overall lifetime risk of developing the disease of 1:400.[118] The inherited form, familial ALS, accounts for approximately 5% of all cases and is associated with hundreds of gene mutations,[119] with over 100 mutations of the human superoxide dismutase (SOD1) gene linked with ALS. Mitochondrial dysfunction, the generation of free radicals, and impaired calcium handling are thought to be important mechanisms in ALS; more recently, two specific mutations in mitochondrial genes, COX1 and IARS2, have also been reported to cause ALS-like syndromes.[119] The extent of mitochondrial dysfunction within spinal neurons in ALS was reported by Keeney and Bennett,[120] who demonstrated that within ALS spinal neurons, there are reduced mtDNA gene copy numbers and increased mtDNA gene deletions.

MR spectra can reliably be obtained from the cervical spinal cord in ALS and have been proposed as a potential biomarker of disease progression.[39,40] Clinical MRS studies on 3 T clinical scanners have reported a number of neurometabolic abnormalities, giving insights into pathogenesis. Reductions in NAA:Ins and NAA:Cho ratios have been reported in the cervical spines of patients with ALS, as well as presymptomatic individuals with a mutation in the SOD1 susceptibility gene.[39,40] Similar MRS abnormalities have also been detected within the spinal cord of SOD1 mice prior to disease development.[121] Clinically, direct correlations between metabolite ratios and patient functions have been observed, with reductions in NAA:Ins and NAA:Cho being associated with smaller forced vital capacity (FVC) measurements.[40] Reductions in NAA ratios seen in the spectroscopy studies reflect the axonal loss seen histopathologically in ALS, but they may also, in part at least, be related to the mitochondrial dysfunction known to occur in ALS.[120,122] In the SOD1 mouse model of ALS, there is a decline in estimated motor neurone numbers prior to the development of clinical signs,[123] and neurophysiological data from healthy SOD1-positive humans show a reduction in estimated motor unit numbers several months in advance of symptom onset.[124] The presence of metabolite abnormalities in presymptomatic patients is highly suggestive that the subclinical phase precedes the onset of clinical signs and symptoms in ALS.

Patient numbers in these MRS studies so far have been small, and further longitudinal studies are required to validate such techniques as biomarkers of disease progression in ALS. However, the relative rarity of the disease makes studies with large numbers of patients from single centers difficult, while the absence of acquisition standardization and the technical expertise needed to perform high-quality MRS have presented barriers to multicenter collaborations.[125]

DTI studies in ALS have largely focused on the brain and consistently report a reduction in FA and an increase in MD.[126–129] In a small, 3 T DTI study of the cervical spinal cord comparing patients with ALS to healthy controls, the authors found a similar reduction in FA across the C1–C6 spinal segments.[38] The reduction in FA correlated with lower average finger- and foot-tapping speeds. An increase in RD was seen at the

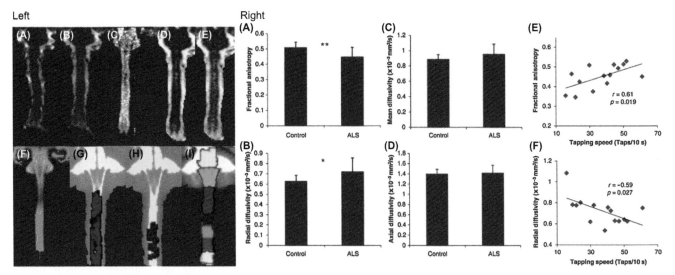

FIGURE 1.1.4 (Left) DTI of cervical spinal cord. (A) A single coronal B0 slice (2 averages) from a representative healthy control subject depicting susceptibility distortion. The cord moves out of the imaging slice at approximately the C6 vertebral body. (B) Distortion-corrected B0 slice from the same subject. (C) Representative FA (range 0–0.9), (D) MD (range $0–2.3 \times 10^{-3}$ mm^2/s), and (E) RD (range $0–2.1 \times 10^{-3}$ mm^2/s) maps of the brainstem and spinal cord. (F) White matter skeleton (in green) overlaid on corresponding mean FA slice. Volume-rendered image (slightly magnified) showing regions with (G) a significant reduction in FA (in red; $p < 0.1$), and (H) a significant increase in RD (in green; $p < 0.1$) in ALS patients compared to age-matched healthy controls. (I) Volume-rendered image showing ROIs drawn along the corticospinal tract starting superiorly at the region of the pons (yellow), pyramids (cyan), C1 and C2 region (red), C3 (blue), C4 (green), C5 (violet), and C6 (yellow). (Right) The decreased diffusion anisotropy seen in the cervical cord of ALS correlates with disease severity. ROI drawn over the WM in cervical cord (C1 through C6) reveals (A) decreased FA ($p = 0.003$), and (B) increased RD ($p = 0.027$) in ALS patients compared to controls. (C) MD approaches statistical significance ($p = 0.089$), but (D) AD was no different between the two groups. There is significant correlation between DTI measures in ALS patients and clinical measures of disease progression, such as (E) RD and (F) FA with the average tapping speed of limbs, among others (*$p < 0.05$; **$p < 0.01$). *Source: Adapted from Ref. 38 with permission from NeuroImage.*

C3–C5 levels, and a negative correlation was seen between RD and finger and foot tapping, respiratory function, as measured by FVC (Figure 1.1.4) and the ASL Functional Rating Scale-R.[38] Interestingly, unlike studies in the brain, no differences in MD and AD were observed between healthy subjects and the ALS group, which is in keeping with a similar finding by Cohen-Adad et al.[130] Larger differences in FA and RD between patients and controls were observed at more distal cervical segments than in the upper cervical cord, supporting the hypothesis that neurodegeneration in ALS starts distally in the motor neuron terminals and then proceeds to involve the cell body (the "dying-back" phenomenon). From a clinical perspective, longer patient survival and the absence of lower motor neurone signs on clinical examination differentiate primary lateral sclerosis (PLS) from ALS.[131] Although much fewer studies have been carried out in patients with PLS, a single DTI study of the brain showed reductions in FA and increased MD in the corpus callosum and intracranial corticospinal tracts.[132] Whether similar changes in DTI metrics are seen in the spinal cord in PLS is unknown and still needs to be determined. PLS is histopathologically distinct from ALS in the brain and spinal cord, and further clinical MRI studies of the spinal cord in this patient group are therefore needed.[133]

1.1.3.7 Quantitative MRI of Structural Spinal Cord Lesions

1.1.3.7.1 *Spinal Cord Tumors*

Intramedullary spinal cord tumors are rare, with an incidence of 1.1/100,000 persons. They can occur anywhere along the length of the spine, but they are most commonly seen in the cervical spine. The most frequent histological types are ependymomas, astrocytomas, and hemangiomas.[134] Although they can often be visualized using conventional MRI on T2-weighted sequences, the effects of the tumors on the long tracts cannot be completely characterized using conventional imaging alone. Hemangioblastomas and ependymomas do not typically infiltrate neighboring tissues and are, therefore, regarded as surgically resectable; conversely, fibrillary astrocytomas often infiltrate surrounding tissue, which poses difficulties for their surgical management. Modern surgical procedures have made fine tumor excision possible, and the surgical outcome can be aided through clear tissue discrimination. Therefore, the development of imaging techniques that are capable of accurately predicting the course of white matter tracts within the spinal cord has the potential to improve surgical planning and patient outcomes.

Vargas et al. demonstrated that in three cases of spinal ependymoma, one case of myeloma, and one case of astrocytoma, DTI with tractography reconstruction showed the displacement of fiber tracts surrounding the tumors.[41] Three of the five tumors studied in the case series showed an increase in the ADC. FA values derived from the site of the tumor were reduced in all cases. In a similar study of five patients with spinal cord astrocytomas,[42] FA values were calculated from the tumor site and were found to be lower than in healthy controls. The FA data from both studies might be explained by an increase in extracellular water volume as a result of vasogenic edema or loss of axonal fibers, with subsequent loss of fiber density. Data from preliminary surgical trials suggest that DTI-derived tractography can be used to plan spinal cord tumor resection since it is capable of predicting the resectability of lesions.[135] However, the numbers of patients recruited in trials have so far been low, and further prospective work is required.

In clinical practice, MR spectroscopy of brain tumors is now commonly used in specialist neurological units; it can be useful diagnostically, and in some situations it helps avoid the need for a biopsy. However, MRS studies characterizing the metabolic profiles of spinal cord tumors, or showing the reliability of the technique, are currently lacking due to the technical challenges associated with spinal cord spectroscopy, as discussed in this chapter (also see Chapter 5.1).

1.1.3.7.2 Spinal Vascular Anomalies

Spinal arteriovenous malformations (AVMs) are congenital abnormalities of the vasculature within the spinal cord that are characterized by a compact intramedullary nidus, with feeding vessels most commonly arising from the anterior or posterior spinal arteries, or both, and draining into an arterialized coronal venous plexus. Typically, spinal AVMs produce a progressive myelopathy with periods of acute neurological worsening secondary to hemorrhage. Spinal AVMs may be associated with an increase of the extracellular fluid compartment because of venous congestion and loss of white matter in the normal-appearing cord distant to the nidus.[136,137] A small patient series by Ozanne et al. demonstrated that DTI of the spinal cord is possible in the presence of AVMs.[43] Interruption of fibers close to the nidus, loss of fibers distant to the lesion, and reduction in FA values were associated with clinical disability scores. Although their study includes a heterogeneous group of patients with AVMs with differing radiological characteristics, which makes it difficult to assign DTI changes to specific subgroups of patients, it suggests the possibility of mechanical effects of AVMs on surrounding tracts. At the level of the nidus, AVMs can interrupt, displace, or separate the fiber tracts, whereas, distant to the nidus, the effects of congestion or gliosis on the tracts can be inferred.

1.1.3.8 Application of Quantitative MRI Techniques as a Screening Tool for Occult Spinal Cord Disease

Spinal cord injury causing myelopathic symptoms can occur in a large number of systemic disorders, including human immunodeficiency virus (HIV), syphilis, systemic lupus erythematosis (SLE), Sjogrens syndrome, and deficiencies in vitamins E and B_{12}, among others. A small number of exploratory studies including only a few patients have attempted to apply qMRI techniques to detect pathology that is radiologically or clinically occult.

In a study of 20 patients with neuroborreliosis, where 12 patients had visible lesions in the brain on PD and T2 scans but none had lesions in the cord, MTR maps and MTR histograms found no differences between patients and controls in average cord MTR.[138]

In patients with neuropsychiatric SLE, Benedetti et al. found that peak height of cervical cord MD histograms were significantly lower in the 11 patients studied, compared to controls, but that average cord MD values were similar between patients and controls.[139] These results imply that some imaging voxels within the region studied had low MD values, but that this wasn't sufficient to affect the overall mean values significantly. There was no difference in FA histograms metrics between patients and controls. The occurrence of MD changes, in the absence of FA changes, has been suggested to reflect the consequences of Wallerian degeneration of long fiber tracts passing through diseased brain areas, because prior studies have shown that Wallerian degeneration first occurs in the axonal membranes and myelin sheaths, thus causing MD changes, but only minor or no changes to the measured FA.[50]

More recently, a comparison of DTI metrics of the cervical spinal cord between a cohort of asymptomatic patients with HIV and normal-appearing spinal cords aimed to screen for HIV- myelopathy-related changes that usually become clinically manifest only in advanced stages of infection.[140] In patients with HIV, there was a trend toward lower mean FA and higher mean MD in each of the measured ROIs within the spinal cord compared to healthy controls, which did not reach statistical significance.

Men with adrenomyeloneuropathy (AMN) usually develop spinal cord atrophy in the advanced stages of the disease. Fatemi et al. assessed patients using MT imaging and showed that they were able to visualize, localize, and quantify damage within the dorsal and lateral columns of patients and that MT hyperintensity in the dorsal column correlated with clinical scores, as assessed by the EDSS, and vibratory sense and postural sway.[141]

1.1.4 CONCLUSIONS AND FUTURE DIRECTIONS

Spinal cord pathology in neurological diseases often causes severe clinical disability, because important neurological functions are conveyed by densely arranged fibers. Quantitative MRI techniques have huge potential to provide information about this pathology, from both microstructural and functional perspectives at the site of spinal injury and distant from it. Changes in qMRI measures have been shown to differentiate patients from controls, and correlate well with clinical disability in a wide range of degenerative spinal cord diseases. Interestingly, in some diseases, such as spondylotic myelopathy, spinal cord diffusion may be able to predict patients who show a poor clinical recovery after surgery,[77] suggesting that qMRI may in future have value in predicting prognosis. However, the imaging studies of patients with spinal cord diseases that we discussed in this chapter are overall few when compared with brain studies carried out for the same diseases, and the former have often included small numbers of patients. Additionally, longitudinal spinal cord qMRI studies are lacking, and therefore it is currently unknown whether qMRI measures change over time. However, advanced spinal cord imaging potentially provides the detection of subclinical disease for earlier diagnosis and management. Spinal cord clinical trials generally employ conventional spinal cord MRI to confirm the safety of the new procedure or drug. Conversely, spinal cord qMRI may provide imaging biomarkers that can be used in clinical trials as outcome measures and to monitor disease progression. After standardization of spinal cord protocols and analysis methods across centers, spinal cord qMRI may even be used in multicenter clinical trials, which are crucial for rarer diseases.

References

1. Wingerchuk DM, Hogancamp WF, O'Brien PC, Weinshenker BG. The clinical course of neuromyelitis optica (Devic's syndrome). *Neurology.* September 22, 1999;53(5):1107–1114.
2. Brooks BR, Miller RG, Swash M, Munsat TL. El Escorial revisited: revised criteria for the diagnosis of amyotrophic lateral sclerosis. *Amyotrophic Lateral Scler.* 2000;1(5):293–299.
3. Bot JC, Barkhof F, Polman CH, et al. Spinal cord abnormalities in recently diagnosed MS patients: added value of spinal MRI examination. *Neurology.* January 27, 2004;62(2):226–233.
4. Soong BW, Paulson HL. Spinocerebellar ataxias: an update. *Curr Opin Neurol.* August 2007;20(4):438–446.
5. Wheeler-Kingshott CA, Hickman SJ, Parker GJ, et al. Investigating cervical spinal cord structure using axial diffusion tensor imaging. *NeuroImage.* May 2002;16(1):93–102.
6. Elshafiey I, Bilgen M, He R, Narayana PA. In vivo diffusion tensor imaging of rat spinal cord at 7 T. *Magn Reson Imaging.* April 2002;20(3):243–247.
7. Ciccarelli O, Altmann DR, McLean MA, et al. Spinal cord repair in MS: does mitochondrial metabolism play a role? *Neurology.* March 2, 2010;74(9):721–727.
8. Miller DH, Altmann DR, Chard DT. Advances in imaging to support the development of novel therapies for multiple sclerosis. *Clin Pharmacol Ther.* April 2012;91(4):621–634.
9. Harrison DM, Caffo BS, Shiee N, et al. Longitudinal changes in diffusion tensor-based quantitative MRI in multiple sclerosis. *Neurology.* January 11, 2011;76(2):179–186.
10. Brex PA, Leary SM, O'Riordan JI, et al. Measurement of spinal cord area in clinically isolated syndromes suggestive of multiple sclerosis. *J Neurol Neurosurg Psychiatry.* April 1, 2001;70(4):544–547.
11. Losseff NA, Webb SL, O'Riordan JI, et al. Spinal cord atrophy and disability in multiple sclerosis. A new reproducible and sensitive MRI method with potential to monitor disease progression. *Brain.* June 1996;119(Pt 3):701–708.
12. Ingle GT, Stevenson VL, Miller DH, Thompson AJ. Primary progressive multiple sclerosis: a 5-year clinical and MR study. *Brain.* November 2003;126(Pt 11):2528–2536.
13. Kendi AT, Tan FU, Kendi M, Yilmaz S, Huvaj S, Tellioglu S. MR spectroscopy of cervical spinal cord in patients with multiple sclerosis. *Neuroradiology.* September 2004;46(9):764–769.
14. Ciccarelli O, Wheeler-Kingshott CA, McLean MA, et al. Spinal cord spectroscopy and diffusion-based tractography to assess acute disability in multiple sclerosis. *Brain.* August 2007; 130(Pt 8):2220–2231.
15. Blamire AM, Cader S, Lee M, Palace J, Matthews PM. Axonal damage in the spinal cord of multiple sclerosis patients detected by magnetic resonance spectroscopy. *Magn Reson Med.* 2007;58(5): 880–885.
16. Henning A, Schar M, Kollias SS, Boesiger P, Dydak U. Quantitative magnetic resonance spectroscopy in the entire human cervical spinal cord and beyond at 3T. *Magn Reson Med.* June 2008;59(6):1250–1258.
17. Marliani AF, Clementi V, Albini Riccioli L, et al. Quantitative cervical spinal cord 3T proton MR spectroscopy in multiple sclerosis. *AJNR Am J Neuroradiol.* January 2010;31(1):180–184.
18. Ciccarelli O, Toosy AT, De Stefano N, Wheeler-Kingshott CA, Miller DH, Thompson AJ. Assessing neuronal metabolism in vivo by modeling imaging measures. *J Neurosci.* November 10, 2010;30(45):15030–15033.
19. Ciccarelli O, Thomas D, De Vita E, et al. Low myo-inositol indicating astrocytic damage in a case series of NMO. *Ann Neurol.* April 3, 2013.
20. Valsasina P, Rocca MA, Agosta F, et al. Mean diffusivity and fractional anisotropy histogram analysis of the cervical cord in MS patients. *NeuroImage.* July 1, 2005;26(3):822–828.
21. Oh J, Zackowski K, Chen M, et al. Multiparametric MRI correlates of sensorimotor function in the spinal cord in multiple sclerosis. *Mult Scler.* April 2013;19(4):427–435.
22. Oh J, Saidha S, Chen M, et al. Spinal cord quantitative MRI discriminates between disability levels in multiple sclerosis. *Neurology.* February 5, 2013;80(6):540–547.
23. Agosta F, Absinta M, Sormani MP, et al. In vivo assessment of cervical cord damage in MS patients: a longitudinal diffusion tensor MRI study. *Brain.* August 2007;130(Pt 8):2211–2219.
24. Agosta F, Pagani E, Caputo D, Filippi M. Associations between cervical cord gray matter damage and disability in patients with multiple sclerosis. *Arch Neurol.* September 2007;64(9):1302–1305.

25. Freund P, Wheeler-Kingshott C, Jackson J, Miller D, Thompson A, Ciccarelli O. Recovery after spinal cord relapse in multiple sclerosis is predicted by radial diffusivity. *Mult Scler.* October 2010;16(10):1193–1202.

26. Rovaris M, Bozzali M, Santuccio G, et al. In vivo assessment of the brain and cervical cord pathology of patients with primary progressive multiple sclerosis. *Brain.* December 2001;124(Pt 12): 2540–2549.

27. Filippi M, Bozzali M, Horsfield MA, et al. A conventional and magnetization transfer MRI study of the cervical cord in patients with MS. *Neurology.* January 11, 2000;54(1):207–213.

28. Rovaris M, Judica E, Ceccarelli A, et al. Absence of diffuse cervical cord tissue damage in early, non-disabling relapsing--remitting MS: a preliminary study. *Mult Scler.* July 2008;14(6): 853–856.

29. Rovaris M, Gallo A, Riva R, et al. An MT MRI study of the cervical cord in clinically isolated syndromes suggestive of MS. *Neurology.* August 10, 2004;63(3):584–585.

30. Charil A, Caputo D, Cavarretta R, Sormani MP, Ferrante P, Filippi M. Cervical cord magnetization transfer ratio and clinical changes over 18 months in patients with relapsing-remitting multiple sclerosis: a preliminary study. *Mult Scler.* October 2006;12(5):662–665.

31. Cheran S, Shanmuganathan K, Zhuo J, et al. Correlation of MR diffusion tensor imaging parameters with ASIA motor scores in hemorrhagic and nonhemorrhagic acute spinal cord injury. *J Neurotrauma.* September 2011;28(9):1881–1892.

32. Shanmuganathan K, Gullapalli RP, Zhuo J, Mirvis SE. Diffusion tensor MR imaging in cervical spine trauma. *AJNR Am J Neuroradiol.* April 2008;29(4):655–659.

33. Elliott JM, Pedler AR, Cowin G, Sterling M, McMahon K. Spinal cord metabolism and muscle water diffusion in whiplash. *Spinal Cord.* March 8, 2011.

34. Kachramanoglou C, De Vita E, Thomas DL, et al. Metabolic changes in the spinal cord after brachial plexus root re-implantation. *Neurorehabil Neural Repair.* February 2013;27(2):118–124.

35. Kara B, Celik A, Karadereler S, et al. The role of DTI in early detection of cervical spondylotic myelopathy: a preliminary study with 3-T MRI. *Neuroradiology.* August 2011;53(8):609–616.

36. Holly LT, Freitas B, McArthur DL, Salamon N. Proton magnetic resonance spectroscopy to evaluate spinal cord axonal injury in cervical spondylotic myelopathy. *J Neurosurg Spine.* March 2009; 10(3):194–200.

37. Hatem SM, Attal N, Ducreux D, et al. Assessment of spinal somatosensory systems with diffusion tensor imaging in syringomyelia. *J Neurol Neurosurg Psychiatry.* December 2009;80(12): 1350–1356.

38. Nair G, Carew JD, Usher S, Lu D, Hu XP, Benatar M. Diffusion tensor imaging reveals regional differences in the cervical spinal cord in amyotrophic lateral sclerosis. *NeuroImage.* November 1, 2010;53(2):576–583.

39. Carew JD, Nair G, Andersen PM, et al. Presymptomatic spinal cord neurometabolic findings in SOD1-positive people at risk for familial ALS. *Neurology.* October 4, 2011;77(14):1370–1375.

40. Carew JD, Nair G, Pineda-Alonso N, Usher S, Hu X, Benatar M. Magnetic resonance spectroscopy of the cervical cord in amyotrophic lateral sclerosis. *Amyotroph Lateral Scler.* May 2011;12(3): 185–191.

41. Vargas MI, Delavelle J, Jlassi H, et al. Clinical applications of diffusion tensor tractography of the spinal cord. *Neuroradiology.* January 2008;50(1):25–29.

42. Ducreux D, Lepeintre JF, Fillard P, Loureiro C, Tadie M, Lasjaunias P. MR diffusion tensor imaging and fiber tracking in 5 spinal cord astrocytomas. *AJNR Am J Neuroradiols.* January 2006; 27(1):214–216.

43. Ozanne A, Krings T, Facon D, et al. MR diffusion tensor imaging and fiber tracking in spinal cord arteriovenous malformations: a preliminary study. *AJNR Am J Neuroradiol.* August 2007;28(7): 1271–1279.

44. Qian W, Chan Q, Mak H, et al. Quantitative assessment of the cervical spinal cord damage in neuromyelitis optica using diffusion tensor imaging at 3 Tesla. *J Magn Reson Imaging: JMRI.* June 2011;33(6):1312–1320.

45. Song SK, Sun SW, Ramsbottom MJ, Chang C, Russell J, Cross AH. Dysmyelination revealed through MRI as increased radial (but unchanged axial) diffusion of water. *NeuroImage.* November 2002;17(3):1429–1436.

46. Kim JH, Budde MD, Liang HF, et al. Detecting axon damage in spinal cord from a mouse model of multiple sclerosis. *Neurobiol Dis.* March 2006;21(3):626–632.

47. Budde MD, Xie M, Cross AH, Song SK. Axial diffusivity is the primary correlate of axonal injury in the experimental autoimmune encephalomyelitis spinal cord: a quantitative pixelwise analysis. *J Neurosci.* March 4, 2009;29(9):2805–2813.

48. Zhang J, Jones M, DeBoy CA, et al. Diffusion tensor magnetic resonance imaging of Wallerian degeneration in rat spinal cord after dorsal root axotomy. *J Neurosci.* March 11, 2009;29(10): 3160–3171.

49. Basser PJ, Mattiello J, LeBihan D. MR diffusion tensor spectroscopy and imaging. *Biophysical J.* January 1994;66(1):259–267.

50. Pierpaoli C, Barnett A, Pajevic S. Water diffusion changes in Wallerian degeneration and their dependence on white matter architecture. *NeuroImage.* June 2001;13(6 Pt 1):1174–1185.

51. Basser PJ, Pierpaoli C. Microstructural and physiological features of tissues elucidated by quantitative-diffusion-tensor MRI. *J Magn Reson B.* June 1996;111(3):209–219.

52. Gass A, Niendorf T, Hirsch JG. Acute and chronic changes of the apparent diffusion coefficient in neurological disorders—biophysical mechanisms and possible underlying histopathology. *J Neurol Sci.* 2001;186(suppl 1):S15–S23.

53. Mamata H, Jolesz FA, Maier SE. Apparent diffusion coefficient and fractional anisotropy in spinal cord: age and cervical spondylosis-related changes. *J Magn Reson Imaging: JMRI.* July 2005;22(1):38–43.

54. Gomez-Anson B, MacManus DG, Parker GJ, et al. In vivo ¹H-magnetic resonance spectroscopy of the spinal cord in humans. *Neuroradiology.* July 2000;42(7):515–517.

55. Marliani AF, Clementi V, Albini-Riccioli L, Agati R, Leonardi M. Quantitative proton magnetic resonance spectroscopy of the human cervical spinal cord at 3 Tesla. *Magn Reson Med.* 2007; 57(1):160–163.

56. Solanky BS, Abdel-Aziz K, Yiannakas MC, Berry AM, Ciccarelli O, Wheeler-Kingshott CA. In vivo magnetic resonance spectroscopy detection of combined glutamate-glutamine in a healthy upper cervical cord at 3 T. *NMR Biomed.* 2013;26(3): 357–366.

57. Patel TB, Clark JB. Synthesis of *N*-acetyl-L-aspartate by rat brain mitochondria and its involvement in mitochondrial/cytosolic carbon transport. *Biochem J.* December 15, 1979; 184(3):539–546.

58. De Stefano N, Matthews PM, Antel JP, Preul M, Francis G, Arnold DL. Chemical pathology of acute demyelinating lesions and its correlation with disability. *Ann Neurol.* December 1995; 38(6):901–909.

59. Davie CA, Hawkins CP, Barker GJ, et al. Detection of myelin breakdown products by proton magnetic resonance spectroscopy. *Lancet.* March 6, 1993;341(8845):630–631.

60. Petroff OA, Graham GD, Blamire AM, et al. Spectroscopic imaging of stroke in humans: histopathology correlates of spectral changes. *Neurology.* July 1992;42(7):1349–1354.

61. Alger JR, Frank JA, Bizzi A, et al. Metabolism of human gliomas: assessment with H-1 MR spectroscopy and F-18 fluorodeoxyglucose PET. *Radiology.* December 1990;177(3):633–641.

62. Matthews PM, Andermann F, Silver K, Karpati G, Arnold DL. Proton MR spectroscopic characterization of differences in regional brain metabolic abnormalities in mitochondrial encephalomyopathies. *Neurology.* December 1, 1993;43(12):2484.

63. Edden RA, Bonekamp D, Smith MA, Dubey P, Barker PB. Proton MR spectroscopic imaging of the medulla and cervical spinal cord. *J Magn Reson Imaging: JMRI.* October 2007;26(4):1101–1105.

64. Schmierer K, Scaravilli F, Altmann DR, Barker GJ, Miller DH. Magnetization transfer ratio and myelin in postmortem multiple sclerosis brain. *Ann Neurol.* September 2004;56(3):407–415.

65. van Waesberghe JH, Kamphorst W, De Groot CJ, et al. Axonal loss in multiple sclerosis lesions: magnetic resonance imaging insights into substrates of disability. *Ann Neurol.* November 1999; 46(5):747–754.

66. Zackowski KM, Smith SA, Reich DS, et al. Sensorimotor dysfunction in multiple sclerosis and column-specific magnetization transfer-imaging abnormalities in the spinal cord. *Brain.* May 2009;132(Pt 5):1200–1209.

67. Inglese M, van Waesberghe JH, Rovaris M, et al. The effect of interferon beta-1b on quantities derived from MT MRI in secondary progressive MS. *Neurology.* March 11, 2003;60(5):853–860.

68. Filippi M, Rocca MA, Pagani E, et al. European study on intravenous immunoglobulin in multiple sclerosis: results of magnetization transfer magnetic resonance imaging analysis. *Arch Neurol.* September 2004;61(9):1409–1412.

69. Compston A, Coles A. Multiple sclerosis. *Lancet.* April 6, 2002; 359(9313):1221–1231.

70. Lublin FD, Reingold SC. Defining the clinical course of multiple sclerosis: results of an international survey. National Multiple Sclerosis Society (USA) Advisory Committee on Clinical Trials of New Agents in Multiple Sclerosis. *Neurology.* April 1996;46(4): 907–911.

71. Barkhof F, Filippi M, Miller DH, et al. Comparison of MRI criteria at first presentation to predict conversion to clinically definite multiple sclerosis. *Brain.* November 1997;120(Pt 11):2059–2069.

72. McDonald WI, Compston A, Edan G, et al. Recommended diagnostic criteria for multiple sclerosis: guidelines from the International Panel on the diagnosis of multiple sclerosis. *Ann Neurol.* July 2001;50(1):121–127.

73. Polman CH, Reingold SC, Banwell B, et al. Diagnostic criteria for multiple sclerosis: 2010 revisions to the McDonald criteria. *Ann Neurol.* February 2011;69(2):292–302.

74. Polman CH, Reingold SC, Edan G, et al. Diagnostic criteria for multiple sclerosis: 2005 revisions to the "McDonald Criteria". *Ann Neurol.* December 2005;58(6):840–846.

75. Kidd D, Thorpe JW, Thompson AJ, et al. Spinal cord MRI using multi-array coils and fast spin echo: II. Findings in multiple sclerosis. *Neurology.* December 1, 1993;43(12):2632.

76. O'Riordan JI, Losseff NA, Phatouros C, et al. Asymptomatic spinal cord lesions in clinically isolated optic nerve, brain stem, and spinal cord syndromes suggestive of demyelination. *J Neurol Neurosurg Psychiatry.* March 1998;64(3):353–357.

77. Lycklama a Nijeholt GJ, Uitdehaag BM, Bergers E, Castelijns JA, Polman CH, Barkhof F. Spinal cord magnetic resonance imaging in suspected multiple sclerosis. *Eur Radiol.* 2000;10(2):368–376.

78. Barkhof F. The clinico-radiological paradox in multiple sclerosis revisited. *Curr Opin Neurol.* June 2002;15(3):239–245.

79. Bergers E, Bot JC, De Groot CJ, et al. Axonal damage in the spinal cord of MS patients occurs largely independent of T2 MRI lesions. *Neurology.* December 10, 2002;59(11):1766–1771.

80. Benedetti B, Rocca MA, Rovaris M, et al. A diffusion tensor MRI study of cervical cord damage in benign and secondary

81. Stevenson VL, Leary SM, Losseff NA, et al. Spinal cord atrophy and disability in MS: a longitudinal study. *Neurology.* July 1998; 51(1):234–238.

82. Liu C, Edwards S, Gong Q, Roberts N, Blumhardt LD. Three dimensional MRI estimates of brain and spinal cord atrophy in multiple sclerosis. *J Neurol Neurosurg Psychiatry.* March 1999; 66(3):323–330.

83. Kalkers NF, Barkhof F, Bergers E, van Schijndel R, Polman CH. The effect of the neuroprotective agent riluzole on MRI parameters in primary progressive multiple sclerosis: a pilot study. *Mult Scler.* December 2002;8(6):532–533.

84. Lin X, Tench CR, Turner B, Blumhardt LD, Constantinescu CS. Spinal cord atrophy and disability in multiple sclerosis over four years: application of a reproducible automated technique in monitoring disease progression in a cohort of the interferon beta-1a (Rebif) treatment trial. *J Neurol Neurosurg Psychiatry.* August 2003;74(8):1090–1094.

85. Horsfield MA, Sala S, Neema M, et al. Rapid semi-automatic segmentation of the spinal cord from magnetic resonance images: application in multiple sclerosis. *NeuroImage.* April 1, 2010; 50(2):446–455.

86. Kearney H, Yiannakas MC, Abdel-Aziz K, et al. Improved MRI quantification of spinal cord atrophy in multiple sclerosis. *J Magn Reson Imaging.* April 30, 2013.

87. Yiannakas MC, Kearney H, Samson RS, et al. Feasibility of grey matter and white matter segmentation of the upper cervical cord in vivo: a pilot study with application to magnetisation transfer measurements. *NeuroImage.* November 15, 2012;63(3): 1054–1059.

88. Rocca MA, Valsasina P, Damjanovic D, et al. Voxel-wise mapping of cervical cord damage in multiple sclerosis patients with different clinical phenotypes. *J Neurol Neurosurg Psychiatry.* January 2013;84(1):35–41.

89. Brand A, Richter-Landsberg C, Leibfritz D. Multinuclear NMR studies on the energy metabolism of glial and neuronal cells. *Dev Neurosci.* 1993;15(3–5):289–298.

90. Fernando KT, McLean MA, Chard DT, et al. Elevated white matter myo-inositol in clinically isolated syndromes suggestive of multiple sclerosis. *Brain.* June 2004;127(Pt 6):1361–1369.

91. Rovaris M, Bozzali M, Santuccio G, et al. Relative contributions of brain and cervical cord pathology to multiple sclerosis disability: a study with magnetisation transfer ratio histogram analysis. *J Neurol Neurosurg Psychiatry.* December 2000;69(6): 723–727.

92. Bozzali M, Rocca MA, Iannucci G, Pereira C, Comi G, Filippi M. Magnetization-transfer histogram analysis of the cervical cord in patients with multiple sclerosis. *AJNR Am J Neuroradiol.* November–December 1999;20(10):1803–1808.

93. Gilmore CP, Geurts JJ, Evangelou N, et al. Spinal cord grey matter lesions in multiple sclerosis detected by post-mortem high field MR imaging. *Mult Scler.* February 2009;15(2):180–188.

94. Chan KH, Ramsden DB, Yu YL, et al. Neuromyelitis optica-IgG in idiopathic inflammatory demyelinating disorders amongst Hong Kong Chinese. *Eur J Neurol.* March 2009;16(3):310–316.

95. Rocca MA, Agosta F, Mezzapesa DM, et al. Magnetization transfer and diffusion tensor MRI show gray matter damage in neuromyelitis optica. *Neurology.* February 10, 2004;62(3):476–478.

96. Yu C, Lin F, Li K, et al. Pathogenesis of normal-appearing white matter damage in neuromyelitis optica: diffusion-tensor MR imaging. *Radiology.* January 2008;246(1):222–228.

97. de Seze J, Blanc F, Kremer S, et al. Magnetic resonance spectroscopy evaluation in patients with neuromyelitis optica. *J Neurol Neurosurg Psychiatry.* April 2010;81(4):409–411.

98. Sekhon LH, Fehlings MG. Epidemiology, demographics, and pathophysiology of acute spinal cord injury. *Spine*. December 15, 2001;26(suppl 24):S2–S12.

99. McDonald JW, Sadowsky C. Spinal-cord injury. *Lancet*. February 2, 2002;359(9304):417–425.

100. Wyndaele M, Wyndaele JJ. Incidence, prevalence and epidemiology of spinal cord injury: what learns a worldwide literature survey? *Spinal Cord*. September 2006;44(9):523–529.

101. Poon PC, Gupta D, Shoichet MS, Tator CH. Clip compression model is useful for thoracic spinal cord injuries: histologic and functional correlates. *Spine*. December 1, 2007;32(25):2853–2859.

102. Kwon BK, Tetzlaff W, Grauer JN, Beiner J, Vaccaro AR. Pathophysiology and pharmacologic treatment of acute spinal cord injury. *Spine J*. July–August 2004;4(4):451–464.

103. Flanders AE, Spettell CM, Tartaglino LM, Friedman DP, Herbison GJ. Forecasting motor recovery after cervical spinal cord injury: value of MR imaging. *Radiology*. December 1996; 201(3):649–655.

104. Carlstedt T. Root repair review: basic science background and clinical outcome. *Restor Neurol Neurosci*. 2008;26(2–3):225–241.

105. Koliatsos VE, Price WL, Pardo CA, Price DL. Ventral root avulsion: an experimental model of death of adult motor neurons. *J Comp Neurol*. April 1, 1994;342(1):35–44.

106. Risling M, Ochsman T, Carlstedt T, et al. On acute gene expression changes after ventral root replantation. *Front Neurol*. 2011;1:159.

107. Kachramanoglou C, Li D, Andrews P, et al. Novel strategies in brachial plexus repair after traumatic avulsion. *Br J Neurosurg*. February 2011;25(1):16–27.

108. Shedid D, Benzel EC. Cervical spondylosis anatomy: pathophysiology and biomechanics. *Neurosurgery*. January 2007;60(1 suppl 1):S7–S13.

109. Baptiste DC, Fehlings MG. Pathophysiology of cervical myelopathy. *Spine J*. November–December 2006;6(suppl 6):190S–197S.

110. Baron EM, Young WF. Cervical spondylotic myelopathy: a brief review of its pathophysiology, clinical course, and diagnosis. *Neurosurgery*. January 2007;60(1 suppl 1):S35–S41.

111. Matsuda Y, Miyazaki K, Tada K. Increased MR signal intensity due to cervical myelopathy. Analysis of 29 surgical cases. *J Neurosurg*. June 1991;74(6):887–892.

112. Takahashi M, Yamashita Y, Sakamoto Y, Kojima R. Chronic cervical cord compression: clinical significance of increased signal intensity on MR images. *Radiology*. October 1989;173(1):219–224.

113. Matsumoto M, Toyama Y, Ishikawa M, Chiba K, Suzuki N, Fujimura Y. Increased signal intensity of the spinal cord on magnetic resonance images in cervical compressive myelopathy. Does it predict the outcome of conservative treatment? *Spine*. March 15, 2000;25(6):677–682.

114. Facon D, Ozanne A, Fillard P, Lepeintre JF, Tournoux-Facon C, Ducreux D. MR diffusion tensor imaging and fiber tracking in spinal cord compression. *AJNR Am J Neuroradiol*. June–July 2005; 26(6):1587–1594.

115. Hori M, Okubo T, Aoki S, Kumagai H, Araki T. Line scan diffusion tensor MRI at low magnetic field strength: feasibility study of cervical spondylotic myelopathy in an early clinical stage. *J Magn Reson Imaging*. 2006;23(2):183–188.

116. Hatem SM, Attal N, Ducreux D. Clinical, functional and structural determinants of central pain in syringomyelia. *Brain*. November 2010;133(11):3409–3422.

117. Roser F, Ebner FH, Maier G, Tatagiba M, Nagele T, Klose U. Fractional anisotropy levels derived from diffusion tensor imaging in cervical syringomyelia. *Neurosurgery*. October 2010;67(4): 901–905. Discussion 905.

118. Hardiman O, van den Berg LH, Kiernan MC. Clinical diagnosis and management of amyotrophic lateral sclerosis. *Nat Rev Neurol*. November 2011;7(11):639–649.

119. Pasinelli P, Brown RH. Molecular biology of amyotrophic lateral sclerosis: insights from genetics. *Nat Rev Neurosci*. September 2006;7(9):710–723.

120. Keeney P, Bennett J. ALS spinal neurons show varied and reduced mtDNA gene copy numbers and increased mtDNA gene deletions. *Mol Neurodegener*. 2010;5(1):21.

121. Niessen HG, Debska-Vielhaber G, Sander K, et al. Metabolic progression markers of neurodegeneration in the transgenic G93A-SOD1 mouse model of amyotrophic lateral sclerosis. *Eur J Neurosci*. March 2007;25(6):1669–1677.

122. Duffy LM, Chapman AL, Shaw PJ, Grierson AJ. Review: the role of mitochondria in the pathogenesis of amyotrophic lateral sclerosis. *Neuropathol Appl Neurobiol*. June 2011;37(4):336–352.

123. Azzouz M, Leclerc N, Gurney M, Warter JM, Poindron P, Borg J. Progressive motor neuron impairment in an animal model of familial amyotrophic lateral sclerosis. *Muscle Nerve*. January 1997; 20(1):45–51.

124. Aggarwal A, Nicholson G. Detection of preclinical motor neurone loss in SOD1 mutation carriers using motor unit number estimation. *J Neurol Neurosurg Psychiatry*. August 1, 2002;73(2): 199–201.

125. Turner MR, Grosskreutz J, Kassubek J, et al. Towards a neuroimaging biomarker for amyotrophic lateral sclerosis. *Lancet Neurol*. May 2011;10(5):400–403.

126. Toosy AT, Werring DJ, Orrell RW, et al. Diffusion tensor imaging detects corticospinal tract involvement at multiple levels in amyotrophic lateral sclerosis. *J Neurol Neurosurg Psychiatry*. September 2003;74(9):1250–1257.

127. Abe O, Yamada H, Masutani Y, et al. Amyotrophic lateral sclerosis: diffusion tensor tractography and voxel-based analysis. *NMR Biomed*. October 2004;17(6):411–416.

128. Sach M, Winkler G, Glauche V, et al. Diffusion tensor MRI of early upper motor neuron involvement in amyotrophic lateral sclerosis. *Brain*. February 2004;127(Pt 2):340–350.

129. Sage CA, Peeters RR, Gorner A, Robberecht W, Sunaert S. Quantitative diffusion tensor imaging in amyotrophic lateral sclerosis. *NeuroImage*. January 15, 2007;34(2):486–499.

130. Cohen-Adad J, El Mendili MM, Morizot-Koutlidis R, et al. Involvement of spinal sensory pathway in ALS and specificity of cord atrophy to lower motor neuron degeneration. *Amyotroph Lateral Scler Frontotemporal Degener*. January 2013;14(1): 30–38.

131. Tartaglia MC, Rowe A, Findlater K, Orange JB, Grace G, Strong MJ. Differentiation between primary lateral sclerosis and amyotrophic lateral sclerosis: examination of symptoms and signs at disease onset and during follow-up. *Arch Neurol*. February 1, 2007;64(2):232–236.

132. Iwata NK, Kwan JY, Danielian LE, et al. White matter alterations differ in primary lateral sclerosis and amyotrophic lateral sclerosis. *Brain*. September 2011;134(Pt 9):2642–2655.

133. Pringle CE, Hudson AJ, Munoz DG, Kiernan JA, Brown WF, Ebers GC. Primary lateral sclerosis. Clinical features, neuropathology and diagnostic criteria. *Brain*. April 1992;115(Pt 2): 495–520.

134. Stein BM, McCormick PC. Spinal intradural tumours. In: Wilkins RHR SS, ed. *Neurosurgery*. New York: McGrawHill; 1996: 1769–1789.

135. Setzer M, Murtagh RD, Murtagh FR, et al. Diffusion tensor imaging tractography in patients with intramedullary tumors: comparison with intraoperative findings and value for prediction of tumor resectability. *J Neurosurg Spine*. September 2010;13(3): 371–380.

136. Berenstein ALL P, ter Brugge KG. *Spinal Arteriovenous Malformation. Surgical Neuroangiography*. 2nd ed. Berlin: Springer-Verlag; 2004:737–843.

137. Krings T, Mull M, Gilsbach JM, Thron A. Spinal vascular malformations. *Eur Radiol.* February 2005;15(2):267–278.

138. Agosta F, Rocca MA, Benedetti B, Capra R, Cordioli C, Filippi M. MR imaging assessment of brain and cervical cord damage in patients with neuroborreliosis. *AJNR Am J Neuroradiol.* April 2006;27(4):892–894.

139. Benedetti B, Rovaris M, Judica E, Donadoni G, Ciboddo G, Filippi M. Assessing "occult" cervical cord damage in patients with neuropsychiatric systemic lupus erythematosus using diffusion tensor MRI. *J Neurol Neurosurg Psychiatry.* August 2007; 78(8):893–895.

140. Mueller-Mang C, Law M, Mang T, Fruehwald-Pallamar J, Weber M, Thurnher MM. Diffusion tensor MR imaging (DTI) metrics in the cervical spinal cord in asymptomatic HIV-positive patients. *Neuroradiology.* August 2011;53(8):585–592.

141. Fatemi A, Smith SA, Dubey P. Magnetization transfer MRI demonstrates spinal cord abnormalities in adrenomyeloneuropathy. *Neurology.* May 24, 2005;64(10):1739–1745.

I. QUANTITATIVE BIOMARKERS IN THE SPINAL CORD: WHAT FOR?

1.2

Inflammatory Demyelinating Diseases

Istvan Pirko[1], Charles R.G. Guttmann[2]

[1]Department of Neurology, Mayo Clinic, College of Medicine, Rochester, MN, USA [2]Center for Neurological Imaging, Brigham and Women's Hospital, Harvard Medical School, Boston, MA, USA

1.2.1 INTRODUCTION

The spinal cord is a common site of involvement in inflammatory demyelinating diseases of the central nervous system (CNS). The most common such disease, multiple sclerosis, is the leading cause of nontraumatic disability in young adults, with an enormous socioeconomic impact.[1] Neuromyelitis optica (NMO), an increasingly recognized and recently redefined condition, also has prominent and very characteristic spinal cord involvement, which is typically much more severe than MS-related transverse myelitis. The critical importance of spinal cord imaging in these conditions is also highlighted by the inclusion of spinal cord magnetic resonance imaging (MRI)-derived metrics in the internationally utilized diagnostic criteria of MS and NMO. However, with the constant evolution of the MS diagnostic criteria, new discoveries pertaining to the pathogenesis and biomarkers of NMO, and the evolving definitions of transverse myelitis, acute disseminated encephalomyelitis (ADEM), pediatric MS, and systemic autoimmune disease-associated and paraneoplastic myelopathies, one might feel overwhelmed when attempting to classify, characterize, diagnose, and manage these conditions. Neuroimaging, specifically MRI, plays a key role in the correct diagnosis of these conditions, and it provides a critically important aid for treatment monitoring. With the advent of advanced MRI techniques enabling quantitative analysis methods, MRI provides a reliable tool in monitoring and characterizing disease progression, and it also enables a unique insight into the generally poorly understood pathogenesis of these disorders.

In this chapter, we will discuss the currently available and constantly evolving MRI-based quantitative tools. These will be discussed in the context of the most common forms of acute and subacute inflammatory myelopathies, including MS-related transverse myelitis, longitudinally extensive transverse myelitis (LETM) related to NMO and NMO spectrum disorder, and idiopathic inflammatory transverse myelitis in the context of MS and as a stand-alone condition. The vast majority of the published quantitative MRI literature clearly has focused on MS, with a smaller but growing proportion of studies related to NMO; for that reason, these two diseases are the main focus when we discuss quantitative methods. Finally, we will outline future perspectives and challenges in the evolving field of quantitative MRI in inflammatory myelopathies.

1.2.2 CLASSIFICATION OF INFLAMMATORY MYELOPATHIES

While there is currently no single universally accepted and utilized classification of inflammatory myelopathies, one can consider several features of these conditions to establish clinically useful classifications. One such feature is the lesion location or "lesion type" (Table 1.2.1).[2] In addition, an important classification strategy also followed in the recently published American Academy of Neurology guidelines is whether the TM episode is complete or partial,[3] which is an especially helpful distinguishing feature at first presentation with transverse myelitis.

> **SPINAL CORD INVOLVEMENT IN INFLAMMATORY MYELOPATHIES: KEY POINTS AND FEATURES**
>
> - Multiple sclerosis (MS): Patch-like lesions abutting the surface of the cord; in contact with

22

cerebral spinal fluid (CSF); up to one-half of the axial crosscut surface is involved, but more commonly one-fourth to one-third

- Neuromyelitis optica (NMO): Longitudinally extensive transverse myelitis—three or more segments long, "center of the cord" appearance on axial cuts, often involves more than 50% on axial cuts
- Idiopathic transverse myelitis (TM): May be similar to MS or NMO-like lesions, without meeting the criteria for either; can be a clinically isolated syndrome (CIS) leading to MS, the first manifestation of NMO, or a stand-alone disease
- Paraneoplastic myelopathies: Most commonly present as tractopathy

1.2.3 TRANSVERSE MYELITIS: A PRACTICAL DEFINITION BASED ON MRI

Transverse myelitis is a collective term for segmental inflammatory disorders of the spinal cord. While TM can be seen in the context of infections, which are typically easily recognized given the associated systemic features and/or CSF findings, most cases represent idiopathic inflammatory diseases, including MS, NMO, and less commonly ADEM, paraneoplastic disorders, or sarcoidosis. Metabolic diseases such as vitamin B_{12} or copper deficiency also may look like TM on conventional MRI, but even with conventional imaging usually there are clear clues regarding their noninflammatory nature.

The most important classifying feature of idiopathic TM is based on its MRI appearance on axial and sagittal scans: lesions that encompass one-fourth to one-third of

TABLE 1.2.1   Classification of Inflammatory Myelopathies Based on Lesion Location

Type of Lesion	Tracts Involved	Clinical Signs	Examples
Complete	All tracts	Pyramidal, sensory, and autonomic dysfunction below lesion	Trauma or acute necrotizing viral myelitis
Bown–Séquard hemicord syndrome	Ipsilateral corticospinal, posterior columns; contralateral spinothalamic	Ipsilateral pyramidal weakness and loss of posterior column function; contralateral spinothalamic loss	Multiple sclerosis, compression
Anterior cord syndrome	Bilateral anterior horn cells corticospinal tracts, spinothalamic and autonomic	Acute bilateral flaccid weakness, loss of pain temperature, and sphincter and autonomic dysfunction; preservation of dorsal column modalities such as joint position sense	Anterior spinal artery occlusion
Posterior cord	Bilateral posterior columns	Bilateral loss of light touch, vibration, and joint position	Vitamin B_{12} or copper deficiency (usually chronic)
Central	Crossing spinothalamic, corticospinal, and autonomic fibers	Dissociated sensory loss (loss of pain and temperature with preserved vibration and joint position); pyramidal distribution weakness below lesion; autonomic dysfunction below the lesion	Syrinx, neuromyelitis optica
Conus medullaris	Autonomic outflow and sacral spinal cord segments	Early sphincter dysfunction, sacral sensory loss, and relatively mild motor dysfunction	Postviral myelitis
Cauda equina	Spinal nerve roots of the cauda equina	Early, often asymmetric flaccid weakness of the lower limbs; sensory loss in root distribution followed by autonomic dysfunction	Acute cytomegalovirus polyradiculitis, compression
Tractopathies	Selective tract involvement	Selective pyramidal, posterior column involvement	Paraneoplastic myelopathy, copper deficiency, vitamin B_{12} deficiency

Modified from Ref. 2.

the cord crosscut surface area, typically abut the CSF, have a wedge-like appearance, and on sagittal images rarely extend beyond one or two segments are typical MS lesions. By contrast, lesions that are mostly gray matter centered, encompass one-half or more of the crosscut surface area, are longitudinally extensive usually beyond three segments, and during their acute stage are associated with mass effect are typical NMO lesions. TM lesions with NMO-like characteristics are often labeled as LETM.

1.2.4 THE SIGNIFICANCE OF TM AND ITS RELATIONSHIP TO MS AND NMO

It is important to note that a single idiopathic TM event should be considered a CIS that may evolve into MS or NMO later, or may be a stand-alone disease without conversion to a more disseminated demyelinating disease. From the standpoint of a classic MS-like TM evolving into clinically definite MS (CDMS, defined as MS with more than one clinical event clearly related to demyelinating disease), the most important clue is whether upon presentation more than just the symptomatic cord lesion is visualized. If additional MS-like lesions are seen in either the brain or spinal cord, and especially if these lesions meet the Barkhof–Tintore "dissemination in space" criteria (Table 1.2.2), then the patient would fall into the "high conversion risk group," which has a >80% risk of developing CDMS over the next 20 years, with a hazard ratio of over 6.4[6] and most of them converting early on.[7–9] If, in addition to nonsymptomatic MS-like lesions, the CSF is also positive for common markers of MS (immunoglobulin G (IgG) index elevation and oligoclonal bands positivity), the conversion risk is even higher, and conversion occurs earlier, typically within the first couple of years.[10]

In 2010, a new set of criteria was proposed for MS, which represents the second modification of the original McDonald MS criteria from 2001.[11] Of note, the 2001 McDonald criteria were the first to incorporate MRI characteristics in the diagnosis of MS. The new 2010 criteria further refine the MRI-based *dissemination in space* and *dissemination in time* (DIT) criteria, with special emphasis placed on spinal cord lesions in the dissemination in space criteria (Table 1.2.2) and in the criteria of primary progressive MS (PPMS). The presence of spinal cord lesions in general increases the diagnostic certainty in MS, as many of the "MS mimics" do not lead to cord lesion formation. In PPMS, and in progressive forms of MS in general, the main symptom is that of a slowly progressive myelopathy, which is reflected by the extensive use of cord-derived MRI parameters in the new diagnostic criteria. Advanced MRI methods are becoming especially important in progressive forms of MS, especially in PPMS: in this MS subtype, the most typical clinical presentation is that of a slowly progressive myelopathy, with only minimal if any accompanying MRI activity on conventional MRI despite the ongoing progression. This MS subtype also represents the most universally disabling form of MS (apart from the very rarely seen cases of fulminant MS such as the Marburg variant), and typically PPMS is also the least likely to respond to currently available treatments. Advanced quantitative MRI will likely play a very important role in monitoring PPMS, especially in upcoming tissue restorative treatment trials, and will likely also shed light on the pathogenesis of this very poorly understood entity.

The new DIT criteria (Table 1.2.3) do not have a cord-specific component but enable one single scan at one time point to fulfill DIT: if a scan has both enhancing ("new") and nonenhancing ("old") lesions in the typical configuration for MS, DIT criteria are met.[11,12] While

TABLE 1.2.2   Criteria for Dissemination in Space in MS

DIS Can Be Demonstrated by ≥1 T2 Lesion[1] in At Least 2 of 4 Areas of the CNS

Periventricular

Juxtacortical

Infratentorial

Spinal cord[2]

[1] *Gadolinium enhancement of lesions is not required for DIS.*
[2] *If a subject has a brainstem or spinal cord syndrome, the symptomatic lesions are excluded from the criteria and do not contribute to lesion count.*
MRI = magnetic resonance imaging; DIS = lesion dissemination in space; CNS = central nervous system.
Based on Refs 4 and 5.

TABLE 1.2.3   Criteria for Primary Progressive MS

PPMS May Be Diagnosed in Subjects with

1. One year of disease progression (retrospectively or prospectively determined)
2. Plus 2 of the 3 following criteria[1]
   a. Evidence for DIS in the brain based on ≥1 T2[2] lesions in at least 1 area characteristic for MS (periventricular, juxtacortical, or infratentorial)
   b. Evidence for DIS in the spinal cord based on ≥2 T2[2] lesions in the cord
   c. Positive CSF (isoelectric focusing evidence of oligoclonal bands and/or elevated IgG index)

[1] *If a subject has a brainstem or spinal cord syndrome, all symptomatic lesions are excluded from the criteria.*
[2] *Gadolinium enhancement of lesions is not required.*
MS = multiple sclerosis; PPMS = primary progressive MS; DIS = lesion dissemination in space; CSF = cerebrospinal fluid; IgG = immunoglobulin G.

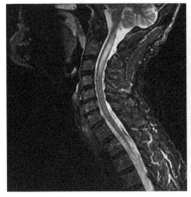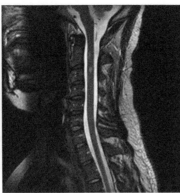

FIGURE 1.2.1 Comparison of longitudinally extensive transverse myelitis (LETM, left panel) and MS-like transverse myelitis (right panel). Note the proximal cervical cord lesion in the NMO-IgG positive LETM case (left panel) associated with a "swollen cord" appearance (mass effect) and mostly *central* cord signal abnormality. Right panel: MS-like transverse myelitis, with small, patchy lesions in the proximal cervical cord. Note the lack of mass effect and lack of a "swollen cord" appearance.

the new DIT criteria certainly will lead to earlier diagnosis and as such may have important treatment ramifications, one must be very cautious with this new development: if more than one pathology is present, such as a one-time demyelinating event intermixed with another pathology that may lead to the presence of enhancing lesions, such as dural AV fistulas in the spinal cord or venous angiomas in the brain, one may encounter cases that do meet DIT criteria but for reasons unrelated to MS. In effect, it can be stated that, as a result of the newly introduced changes, the specificity of the new criteria is lower, while the sensitivity to classify as MS is higher (Figure 1.2.1).

TABLE 1.2.4   NMO Diagnostic Criteria

Mayo Clinic Diagnostic Criteria for Neuromyelitis Optica (NMO)
Definite NMO
Optic neuritis
Acute myelitis
At least two of three supportive criteria
1. Contiguous spinal cord MRI lesion extending over three or more vertebral segments
2. Brain MRI not meeting diagnostic criteria for multiple sclerosis
3. NMO-IgG seropositive status

1.2.5 NEUROMYELITIS OPTICA: THE FIRST DEMYELINATING DISEASE WITH A KNOWN SERUM MARKER

Although NMO was considered for decades an "MS variety" and a "severe form of MS," recent research has completely redefined this inflammatory demyelinating disease and concluded that it has different epidemiology, pathology, CSF findings, radiological features, and response to therapy than classic MS. Dr Vanda Lennon and her colleagues at Mayo Clinic identified a serum marker for this disease: NMO-IgG, an antibody against aquaporin-4 water channels in astrocytic endfeet. NMO-IgG is seen in up to 80% of NMO cases, and when seen, it is virtually pathognomonic to NMO (specificity close to 100%)[13,14] (Table 1.2.4). It is likely that NMO-IgG is actually pathogenic in the right environment, and not just a biomarker.[15] The fact that NMO's marker antibody has nothing to do with myelin or oligodendrocytes, but is for a water channel on astrocytes, is both surprising and very significant from the standpoint of new directions in demyelinating disease research. NMO is now considered a disease that

primarily targets astrocytes. The only remaining link between MS and NMO is the presence of demyelination in both entities; however, in NMO, demyelination is just a small part of the extensive pathology, and it isn't even present in every lesion type that NMO can be associated with.[16,17] Active inflammatory NMO lesions are associated with more extensive tissue damage than MS lesions. NMO pathology also includes uncharacteristic elements for MS, such as eosinophilic infiltration, loss of aquaporin-4 staining in lesions vs. the upregulation of aquaporin-4 immunoreactivity in MS, and nonlesional pathology in normally aquaporin-4-rich areas characterized by aquaporin-4 loss without severe inflammation.[16–19]

From the spine-imaging standpoint, NMO cases are characterized by LETM. It is important to note that a myelitis event associated with LETM does not equal NMO: by definition, NMO must include optic neuritis as well as transverse myelitis[20] (Table 1.2.3). In addition, LETM may be associated with other conditions, such as ADEM or pediatric MS. However, first presentation with LETM may imply that the patient is at risk for the development of the full clinical phenotype of NMO and/or for recurrent myelitis events. This situation, especially when associated with NMO-IgG positivity, is often labeled NMO spectrum disorder (NMO-SD). LETM in NMO-SD can be relapsing; this is similar to the situation of relapsing optic neuritis with NMO-IgG positivity, which is the "other extreme" of NMO-SD.[21,22]

The positivity of autoantibodies related to other autoimmune diseases such as Sjögren's syndrome, rheumatoid arthritis, systemic lupus erythematosus, and others is very common in NMO and rather uncommon in MS. Cases that were previously considered "Sjögren's myelitis" or "lupus myelitis" may also represent NMO-SD, which is an active area of clinical investigations.[23]

It is critically important to differentiate NMO from MS, as NMO not only responds poorly to standard MS disease-modifying agents (including a poor response or even no response to otherwise very effective agents in MS treatment, such as natalizumab)[4,24] but also may actually *worsen* from interferon therapy.[25,26] However, NMO shows a reasonable response to immunosuppressive medications, and to agents that selectively suppress or modify B-cell function and/or antibody production.

From the standpoint of advanced imaging methods, it is very important to note that unlike in MS, normal-appearing white and gray matter (NAWM and NAGM) abnormalities are much more restricted or nonexistent in NMO,[5,27] and they appear to involve only areas "directly hit" by active disease, such as the corticospinal tract as well as the optic radiation.

Paraneoplastic myelopathies, another form of inflammatory myelopathies, are increasingly recognized.[28–32] A characteristic finding is the appearance of *tractopathy*—symmetric T2 hyperintensity along both sides of the cord, usually over several segments, following the distribution of specific tracts. This finding commonly demonstrates faint gadolinium enhancement as well. Specific paraneoplastic antibodies may be associated with a variety of clinical presentations, and the antibodies typically predict the underlying cancer type and not the associated neurological syndrome. Therefore, in our view, testing just one or two antibodies while thinking that others are unlikely to be associated with the given neurological condition is an outdated approach; instead, a full panel of paraneoplastic antibodies should be tested. CRMP-5, amphiphysin IgG, GAD-65, VGKC, P/Q or *N*-type calcium channel, PCA-2, ANNA-2, and neuronal acetylcholine receptor antibodies have all been detected in myelopathy cases. CRMP-5 is in the differential diagnosis of NMO as both myelopathy and optic neuropathy can be observed in the presence of this antibody; this antibody is most commonly associated with small-cell lung cancer.[33]

1.2.6 MRI OF THE SPINAL CORD: QUALITATIVE VERSUS QUANTITATIVE IMAGING

Although all of the diagnostic features of the various inflammatory myelopathies discussed here are based on *qualitative imaging characteristics*, advanced MRI methods allow for quantitative MR analysis as well. Quantitative MRI in general is mostly utilized in clinical and basic research; however, as alluded to in this chapter, quantitative MRI metrics of the spinal cord may be especially helpful in monitoring progressive MS cases, where classic MRI measures show poor correlation with the clinical status.[34] Quantitative MRI metrics also play an important role as outcome measures in clinical trials, although the significance of these has recently been questioned.[35]

Even from the standpoint of the acquisition of "classic" qualitative spinal cord images, more recent advances in MRI methodology have resulted in increased sensitivity for lesion detection. Magnetization transfer gradient echo (MT-GE) images[36] and fast-STIR (short tau inversion recovery) sequences were found to depict more cervical cord MS lesions than the classic fast spin echo (FSE) sequence, with fast-STIR having the best sensitivity.[37]

TYPICAL MINIMAL CLINICAL PROTOCOL FOR THE SPINAL CORD IN DEMYELINATING DISEASES

- T$_1$-weighted sagittal FSE or turbo spin echo
- T$_2$-weighted sagittal FSE or turbo spin echo
- STIR sagittal
- Postgadolinium T1-weighted sagittal FSE or turbo spin echo

1.2.7 MAGNETIZATION TRANSFER MRI STUDIES OF THE SPINAL CORD

Magnetization transfer (MT) imaging (see chapter 3.4) provides a quantifiable parameter that can be applied with high resolution even to delicate structures, such as the spinal cord and the optic nerve. Both two-dimensional (2D) and three-dimensional (3D) acquisition methods are available.[38] The generation of MT ratio maps is computationally very straightforward and does not require complex postprocessing methods; image acquisition is also easily available on virtually every clinical system. The MT ratio provides an excellent measure for overall tissue integrity from the standpoint of the macromolecular environment. MT imaging has been successfully applied to patients with MS, showing lesion heterogeneity, subtle changes in the NAWM, and a better correlation with disability in comparison to conventional T2-weighted images. The MT ratio was reduced in the cervical cord, compared with healthy controls. Clinical disability may correlate with MTR independent of cord atrophy, which may in turn relate to preliminary findings of a correlation between axonal loss and MTR in the spinal cord.[39]

MT is especially powerful in assessing NAWM and NAGM. In a study of 8 NMO and 10 MS patients compared to nine healthy volunteers, no significant difference was found for any of the normal-appearing MTR histogram metrics between NMO patients and controls, while MS patients had a significantly lower histogram average MTR and peak height, suggestive of lack of pathology in the normal-appearing cord and brain areas in NMO. The cervical cord MTR histogram metrics, including lesional areas between NMO and MS patients, were otherwise not statistically different.[5]

A larger study of 90 MS patients and 20 matched healthy controls compared MTR histograms obtained using axial, contiguous, 5 mm thick slices and sagittal 3 mm slices. On the axial slices, MS patients had significantly lower average cervical cord MTR and peak height compared to controls. When comparing MTR histograms using sagittal slices, MS patients also had significantly lower average cervical cord MTR and peak location (but not height) than did control subjects. Patients with motor symptoms had significantly lower average cord MTR and peak location than those without.[40]

The different MS subtypes may demonstrate slightly but significantly different MT-MRI characteristics. In a study comparing 52 relapsing-remitting MS (RRMS), 33 secondary progressive MS (SPMS), and 11 PPMS cases vs. 21 controls, patients with SPMS had more cervical cord lesions and more images with visible cervical cord damage than did patients with RRMS or PPMS ($p = 0.04$). MS patients as a group had significantly lower average MTR of the cervical cord ($p = 0.006$) than control subjects. Compared to controls, patients with RRMS had similar MTR histogram-derived measures, whereas those with PPMS had lower average MTR ($p = 0.01$) and peak height ($p = 0.02$). Patients with SPMS had lower histogram peak height than did those with RRMS ($p = 0.03$). The peak position and height of the cervical cord MTR histogram were independent predictors of motor disability. Interestingly, brain T2 lesion load did not correlate with any of the cervical cord MTR histogram metrics.[41] This study overall demonstrated that progressive forms of MS are in general associated with more severe MT-MRI detectable tissue damage in the cord than RRMS, consistent with the clinical fact that most forms of progressive MS present with an insidiously progressive myelopathy.

The correlation between MTR and cord atrophy remains controversial, with some studies demonstrating correlation, while others do not. In a study of 65 MS cases (14 RRMS, 34 SPMS, and 17 PPMS) and nine healthy volunteers, MTR decrease was again demonstrated in MS patients, with weak but significant correlation with EDSS,[42] the most commonly used functional outcome measure in MS-related clinical trials ($r = -0.25$, $p < 0.05$). Correlation between EDSS and spinal cord surface area (its cross-sectional area, or CSA) was better (SRCC $= -0.40$, $p < 0.01$).[43] Interestingly, CSA, a commonly used numerical measure of cord atrophy, did not correlate with MTR ($r = 0.1$, $p = 0.4$), but combining MTR with CSA improved correlation with EDSS ($r = -0.46$, $p < 0.001$), suggesting an independent correlation between disability and these MR-derived parameters. EDSS was higher (suggesting increased disability) in patients with diffuse spinal cord abnormality regardless of focal lesions compared to patients without such abnormalities, and CSA was also lower in patients with diffuse cord abnormality. MTR was also slightly but significantly lower in patients with diffuse cord abnormalities.[43] This study not only highlights the fact that both MTR and CSA may independently capture different but synergistic substrates of disability measures, but also demonstrates that nonlesional cord abnormalities can be critically important determinants of overall disability, independent of and unrelated to lesion load. This diffuse pathology, external to classic focal lesions, is largely undetectable on conventional MRI and is an especially important determinant in PPMS and SPMS patients. Quantitative MT-MRI detectable spinal cord damage appears to correlate very well with disability measures in these patients.[44]

MT-derived measures have also been applied to CIS presenting as transverse myelitis. In a study of 45 such cases, the mean values of MTR histogram-derived metrics were not different between CIS patients and healthy controls subjects. Only three patients showed significantly lower cord MTR values than control subjects. These findings either suggest a sensitivity issue for detection of changes at the CIS stage with MT-MRI, or the absence of demyelination in the cervical cord soon after the onset of MS-like CIS, even in patients with subsequent evolution to MS.[45]

Longitudinal follow-up studies have also been performed to validate the clinical utility of MT imaging derived measures. In 14 untreated patients with RRMS over 18 months, the average cervical cord MTR was correlated with relapse rate ($r = -0.56$,

$P = 0.037$). A moderate correlation (r values ranging from -0.33 to -0.36) between baseline cervical cord MTR metrics and EDSS changes over 18 months was also noted, but this wasn't significant ($p = 0.26$ and 0.21, respectively), perhaps due to the relatively small sample size. It is intriguing, though, that a "snapshot" quantitative MT imaging assessment of the cervical cord may be indicative of short-term disease evolution in RRMS.[46]

One of the largest scale MT imaging-based studies in PPMS to date utilized MRI data from multiple centers, including 226 cases and 84 controls. This study confirmed the role and significance of MT imaging in assessing cord pathology in MS. In addition to providing disease-related data, another goal of this project was to compare and standardize data derived from different scanners at various centers. Mean CSA and MTR-derived metrics showed significant intercenter heterogeneity. After correcting for the center, pooled average MTR and histogram peak height values were significantly different between PPMS patients and controls in all tissue classes, including the spinal cord. More severe cord atrophy and MT-MRI detectable NAGM damage were demonstrated in patients requiring walking aids. PPMS severity therefore can be sensitively assessed by MT imaging, and atrophy-related measures may further aid in the assessment of spinal cord damage in these cases.[47]

In a study utilizing a novel MT-weighted imaging approach, the authors measured CSF-normalized MT signals in the dorsal and lateral columns and gray matter of the cervical cord in 42 MS cases. They also acquired other measures, including brain lesion volume, cervical spinal cord lesion number and cross-sectional area, vibration sensation, strength, walking velocity, and standing balance. They found that dorsal column CSF-normalized MT signal specifically correlated with vibration sensation ($R = 0.58$, $P < 0.001$), and the lateral column signal with strength ($R = -0.45$, $P = 0.003$), in full correlation with the functional anatomy of these cord regions. A stepwise multiple regression analysis revealed that dorsal column signal and diagnosis subtype alone explained a significant portion of variance in sensation ($R^2 = 0.54$, $P < 0.001$), whereas lateral column signal and diagnosis subtype explained a significant portion of variance in strength ($R^2 = 0.30$, $P < 0.001$). This study demonstrates that functionally compartmentalized MT-MRI data are very helpful in the analysis of specific types of disability in MS, and it suggests that quantitative assessment of selected forms of disability with MRI is feasible[48] (Figure 1.2.2).

The above MT-MRI studies clearly demonstrate the sensitivity of this method to nonlesional disability determinants in MS, especially in progressive forms of MS that are typically very hard (or impossible) to monitor using just conventional MRI. In addition to more accurate clinical follow-up, these metrics will be very important in future clinical trials of enhanced tissue restoration.

1.2.8 DIFFUSION-WEIGHTED IMAGING STUDIES IN THE SPINAL CORD

Diffusion tensor imaging (DTI) (see chapter 3.1) is an advanced imaging modality enabling voxel-based visualization of tract orientation, providing well-defined quantitative measures such as fractional anisotropy (FA), axial diffusivity (AD), radial diffusivity (RD), and mean diffusivity (MD).

FA and MD typically change in opposite directions as a result of MS-related white matter pathology. In 24 PPMS cases and 13 healthy controls, PPMS patients were found to have cervical cord cross-sectional area consistent with cord atrophy and decreased average cord fractional anisotropy ($p = 0.007$) with increased mean diffusivity ($p = 0.024$).[49] No correlations were found between DT-MRI metrics of the cord and quantities obtained from conventional MRI and DT-MRI of the brain, suggesting that changes in the cord are likely independent of brain damage in PPMS. Similarly to these observations, the average cervical cord FA was found to be significantly lower in 44 MS cases with various phenotypes compared to 17 controls.[50] Cord cross-sectional area, average FA, and average MD were all significantly correlated with the degree of disability (r values ranging from 0.36 to 0.51). With multivariate linear regression, the applied model retained average cord FA and average brain MD as variables independently associated with disability, with a correlation coefficient of 0.73 ($P < 0.001$). Similar findings were also documented in other cohorts.[51]

DTI changes were specifically scrutinized in different normal-appearing spinal cord regions (NASCs) in RRMS. DTI metrics in areas of NASC in MS were significantly different in the 24 patients compared with the equal number of matched control subjects: FA was lower in the lateral ($p < 0.0001$), posterior ($p < 0.0001$), and central ($p = 0.049$) NASC regions of interest (ROIs), consistent with nonlesional diffuse damage to mainly WM (lateral and posterior) but also GM (central) areas.[52]

DTI of the cord may also be capable of characterizing the differences between benign MS and disabling forms such as SPMS. In a study of 40 benign MS patients, 28 SPMS patients, and 18 controls, 92% of benign patients and all SPMS cases demonstrated cervical cord lesions. Compared with healthy individuals, benign MS patients had higher average cord MD, while SPMS patients had not only higher average cord MD but also lower average cord FA and lower CSA. EDSS was correlated with CSA

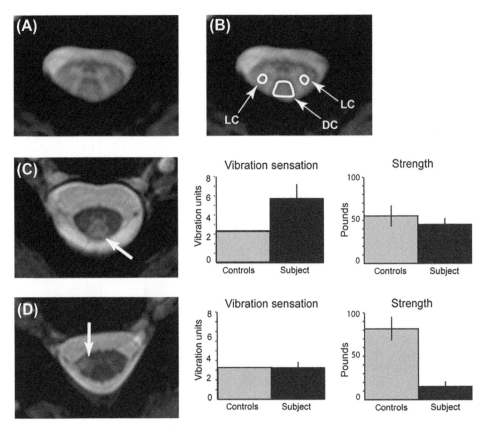

FIGURE 1.2.2 Magnetization transfer imaging of the spinal cord. Representative MT CSF axial spinal cord slices for one healthy participant and two individuals with multiple sclerosis with a lesion in either the dorsal column or lateral column. (A–B) 50-year-old healthy control with clear delineation of spinal cord gray and white matter; (B) outlines of regions of interest drawn for dorsal and lateral columns; (C) 43-year-old MS patient with a dorsal column lesion showing significantly decreased vibration sensation (6.5 vibration units); and (D) 47-year-old MS patient with lesion in the right corticospinal tract, resulting in significantly decreased strength in both ankles (right = 15.0 lb, left = 37.5 lb) and decreased walking speed (0.57 m/s), but normal vibration sensation. *Source: Adapted from Ref. 48.*

($r = -0.47$, $p < 0.0001$), average cord FA ($r = -0.37$, $p = 0.002$), and brain T2 lesion volume (LV) ($r = 0.34$, $p = 0.005$). A multivariate regression model identified CSA, average cord FA, and brain T2 LV as variables independently influencing the EDSS score ($r = 0.58$, $p < 0.0001$). These findings suggest that cervical cord damage outside focal macroscopic lesions is limited in patients with benign MS, and that FA, the measure of overall tissue organization, is indistinguishable between benign cases and healthy controls.[53]

DTI data enable analysis based on ROIs, or in a tract-based fashion. Twenty-one healthy subjects, 11 MS patients with spinal cord lesions, and 10 MS patients without spinal cord lesions were studied by both ROI and tract-based DTI-derived measures. FA, RD, and the ratio between AD and RD were significantly lower in the spinal cords of MS patients with lesions compared with the control subjects using both the ROI method and the tractography-based approach. With both image analysis methods, the FA and the ratio of the longitudinal and transverse diffusivities were significantly different between the control group and the MS patient group

without cord lesions ($P = 0.013$), suggesting that nonlesional cord areas also display similar damage as ones with lesions.[54]

RD and AD capture different tissue characteristics, which as per animal experiments may represent axonal (axial) and myelin (radial) integrity; however, this remains controversial.[55,56] In MS patients, lower radial diffusivity of the cortico-spinal tract at baseline was associated with better clinical outcome following relapses affecting such tracts. As patients improved clinically during the follow-up, they showed further decrease in radial diffusivity in these areas.[57]

DTI, similarly to MTR, is also capable of capturing the differences between NMO, MS, and controls. Three groups of 10 cases each differed in terms of average mean diffusivity ($p = 0.008$) and average fractional anisotropy ($p = 0.04$), with good correlation between EDSS and cord average mean diffusivity in both patient cohorts ($r = 0.52$, $p = 0.02$).[58] In 32 MS, 8 NMO cases, and 17 controls, the FA value was decreased in NMO patients in the anterior column at C2 compared to MS patients and controls. Also in this column, the radial diffusivity value showed increased NMO compared to MS and to controls. The FA value of the posterior column was decreased in NMO in comparison to controls. At C7, axial and mean diffusivity were higher in NMO than in MS and controls. This suggests more extensive cord damage in NMO, which is well along the lines of what is known from ex vivo pathology studies.[59] Another study of MS vs. NMO concentrated on lesional areas of the cord, and it demonstrated increased radial diffusivity in both NMO and MS compared with healthy controls ($p < 0.001$), but to a greater extent in NMO when compared with MS ($p < 0.001$). Axial diffusivity was decreased in T2 lesions in both NMO and MS compared with controls ($p < 0.001$, $p = 0.001$), but it did not differ between the two diseases. Radial diffusivity and

fractional anisotropy within white matter regions upstream and downstream of T2 lesions were different from controls in each disease.[60]

DTI imaging of the spinal cord is expected to become more readily available for research studies in the near future. It may play an important role in assessing tract integrity, in attempting to differentiate axonal vs. myelin pathology in vivo, and in monitoring tissue restoration in future clinical trials of remyelinating or axonal protective and/or restorative agents.

Q-space analysis (see chapter 3.2) is an alternative analysis technique for diffusion-weighted imaging data in which the probability density function (PDF) for molecular diffusion is estimated without the need to assume a Gaussian shape[61] (Figure 1.2.3). A team

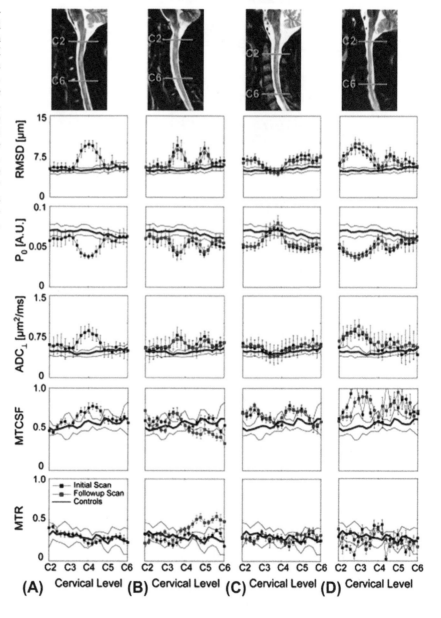

FIGURE 1.2.3 Quantitative high b-value q-space diffusion weighted imaging of the spinal cord. RMSD, P_0, ADC, MTCSF, and MTR within regions of interest in the dorsal column WM (mean ± standard deviation over the voxels in the ROI), plotted as a function of cervical level. Results for four patients—(A) 25-year-old male with RRMS, (B) 31-year-old female with RRMS, (C) 43-year-old female with SPMS, and (D) 41-year-old male with SPMS—are compared with the average results (solid black line, ± one standard deviation) from eight healthy controls. Initial and follow-up results are shown for three of the MS patients. Sagittal STIR images show slice and lesion localization for the initial exam of each patient. PDF: probability density function; RMSD: root mean square displacement. *Source: Modified from Ref. 61.*

of investigators from Johns Hopkins University demonstrated the feasibility of performing q-space imaging in the cervical spinal cord of eight healthy volunteers and four MS patients. In the dorsal column white matter, q-space contrasts showed a significant ($p < 0.01$) increase in the width and a decrease in the height of the PDF in lesions, the result of increased diffusion. The observed q-space contrast exhibited improved detection of abnormal diffusion compared to perpendicular apparent diffusion coefficient measurements. The conspicuity of lesions compared favorably with MT-weighted images and quantitative CSF-normalized MT measurements. Thus, q-space DWI can be used to study water diffusion in the human spinal cord in vivo and is well suited to assess white matter damage.

1.2.8.1 Functional MRI of the Spinal Cord in Inflammatory Myelopathies

Functional MRI (see chapter 4.1) investigations involving the cord in MS are relatively new additions to the field of functional MRI (fMRI) research.[62] Investigators from Milan studied tactile-associated cord fMRI changes between different clinical stages of relapse-onset multiple sclerosis in 49 MS patients (30 RRMS and 19 SPMS) and 19 controls during a tactile stimulation of the right hand. Both MS groups showed a significantly higher cord fMRI activity, with no difference between patient groups. The enrolled 26 severely disabled patients showed cord overactivation relative to controls ($p = 0.004$) and to patients with mild disability ($p = 0.04$). Both controls and cases showed functional lateralization of cord activity, which was predominant in the cord side ipsilateral to the stimulus, and a more frequent activation of the posterior than of the anterior cord quadrants.

The same team of investigators also studied tactile-associated cervical spinal cord activation in 23 patients with primary progressive MS vs. 18 healthy controls during tactile stimulation of the right hand[63] (Figure 1.2.4). They concluded that patients with PPMS had higher mean spinal cord activity on functional MR images than did controls. A higher occurrence of functional MR activation in the right vs. left side of the spinal cord and in the posterior vs. anterior section of the spinal cord was found in both control subjects and patients with PPMS; it is unclear if the laterality correlated with handedness or not. The mean spinal cord fMRI signal intensity change also correlated with regional spinal cord FA.

fMRI was also used to assess cervical cord activity associated with proprioception in 24 relapsing MS patients and 10 controls.[64] fMRI was performed using a block design during a proprioceptive stimulation consisting of a passive flexion-extension of the right upper limb. MS patients had higher average cord fMRI signal changes than controls (3.4% vs. 2.7%, $P = 0.03$). Compared to controls, MS patients also had a higher average signal change in the anterior section of the right cord at C5 ($P = 0.005$) and left cord at C5–C6 ($P = 0.03$), whereas no difference was found in the other cord sections.

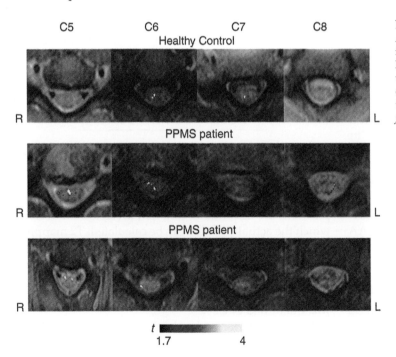

FIGURE 1.2.4 Functional MRI of spinal cord activation. Activation maps (colored by *t* value) of cervical spinal cord from C5 to T1 on axial intermediate-weighted spin echo MRI of a healthy control subject (top) and two patients with PPMS (middle and bottom) during tactile stimulation of the right palm. Note the different activation pattern between cases and controls. L = left; R = right. *Source: Modified from Ref. 63.*

While the number of fMRI studies in the cord is relatively low, it is important to further these investigations because this technique may enable efficient monitoring of functional recovery in the context of treatment.

1.2.9 MR SPECTROSCOPY

MR spectroscopy[65,66] (MRS; see chapter 5.1) enables one to measure the concentration of metabolites that are relevant in demyelinating diseases, because of their involvement in pathological processes such as axonal loss, gliosis, and neurotoxicity. The utilization of MRS in cord studies is relatively new. A study performed in 2004 was the first to report MRS findings of normal-appearing cervical spinal cords in multiple sclerosis patients and in healthy controls.[67] The Turkish team of investigators demonstrated reduced NAA within the cervical spinal cord compared with healthy controls, suggesting axonal loss and damage within even normal-appearing spinal cords of MS patients. Other investigators of an animal model of MS reported that brainstem MRS is a useful marker of spinal cord-centered demyelination and remyelination.[68]

In a feasibility study performed at 3 T,[69] investigators from Bologna reported LCModel-based quantitative MRS in 10 healthy volunteers. They demonstrated that MR spectra can be acquired in a fashion that enables quantification via LCModel, and presented tNAA, Cholin (Cho), Creatin (Cre), and myo-inositol concentrations in the studied volunteers.

A study investigating the correlations of EDSS-based outcome measures with spinal cord MRS and brain and cord atrophy measures in 11 patients with MS and 11 controls demonstrated that the concentration of NAA was reduced in the spinal cord in MS patients relative to controls (by 32%, $P < 0.05$), indicating significant axonal and/or neuronal damage.[70] Additionally, the spinal cord was significantly atrophied based on surface area measurement (15%, $P < 0.001$). It is unclear whether any of the patients had active lesions at the time of this study, or whether cord lesions were seen in the area studied for atrophy and in the MRS voxel. No significant reduction in brain NAA was seen in this MS group. No correlations between functional outcome measures and volumetric atrophy measurements were demonstrated; however, spinal cord NAA correlated with the cerebellar subscore of neurological assessment ($P < 0.005$), and brain NAA correlated with disease duration ($P < 0.05$).

A time-course study at 1, 3, and 6 months involving 14 MS cases undergoing a spinal cord relapse and 13 controls demonstrated that patients who recovered from their relapse showed a sustained increase in NAA after 1 month.[71] Among MS cases, a greater increase of NAA after 1 month was associated with greater recovery. Interestingly, patients showed significant cord atrophy during follow-up, likely as a result of the resolution of inflammatory edema and infiltrates ("pseudoatrophy"), which did not correlate with clinical changes. A worse recovery was predicted by longer disease duration at study entry. The authors hypothesize that the partial recovery of N-acetyl-aspartate levels after the acute event may be driven by increased axonal mitochondrial metabolism. The purported repair mechanism is associated with clinical recovery, and it is less efficient in patients with longer disease duration.

In the same study cohort of 14 cases vs. 13 controls, probabilistic tractography was performed at C1–C3 to track the lateral cortico-spinal tracts in the lateral columns, the anterior cortico-spinal tracts and the anterior spino-thalamic fasciculi in the anterior columns, and the bilateral fasciculus gracilis and cuneatus in the posterior columns[72] (Figure 1.2.5). Patients showed lower NAA of the cervical cord, and lower voxel-based probabilistic connectivity and lower fractional anisotropy of the lateral cortico-spinal tracts and posterior tracts, than controls. In patients, significant correlations were confirmed between EDSS and myo-inositol, Cho, Cre, and radial diffusivity of the lateral cortico-spinal tracts. The 9-hole peg test correlated with Cre, radial diffusivity of the lateral cortico-spinal tracts, connectivity and fractional anisotropy of the posterior tracts, and connectivity of the anterior tracts.

MRS remains an interesting experimental tool in a variety of CNS diseases, but because of inherent technical limitations and low sensitivity and specificity, further development is needed for this technique to play a major role in the diagnosis and monitoring of inflammatory myelopathies.

1.2.10 RELAXOMETRY IN THE SPINAL CORD: T1 MAPPING

Relaxometry represents another method of quantitative MR analysis, deriving voxel-based numerical values for the actual spin relaxation times. In most cases, single slice methods are used, and for T1 measurement, multiple scans are acquired at different inversion times from which the actual T1 value can be calculated. T2 mapping and especially short T2 component analysis[73] have also been extensively utilized in demyelinating disease research of the brain, including one feasibility study[74] and one study of in PPMS where myelin water fraction was quantified at C2–C3.[75]

In a study performed by investigators in Nottingham, United Kingdom, cervical cord T1 relaxometry was assessed and compared in eight RRMS and seven

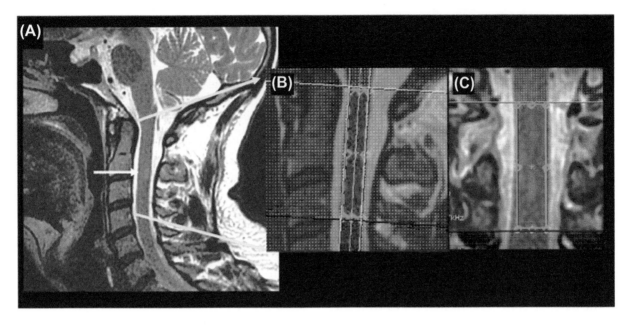

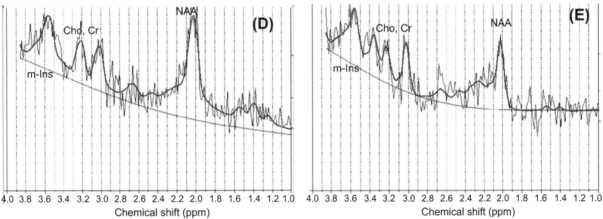

FIGURE 1.2.5 MR spectroscopy of the spinal cord. (A) Sagittal T2-weighted image of the spinal cord of a patient that shows a posterior lesion at C2–C3 (white arrow). Location of a PRESS volume of interest between C1 and C3 on the sagittal (B) and coronal (C) images. (D and E) Spectra obtained by LCModel analyses of a control (D) and MS case (E). The tNAA of the control was NAA 6.7 mM/l (%SD 9), and that of the patient was 4.9 mM/l (%SD 13). *Source: Adapted from Ref. 72.*

SPMS patients and six healthy controls, and correlated with normalized upper cervical cord area, brain white matter T1 maps, T2 lesion load, along with disability measures.[76] Median cervical cord T1 values were significantly increased in RRMS ($p = 0.0006$) and SPMS ($p < 0.0001$) compared with controls, and were also increased in SPMS compared to RRMS cases ($p = 0.002$). In the overall patient cohort, cord-based T1 relaxation times correlated significantly with median cerebral white matter T1 ($r = 0.7$, $p = 0.0046$) and cord atrophy ($r = -0.87$, $p < 0.0001$), but not with T2 lesion load. Cervical cord T1 and cord atrophy also correlated significantly with functional outcome measures. While this technology has not been extensively utilized in cord imaging, the data discussed here suggest that

relaxometry can become a relevant tool in this area of investigation.

1.2.11 MEASUREMENTS AND SIGNIFICANCE OF SPINAL CORD ATROPHY

Several of the studies discussed here utilized cord atrophy as an outcome measure, and found that atrophy contributes very significantly to disability. Spinal cord atrophy (see chapter 3.6) and its MRI measurement were the topics of a recent comprehensive review.[77]

The desire to quantify cord atrophy is not new: a study from London in 1996 that already aimed at developing a highly reproducible and accurate method for the quantification of spinal cord atrophy reported an intraobserver coefficient of variation of only 0.8%.[78] The excellent reproducibility was later further confirmed.[79] This semiautomated technique measures the CSA of the cord at the C2 level. When applied to 60 patients with clinically definite MS, a strong correlation between CSA and EDSS was also demonstrated ($r = -0.7$, $P < 0.001$).

The same team performed a serial study of 13 healthy control subjects and 28 MS cases, confirming that patients have significantly smaller cords than control subjects at baseline and established that patients have a significant loss in cord cross-sectional area during 12 months, which was not seen in control subjects ($p < 0.001$).[80] This reduction in cord size was especially prominent in PPMS and may allow for more accurate monitoring of disease evolution in that cohort of MS patients. The baseline cord cross-sectional area correlated strongly with the EDSS ($r = -0.52$, $p = 0.005$) and with disease duration ($r = -0.75$, $p < 0.001$); however, there was no significant difference in absolute cord area or change in cord area between those patients with a definite increase in EDSS and those without. The same data set was also reanalyzed using a B-spline active surface technique, which was found to be less sensitive at detecting small serial changes compared with their previously established method.[81]

In 27 early RRMS patients with less than 3 years of disease duration, yearly assessment of upper cervical cord atrophy for 3 years was performed.[82] Longitudinal analysis showed a significant decrease in cord surface area within the patient cohort ($p < 0.001$) and in comparison with controls ($p = 0.001$).

A Sobel edge detection-based technique was also developed to determine upper cervical cord surface area using 3D volume acquisition images of the cord to increase accuracy.[83] Nottingham-based investigators reported a study in 31 healthy controls, 20 RRMS cases, and 18 SPMS cases, with serial imaging at baseline and at 6, 12, 18, and 48 months during two treatment trials of high-dose subcutaneous interferon beta-1a. The intraobserver coefficient of variation of the method was 0.42%. A significant reduction in cord surface area was detected at month 6 in the placebo group ($p = 0.04$) and at month 12 for the treatment group ($p = 0.03$). The change in upper cord surface area was significantly correlated with EDSS change at months 12, 18, and 48. While possible confounding effects of interferon treatment cannot be excluded, this study clearly showed that edge detection is reproducible and sensitive to changes in spinal cord area, and that this change is related to clinical disability.

More recently, 3D analysis techniques of cord atrophy have also been demonstrated and validated.

Investigators at the University of Buffalo studied three different measures of cervical cord atrophy in 66 MS patients of all subtypes and 19 controls.[84] The outcome measures included cervical cord absolute volume (CCAV) in cubic millimeters and two normalized cervical cord measures: cervical cord fraction (CCF) = CCAV/thecal sac absolute volume, and cervical cord to intracranial volume (ICV) fraction (CCAV/ICV). CCAV itself and CCF demonstrated the largest differences between cases and controls, and between different disease subtypes. In regression analysis predicting disability, CCAV was retained first, followed by BPF, a commonly used brain atrophy measure. In full agreement with what is known clinically—and that is that features of myelopathy, when seen in MS cases, tend to be disabling—cervical cord atrophy measurement compared with brain-derived measures provided valuable additional information related to disability.

In a study by Harvard investigators utilizing 3 T MRI of the whole brain and whole spinal cord, 21 patients with MS (18 with RRMS, one with SPMS, one with PPMS, and one with a CIS) were studied to determine the relationship between disability and MRI-derived volumetric measures.[85] All were on treatment and had mild disability. Importantly, in this study all CNS volumes were normalized by the intracranial volume. Spinal cord volume was segmented using a semiautomated method with bins assigned to either the cervical or thoracic regions. Among all MRI measures, only upper cervical spinal cord volume correlated significantly with EDSS score ($r = -0.515$, $P = 0.020$). The authors concluded that the weak relationship between spinal cord and brain lesions and atrophy might suggest that they progress at least partially independently in MS patients.

In studies of CNS atrophy related to inflammatory demyelinating diseases, one needs to consider that volume changes not only are directly determined by "tissue loss" as a result of the progressive disease, but also represent an interplay between tissue loss, inflammatory infiltration, edema, and potential toxic effects of the utilized disease-modifying agents. In a study aimed at identifying the levels most susceptible to atrophy in MS patients, 35 MS cases and 27 healthy controls were studied with volumetric whole cord 3 T MRI by Harvard-based investigators.[86] The spinal cord was segmented, and the volumes were normalized and assigned to bins representing each vertebral level. A trend toward increased spinal cord volume throughout the cervical and thoracic cord in RRMS and CIS reached statistical significance at the T10 vertebral level. A statistically significant decrease was found in spinal cord volume at the upper cervical levels in PPMS and SPMS vs. RRMS and CIS. Patients with PPMS demonstrated a trend toward upper cervical cord atrophy. The trend toward increased volume at the cervical and thoracic levels in RRMS most likely represents the inflammation or edema-related cord expansion discussed here. The team of investigators concluded that with the disease causing both expansion and contraction of the cord, the specificity of spinal cord volume measures for neuroprotective therapeutic effect may be limited and may be applicable only to chronic cases of PPMS as opposed to other forms of MS.

Finally, another study from the same group of Harvard investigators proposed to measure the subolivar portion of the medulla oblongata, the intracranial prolongation of the spinal cord, to assess whether this measure could serve as a surrogate for actual measurements of upper cervical cord atrophy.[87] Since longitudinal MRI assessment of the spinal cord is performed much less frequently than head imaging, these investigators proposed that an indirect assessment of spinal cord atrophy through medulla oblongata measures on routinely acquired head images would be of great practical value. This study compared medulla oblongata and upper cervical cord cross-sectional measures in 45 MS patients (32 RRMS, eight SPMS, and five PPMS patients) with both a head and spinal cord MRI examination performed on the same day, paired with a clinical visit less than 30 days before or after the MRI scan. Twenty-nine age-matched and sex-matched healthy control subjects with head MRI were also included in this study. In the patients, medulla oblongata volume (MOV) over a standardized 9 mm subolivar segment correlated significantly with upper cervical cord volume (UCCV) ($r = 0.67$), BPF ($r = 0.45$), disease duration ($r = -0.64$), age ($r = -0.47$), EDSS score ($r = -0.49$), and ambulation index (AI) ($r = -0.52$). Volume loss of the medulla oblongata was $-0.008 \, cm^3$/year of age in patients with MS, but no significant linear relationship with age was found for healthy control subjects. The patients had a smaller MOV (mean $\pm$ SD, $1.02 \pm 0.17 \, cm^3$) than healthy control subjects ($1.15 \pm 0.15 \, cm^3$), although BPF was unable to distinguish between these two groups. MOV was smaller in patients with progressive MS (SPMS: $0.88 \pm 0.19 \, cm^3$; PPMS: $0.95 \pm 0.30 \, cm^3$) than in patients with RRMS ($1.08 \pm 0.15 \, cm^3$). A model including both MOV and BPF predicted AI better than BPF alone ($P = 0.04$). Good reproducibility in MOV measurements was demonstrated for intrarater (intraclass correlation coefficient: 0.97), interrater (0.79), and scan rescan data (0.81). The authors concluded that intracranial medulla oblongata measurements could indeed serve as a biomarker of spinal cord damage. This approach could clearly be of great interest for application in routine clinical practice.

THE ROLE OF QMRI IN DEMYELINATING DISEASES IN THE SPINAL CORD

- Differential diagnosis: MS, NMO, TM, and LETM characterization
- Sensitivity to alterations in spinal cord NAWM and NAGM
- Increased specificity to pathology (demyelination vs. degeneration)
- Quantifies metabolic features
- Stronger correlation with disability

1.2.12 CONCLUSIONS

The spinal cord is a frequent target of neuroinflammatory diseases affecting the CNS. MRI of the brain and spinal cord has become the single most important paraclinical marker of demyelinating diseases, with MRI-based markers routinely used in the diagnosis, differential diagnosis, prognosis, and monitoring of common inflammatory demyelinating diseases. MRI also provides a very useful aid to treatment monitoring and planning. In MRI research, a growing number of advanced techniques have truly revolutionized our understanding of MS and other inflammatory demyelinating diseases. Advanced qMRI methods of spinal cord involvement are of especial importance, given that these studies at least partially resolve the poor correlation between disability and conventional MRI-derived lesion load. qMRI enables the monitoring of progressive forms of MS, where much of the disability is known to be spinal cord related, but conventional imaging cannot sensitively capture the ongoing pathology. The presented quantitative metrics are also expected to enable monitoring of upcoming clinical trials aiming to restore tissue integrity. In addition to the already-published techniques presented here, it is likely that newer techniques will become available to monitor spinal cord involvement, and existing methods will be further refined. While most of the advanced techniques are currently only utilized for research, some of the techniques requiring relatively minimal postprocessing such as MTR maps or MTR histograms may gain ground in standard patient care, similar to the now universal utilization of MD maps in brain imaging. Spinal cord imaging and related quantitative analysis methods are expected to remain a dynamically expanding field in inflammatory demyelinating CNS disease research.

81. Hickman SJ, Coulon O, Parker GJ, et al. Application of a B-spline active surface technique to the measurement of cervical cord volume in multiple sclerosis from three-dimensional MR images. *J Magn Reson Imaging*. 2003;18(3):368–371.

82. Rashid W, Davies GR, Chard DT, et al. Increasing cord atrophy in early relapsing-remitting multiple sclerosis: a 3 year study. *J Neurol Neurosurg Psychiatry*. 2006;77(1):51–55.

83. Lin X, Tench CR, Turner B, Blumhardt LD, Constantinescu CS. Spinal cord atrophy and disability in multiple sclerosis over four years: application of a reproducible automated technique in monitoring disease progression in a cohort of the interferon beta-1a (Rebif) treatment trial. *J Neurol Neurosurg Psychiatry*. 2003; 74(8):1090–1094.

84. Zivadinov R, Banas AC, Yella V, Abdelrahman N, Weinstock-Guttman B, Dwyer MG. Comparison of three different methods for measurement of cervical cord atrophy in multiple sclerosis. *AJNR Am J Neuroradiol*. 2008;29(2):319–325.

85. Cohen AB, Neema M, Arora A, et al. The relationships among MRI-defined spinal cord involvement, brain involvement, and disability in multiple sclerosis. *J Neuroimaging*. 2012;22(2):122–128.

86. Klein JP, Arora A, Neema M, et al. A 3T MR imaging investigation of the topography of whole spinal cord atrophy in multiple sclerosis. *AJNR Am J Neuroradiol*. 2011;32(6):1138–1142.

87. Liptak Z, Berger AM, Sampat MP, et al. Medulla oblongata volume: a biomarker of spinal cord damage and disability in multiple sclerosis. *AJNR Am J Neuroradiol*. 2008;29(8):1465–1470.

Traumatic Spinal Cord Injury
Acute Spinal Cord Injury and Prognosis

David W. Cadotte, Michael G. Fehlings

Division of Neurosurgery, Department of Surgery, University of Toronto; Krembil Neuroscience Center, Toronto Western Hospital, University Health Network, ON, Canada

1.3A.1 INTRODUCTION

Prior to the 1980s a diagnosis of trauma to the spinal cord was largely inferred based on either X-rays showing misalignment of the spinal column or myelography whereby interruption of the flow of contrast medium in the cerebral spinal fluid (CSF) space indicated impingement of the spinal cord. With the widespread adoption of MRI came the visualization of the spinal cord itself, and along with it a revolution in the diagnosis and treatment of traumatic spinal cord injury. It wasn't long after the implementation of MR imaging that numerous research groups began to study the ability of MRI to determine both neurological function and prognosis following spinal cord injury. Numerous studies were undertaken with an aim of understanding the limitations of MRI to aid clinicians in treating their patients. These studies, reviewed and summarized here, introduced a host of new questions to the field such as the meaning of different signal characteristics with respect to pathological changes in the spinal cord tissue and the ability of these signal characteristics to yield meaningful clinical information such as the degree of damage to the spinal cord in terms of neurological function and the potential prognostic implications.

The advantages of being able to both determine neurological function and predict prognosis after acute traumatic spinal cord injury by reviewing MRI scans are numerous. While determining function and prognosis may seem beyond the limits of structural MR imaging, significant progress has been made in this direction. Benefits include distinguishing subclasses of patients that would benefit from different treatment options; for example, persons with severe spinal cord compression may benefit most from urgent decompressive surgery. Others, with no spinal cord compression, may benefit from delivery of neuroprotective agents, either systemically or locally. Accurate diagnostic and prognostic information could be conveyed to patients, family members, and the rehabilitation team such that efforts can be coordinated to plan and execute the best rehabilitation strategy.

Other modalities have certainly been used to predict prognosis following spinal cord injury, each with its own limitation. Physical examination, electrophysiology, computed tomography, and myelography have been studied.[1-3] Of these, neurological examination has maintained its position as the gold standard for assessing patients both in the acute stage and at long-term follow-up. There are however two factors that make an alternate test worth seeking. The first is that patients who suffer from traumatic spinal cord injury often have other associated injuries, are intoxicated or are medically unstable making a thorough examination impossible. The second is that a neurological examination taken immediately after injury is often not a good indicator of prognosis.[4-7]

In this chapter we aim to convey three messages. The first will describe the meaning of different MRI signal characteristics relative to the pathobiology of spinal cord injury as elucidated in animal imaging models. We will place an emphasis on animal imaging models that use MRI as a prognostic tool after traumatic spinal cord injury. The second message is to describe how quantitative measurements of maximum spinal cord compression (MSCC) and maximum canal compromise (MCC) can be used as a tool to describe the degree of spinal cord damage in a patient. The third message of this chapter is to describe how intramedullary MRI signal characteristics have been used as a diagnostic and prognostic tool. To accomplish this, we have conducted a meta-analysis of published papers and constructed receiver operator characteristics to describe the sensitivity and specificity of different MR signal characteristics.

1.3A.2 MESSAGE 1: ANIMAL MODELS THAT LINK PATHOLOGY OF ACUTE SPINAL CORD INJURY TO MR SIGNAL CHARACTERISTICS

Table 1.3A.1 summarizes the animal literature regarding the use of MRI as a prognostic tool in spinal cord injury. Of the eight animal studies identified, five were performed in a rat model and three in a mouse model. Each study involved a surgical procedure to induce spinal cord injury followed by serial clinical examinations and MRI studies. Attempts were then made to correlate clinical status with MRI findings.

Six of the eight studies showed a positive correlation between prognosis and MRI characteristics.[15–20] Two of

the eight studies showed no such correlation.[9,21] These discrepancies can easily be explained by the fact that each of these studies examined novel ways of imaging the injured animal spinal cord. The negative studies examined the use of diffusion tensor metrics[9] and high magnetic field strength[21] (9.4 T) on recovery. Establishing these novel methods in an animal model must take place prior to using them to predict either neurological function or prognosis.

Of the studies that showed a positive correlation, two focused on vascular effects, two focused on neuronal structure and function, and two simply reported MRI characteristics as they relate to functional recovery.

1.3A.2.1 Vascular Effects

Bilgen et al.[15] focus on the disruption of the blood–spinal cord barrier (BSCB) following injury. The degree of MR contrast directly correlated with neurological outcome (higher contrast uptake relates to poor outcome). Followed over time, neurological

TABLE 1.3A.1 Experimental Studies Assessing the Relationship between MRI Imaging and Prognosis in Animal Models of SCI

Investigators (y)	Species	Injury Model	MRI[a] Measure	Conclusion
Bilgen et al.[8]	Rat	Contusion injury to mid-thoracic cord	Gd[b]-enhanced T1 weighted images	T1 contrast enhancement correlates with the degree of NR[f]
Narayana et al.[9]	Rat	Contusion injury to mid-thoracic cord	T1, T2, and density-weighted images	Return of gray-white differentiation correlates with NR
Deo et al.[10]	Rat	Contusion injury to mid-thoracic cord	Diffusion tensor imaging	DTI[c] metrics do not consistently correlate with NR
Stieltjes et al.[11]	Mouse	Spinal cord transection (80%) at the mid-thoracic level	Manganese-enhanced MRI images	Manganese enhanced MRI correlates with NR in animals treated with novel therapeutic agents
Bilgen et al.[12]	Mouse	Contusion injury to mid-thoracic cord	High resolution (9.4 T) images	Differential MRI characteristics did not correlate with NR
Nossin-Manor et al.[13]	Rat	Hemi-crush injury to mid-thoracic cord (mild vs. severe)	Diffusion-weighted MRI (high b-value, q-space)	Novel DWI[d] characteristics correlate with NR
Nishi et al.[5]	Mouse	Contusion injury to mid-thoracic level (mild, moderate, severe)	T1 and T2 images at 7 Tesla	Lesion volume (T1 images) correlates with NR
Mihai et al.[14]	Rat	Contusion injury to cervical cord (unilateral C5)	T1, T2, and proton density images (±Gad[e])	Hypodense T1 signal and lesion length correlates with NR

[a] Magnetic resonance imaging.
[b] Gadopentate dimeglumine.
[c] Diffusion tensor imaging.
[d] Diffusion weighted imaging.
[e] Gadodiamide.
[f] Neurological recovery.

improvement comes at a point when contrast uptake into the lesion diminishes. This suggests that reformation of the BSCB is important for regain of neurological activity. In a similar longitudinal study that combines clinical, MRI, and histological data,[17] the authors demonstrate that spontaneous recovery occurs between two and eight weeks. As neurological function returns, there is a gradual return of gray-white differentiation adjacent to cord contusion (noted by areas of hypo- and hyperintense T2W images).

1.3A.2.2 Neuronal Structure and Function

Two of the animal studies investigated neuronal function via MR imaging after injury. Stieltjes et al.[20] used manganese (a surrogate marker for neuronal activity) as a contrast agent. They detected changes in neuronal structure and function following injury and compared this with recovery. Using an antibody to CD95 ligand, a neutralizing antibody shown to prevent apoptotic cell death and promote neuronal recovery in animal models,[14] the authors compared functional tests with MRI findings. There was a strong correlation between manganese uptake, especially caudal to the level of injury, and functional recovery after treatment with the antibody. Also investigating neuronal function, Nossin-Manor et al.[19] used a novel MRI sequence (high b-value q-space diffusion MRI) that provides information about the integrity of white matter tracts. The authors subjected rats to either a mild or severe hemi-crush injury to the mid-thoracic cord and followed the evolution of injury with both MRI and behavioral testing. Subsequent histological analysis was carried out. Functional recovery occurred in the mild injury group but not in the severe injury group. When comparing the mild and severe injury group at five days post injury, the diffusion weighted imaging (DWI) characteristics were similar at the lesion site. As the distance from the injury site increased, the differences in DWI characteristics became apparent between the mild and severely injured groups. Over the course of six weeks, there was improvement in the DWI characteristics of the mild injury group but not the severe injury group. The improvement in MRI characteristics correlated with neurological recovery.

1.3A.2.3 MRI Characteristics as they Relate to Functional Recovery in Animals

Both Nishi et al.[18] and Mihai et al.[16] carried out longitudinal studies that involved spinal lesions, with varying degrees of force, followed by clinical testing, MRI studies, and histological analysis. Ex vivo MRI[18] revealed lesion volumes that correlated with both the force of injury and behavioral improvement following injury. In vivo MRI[16] revealed cord swelling (increased cord volume), cord edema (hypointense T1 and hyperintense T2 signal), and lesion length to be the most valuable parameters as these were highly correlated to behavioral outcomes and histopathological characteristics of the lesion.

As a final point, Bilgen et al.[21] used a contusion model to the mid-thoracic spinal cord and followed the injury with serial MRI scans, behavioral testing, and histological analysis. Despite receiving the same contusion injury, two different MRI injury patterns were noted in the animals: focal and diffuse. The neurological recovery in each of these subgroups was not statistically different. The authors attribute the different MRI characteristics to a vascular and inflammatory phenomenon. In this sense, the different MRI characteristics did not reflect different neurological improvement.

Each of the previous eight studies was carried out using a similar injury model and a wide variety of MR imaging techniques. While each study focused on unique aspects of spinal cord injury pathophysiology, ranging from vascular phenomena to neuronal function, all attempted to correlate behavioral improvement with imaging characteristics.

1.3A.3 MESSAGE 2: QUANTITATIVE MSCC AND MCC

In an attempt to delineate the precise cause of neurological dysfunction following acute, traumatic spinal cord injury, researchers have divided the temporal sequence of destructive events into primary and secondary injury. Primary injury refers to the destructive forces that directly damage the neural structures such as the shear force tearing an axon or the direct compressive force occluding a blood vessel resulting in ischemia. These destructive primary mechanisms not only result in instantaneous damage to neurons and blood vessels but also initiate a cascade of cellular mechanisms that result in ongoing damage to the neural structures, termed secondary injury. In fact, in cases of ongoing primary injury, for example in the setting of a fracture dislocation where the bony spinal column is displaced and physically pushed up against the spinal cord, these cellular mechanisms are thought to be locked into the "on" position until such physical forces are removed either by closed reduction or surgically. A detailed explanation of the secondary injury hypothesis of traumatic spinal cord injury can be found in the seminal publication by Tator and Fehlings.[22]

In order to account for the ongoing forces of spinal cord compression that may exacerbate the initial injury, the Fehlings research team established a quantitative method for evaluating and reporting spinal canal compromise and spinal cord compression.[23] Through a multicenter study, the authors established the following criteria.

1.3A.3.1 Maximum Canal Compromise

Using mid-sagittal CT reconstructions or MRI images and the respective axial slices, one should identify the level of maximum spinal canal compromise (MCC) and compare this with the normal canal diameter at the mid-vertebral body level above and below the lesion. This is quantified using the formula shown in Figure 1.3A.1 where D_i is the anteroposterior canal distance at the level of maximum injury, D_a is the anteroposterior canal distance at the nearest normal level above the level of injury, and D_b is the anteroposterior canal distance at the nearest normal level below the level of injury.

1.3A.3.2 Maximum Spinal Cord Compression

The anteroposterior cord diameter on mid-sagittal and axial T2 MRI images at the level of maximum compression should be compared with the anteroposterior cord diameter at the normal levels immediately above and below the level of injury. If cord edema is present, measurements of normal anteroposterior cord diameter should be made at mid-vertebral body levels just beyond the rostral and caudal extent of the cord edema at the levels where the cord appears normal. These values are quantified using the formula depicted in Figure 1.3A.2 where d_i is the anteroposterior cord distance at the level of maximum injury, d_a is the anteroposterior cord distance at the nearest normal level above the level of injury, and d_b

is the anteroposterior cord distance at the nearest normal level below the level of injury.

In their analysis of 100 acute SCI patients, Miyanji et al.[23] determined that both MSCC and MCC predicted the baseline ASIA motor score but only MSCC was a predictor of neurologic recovery after traumatic SCI. The authors note that obtaining a static MR image after the moment of impact does not take into account the dynamic forces at play that account for the traumatic injury. As such, one can expect limited information from a single scan within 72 h of injury. It may be prudent to obtain repeat images within the first several weeks after injury to gain a better appreciation of ongoing changes to the spinal cord. In fact, Shimada and Tokioka found that prognostic images are best obtained two to three weeks after the initial injury.[24]

TYPICAL CLINICAL PROTOCOL FOR SPINAL CORD IN ACUTE SCI

- T_1-weighted sagittal
- T_2-weighted sagittal
- Short-tau inversion recovery (STIR) sagittal + axial (or equivalent fat-suppressed sequence)
- Fluid attenuated inversion recovery (FLAIR) sagittal
- Other as needed (example MRA to assess vertebral artery integrity if injury or dissection is suspected)

FIGURE 1.3A.1   Preoperative T2 (A) and postoperative T1 (B) and T2 (C) spine MRI images of an 18-year-old male that sustained a spinal cord injury after being involved in a motor vehicle accident. (A) Illustrates how to calculate maximum canal compromise (MCC). D_i is the anteroposterior canal diameter at the level of maximum injury, D_a is the anteroposterior canal diameter at the nearest normal level above the level of injury, and D_b is the anteroposterior canal diameter at the nearest normal level below the level of injury. Panels (B) and (C) illustrate the effect of decompressive surgery on relieving canal compromise and restoring normal alignment.

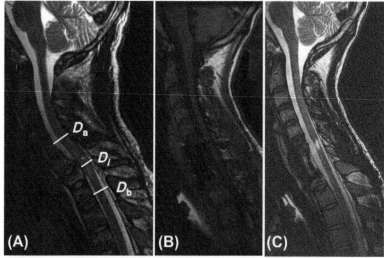

Maximum canal compromise (MCC)

$$\left(1 - \frac{D_i}{(D_a + D_b)/2}\right) \times 100\%$$

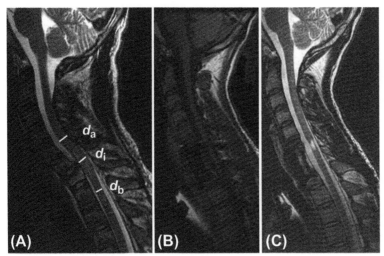

FIGURE 1.3A.2 Preoperative T2 (A) and postoperative T1 (B) and T2 (C) spine MRI images of an 18-year-old male that sustained a spinal cord injury after being involved in a motor vehicle accident. (A) Illustrates how to calculate the maximum spinal cord compression (MSCC). Where d_i is the anteroposterior cord distance at the level of maximum injury, d_a is the anteroposterior cord distance at the nearest normal level above the level of injury, and d_b is the anteroposterior cord distance at the nearest normal level below the level of injury. Panels (B) and (C) illustrate the effect of decompressive surgery on relieving canal compromise and restoring normal alignment.

Maximum spinal cord compression (MSCC)

$$\left(1 - \frac{d_i}{(d_a + d_b)/2}\right) \times 100\%$$

1.3A.4 MESSAGE 3: MRI SIGNAL CHARACTERISTICS AFTER ACUTE TRAUMATIC SPINAL CORD INJURY: WHAT IS THE SENSITIVITY AND SPECIFICITY OF DETERMINING NEUROLOGIC FUNCTION AT THE TIME OF INJURY AND FOR PREDICTING LONG-TERM PROGNOSIS?

Through a systematic review we identified a total of 39 clinical studies: 10 reported solely on clinical assessment[11,12,25–32] and 29 reported on MRI findings in addition to clinical characteristics both at presentation after acute SCI and follow-up.[8,13,23,24,33–56] The total number of patients represented in these studies was 4804.

We compared the initial clinical grade or MRI imaging characteristic with follow-up clinical grade. In order to determine the sensitivity and specificity by which spinal MRI can predict prognosis after acute traumatic SCI, we defined a "positive" test as one whereby the patient does not recover neurological function. In other words, a positive test reflects the clinicians' ability to use MRI signal characteristics to inform a patient that recovery is unlikely. Using this as a base definition, we calculated the sensitivity and specificity of MRI to predict outcome and constructed receiver operator characteristic curves.[57] We did so by using the maximum likelihood estimation assuming a binomial distribution. We used the statistical software ROC-kit (Windows version 1.0.1 Beta 2; available from the University of Chicago)[58] to fit the curve and estimate the area under the curve.[59] Graphs were created using MS Excel (2008 for Mac).

Clinical examination and MRI characteristics exist along a spectrum. Clinical examination occurs along the American spinal injury association (ASIA) grade A through E or Frankel grade A through D. In both cases an "A" grade represents a more severe neurological deficit in comparison to a "D" or "E" grade. MRI characteristics occur as follows: normal, T2-weighted signal intensity, cord compression, cord swelling, evidence of intramedullary hemorrhage, and cord transection. Receiver operator characteristic (ROC) plots were constructed to illustrate the sensitivity and specificity of each measure. ROC plots provide a graphical representation of the sensitivity and specificity of a particular test and allow a clinician or radiologist to perform a cost–benefit analysis of the diagnostic decision they are making. In other words, one is able to quantify how reliable the test is at diagnosing a certain condition or predicting a certain prognosis. As stated in the previous methods section, we defined a positive test as one in which a clinician predicts that an SCI patient will not recover.

Figure 1.3A.3 demonstrates the ROC curve for the accuracy of clinical examination, when conducted within 72 h of SCI, to predict prognosis, and Figure 1.3A.4 demonstrates the ROC curve for the accuracy of MRI, when conducted within 72 h of SCI, to predict prognosis.

When performed within 72 h, clinical examination has an area under the curve (AUC) = 0.86 (95% confidence interval: 0.82, 0.87). MRI has an AUC = 0.78 (95% confidence interval: 0.71, 0.83). Empirical data reveals that an initial clinical assessment of ASIA D has a sensitivity of 93% and a specificity of 25% to predict prognosis (defined as: no recovery), whereas an

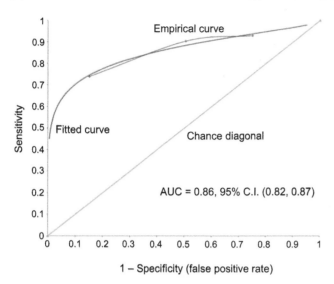

FIGURE 1.3A.3   Receiver operator characteristics are displayed for clinical examination carried out within 72 h of SCI where a "positive test" is defined as no change in clinical examination at follow-up. Shown are the empirical curve (blue line), the fitted curve (red line), and the chance diagonal (green line). The area under the curve (AUC), when the empirical data is fitted to a binomial distribution, is 0.86 (95% confidence interval: 0.82, 0.87) where 1 represents a perfectly sensitive and specific test. *Source: Originally published in Ref. 60.*

initial clinical assessment of ASIA A has a sensitivity of 74% and a specificity of 85% to predict prognosis (defined as: no recovery). Similarly, an MRI with no signal changes (normal) has a sensitivity of 100% and a specificity of 19% to predict prognosis (defined as:

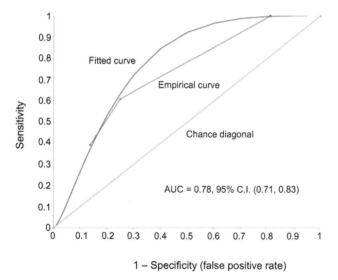

FIGURE 1.3A.4   Receiver operator characteristics are displayed for MRI carried out within 72 h of SCI where a "positive test" is defined as no change in clinical examination at follow-up. Shown are the empirical curve (blue line), the fitted curve (red line), and the chance diagonal (green line). The area under the curve (AUC), when the empirical data is fitted to a binomial distribution, is 0.78 (95% confidence interval: 0.71, 0.83) where 1 represents a perfectly sensitive and specific test. *Source: Originally published in Ref. 60.*

no recovery), whereas an MRI revealing evidence of intramedullary hemorrhage has a sensitivity of 39% and a specificity of 86% to predict prognosis (defined as: no recovery).

These data can also be represented in terms of a likelihood ratio. As an example: if a physician were to tell a patient who presented with an ASIA A SCI (examination conducted <72 h after injury) that he or she would not recover, this statement would be accurate with a sensitivity of 74% and a specificity of 85% (data extracted from empirical curve). This translates into a likelihood ratio of 4.93. In other words, a patient who presents with an ASIA A exam (conducted within 72 h) is 4.93 times more likely to *not recover* rather than recover.

Figure 1.3A.5 illustrates two case examples whereby each individual had an MRI within 72 h of injury. Selective mid-sagittal T2-weighted images are provided. The interpretation of intramedullary signal characteristics can be difficult, and we have therefore included a summary of how the T1 and T2 signal characteristics of blood change over time. The left image was obtained from a 32-year-old male who was involved in a motor vehicle accident and presented with an ASIA B incomplete injury with a motor level at C6 and a sensory level at C8. Note the T2-weighted hyperintensity in the spinal cord. The right image was obtained from a 26-year-old female who fell from a height of >10 m. She presented with a C5 ASIA A injury. Note the mixed T2 hypointensity (white arrow) and hyperintensity indicating hemorrhage within the cord. In addition, there is severe spinal cord compression. On follow-up, the 32-year-old male (left image) had recovered both motor and sensory function to a certain degree, whereas the young female (right image) did not.

The use of MRI to predict outcome after SCI theoretically overcomes many of the limitations identified for the use of clinical exam. For instance, as long as the patient is able to remain still within the scanner, the predictive capacity of MRI is independent of patients' effort, level of consciousness, or ability to cooperate, hence reducing the influence of patient- and injury-related confounders. In addition, the influence of bias is reduced, since MRI will invariably identify gross macroscopic details and anatomic disruptions present within the spinal cord post injury. However, MRI as a predictive tool has its own set of limitations. As mentioned, conventional MRI gives clinicians a static macroscopic anatomical picture without providing any direct information regarding neurologic function. Although we can clearly see tissue disruptions such as spinal cord hematoma, significant edema formation, or complete transection, we are unable to visualize evidence of microscopic injury at an axonal or cellular level. After primary spinal cord compression or injury, animal

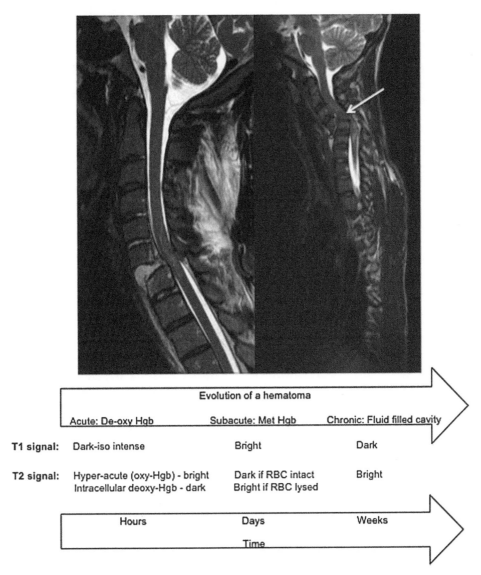

FIGURE 1.3A.5 Two case examples are illustrated along with a guide to the interpretation of intramedullary signal characteristics. The left image is a mid-sagittal T2-weighted MRI that was obtained within 72 h of a 32-year-old male sustaining a traumatic spinal cord injury in a motor vehicle collision; note the T2-weighted hyperintensity within the spinal cord. The right image is a mid-sagittal T2-weighted MRI that was obtained within 72 h of a 26-year-old female sustaining a traumatic spinal cord injury due to a fall from >10 m; the white arrow points to mixed T2-weighted hypo- and hyperintensity, indicating hemorrhage within the cord. In addition, there is a significant amount of spinal cord compression. *Source: Originally published in Ref. 60.*

models of SCI have proven the existence of secondary injury mechanisms at a microscopic level that potentiate the ultimate degree of neurologic deficit. It is therefore possible to have ongoing secondary injury and tissue destruction without visualizing a corresponding change in the MR image. The results of the current study underscore these observations. For instance, when MRI revealed a spinal cord hematoma, the sensitivity of this finding in predicting long-term outcome was poor. This can be attributed to a high degree of false negative results, whereby the absence of a cord hematoma on initial MRI scans may be expected to predict positive neurologic improvement over time but other unseen factors are at play. This disconnect between the absence of spinal cord hemorrhage and positive neurologic improvement underscores the inability of standard MRI techniques to detect ongoing, microscopic injury mechanisms that attenuate potential for neurologic recovery. Quantitative techniques such as diffusion-weighted imaging, magnetization transfer, and T2 relaxation have the potential to bring additional insights into microscopic injury.

1.3A.5 CONCLUSIONS

In this chapter we have provided an overview of the following: (1) Animal imaging models that aim to correlate pathological changes after traumatic spinal cord injury with specific MR signal characteristics. (2) A quantitative means of measuring maximum spinal cord compression and maximum spinal canal compromise, values that aim to quantify the degree of ongoing compression of the spinal cord and reflect secondary injury mechanisms. (3) We report the sensitivity and specificity of clinical examination in comparison to conventional MRI as a diagnostic and prognostic tool following acute traumatic SCI. Through a meta-analysis of previously published studies, we demonstrate that an absence of signal change in the spinal cord or mild T2-weighted hyperintensity is associated with a favorable prognosis, whereas evidence of hemorrhage in the spinal cord and spinal cord transection is associated with a poor prognosis.

MRI has considerably advanced since its adoption into the world of clinical medicine at the end of the twentieth century. Initial low-field strength magnets have been replaced by higher-and-higher field strengths with advanced coils and more sophisticated pulse sequences allowing for improved signal-to-noise ratio and better visualization of tissue.[10] One can only imagine the excitement that clinicians had in the 1980s when they first visualized the human spinal cord. Today we are advancing far beyond this initial success and are able to visualize gray matter–white matter boundaries and infer the integrity of white matter tracts with fractional anisotropy values acquired with diffusion imaging.[61] Similarly, magnetization transfer-derived quantities have been used to assess macromolecular tissue damage.[62] The ultimate goal with regard to quantitative MRI (qMRI) in the setting of spinal cord injury will be to integrate advanced imaging methods (DTI, MT, fMRI, and MRS) in order to precisely define both the structural and functional consequences of injury. The completion of a number of large clinical trials in this field has demonstrated the heterogeneity of both structural and functional damage to the spinal cord across patients. If novel therapeutic strategies are hoped to improve the lives of individual patients, it will be important to accurately diagnose and tailor treatments to specific pathologies. For example, persons who suffer from neuropathic pain may benefit from spinal fMRI studies to delineate the pain generator. To outline the integrity of specific spinal circuits and how these circuits may be disrupted after SCI will provide another great advance in our understanding of spinal cord injury and will certainly aid our ability to deliver novel treatment options.

WHAT ADDITIONAL INFORMATION CAN QMRI BRING IN ACUTE SCI?

- *DWI, MT, T2 relaxation*: impairment of WM tracts, detecting early Wallerian degeneration, gliosis
- *Ultra high field*: high spatial resolution to delineate the extension of the lesion (volume) and the effect of novel treatments aimed at halting progression of secondary injury
- *fMRI*: delineation of resting spinal circuits, circuit responses to either motor or sensory stimuli and how injury may result in maladaptive plasticity and clinical symptoms such as neuropathic pain or spasticity

References

1. Brant-Zawadzki M, Miller EM, Federle MP. CT in the evaluation of spine trauma. *AJR Am J Roentgenol*. 1981;136(2):369–375.
2. Virapongse C, Kier EL. Metrizamide myelography in cervical spine trauma: a modified technique using lateral fluoroscopy. *Radiology*. 1982;144(3):636–637.
3. York DH, Watts C, Raffensberger M, Spagnolia T, Joyce C. Utilization of somatosensory evoked cortical potentials in spinal cord injury. Prognostic limitations. *Spine (Phila Pa 1976)*. 1983;8(8):832–839.
4. Bedbrook G. Recovery of spinal cord function. *Paraplegia*. 1980;18(5):315–323.
5. Ducker TB, Russo GL, Bellegarrique R, Lucas JT. Complete sensorimotor paralysis after cord injury: mortality, recovery, and therapeutic implications. *J Trauma*. 1979;19(11):837–840.
6. Suwanwela C, Alexander Jr E, Davis Jr CH. Prognosis in spinal cord injury, with special reference to patients with motor paralysis and sensory preservation. *J Neurosurg*. 1962;19:220–227.
7. Young JS, Dexter WR. Neurological recovery distal to the zone of injury in 172 cases of closed, traumatic spinal cord injury. *Paraplegia*. 1978;16(1):39–49.
8. Dai L. Magnetic resonance imaging of acute central cord syndrome: correlation with prognosis. *Chin Med Sci J*. 2001;16(2):107–110.
9. Deo AA, Grill RJ, Hasan KM, Narayana PA. In vivo serial diffusion tensor imaging of experimental spinal cord injury. *J Neurosci Res*. 2006;83(5):801–810.
10. Fries P, Runge VM, Kirchin MA, Watkins DM, Buecker A, Schneider G. Magnetic resonance imaging of the spine at 3 Tesla. *Semin Musculoskelet Radiol*. 2008;12(3):238–252.
11. Folman Y, el Masri W. Spinal cord injury: prognostic indicators. *Injury*. 1989;20(2):92–93.
12. Frankel HL, Hancock DO, Hyslop G, et al. The value of postural reduction in the initial management of closed injuries of the spine with paraplegia and tetraplegia. I. *Paraplegia*. 1969;7(3):179–192.
13. Flanders AE, Spettell CM, Tartaglino LM, Friedman DP, Herbison GJ. Forecasting motor recovery after cervical spinal cord injury: value of MR imaging. *Radiology*. 1996;201(3):649–655.
14. Demjen D, Klussmann S, Kleber S, et al. Neutralization of CD95 ligand promotes regeneration and functional recovery after spinal cord injury. *Nat Med*. 2004;10(4):389–395.

15. Bilgen M, Abbe R, Narayana PA. Dynamic contrast-enhanced MRI of experimental spinal cord injury: in vivo serial studies. *Magn Reson Med.* 2001;45(4):614–622.

16. Mihai G, Nout YS, Tovar CA, et al. Longitudinal comparison of two severities of unilateral cervical spinal cord injury using magnetic resonance imaging in rats. *J Neurotrauma.* 2008;25(1):1–18.

17. Narayana PA, Grill RJ, Chacko T, Vang R. Endogenous recovery of injured spinal cord: longitudinal in vivo magnetic resonance imaging. *J Neurosci Res.* 2004;78(5):749–759.

18. Nishi RA, Liu H, Chu Y, et al. Behavioral, histological, and ex vivo magnetic resonance imaging assessment of graded contusion spinal cord injury in mice. *J Neurotrauma.* 2007;24(4):674–689.

19. Nossin-Manor R, Duvdevani R, Cohen Y. Spatial and temporal damage evolution after hemi-crush injury in rat spinal cord obtained by high b-value q-space diffusion magnetic resonance imaging. *J Neurotrauma.* 2007;24(3):481–491.

20. Stieltjes B, Klussmann S, Bock M, et al. Manganese-enhanced magnetic resonance imaging for in vivo assessment of damage and functional improvement following spinal cord injury in mice. *Magn Reson Med.* 2006;55(5):1124–1131.

21. Bilgen M, Al-Hafez B, Alrefae T, et al. Longitudinal magnetic resonance imaging of spinal cord injury in mouse: changes in signal patterns associated with the inflammatory response. *Magn Reson Imaging.* 2007;25(5):657–664.

22. Tator CH, Fehlings MG. Review of the secondary injury theory of acute spinal cord trauma with emphasis on vascular mechanisms. *J Neurosurg.* 1991;75(1):15–26.

23. Miyanji F, Furlan JC, Aarabi B, Arnold PM, Fehlings MG. Acute cervical traumatic spinal cord injury: MR imaging findings correlated with neurologic outcome—prospective study with 100 consecutive patients. *Radiology.* 2007;243(3):820–827.

24. Shimada K, Tokioka T. Sequential MR studies of cervical cord injury: correlation with neurological damage and clinical outcome. *Spinal Cord.* 1999;37(6):410–415.

25. Coleman WP, Geisler FH. Injury severity as primary predictor of outcome in acute spinal cord injury: retrospective results from a large multicenter clinical trial. *Spine J.* 2004;4(4):373–378.

26. Crozier KS, Graziani V, Ditunno Jr JF, Herbison GJ. Spinal cord injury: prognosis for ambulation based on sensory examination in patients who are initially motor complete. *Arch Phys Med Rehabil.* 1991;72(2):119–121.

27. Geisler FH, Coleman WP, Grieco G, Poonian D. The Sygen multicenter acute spinal cord injury study. *Spine (Phila Pa 1976).* 2001;26(suppl 24):S87–S98.

28. Katoh S, el Masry WS. Motor recovery of patients presenting with motor paralysis and sensory sparing following cervical spinal cord injuries. *Paraplegia.* 1995;33(9):506–509.

29. Marino RJ, Ditunno Jr JF, Donovan WH, Maynard Jr F. Neurologic recovery after traumatic spinal cord injury: data from the Model Spinal Cord Injury Systems. *Arch Phys Med Rehabil.* 1999;80(11):1391–1396.

30. Maynard FM, Reynolds GG, Fountain S, Wilmot C, Hamilton R. Neurological prognosis after traumatic quadriplegia. Three-year experience of California Regional Spinal Cord Injury Care System. *J Neurosurg.* 1979;50(5):611–616.

31. Sannohe A, Harata S, Ueyama K, et al. The prognosis and the treatment of patients with a C3/4 spinal cord injury. *Spinal Cord.* 1996;34(8):486–487.

32. van Middendorp JJ, Hosman AJ, Pouw MH, Van de Meent H. ASIA impairment scale conversion in traumatic SCI: is it related with the ability to walk? A descriptive comparison with functional ambulation outcome measures in 273 patients. *Spinal Cord.* 2009;47(7):555–560.

33. Andreoli C, Colaiacomo MC, Rojas Beccaglia M, Di Biasi C, Casciani E, Gualdi G. MRI in the acute phase of spinal cord traumatic lesions: relationship between MRI findings and neurological outcome. *Radiol Med.* 2005;110(5–6):636–645.

34. Boldin C, Raith J, Fankhauser F, Haunschmid C, Schwantzer G, Schweighofer F. Predicting neurologic recovery in cervical spinal cord injury with postoperative MR imaging. *Spine (Phila Pa 1976).* 2006;31(5):554–559.

35. Bondurant FJ, Cotler HB, Kulkarni MV, McArdle CB, Harris Jr JH. Acute spinal cord injury. a study using physical examination and magnetic resonance imaging. *Spine (Phila Pa 1976).* 1990;15(3):161–168.

36. Ishida Y, Tominaga T. Predictors of neurologic recovery in acute central cervical cord injury with only upper extremity impairment. *Spine (Phila Pa 1976).* 2002;27(15):1652–1658. Discussion 1658.

37. Mahmood NS, Kadavigere R, Avinash KR, Rao VR. Magnetic resonance imaging in acute cervical spinal cord injury: a correlative study on spinal cord changes and 1 month motor recovery. *Spinal Cord.* 2008;46(12):791–797.

38. Marciello MA, Flanders AE, Herbison GJ, Schaefer DM, Friedman DP, Lane JI. Magnetic resonance imaging related to neurologic outcome in cervical spinal cord injury. *Arch Phys Med Rehabil.* 1993;74(9):940–946.

39. Mascalchi M, Dal Pozzo G, Dini C, et al. Acute spinal trauma: prognostic value of MRI appearances at 0.5 T. *Clin Radiol.* 1993;48(2):100–108.

40. Miranda P, Gomez P, Alday R, Kaen A, Ramos A. Brown-Sequard syndrome after blunt cervical spine trauma: clinical and radiological correlations. *Eur Spine J.* 2007;16(8):1165–1170.

41. Nidecker A, Kocher M, Maeder M, et al. MR-imaging of chronic spinal cord injury. Association with neurologic function. *Neurosurg Rev.* 1991;14(3):169–179.

42. O'Beirne J, Cassidy N, Raza K, Walsh M, Stack J, Murray P. Role of magnetic resonance imaging in the assessment of spinal injuries. *Injury.* 1993;24(3):149–154.

43. Ramon S, Dominguez R, Ramirez L, et al. Clinical and magnetic resonance imaging correlation in acute spinal cord injury. *Spinal Cord.* 1997;35(10):664–673.

44. Sato T, Kokubun S, Rijal KP, et al. Prognosis of cervical spinal cord injury in correlation with magnetic resonance imaging. *Paraplegia.* 1994;32(2):81–85.

45. Schaefer DM, Flanders AE, Osterholm JL, Northrup BE. Prognostic significance of magnetic resonance imaging in the acute phase of cervical spine injury. *J Neurosurg.* 1992;76(2):218–223.

46. Selden NR, Quint DJ, Patel N, d'Arcy HS, Papadopoulos SM. Emergency magnetic resonance imaging of cervical spinal cord injuries: clinical correlation and prognosis. *Neurosurgery.* 1999;44(4):785–792. Discussion 792–793.

47. Shepard MJ, Bracken MB. Magnetic resonance imaging and neurological recovery in acute spinal cord injury: observations from the National Acute Spinal Cord Injury Study 3. *Spinal Cord.* 1999;37(12):833–837.

48. Shin JC, Kim DY, Park CI, Kim YW, Ohn SH. Neurologic recovery according to early magnetic resonance imaging findings in traumatic cervical spinal cord injuries. *Yonsei Med J.* 2005;46(3):379–387.

49. Silberstein M, Brown D, Tress BM, Hennessey O. Suggested MRI criteria for surgical decompression in acute spinal cord injury. Preliminary observations. *Paraplegia.* 1992;30(10):704–710.

50. Silberstein M, Hennessy O. Implications of focal spinal cord lesions following trauma: evaluation with magnetic resonance imaging. *Paraplegia.* 1993;31(3):160–167.

51. Silberstein M, Tress BM, Hennessy O. Prediction of neurologic outcome in acute spinal cord injury: the role of CT and MR. *Am J Neuroradiol.* 1992;13(6):1597–1608.

52. Takahashi M, Harada Y, Inoue H, Shimada K. Traumatic cervical cord injury at C3-4 without radiographic abnormalities:

correlation of magnetic resonance findings with clinical features and outcome. *J Orthop Surg (Hong Kong)*. 2002;10(2):129–135.

53. Takahashi M, Izunaga H, Sato R, et al. Correlation of sequential MR imaging of the injured spinal cord with prognosis. *Radiat Med*. 1993;11(4):127–138.

54. Tewari MK, Gifti DS, Singh P, et al. Diagnosis and prognostication of adult spinal cord injury without radiographic abnormality using magnetic resonance imaging: analysis of 40 patients. *Surg Neurol*. 2005;63(3):204–209. Discussion 209.

55. Tsuchiya K, Fujikawa A, Honya K, Tateishi H, Nitatori T. Value of diffusion-weighted MR imaging in acute cervical cord injury as a predictor of outcome. *Neuroradiology*. 2006;48(11):803–808.

56. Yamashita Y, Takahashi M, Matsuno Y, et al. Acute spinal cord injury: magnetic resonance imaging correlated with myelopathy. *Br J Radiol*. 1991;64(759):201–209.

57. Obuchowski NA. Receiver operating characteristic curves and their use in radiology. *Radiology*. 2003;229(1):3–8.

58. Pesce LL, Papaioannu J, Metz CE. *ROC-kit Windows 1.0.1 Beta 2*. University of Chicago; 2011.

59. Park SH, Goo JM, Jo CH. Receiver operating characteristic (ROC) curve: practical review for radiologists. *Korean J Radiol*. 2004;5(1):11–18.

60. Cadotte DW, Wilson JR, Mikulis D, Stroman PW, Brady S, Fehlings MG. Conventional MRI as a diagnostic and prognostic tool in spinal cord injury: a systemic review of its application to date and an overview on emerging MRI methods. *Exp Opin Med Diagn*. 2011;5(2):121–133.

61. Onu M, Gervai P, Cohen-Adad J, et al. Human cervical spinal cord funiculi: investigation with magnetic resonance diffusion tensor imaging. *J Magn Reson Imaging*. 2010;31(4):829–837.

62. Smith SA, Jones CK, Gifford A, et al. Reproducibility of tract-specific magnetization transfer and diffusion tensor imaging in the cervical spinal cord at 3 tesla. *NMR Biomed*. 2010;23(2):207–217.

1.3B

Traumatic Spinal Cord Injury
Chronic Spinal Cord Injury and Recovery

John Kramer, Patrick Freund, Armin Curt

Spinal Cord Injury Center, University Hospital Balgrist, University of Zürich, Zürich, Switzerland

1.3B.1 INTRODUCTION

The introduction of magnetic resonance imaging (MRI) to the field of spine trauma has vastly improved the clinical diagnosis of spinal cord injury (SCI). MRI has advantages over conventional X-ray and computer tomography (CT) as it more precisely details posttraumatic compression of the spinal cord, either due to soft tissue (i.e., traumatic disc herniation or bleeding within the spinal canal) or spinal canal encroachment (e.g., following a burst fracture or vertebral misalignment). Also in cases where an SCI is clinically suspected, but without obvious vertebral column fracture or discoligamentary injury (SCIWORA = spinal cord injury without obvious radiological abnormality), MRI is essential for the diagnosis of injury and planning of appropriate surgical interventions. In addition, MRI studies in acute SCI are applied in order to estimate long-term outcomes (i.e., prognosis) and as a postsurgical outcome measure in selected cases to confirm that the spinal cord is indeed sufficiently decompressed.

With the advent of novel treatment options aiming at the repair of the injured spinal cord, insights into disease mechanisms paralleling functional recovery are essential in order to distinguish treatment-induced changes from spontaneous recovery (i.e., pattern and extent of repair/regeneration beyond spontaneous recovery). Regardless if applied during spontaneous or therapeutically derived recovery, changes in anatomical substrates in the spinal cord may be subthreshold to detection compared to other clinical measurement instruments. However, compared to the brain, MRI of the spinal cord faces a number of technical (i.e., artifacts) and anatomical (i.e., small size) challenges that limit conventional approaches for cross-sectional and longitudinal studies. Consequently, fewer advanced MRI techniques

have reached the level of clinical (i.e., routine and robust) applicability to evaluate damage/integrity at the level of the spinal cord lesion. The primary aims of this chapter will be to describe: (1) the current state of MRI as a complementary tool to the neurophysiological examination of SCI for the purpose of monitoring changes during the course of recovery during standard rehabilitation, and (2) future MRI applications to disclose anatomical regeneration/repair due to novel treatment (medical or surgical) and/or rehabilitation interventions.

1.3B.2 NEUROPHYSIOLOGY AND MRI: COMPLEMENTARY APPROACHES

At present, most clinical applications of MRI to assess the injured spinal cord are rather qualitative (i.e., defining the localization, size, and type of damage, such as bleeding and compression). Therefore, MRI findings of the injured spinal cord need to be complemented by clinically meaningful readouts as well as quantitative neurophysiological measures that provide additional insights into spinal cord function. Neurophysiological approaches commonly adopted after SCI include those that objectively examine spinal conduction in specific ascending and descending pathways.[1] Ascending fibers in the dorsal columns, which convey light touch sensation and proprioception, are most frequently studied by measuring somatosensory evoked potentials (SSEPs) using electroencephalography (EEG) techniques following surface electrical stimulation of mixed nerves in the periphery (e.g., tibial nerves). The other major ascending sensory pathway, conveying pain and temperature sensation (i.e., spinothalamic tract), can likewise be investigated monitoring evoked EEG responses to contact or radiant heat stimulation (contact heat evoked potentials, CHEPs, or laser evoked potentials, LEPs, respectively).[2] Descending pathways (e.g., corticospinal tract) are routinely examined by measuring motor evoked potentials (MEPs) following noninvasive stimulation of the motor cortex (i.e., transcranial magnetic stimulation or TMS) and recording electromyography (EMG) in the periphery. Whether ascending or descending pathways are examined, neurophysiological outcomes provide an objective readout of spinal conduction based on latency and amplitude of the measured cortical or muscle responses. Therefore, sensory (SSEP) and motor (MEPs) evoked potentials are principally important for detecting lesions in affecting spinal white matter.

The primary objective of implementing neurophysiology after SCI is to assess the severity of sensory and motor deficits related to the damaged area of spinal cord (i.e., localization and density of damage), independent of complex sensorimotor function (i.e., motor task or rating of sensory perception). The goal of coupling neurophysiological outcomes with MRI is not to provide redundant information regarding the severity of damage of the spinal cord (as revealed by SSEPs, CHEPs/LEPs, or MEPs) but rather as a complementary assessment relating morphological and functional changes. Although there is a relationship between functional and anatomical findings (i.e., in complete cord damage and absence of SSEPs/LEPs/MEPs), the functional impact of morphological changes (e.g., swelling and edema of the cord or hemorrhage) on the performance of complex sensorimotor tasks may vary considerably between subjects. This could be related to a number of factors, including the heterogeneity of the lesion area in the white and gray matter.

CLINICAL ASSESSMENT TOOLS IN SCI

- International Standards for the Neurological Classification of SCI light touch and pinprick, and motor scores
- Electrophysiology (somatosensory and motor evoked potentials, contact heat evoked potentials, nerve conduction)
- T1- and T2-weighted MRI

1.3B.3 MORPHOLOGICAL CHANGES IN THE SPINAL CORD AFTER SCI

The primary strength of MRI in the acute stages of SCI is to objectively assess the localization and extent of morphological damage in the spinal cord, from which surgical interventions can be planned. During the transition from the acute to chronic stage of SCI, the role of MRI changes, with the emphasis to disclose secondary morphological changes ongoing in the spinal cord. Therefore, it is important to understand the typical evolution of spinal cord damage according to clinical MRI findings and the extent to which observed changes can be related to clinical outcome. From the perspective of a clinical trial, an understanding of the dynamic temporal and spatial pattern of the changes in the gross damage and eventual formation of the posttraumatic (i.e., consolidated) lesion area is required to distinguish potential effects of interventions on the lesion area.

While the acquisition of MRI after SCI is routinely performed in the acute stages of injury, there are no studies that have systematically tracked (prospective longitudinal follow-up) changes in the spinal cord during the course of recovery. This is likely due, in part, to some of the challenges of spinal cord MRI. However, based on clinical observations of T1- and T2-weighted anatomical images collected serially in the first year after SCI in patients demonstrating representative patterns of spontaneous recovery, and where surgical instrumentation was either not implanted or not resulting in significant MRI artifacts, SCI are often characterized by three prominent morphological stages (Figure 1.3B.1).

The first stage corresponds to the acute onset of edema and hemorrhage spreading rostrally and caudally from the injury epicenter. T1-weighted images are generally more sensitive to detecting hemorrhage, whereas T2-weighted images are sensitive to edema. An intramedullary high intensity signal change can be observed on sagittal images in the early hours after SCI and may extend across a number of segments (Figure 1.3B.1(A)). The signal change at this point is generally diffuse, and it may be difficult to define the most rostral and caudal boundaries.

The second stage is marked by ongoing resolution of posttraumatic edema and hemorrhage,[3] evident by an apparent shrinking of the rostral-caudal extent of the high intensity intramedullary signal change (Figure 1.3B.1(B–C)). Lastly, the formation of a posttraumatic cyst, the rostral-caudal and ventral-dorsal boarders of which are generally well defined, represents the final morphological stage of SCI. Atrophic shrinking of the affected area of spinal cord in the sagittal plane (i.e., rostral-caudal) becomes obvious at this stage. At this point, the area of the posttraumatic cyst is generally stable, and further changes in size are not expected. Although the specific timing stages 1 and 2 are likely to vary considerably between subjects, the formation of the cyst should be complete within the first year after injury (Figure 1.3B.1(C and D)).

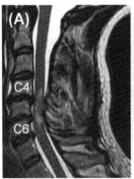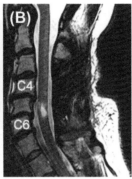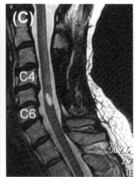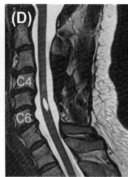

FIGURE 1.3B.1 Morphological changes in the spinal cord can be serially examined by clinical MRI techniques. In this example, the characteristic stages of morphological changes in the spinal cord are apparent based on T2-weighted anatomical images during the transition from acute to chronic stages of injury. Note the rather diffuse damage imaged during the acute phase of SCI (A) with extensive edema spreading from the lesion area, followed by the shrinking of the rostral-caudal boundary ((B–C); 3–6 months post SCI), and the eventual formation of a posttraumatic cyst combined with a focal spinal cord atrophy ((D); 6–24 months post SCI).

STAGES OF SCI BASED ON CLINICAL MRI

- Stage 1: Rostral and caudal spread of edema and hemorrhage
- Stage 2: Resolution of edema and hemorrhage
- Stage 3: Formation of posttraumatic cyst and spinal cord atrophy rostral and caudal to injury epicenter

1.3B.4 RELATIONSHIP BETWEEN NEUROLOGICAL RECOVERY AND MORPHOLOGICAL CHANGES

Some changes in clinical MRI findings may correspond with obvious features of spontaneous neurological recovery. For example, the greatest period of spontaneous neurological recovery according to clinical sensory and motor testing outcomes is expected in the initial months after injury, begins to plateau at approximately 4–6 months, and remains relatively stable thereafter.[4] Therefore, spontaneous recovery roughly occurs in parallel with some of the morphological changes described before. However, the relationship between morphological changes and spontaneous recovery is poorly understood. Even in patients where gross morphological changes are observed (e.g., enlargement of the posttraumatic cyst), the severity of injury may not change and the patient remains clinically stable. While this represents an apparent discrepancy between MRI and functional outcomes in longitudinal pathways traversing the lesion epicenter, this underscores the importance of coupling MRI with neurophysiological outcomes to assess function. Indeed, neurophysiological outcomes assessing conduction in ascending and descending pathways traversing through the lesion level generally remain unchanged during recovery.[4,5]

Although the majority of individuals with SCI are expected to moderately improve from their initial sensory and motor deficits, the trajectory of spontaneous recovery can take a deleterious turn of events in the months and years following SCI. In fact, the role of clinical MRI techniques in disclosing neurological complications (e.g., posttraumatic tethering and/or progressive syrinx formation) associated with SCI is much better defined than the role of monitoring spontaneous neurological recovery.[6] The incidence of the development of posttraumatic syringomyelia after SCI has been reported between 5% and 8%.[7] Particularly when coupled with obvious signs of descending neurological deficits (e.g., loss of muscle strength in myotomes rostral to the initial level of injury), the appearance of posttraumatic tethering and/or progressive syrinx formation according to MRI often warrants surgical intervention to prevent further deterioration. In some cases where a posttraumatic cyst develops, surgical intervention is potentially warranted based solely on MRI findings if further increases in rostral-caudal boundary threaten vital brainstem functions (i.e., breathing). The onset of symptoms related to syrinx formation can be rapid, thus imaging the spinal cord for morphological changes to confirm the diagnosis is paramount. In the majority of cases, following surgical intervention collapsing of the syrinx can be imaged by T2-weighted MRI. Neurophysiology coupled with MRI has an important role in confirming that the developing cyst is altering conduction in the spinal cord. Owing to the fact that small diameter afferent fibers conveying temperature sensation decussate across spinal segments before ascending in the spinothalamic tract, CHEPs/LEPs are particularly useful to examine the functional significance of lesions localized or developing in the central gray matter. This can be achieved by stimulating dermatomes corresponding to segments adjacent to the imaged level of pathology.

1.3B.5 THE MRI PARADOX: WHEN ANATOMICAL CHANGES DO NOT CORRESPOND TO FUNCTIONAL CHANGES

The "MRI paradox", whereby gross morphological changes are observed according to MRI in the absence of any or severe functional deterioration in the spinal cord or vice versa, continues to puzzle clinicians and researchers.[8] Some of the most complex and interesting cases that highlight the MRI paradox involve patients with posttraumatic holocord syringomyelia. In the example shown in Figure 1.3B.2, the neurophysiological readouts indicate that spinal conduction is, in fact, almost completely normal in the upper limbs. Thus, despite a gross morphological change in the spinal cord affecting cervical segments, function in ascending and descending pathways remains nearly completely intact.

The reason for such gross morphological changes unaccompanied by severe functional changes or neurological deterioration is not well understood. However, this paradox is not unique to MRI; histological studies of the spinal cord also illustrate that function may not accurately correspond to the anatomical neuropathology after injury. Indeed, the spinal cord is rarely completely transected even in cases with complete sensory and motor loss, and spared white matter traverses the injury epicenter.[9,10] In part, the discrepancy between anatomical and functional changes may be related to the low resolution and/or low specificity/sensitivity of clinical MRI techniques to distinguish differences in pathology (e.g., demyelination).[8] Implementing a neurophysiological approach is therefore important in order to determine if subtle changes in spinal conduction may be present in the white matter, as changes in latency and amplitude of evoked potentials (sensory and motor) may also precede the onset of measurable clinical deficits.

1.3B.6 CONVENTIONAL MRI APPROACHES IN SCI CLINICAL TRIAL MANAGEMENT

At present, there is no effective treatment option to resolve the sensory loss and motor paralysis associated with SCI. However, there are a number of potential strategies that might translate to patient benefits, and implementing valid and reliable outcome measures to assess safety and efficacy of interventional strategies is paramount. Since small treatment effects may accompany initial approaches to resolve sensorimotor deficits, it is important that outcomes are sensitive to detect subtle changes (i.e., responsive). Therapeutic options in SCI generally fall into one of two categories: neuroprotective or neurorestorative. Whereas neuroprotection aims to prevent secondary damage caused by the cascade of biochemical events in the central nervous system triggered by SCI, including hemorrhagic events and edema, neurorestorative strategies intend to reconstitute partial or complete loss of function in neural circuitry affected by SCI. The latter category includes regeneration and remyelination of axons across or around a lesion site in the spinal cord. Regardless of the treatment strategy employed, the changes in neurological structures are expected to occur over time, often during spontaneous recovery, and therefore require longitudinal investigation. The capability of conventional MRI to noninvasively examine gross morphological changes in the spinal cord represents a potentially powerful outcome measure on which to determine therapeutic safety and efficacy of

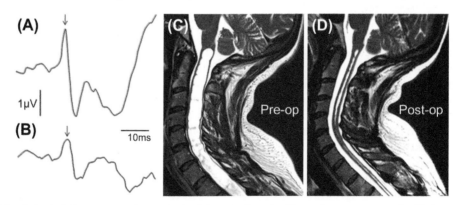

FIGURE 1.3B.2 Morphological changes according to MRI of the spinal cord will not always correspond with functional outcomes. In this example, contrary to normal median (A) and ulnar (B) somatosensory evoked potentials (arrows indicate potentials used in evaluating latency and amplitude, which are well within normal values for this example), T2-weighted anatomical images demonstrate the presence of a posttraumatic holocord syringomyelia (C). Following surgical intervention, collapsing of the syringomyelia can be readily observed (D). This example highlights the utility of MRI to disclose changes in spinal cord morphology while this patient did not suffer from severe neurological deterioration at the time of imaging (she reported only with mild sensory disturbances without changes in dexterity) and surgical intervention was performed to prevent further increases in the size of the syringomyelia that eventually might affect vital brainstem areas.

a given treatment. The use of MRI in this way goes beyond most current clinical trial applications, which have employed MRI criteria for the purposes of reducing subject heterogeneity (i.e., inclusion/exclusion criteria).[11]

The advantage of employing MRI as a surrogate of safety and efficacy is that clinical neuroimaging outcomes are objective and may be sensitive to morphological changes that are subthreshold for detection according to other neurological outcomes (including neurophysiological outcomes). In the context of demonstrating the safety of a therapeutic intervention, MRI may have an important role in revealing potentially deleterious morphological changes in the spinal cord resulting from treatment that are not yet functionally meaningful. This is not unlike the current applications of MRI to assess spontaneously derived posttraumatic syringomyelia. Using MRI as a measure of safety could be chiefly important for restorative strategies, including those cell-based therapies that will be injected into the spinal cord in order to regenerate lost axons, but which may also result in cystic formation due to uncontrolled growth. MRI may also be useful to assess the preliminary biological activity of a given therapeutic in a neuroprotective study. To this end, the effects on hemorrhage and edema may be studied as a marker of biological efficacy.[12] However, for more detailed information, including if a therapeutic remyelinates spared axons after SCI, changes in spinal conduction based on neurophysiological outcomes may be a more appropriate surrogate than conventional MRI.

There are two primary problems with the use of current clinical MRI techniques as outcome measures in clinical SCI trials. Firstly, as already stated, conventional MRI represents a surrogate biomarker of function (i.e., indirect measure related to anatomy, not necessarily functional outcomes) and, as such, cannot be adopted as a primary endpoint in a pivotal phase III clinical study designed to determine the efficacy of a given therapeutic. Most importantly, changes in the neuroanatomical structures within the spinal cord would not necessarily equate to changes in functional connectivity in the spinal cord. Whereas observed improvements in neurological structures according to MRI are not sufficient alone to conclude that a therapeutic is effective, deleterious changes (i.e., increase in the area of the posttraumatic cyst) are likely enough to be considered an adverse event.

Secondly, clinical MRI techniques presently suitable to assess therapeutic efficacy and safety (T1- and T2-weighted images) lack standardized outcomes on which to quantify the damage in the injured spinal cord. At this point, the interpretation of MRI remains largely qualitative and therefore depends largely on the experience of the individual examiner. In the context of assessing anatomical changes in the spinal cord during spontaneous or treatment-induced recovery, it is important that the reliability of objective clinical MRI outcomes be adequately validated.

USE OF MRI IN CLINICAL SCI TRIALS

- Inclusion/Exclusion criteria (e.g., individuals with complete cord transections or rostral caudal lesions exceeding a set number of segments)
- Monitor changes in morphological structures associated with or independent of a therapy
- Detect deleterious changes in the spinal cord—paramount to establish safety of a therapy

---

1.3B.7 FUTURE DIRECTIONS OF MRI AND SCI

The use of MRI to serially evaluate pathological events within the spinal cord in neurological conditions, such as multiple sclerosis (MS), is well established.[13] Despite recent and numerous advances in MRI techniques, it remains technically challenging to obtain meaningful MRI results at the level of the injured spinal cord. As previously discussed, this is partially due to artifacts from fractured disks and fixative vertebral implants near the level of injury.

A promising strategy to overcome the issues related to surgical instrumentation is to focus on areas rostral to the injury site initially unaffected by the lesion area. A valid and established MRI tool is the assessment of cross-sectional spinal cord area. Usually, the cross-sectional spinal cord area is estimated on reformatted axial slices at cervical level C2/C3 on 3D T1-weighted anatomical scans.[14] In individuals with SCI and instrumentation fixating the spinal column, this is generally well above the injury level and thus artifact free. In MS, cross-sectional spinal cord area measurement has proven to be sensitive toward changes in disease state[15] and has been employed to track potential treatment effects associated with a therapeutic intervention.[16]

Only recently was the measure of cross-sectional spinal cord area introduced to the field of SCI[17] (Figure 1.3B.3). In chronic SCI, marked cord atrophy at the C2/C3 level has been demonstrated in para- and tetraplegic patients.[18–20] Cord atrophy, an endpoint of neurodegeneration resulting from SCI, could be mediated through the accumulation of multiple microstructural events over time, including axonal degeneration and demyelination, axonal dieback, and neuronal loss.[21]

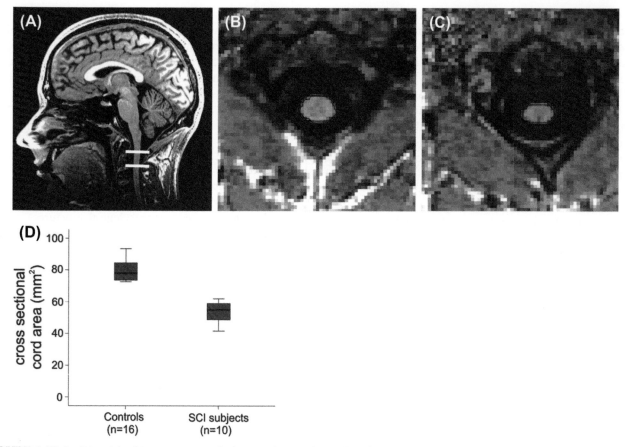

FIGURE 1.3B.3   T1-weighted image covering the brain and cervical spinal cord to simultaneously assess the cross-sectional cord area and cortical gray and white matter volume using voxel-based morphometry (A). (B) and (C) show one representative reformatted axial slice of the cervical cord (C2/C3 level) in one control and one chronic tetraplegic patient, respectively. (D) Cross-sectional cord area comparison between 16 healthy controls and 10 chronic tetraplegic patients. Note significant cord area shrinkage of more than 30% in SCI patients.[19] *Source: Figures are reproduced with permission from Ref. 19.*

However, due to relatively low imaging resolution, it has not been possible to distinguish trauma-related changes between spinal gray (e.g., motor neuron death) and white matter integrity (e.g., axonal degeneration and demyelination). Moreover, it is unclear whether cord atrophy is related to the lesion level or time post injury.[18] However, recent improvement in spatial resolution and image contrast at 3T (Yinnakas et al., in press *NeuroImage*) and 7T (Sigmund et al., 2012 *NMR Biomed*) enabled measurements of gray and white matter fraction in healthy controls. These developments might be applicable to the SCI population. Crucially, lower cross-sectional spinal cord area is associated with lower clinical scores and impaired manual dexterity. The link between cord atrophy and disability suggests that cross-sectional spinal cord area may be useful to track changes in the spinal cord in longitudinal studies. In order to obtain more clinically relevant and detailed information, further improvements in imaging techniques providing reliable and high-resolution images are required.

1.3B.7.1 Diffusion Weighted and Magnetization Transfer Imaging

Characterizing microstructural alteration of spinal white matter integrity with diffusion tensor imaging (DTI) can further improve our understanding between central tract specific changes to clinical impairment. During acute SCI, DTI has been shown to be predictive of long-term functional recovery.[22,23] In chronic SCI, DTI is correlated with clinical measures of injury severity.[24] The reproducibility of DTI has also recently been demonstrated in children.[25] DTI indexes are altered at the lesion site and rostral to it suggesting trauma-induced degenerative processes in ascending and descending central pathways. Importantly, reduced white matter integrity of specific central pathways was linked to clinical disability. Thus, DTI holds promise to quantify the degree of white matter integrity, to predict recovery, and to monitor the effects of therapeutic interventions. Similarly, magnetization transfer imaging has shown potential for detecting pathology in the white matter associated with demyelination[20] and could be a potential avenue for probing the effect of remyelinating therapies in SCI.

1.3B.8 CONCLUSIONS

At present, MRI findings after SCI should be primarily interpreted as evidence of anatomical damage in the spinal cord. For the purposes of assessing function in the injured spinal cord, MRI needs to be coupled with clinical and neurophysiological studies (e.g., SSEPs and MEPs). Few research studies have assessed changes in the spinal cord according to MRI after injury in a longitudinal study, but a clear evolution of the damaged spinal cord area can be observed using clinical techniques (e.g., T1- and T2-weighted images). However, the relationship between these morphological changes and functional recovery remains to be determined. Additional studies are needed to establish valid and sensitive outcomes to objectively assess the injured spinal cord, as well as overcome the limitations of imaging at the area of lesion. At present, clinical MRI represents a suitable trial endpoint to assess safety for therapies aimed at regenerating the damaged spinal cord. The success of implementing novel MRI techniques (e.g., cross-sectional spinal cord area rostral to the lesion level and DTI) to assess changes in the spinal cord during spontaneous recovery will ultimately decide the utility of MRI as a marker of therapeutic efficacy.

References

1. Curt A, Dietz V. Electrophysiological recordings in patients with spinal cord injury: significance for predicting outcome. *Spinal Cord*. 1999;37(3):157–165.
2. Pazzaglia C, Valeriani M. Brain-evoked potentials as a tool for diagnosing neuropathic pain. *Expert Rev Neurother*. 2009;9(5):759–771.
3. Miyanji F, Furlan JC, Aarabi B, Arnold PM, Fehlings MG. Acute cervical traumatic spinal cord injury: MR imaging findings correlated with neurologic outcome—prospective study with 100 consecutive patients. *Radiology*. 2007;243(3):820–827.
4. Curt A, Van Hedel HJ, Klaus D, Dietz V. Recovery from a spinal cord injury: significance of compensation, neural plasticity, and repair. *J Neurotrauma*. 2008;25(6):677–685.
5. Spiess M, Schubert M, Kliesch U, Halder P. Evolution of tibial SSEP after traumatic spinal cord injury: baseline for clinical trials. *Clin Neurophysiol*. 2008;119(5):1051–1061.
6. Falci SP, Indeck C, Lammertse DP. Posttraumatic spinal cord tethering and syringomyelia: surgical treatment and long-term outcome. *J Neurosurg Spine*. 2009;11(4):445–460.
7. Edgar R, Quail P. Progressive post-traumatic cystic and non-cystic myelopathy. *Br J Neurosurg*. 1994;8(1):7–22.
8. Barkhof F. The clinico-radiological paradox in multiple sclerosis revisited. *Curr Opin Neurol*. 2002;15(3):239–245.
9. Kakulas BA. Pathology of spinal injuries. *Cent Nerv Syst Trauma*. 1984;1(1):117–129.
10. Hayes KC, Kakulas BA. Neuropathology of human spinal cord injury sustained in sports-related activities. *J Neurotrauma*. 1997;14(4):235–248.
11. Jones LA, Lammertse DP, Charlifue SB, et al. A phase 2 autologous cellular therapy trial in patients with acute, complete spinal cord injury: pragmatics, recruitment, and demographics. *Spinal Cord*. 2010;48(11):798–807.
12. Leypold BG, Flanders AE, Schwartz ED, Burns AS. The impact of methylprednisolone on lesion severity following spinal cord injury. *Spine (Phila Pa 1976)*. 2007;32(3):373–378. Discussion 9–81.
13. Miller DH, Barkhof F, Frank JA, Parker GJ, Thompson AJ. Measurement of atrophy in multiple sclerosis: pathological basis, methodological aspects and clinical relevance. *Brain*. 2002;125(Pt 8):1676–1695.
14. Losseff NA, Webb SL, O'Riordan JI, et al. Spinal cord atrophy and disability in multiple sclerosis. A new reproducible and sensitive MRI method with potential to monitor disease progression. *Brain*. 1996;119(Pt 3):701–708.
15. Stevenson VL, Leary SM, Losseff NA, et al. Spinal cord atrophy and disability in MS: a longitudinal study. *Neurology*. 1998;51(1):234–238.
16. Kalkers NF, Barkhof F, Bergers E, van Schijndel R, Polman CH. The effect of the neuroprotective agent riluzole on MRI parameters in primary progressive multiple sclerosis: a pilot study. *Mult Scler*. 2002;8(6):532–533.
17. Freund PA, Dalton C, Wheeler-Kingshott CA, et al. Method for simultaneous voxel-based morphometry of the brain and cervical spinal cord area measurements using 3D-MDEFT. *J Magn Reson Imaging*. 2010;32(5):1242–1247.
18. Lundell H, Barthelemy D, Skimminge A, Dyrby TB, Biering-Sorensen F, Nielsen JB. Independent spinal cord atrophy measures correlate to motor and sensory deficits in individuals with spinal cord injury. *Spinal Cord*. 2011;49(1):70–75.
19. Freund P, Weiskopf N, Ward NS, et al. Disability, atrophy and cortical reorganization following spinal cord injury. *Brain*. 2011;134(Pt 6):1610–1622.
20. Cohen-Adad J, El Mendili MM, Lehericy S, et al. Demyelination and degeneration in the injured human spinal cord detected with diffusion and magnetization transfer MRI. *NeuroImage*. 2011;55(3):1024–1033.
21. Dusart I, Schwab ME. Secondary cell death and the inflammatory reaction after dorsal hemisection of the rat spinal cord. *Eur J Neurosci*. 1994;6(5):712–724.
22. Cheran S, Shanmuganathan K, Zhuo J, et al. Correlation of MR diffusion tensor imaging parameters with ASIA motor scores in hemorrhagic and nonhemorrhagic acute spinal cord injury. *J Neurotrauma*. 2011;28(9):1881–1892.
23. Kim JH, Loy DN, Wang Q, et al. Diffusion tensor imaging at 3 hours after traumatic spinal cord injury predicts long-term locomotor recovery. *J Neurotrauma*. 2010;27(3):587–598.
24. Petersen JA, Wilm BJ, von Meyenburg J, et al. Chronic cervical spinal cord injury: DTI correlates with clinical and electrophysiological measures. *J Neurotrauma*. 2012;29(8):1556–1566.
25. Mulcahey M, Samdani A, Gaughan J, et al. Diffusion tensor imaging in pediatric spinal cord injury: preliminary examination of reliability and clinical correlation. *Spine (Phila Pa 1976)*. 2011;37(3):E797–803.

Further Reading

1. Ashburner J, Friston KJ. Voxel-based morphometry—the methods. *NeuroImage*. 2000;11(6 Pt 1):805–821.
2. Basser PJ, Mattiello J, LeBihan D. MR diffusion tensor spectroscopy and imaging. *Biophys J*. 1994;66(1):259–267.

PART II

PHYSICS OF MRI

Array Coils

Julien Cohen-Adad[1,2], *Lawrence L. Wald*[3,4]

[1]Institute of Biomedical Engineering, Polytechnique Montreal; Functional Neuroimaging Unit, CRIUGM, Université de Montréal, Montreal, QC, Canada [2]Functional Neuroimaging Unit, CRIUGM, Université de Montréal, Montreal, QC, Canada [3]A.A. Martinos Center for Biomedical Imaging, Massachusetts General Hospital, Harvard Medical School, Charlestown, MA, USA [4]Harvard-MIT Division of Health Sciences and Technology, MIT, Cambridge, MA, USA

2.1.1 INTRODUCTION

Essential parts of a magnetic resonance imaging (MRI) system, radiofrequency (RF) coils or antennas are used to transmit and/or receive signal. Phased-array coils combine multiple small coil elements to transmit or receive signal using independent channels. Array coils were first described in a seminal paper by Roemer et al., and proof-of-concept was demonstrated in the spine. Since then, array coils have become the standard for multiple body parts in research and clinical MRI. The two main advantages are their increased sensitivity and the possibility of faster acquisition via parallel imaging. Several concepts related to array coils need to be understood to appreciate their full benefits and optimize their use, notably the B_1 magnetic field, the so-called geometric factor (g-factor), and the signal-to-noise ratio (SNR).

This chapter will first introduce theoretical concepts related to RF coils, then will cover array coils and their advantages and limitations. We will review some of the existing array coils for human spinal cord imaging. We will then present design and building considerations, including safety aspects. Finally, we will look at how to evaluate transmit (Tx) and receive (Rx) coils (including the SNR and g-factor).

2.1.2 COIL THEORY

The basic principle of RF coils is to create a B_1 magnetic field that rotates the magnetization of the nuclei (Tx coils) or to measure signal emitted by the resonating nuclei in the transverse plane (Rx coils). Both Tx and Rx

coils are tuned to the Larmor frequency (ω), at which particles can exchange energy. The Larmor frequency depends on the gyromagnetic ratio of the particle (γ) and on the magnetic field strength they are submitted to (B), according to $\omega = \gamma B$. For example at 3 tesla, the Larmor frequency of water protons is about 127 MHz.

Coils consist of a set of inductive (L) and capacitive (C) elements that are chosen to make the coil resonate at the Larmor frequency, according to:

$$\omega = \frac{1}{2\pi\sqrt{LC}}$$

Coils are designed for transmitting, receiving, or performing both functions. The geometry of the coil can be optimized for its purpose. Typically, for transmitting coils, B_1 homogeneity should be high in order to obtain similar excitation (flip angle) over the region of interest. Conversely, for receiving, the ability to detect small magnetic flux generated by the resonating spins becomes more important than homogeneity, therefore sensitivity will be optimized. Thus, several coil geometries exist that achieve either good homogeneity or good sensitivity (sometimes both). Examples of volume and surface coils associated with their respective B_1 field are shown in Figure 2.1.1. Typically, volume coils are used for transmission since they are made up of large elements and can achieve good B_1 homogeneity. Conversely, small surface coils are preferred for reception since they achieve high sensitivity. In standard MRI systems, the Tx coil is usually integrated into the scanner (also called the "body coil"), while the Rx coil is manually plugged into the system (either the patient's table or the body of the scanner).

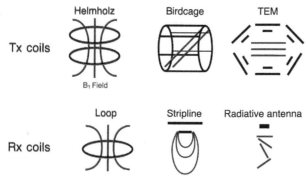

FIGURE 2.1.1 Illustration of typical Tx (top) and Rx (bottom) coils in MRI, including the direction of its B_1 field (in red). Volume coils (such as birdcage coils) provide homogeneous excitations (adequate for Tx), while small surface coils provide high SNR (adequate for Rx). Stripline and radiative antennas are of particular interest at ultrahigh fields (>7 T).

To understand how receive coils work, let's consider a simple loop coil. According to Faraday's law, the alternating magnetic field produced by the nearby rotating nuclei induces an alternating current in the loop. This principle is similar to the bicycle dynamo from which a current is generated via a rotating small magnet nearby a solenoid coil. The sensitivity of a single loop can be obtained from the Biot–Savart law. The larger the loop, the deeper it can capture signal from, but also the higher the amount of noise it will capture from the object scanned. Hence, optimal loop size should be designed depending on the desired penetration depth. For example, to achieve optimal sensitivity at 8 cm deep, a loop of approximately 8 cm is desired.

2.1.2.1 Q-Factor

The coil has resistive losses (R) within its conducting wires and various connections. The quality factor of the coil (Q) can be calculated as $Q = \omega L/R$. The higher the Q, the higher the SNR and hence the sensitivity of the coil. If the coil is loaded with biological tissue, some energy from the tissue is also captured by the coil via capacitive coupling. The fraction of loss dissipated in the tissue relative to the coil is evaluated by the so-called Q ratio, which is the ratio between Q while the coil is unloaded (Q_U) and Q when the coil is loaded (Q_L). Hence, Q_U is necessarily bigger than Q_L given that the body contributes to the measured noise. The goal when designing a coil is therefore to have Q_U/Q_L that is maximized, so that the coil is dominated by body noise with minimal electronic noise contribution.

2.1.3 ARRAY COILS

2.1.3.1 Sensitivity

As mentioned in this chapter, a large loop can cover a large region but captures more thermal and physiological noise from the body. Contrariwise, a small loop captures less noise, as its sensitivity profile is restricted to a very small region close to the loop. The idea of having multiple small loops next to each other is to combine them in order to gain penetration in the sensitivity profile, while only capturing a small amount of noise coming from each individual coil element. This gives the rationale for designing coil arrays.[1]

It is often mistakenly thought that in deep tissue, the sensitivity of phased-array coils with lots of small coils is poorer than that of coils with less but bigger elements. Although it is true that the penetration of each individual element of a phased-array coil is reduced, when combining several smaller elements into a phased-array coil, the sensitivity in deep tissue is similar to that of a coil with fewer elements. However, closer to the coil, the sensitivity of a phased-array coil is significantly higher. This was notably demonstrated using theoretical analyses[2] and experiments.[3] Figure 2.1.2 illustrates this point by comparing different coil arrangements.

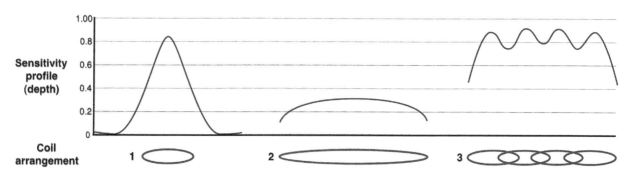

FIGURE 2.1.2 Sensitivity profiles at a depth of 8 cm for three different surface coil arrangements: (1) a single 8 cm square coil, (2) a single large 30 × 15 cm rectangular coil, and (3) a phased array made of 8 cm square coils. An SNR of 1 corresponds to a theoretical upper limit SNR variance given for linear reception array coils with the sensitivity profile given in (1). *Adapted from*[1].

2.1.3.2 Parallel Imaging

Another benefit of array coils—in addition to higher sensitivity—is that simultaneous reception from the coils enables parallel imaging reconstruction methods. Parallel acquisition consists of skipping lines of k-space in the phase-encoding direction, which reduces the effective echo spacing, resulting in less image distortions in echo planar imaging (EPI) sequences (also see Chapter 2.3). The signal recorded by each independent coil is then used to reconstruct an unaliased image by either filling missing lines of k-space (the SMASH[4] or GRAPPA[5] methods) or unaliasing pixels in the image domain (the SENSE method).[6] The performance of the coil regarding acceleration capabilities is therefore dictated by the geometry of the coil, or the so-called g-factor. The lower the g-factor, the better the coil performance is with respect to parallel acquisition, with the lowest g-factor being 1.

To qualitatively assess a coil capability for parallel imaging, one first needs to consider what will be the typical direction for phase encoding (i.e., direction of acceleration). For example, if a coil consists of 16 elements disposed around a cylinder (see Figure 2.1.3(A)), the g-factor will be low in the X and Y directions, while it will be high along the Z direction. This means that the coil will perform better when acceleration occurs along the X or Y direction. In contrast, Figure 2.1.3(B) shows an arrangement that favors acceleration in the Z direction but not in the X or Y direction. Hence, optimal design of a coil should take into consideration acceleration capabilities. That is, if spinal cord imaging is typically performed with phase encoding in the antero-posterior direction, there should be enough individual coil coverage along this direction in order to reduce the g-factor. If this were not the case, reconstruction artifacts would occur and SNR would be substantially reduced (SNR is inversely proportional to the g-factor, as described later in this chapter). For a comprehensive review on parallel imaging, the reader is referred to Ref. 7.

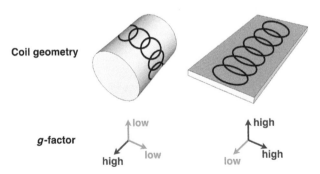

FIGURE 2.1.3 Relationship between coil geometry and the g-factor. A low g-factor means good acceleration capabilities, while a high g-factor means poor acceleration capabilities. Quantitative evaluation of the g-factor is described later in this chapter.

RECOMMENDATIONS FOR ACCELERATION[a]

- *Twelve-channel (12-ch) head coil* (upper cervical): maximum of 3× acceleration along the antero-posterior (A-P) or right-left (R-L) direction
- *4-ch neck coil* (cervical): maximum of 2× acceleration along the A-P or R-L direction
- *24-ch spine array* (thoracic and lumbar): maximum of 2× acceleration along the A-P or R-L direction, 3× acceleration along the superior-inferior (S-I) direction

[a] With some vendors, it is possible to manually set the number of channels used with particular coils; for example, the spine array matrix can be used as *single* (CP), *dual*, or *triple mode*. For the highest parallel imaging capabilities, *triple mode* should be set.

2.1.3.3 Design and Building Considerations

2.1.3.3.1 Geometry

When designing RF coils, some key aspects need to be considered. One of the most important aspects is that the Tx coil should have excellent B_1 homogeneity, while the Rx coil should have excellent sensitivity. Hence, for Rx coils, elements need to be close to the region of interest (e.g., the spinal cord). A morphological model in combination with B_1 field simulations are helpful for designing the final shape of the coil former and the layout of each element.

For the cervical spinal cord, the geometry of the body allows elements to be placed around the neck to improve sensitivity. In typical state-of-the-art clinical coils, the head coil is compatible with the spine array and an anterior neck coil, and all elements can be selected simultaneously for imaging the head and spinal cord. Additionally, commercially available head and cervical arrays are typically designed for comfort and to be used with nearly 100% of the population, and hence they are generally not made to fit as tightly to the body as might be desired in a research setting where sensitivity is the primary concern.

For the thoracic, lumbar, and sacral spinal cord, elements need to be placed posteriorly to the body. Placing elements anteriorly could be considered, given the almost central location of the spinal cord in the A-P direction. An advantage of placing elements anteriorly is to lower the g-factor in the A-P direction, enabling at least twofold acceleration in this direction, which is difficult to achieve with coils placed only posteriorly. Of course, superior-inferior or right-left acceleration is still possible with phased-array coils placed posteriorly, although these phase-encoding directions are less commonly used with spinal cord EPI. One disadvantage of having elements anteriorly is that signal from the heart (for thoracic) and/or chest (for thoraco-lumbar) would be picked up. These regions are prone to severe motion artifacts and therefore can result in severe ghosting artifacts that can overlap the spinal cord. Another disadvantage of placing elements anteriorly is that using reduced field-of-view (FOV) techniques requires further saturation (or two-dimensional selective RF excitation) to null the signal coming anteriorly from the cord. If no anterior coil is used, very little signal is picked up from regions anterior to the cord, making it easier to apply reduced FOV techniques.

An original design of a thoraco-lumbar 7 T phased-array coil has been proposed by Vossen et al.[8] There, the Tx coil is placed anteriorly, and the Rx coil posteriorly. One advantage of doing so is that the total power deposited in the body is lower if the RF energy is transmitted through the lungs from the anterior side to the centrally located spinal cord, compared to the case where the Tx coil is placed on the posterior side of the body, where the RF field must propagate through a large muscle mass with high conductivity.

2.1.3.4 Review of Array Coils for the Spinal Cord

Although receive arrays were originally developed and demonstrated for spinal cord imaging,[1] most highly parallel detectors (≥ 32 elements) have focused on being developed for the brain and heart.

For 1.5 and 3 T systems, several array designs have been proposed for the spinal cord.[9–13] These include arrays designed for full coverage of the spine, with up to 24 channels,[10] and those designed specifically for the cervical spine, with up to 16 channels.[9] Given that these designs are typically not compatible with manufacturers' head coils, recent designs have included the brain for full coverage of the head and cervical spinal cord, using for example 32 elements[13] or 64 elements.[14]

For 7 T systems, mostly Tx and Rx coils have been developed, including 4-ch and 6-ch coils using nonoverlapping elements,[15] an 8-ch coil (two rows of four overlapped elements),[16] and a 4-ch coil.[17] Using the latter coil, the SNR benefit of 7 T over 3 T was notably shown by comparing data acquired in the same subject. At 7 T, separate Tx and Rx coils have also been designed. For example, a 2-ch Tx was combined with an 8-ch Rx coil (one row of overlapped elements for a total length of 90 cm),[8] where simulations were used to find the best location for excitation (anteriorly versus posteriorly). In another work, a 4-ch Tx was combined with a 19-ch Rx coil.[18] In this design, Zhao et al. used the 4-ch Tx coil with a single-channel Tx mode where the Tx signal was split using a butler matrix (with the 45° phase incrementally added in each element to optimize B_1 homogeneity). More recently, a 30-ch Rx coil demonstrated high-quality magnetic resonance spectroscopy in the spinal cord.[19]

Multiple groups opted for a flat design. These coils are easier to build, and they can be used for any level of the spine. One disadvantage, however, is that they are not optimized for the cervical region, where elements could also be placed around the neck, thereby potentially increasing the sensitivity and *g*-factor. Picture samples of spine coils for 3 T and 7 T systems are shown in Figure 2.1.4.

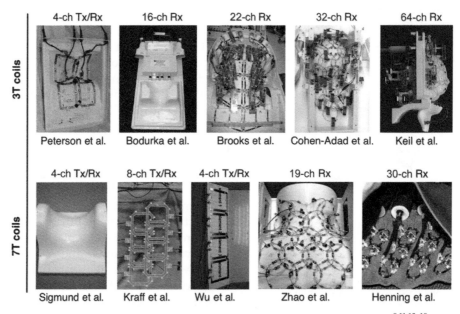

FIGURE 2.1.4   Pictures of spine array coils for 3 T (top) and 7 T (bottom).[9,11,13–19]

2.1.4 EVALUATION OF Tx ARRAY COILS

2.1.4.1 SAR Calculation

For Tx coils, the main safety assessment is the energy deposited to the tissue during excitation. It is measured by the specific absorption rate (SAR), defined as the RF power absorbed per unit of mass of an object (in W/kg). Limits of maximum SAR are fixed by country authorities and cannot exceed certain values. For example, in the United States, during normal operation mode over a period of 6 min, the maximum SAR allowed is 4 W/kg (whole body average over 15 min) or 8 W/kg (in the head or trunk over 10 min).[20]

Hence, when building a coil, SAR is calculated as a function of the voltage submitted to the coil, in order to get an estimate of the maximum voltage that is allowed. To predict SAR from a particular design, electromagnetic simulations are required. Using finite-difference time domain (FDTD) or finite element method (FEM) modeling of Maxwell's equation, and using models of human tissue, it is possible to predict conductivity. Simulation software packages include Remcom, Semcad and HFSS. Figure 2.1.5 shows an example of 4-ch Tx coil simulations for estimating the B_1 field, as well as the SAR in a human model. Simulations, however, can be quite computer-intensive and results are very sensitive to the input parameters (geometry and placement of the coils, modeling of the gradient cylinder, choice of gridding, and choice of human model). Hence, it is often the case that SAR simulations can be off compared to the real situation, given the inaccuracies of simulations and the nonperfect reproduction of the design on the bench. For this reason, it is advisable to perform additional temperature tests on a phantom and be conservative on the maximum voltage allowed.

2.1.5 EVALUATION OF Rx ARRAY COILS

2.1.5.1 Image SNR

Although SNR can easily be calculated by dividing the mean signal intensity by the standard deviation in the image background, this method is no more correct when using phased-array coils, given that both the statistical and the spatial distribution of noise are different than that with a single-channel coil. For example, the sum-of-squares reconstruction changes the statistical distribution of background noise,[21] and some filters applied during reconstruction can influence the spatial distribution of the noise.[22]

Hence, for quantifying SNR in a phased-array coil, other methods should be employed based on the true calculation of noise in each voxel.[23] One method is to acquire a proton density weighted gradient echo image, then measure noise covariance in each channel using the same sequence without RF excitation. Given a signal vector S (a vector of image intensities at a given pixel across all coils), with S^H being the Hermitian transpose of S, the image SNR for the root-sum-of-squares (rSoS) combination image[2] can be expressed as:

$$\mathrm{SNR}^{\mathrm{rSoS}} = \frac{S^H S}{\sqrt{S^H \Psi S}}$$

If Ψ^{-1} is the inverse of the noise covariance matrix Ψ, the image SNR for the noise covariance weighted rSoS reconstruction (cov-rSoS)[1] is:

$$\mathrm{SNR}^{\mathrm{cov-rSoS}} = \sqrt{S^H \Psi^{-1} S}.$$

Examples of image SNR for different phased-array coils are shown in Figure 2.1.6.

2.1.5.2 G-factor

Several parallel imaging reconstruction techniques exist, such as GRAPPA, which operates in k-space by filling missing phase-encoding lines,[24] and SENSE, which operates in the image domain by unaliasing images.[6] An acceleration factor R (also called iPAT in Siemens systems) means the number of phase-encoding lines is divided by a factor R; therefore, acquisition will be R times faster. Consequently, the SNR will be reduced by a factor $\sqrt{R}$ due to reduced Fourier averaging.

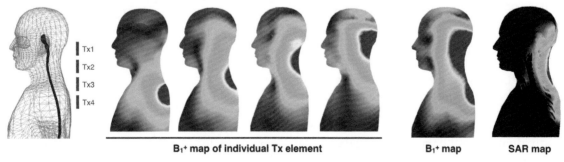

B₁⁺ map of individual Tx element   B₁⁺ map   SAR map

FIGURE 2.1.5 Transmit coil calculation of a B_1^+ field and SAR map using a 3D FEM simulator (HFSS). *Source: Courtesy of Wei Zhao, MGH Martinos Center for Biomedical Imaging.*

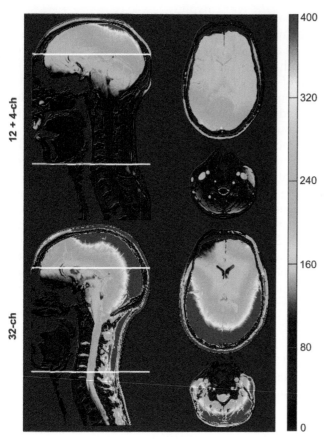

FIGURE 2.1.6   Image SNR for a 12-ch head and 4-ch neck coil (top) and a 32-ch head and spine coil (bottom). The 32-ch coil yields about 2× more SNR in the spinal cord compared to the 12 + 4-ch coil. The SNR unit depends on a few parameters (notably, FFT scaling) but allows direct comparison between coils if the same parameters are used.

SNR will also be influenced by the performance of the parallel reconstruction. When using the SENSE algorithm,[6] SNR relates to the performance in unaliasing pixels in the image domain. This performance directly relates to how different the sensitivity profile of each receive coil (B_1) is for a given pixel, and therefore depends on the geometric placement of each coil with respect to the imaged region. A measure of this parameter is the g-factor. Hence, the SNR in a parallel imaging experiment (SNR_{pi}) can be written as:

$$SNR_{pi} = SNR_{full}/\left(g \cdot \sqrt{R}\right),$$

where SNR_{full} is the SNR without applying parallel imaging (i.e., full k-space is acquired), R is the acceleration factor, and g is the g-factor.

The SENSE g-factor can then be computed voxel-wise from the individual channel data, noise covariance statistics, and coil sensitivity map information by taking the ratio between the $SNR^{cov-rSoS}$ and SENSE SNR maps.[6] We can write:

$$g_p = \sqrt{\left[\left(C^H \Psi^{-1} C\right)^{-1}\right]_{p,p} \left[\left(C^H \Psi^{-1} C\right)\right]_{p,p}}$$

where C is the coil sensitivity, C^H is the Hermitian transpose of C, and Ψ^{-1} is the inverse of the noise covariance matrix Ψ. Figure 2.1.7 shows a comparison of inverse g-factor maps ($1/g$) for 12-ch head, 4-ch neck and 32-ch head and spine coils. From these maps, it becomes clear that the 32-ch coil can be used with a higher acceleration factor without significant loss in SNR.

2.1.5.3 Stability

Diffusion-weighted (see Chapter 1.3A) or functional MRI (fMRI) (see Chapter 1.3B) protocols typically require EPI-based sequences. Yet, EPI sequences impose strong mechanical constraints on the system, due to the fact that encoding gradients are switching at a high rate during the readout of the nuclear magnetic resonance signal. These mechanical vibrations are transmitted from the gradients to the Rx coil via the patient table and can produce artifacts such as ghosting or intensity variations. These artifacts can be the result of poor soldering of some components of the coil or of vibration of cables. The amplitude of these coil-related artifacts varies in time; therefore, it can be a source of additional temporal variance in functional MRI (fMRI) experiments. Assessing the presence of these is therefore an important part of assessing the quality of coils.

Because these artifacts result from mechanical vibrations, one way to assess their presence is to run an EPI time series on an agar phantom. A typical procedure, performed for example at the MGH Martinos Center (Boston, MA, USA), is to use single-shot gradient echo EPI with the following parameters: FOV = 200 mm; repetition time/echo time (TR/TE) = 1000/30 ms; bandwidth = 2298 Hz/pixel; flip angle = 90°; matrix = 64 × 64; 16 slices of 5 mm each; and 500 measurements. Once data are acquired, the peak-to-peak variation in the signal intensity is averaged over a 15-pixel square region of interest positioned in the center of the phantom. Linear and quadratic trends need to be removed from the time series.[25]

2.1.5.4 Applications of Array Coils

A recently developed 32-ch coil[13] is compared with commercially available coils (Siemens Healthcare, Erlangen, Germany): a 12-ch head coil, 4-ch neck coil,

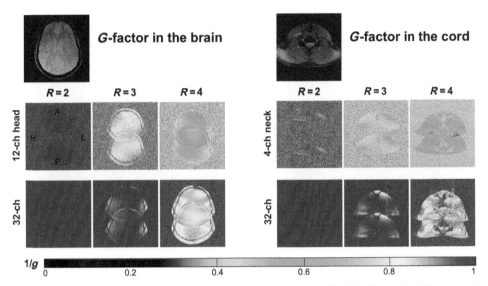

FIGURE 2.1.7 Maps of the inverse g-factor $(1/g)$ at various acceleration factors for the 12-ch head coil, the 4-ch neck coil, and a custom-made 32-ch head and spine coil.[13] Phase encoding was set to A-P. This figure suggests that 2× acceleration is feasible in the brain and spinal cord, with a relatively small hit in SNR for the 4-ch ($g \approx 1.05$), 12-ch ($g \approx 1$), and 32-ch ($g \approx 1$) coils. However, at an $R = 3$ acceleration factor, the 4-ch coil yields a g-factor of about 1.35 in the spinal cord (versus ~1.05 for the 32-ch coil); therefore, it is not advised for most applications (although still possible).

and 24-ch spine coil (only the most rostral three-element row was activated). Figure 2.1.8 shows results for diffusion tensor imaging (DTI) and fMRI.

A recently developed 64-ch head and neck coil demonstrated further improvements in SNR. Figure 2.1.9 shows an example of an anatomical T_1-weighted

MPRAGE acquired at 0.7 mm isotropic resolution in 4:43 min with $R = 3$ acceleration. A readout-segmented diffusion-weighted sequence demonstrated 2 mm isotropic resolution of the whole brain and cervical spinal cord, with successful DTI tractography without the need for distortion correction.

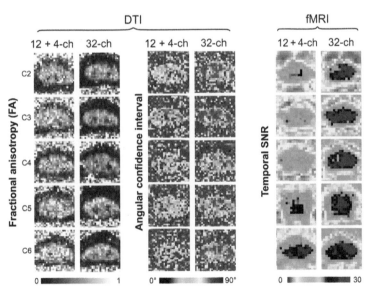

FIGURE 2.1.8 Comparison between a commercial 12 + 4-ch coil and a 32-ch head and spine coil. A DTI comparison shows fractional anisotropy (FA) and maps of 95% angular confidence computed with FSL BedpostX from diffusion-weighted images at 0.6×0.6 mm² in-plane spatial resolution. Overall, the 32-channel coil provides lower angular uncertainty in the cervical cord. Right panel: Temporal SNR (tSNR) comparison. Mean tSNR in the spinal cord was 13.9 for the standard coil and 24.7 for the 32-ch coil. For details on how to compute temporal SNR, see Chapter 4.1.

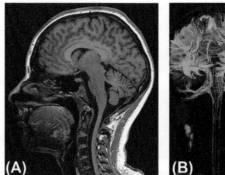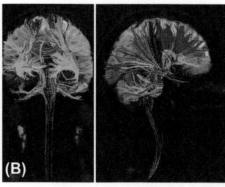

FIGURE 2.1.9   Application of a 64-ch head and spine coil[26] on a Skyra system (Siemens Healthcare). (A) T_1-weighted MPRAGE anatomical image (TR/TE/inversion time (TI): 1.9 s/2.5 ms/900 ms; matrix: 314×320; FOV: 250×250 mm^2; slice thickness: 0.7 mm; BW: 190 Hz/pixel; acceleration factor $= 3$; and acquisition time: 4:43 min). (B) Readout-segmented EPI[27] with the following parameters: five readout segments; TR/TE $= 9500/61$ ms; matrix: 96×128; resolution $= 2$ mm isotropic; number of slices $= 64$ with sagittal orientation; acceleration factor $= 2$; $b = 800$ s/mm^2; 20 diffusion-encoding directions; and BW $= 1100$ Hz/pixel. DW data were motion corrected (FSL FLIRT). No distortion correction was applied. Tractography was performed with TrackVis.

2.1.6 CONCLUSION

Since the introduction of phased-array coils by Roemer et al. in 1990, almost every clinical coil sold today is a phased-array coil. From the initial MRI systems with 4–8 Rx channels, most current clinical systems are now equipped with 16–32 channels, and some of the newest systems can go up to 128 channels. The trend for increasing the number of independent receivers in MR systems is driven by the benefits of highly parallelized Rx coil arrays, which provide a significant increase in sensitivity and acceleration capabilities. Similarly, increasing the number of Tx channels also has advantages for parallel transmission, which facilitates selective excitation and was shown to be appropriate for spinal cord imaging with reduced FOV. Currently, all main MRI scanner manufacturers offer a 32-ch coil for brain imaging as part of their standard product line. Unfortunately, this trend does not apply to the spine, for which the standard commercial coil still has very few elements per surface. However, although challenging to design, there are no fundamental limitations for having such a large amount of elements around the spine, as demonstrated by several groups. For example, a 64-ch head and spine coil showed at least $2\times$ more sensitivity in the spinal cord compared to the current commercial product.[14] One reason for spine arrays lagging behind brain and cardiac coils in terms of number of channels is probably due to the somewhat lower focus on spinal cord research. In fact, advanced quantitative techniques have only recently been applied to the spinal cord. In the future, it is desirable that vendors embrace this need, develop coil technology dedicated to the spine, and widely distribute array coils with higher detection and parallel imaging capabilities.

References

1. Roemer PB, Edelstein WA, Hayes CE, Souza SP, Mueller OM. The NMR phased array. *Magn Reson Med*. 1990;16(2):192–225.
2. Wright SM, Wald LL. Theory and application of array coils in MR spectroscopy. *NMR Biomed*. 1997;10(8):394–410.
3. Wiggins GC, Polimeni JR, Potthast A, Schmitt M, Alagappan V, Wald LL. 96-Channel receive-only head coil for 3 Tesla: design optimization and evaluation. *Magn Reson Med*. 2009;62(3):754–762.
4. Sodickson DK, Manning WJ. Simultaneous acquisition of spatial harmonics (SMASH): fast imaging with radiofrequency coil arrays. *Magn Reson Med*. 1997;38(4):591–603.
5. Griswold MA, Jakob PM, Heidemann RM, et al. Generalized autocalibrating partially parallel acquisitions (GRAPPA). *Magn Reson Med*. 2002;47(6):1202–1210.
6. Pruessmann KP, Weiger M, Scheidegger MB, Boesiger P. SENSE: sensitivity encoding for fast MRI. *Magn Reson Med*. 1999;42(5):952–962.
7. Larkman DJ, Nunes RG. Parallel magnetic resonance imaging. *Phys Med Biol*. 2007;52(7):R15–R55.
8. Vossen M, Teeuwisse W, Reijnierse M, Collins CM, Smith NB, Webb AG. A radiofrequency coil configuration for imaging the human vertebral column at 7T. *J Magn Reson*. 2011;208(2):291–297.
9. Bodurka J, Ledden P, Bandettini P. SENSE optimized sixteen element receive array for cervical spinal cord imaging at 3T. *Proceedings of the 16th Annual Meeting of ISMRM*. Toronto, Canada; 2008: 1078.
10. Matschl V, Reykowski A, Jahns K, Hergt M, Fischer H. 48 Channel body/spine matrix coils for 3 Tesla. *Proceedings of the 13th Annual Meeting of ISMRM*. Miami, USA; 2005: 952.
11. Peterson DM, Duensing GR, Caserta J, Fitzsimmons JR. An MR transceive phased array designed for spinal cord imaging at 3 Tesla: preliminary investigations of spinal cord imaging at 3 T. *Invest Radiol*. 2003;38(7):428–435.
12. Reykowski A, Hemmerlein M, Wolf S, Fischer H. 16 Channel head/neck matrix coils for 3 Tesla. *Proceedings of the 13th Annual Meeting of ISMRM*. Miami, USA; 2005: 908.
13. Cohen-Adad J, Mareyam A, Keil B, Polimeni JR, Wald LL. 32-Channel RF coil optimized for brain and cervical spinal cord at 3 T. *Magn Reson Med*. 2011;66(4):1198–1208.

14. Keil B, Biber S, Rehner R, et al. A 64-channel array coil for 3T head/neck/C-spine imaging. *Proceedings of the 20th Annual Meeting of ISMRM*. Melbourne, Australia; 2012: 1626.

15. Wu B, Wang C, Krug R, et al. *7T Human Spine Arrays with Adjustable Inductive Decoupling*. Honolulu. 2009 April, 2997.

16. Kraff O, Bitz AK, Kruszona S, et al. An eight-channel phased array RF coil for spine MR imaging at 7 T. *Invest Radiol*. 2009;44(11):734–740.

17. Sigmund EE, Suero GA, Hu C, et al. High-resolution human cervical spinal cord imaging at 7 T. *NMR Biomed*. 2012;25:891–899.

18. Zhao W, Cohen-Adad J, Polimeni JR, et al. 19-Channel Rx array coil and 4-channel Tx loop array for cervical spinal cord imaging at 7T MRI. *Proceedings of the 20th Annual Meeting of ISMRM*. Melbourne, Australia; 2012: 310.

19. Henning A, Koning W, Fuchs A, et al. 1H MRS in the human spinal cord at 7T using a combined RF shimming and travelling wave transmit approach. *Proceedings of the 21st Annual Meeting of ISMRM*. Salt Lake City, USA; 2013: 711.

20. Bottomley PA. Turning up the heat on MRI. *J Am Coll Radiol*. 2008; 5(7):853–855.

21. Constantinides CD, Atalar E, McVeigh ER. Signal-to-noise measurements in magnitude images from NMR phased arrays. *Magn Reson Med*. 1997;38(5):852–857.

22. Dietrich O, Raya JG, Reeder SB, Reiser MF, Schoenberg SO. Measurement of signal-to-noise ratios in MR images: influence of multichannel coils, parallel imaging, and reconstruction filters. *J Magn Reson Imaging*. 2007;26(2):375–385.

23. Kellman P, McVeigh ER. Image reconstruction in SNR units: a general method for SNR measurement. *Magn Reson Med*. 2005; 54(6):1439–1447.

24. Griswold MA, Blaimer M, Breuer F, Heidemann RM, Mueller M, Jakob PM. Parallel magnetic resonance imaging using the GRAPPA operator formalism. *Magn Reson Med*. 2005;54(6): 1553–1556.

25. Weisskoff RM. Simple measurement of scanner stability for functional NMR imaging of activation in the brain. *Magn Reson Med*. 1996;36(4):643–645.

26. Keil B, Cohen-Adad J, Porter DA, et al. Simultaneous diffusion-weighted MRI of brain and cervical spinal cord using a 64-channel head-neck array coil at 3T. *Proceedings of the 21st Annual Meeting of ISMRM*. Salt Lake City, USA; 2013: 1210.

27. Porter DA, Heidemann RM. High resolution diffusion-weighted imaging using readout-segmented echo-planar imaging, parallel imaging and a two-dimensional navigator-based reacquisition. *Magn Reson Med*. 2009;62(2):468–475.

B_0 Inhomogeneity and Shimming

Jürgen Finsterbusch

Department of Systems Neuroscience, University Medical Center Hamburg-Eppendorf,
Hamburg, Germany

In the context of magnetic resonance (MR) experiments, "shimming" describes the procedures performed to provide a sufficiently homogeneous field of the magnetic flux density within the sample or a selected subvolume of it. Since the advent of in vivo MR, shimming has always been an important issue for MR imaging (MRI) and MR spectroscopy (MRS). The generation of a homogeneous static magnetic field is technically challenging not only because of the larger magnet bore required, in particular for human whole-body MR systems, but also due to the different susceptibilities of air, bone, and tissues and their distribution within the body, which induce additional field inhomogeneities. These problems increase with the static magnetic field and are still prominent despite the progress achieved in shimming in the past.

More recently, the problem of inhomogeneous radiofrequency (RF) fields has risen in high static magnetic fields for which the wavelength can be comparable to the size of the body part investigated. As a consequence, standing wave effects can become relevant and yield an inhomogeneous flip angle in the object that can hamper acquisitions. The correction of such B_1 inhomogeneities, often referred to as "B_1 shimming", is an evolving field of research and, for instance, has driven the development of parallel transmission techniques. However, this topic is beyond the scope of this chapter, which will focus on shimming of the static magnetic flux density B_0 for applications in humans, in particular in the spinal cord.

So far, only a few studies have been presented that address shimming issues specifically for the human spinal cord. In particular, a detailed evaluation and comparison of the various shim approaches that have been developed and applied previously, such as for the human brain (see Ref. 1 for an overview), has not been performed. Therefore, this chapter will cover not only the standard shim methods that are routinely used for the spinal cord, but also other promising and emerging shim techniques that could provide a benefit for spinal cord applications even if they are currently not commonly available.

The background section (Section 2.2.1) addresses the origins of field inhomogeneities in vivo and the problems that they may cause, and underlines the importance of shimming for MRI and MRS. It is followed by Section 2.2.2 on the field inhomogeneities relevant in the human spinal cord. Then the principles of shimming are presented in detail, covering the required hardware in Section 2.2.3, static and dynamic shim approaches (Section 2.2.4), the measurement of the field distribution (Section 2.2.5), usually a prerequisite of shimming, and the basics of shim algorithms (Section 2.2.6) that aim to determine the optimum setup of the available shim hardware. The subsequent sections will deal with practical issues of shimming (Section 2.2.7) and specific problems and solutions for T_2^*- and diffusion-weighted acquisitions (Sections 2.2.8 and 2.2.9) and MRS (Section 2.2.10). Finally, a short summary is provided in Section 2.2.11.

2.2.1 BACKGROUND

- The MR frequency depends on the magnetic flux density (i.e., on the magnetic field strength and the magnetic susceptibility)
- Accurate spatial encoding and MRS peak identification require a homogeneous field of the flux density

- Field inhomogeneities
  - yield the wrong localization (e.g., geometric slice or image distortions)
  - broaden line widths in MRS and hamper the identification of metabolites
  - cause unwanted signal losses (e.g., in T_2^* weighting) or distort the diffusion weighting
- In human applications, field inhomogeneities usually are dominated by differences in magnetic susceptibility within and around the body
- B_0 shimming aims to minimize the field inhomogeneities in order to improve image and spectra quality and localization

The MR resonance frequency, the Larmor frequency, is proportional to the magnetic flux density. MRI and MRS rely on the assumption that, in the absence of pulsed field gradients, the Larmor frequency of all (magnetically equivalent) spins is virtually identical, independent of their position within the object, slice, or voxel. Only then is the assignment of the Larmor frequencies to specific chemical shifts or, in the presence of pulsed field gradients, to spatial coordinates in the gradient direction unambiguous, accurate, and correct. Any deviation from a perfectly homogeneous field of the flux density, such as an offset, a field gradient, or a more complex field variation, disturbs these assignments and can result in misassigned chemical shifts and a wrong localization.

Spatial encoding with pulsed field gradients is based on the linear increase of the field along the gradient direction.[2] Field inhomogeneities superimpose the field of the pulsed gradient, and the resulting field can be shifted, distorted, rotated, and bended. This can cause a misregistration of slice-selective RF excitations and of the acquired signal, yielding incorrect slice positions, orientations, and thicknesses and geometric distortions of the image (Figure 2.2.1). Slice shifts can also reduce the effective slice thickness, and, thus, the signal intensity in RF refocused acquisitions like spin-echo imaging is diminished if the induced shifts vary between the different RF excitations. These effects are not very pronounced for standard spin-echo and gradient-echo imaging; however, they could hamper quantitative measurements in regions with considerable field inhomogeneities (e.g., close to major air cavities and the body surface or implants and devices). Furthermore, quantitative diffusion-weighting experiments that are also based on pulsed field gradients can also be affected by field inhomogeneities (see Section 2.2.9).

Many fast-imaging techniques, like steady-state free precession (SSFP) or spiral imaging, are very sensitive

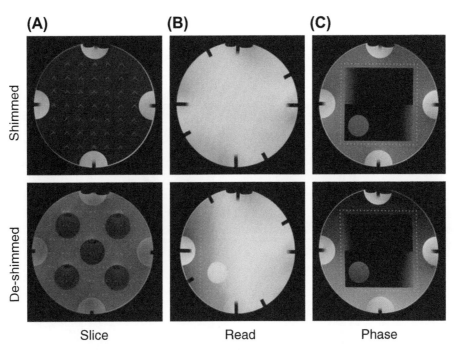

FIGURE 2.2.1 Examples for artifacts induced by field inhomogeneities in standard gradient-echo and spin echo imaging of a phantom. While the upper row shows images obtained with an optimum shim setup, the lower row was acquired with linear field gradients in (A) slice selection, (B) frequency-encoding (left-right), and (C) phase-encoding directions that were realized by an offset on the static shim current of the gradient coil. They yield (A) a shift of the slices, (B, C) a slice tilt around (B) a vertical and (C) a horizontal axis, (B) a compression in the left-right direction, and (C) a shearing in the image plane.

to field inhomogeneities and already exhibit severe image artifacts like banding artifacts and image blurring for moderate field variations. In particular, echo-planar imaging, which is often used for diffusion-weighted and functional neuroimaging, suffers from pronounced geometric distortions in the presence of typical field inhomogeneities, most notably in the phase-encoding direction (Figure 2.2.2).

Because field inhomogeneities broaden the frequency distribution of the spins, they can also cause significant intravoxel dephasing. While this effect vanishes in RF refocused (e.g., spin-echo) imaging, it can reduce the signal amplitude considerably in T_2^*-weighted acquisitions (see Section 2.2.8), as used for functional neuroimaging based on the blood oxygenation level–dependent (BOLD) contrast (Figure 2.2.3). The dephasing increases with the voxel size (Figure 2.2.3) and is usually most pronounced in the slice direction, mainly due to the larger voxel dimension often used in this direction.

In spectroscopy, field inhomogeneities broaden the line width, which reduces the peak amplitudes, distorts the line shape, and can shift the frequency of peaks (Figure 2.2.4). These effects hinder the reliable detection

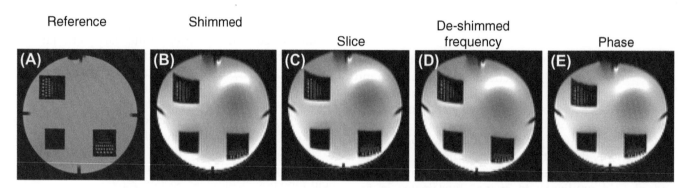

FIGURE 2.2.2 (A) Reference image and (B–E) examples of artifacts induced by field inhomogeneities in spin echo echo-planar imaging of a phantom. The inhomogeneities were linear field gradients that were realized by an offset on the static shim current of the gradient coil in (C) slice-selection, (D) frequency-encoding (left-right), and (E) phase-encoding directions and cause (C) a slight shift of the image in the phase-encoding direction (up-down), (D) a shearing in the image plane, and (E) a compression in the phase-encoding direction. If the shim current offsets and, thus, the linear field inhomogeneities are inverted, the image shift and the shearing occur in opposite directions, while the compression converts to a stretching. It should be emphasized that the field gradients used here were by a factor of 25 lower than those used in Figure 2.2.1. Also note that (B) represents an image that is acquired without additional field inhomogeneities (i.e., an optimized standard shim setup) and also exhibits pronounced geometric distortions.

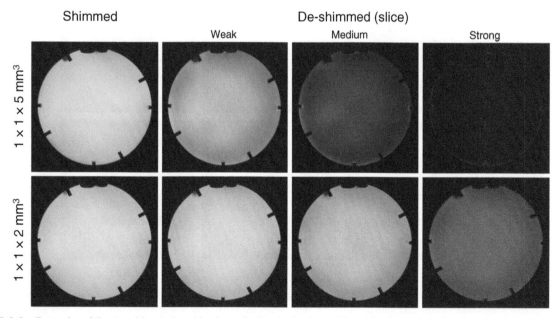

FIGURE 2.2.3 Examples of the signal loss induced by through-slice dephasing in T_2^*-weighted imaging of a phantom with a slice thickness of 5 mm (upper) and 2 mm (lower). A linear field gradient was applied in the slice direction that increases from left to right. The signal loss is much higher for the thicker sections.

(A) Shimmed

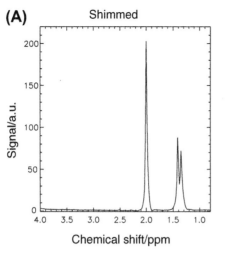

(B) De-shimmed

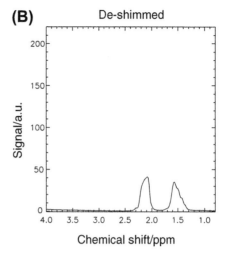

FIGURE 2.2.4 Examples of the artifacts in MRS in the presence of field inhomogeneities (a linear field gradient in one direction) in a phantom. Compared to (A) a spectrum acquired with an optimized shim setup, (B) the spectrum with field inhomogeneities exhibits a shift of the peaks, a broadening of the line width, distortions of the line shape, and reduced peak amplitude. These effects severely hamper the reliable detection and quantification of metabolites.

and unambiguous identification of metabolite-specific peaks, couplings, and patterns (Figure 2.2.4), and they hamper the quantification of metabolite concentrations (see Section 2.2.10). Furthermore, chemical-shift selective excitation or acquisition schemes (e.g., water suppression, fat saturation, or spectral editing) can be disturbed considerably, which may also affect imaging experiments.

Thus, a sufficiently homogeneous field of the magnetic flux density is crucial for MRI and MRS, and the efforts undertaken to shim the field (i.e., to optimize its homogeneity) are an important part of the adjustment procedure prior to the acquisition (see Section 2.2.7) that can improve the image and spectrum quality significantly (see Figures 2.2.1–2.2.4).

The static magnetic flux density effectively reflects the combined effect of (1) the magnetic field generated by electric currents (e.g., in the magnet), and (2) the magnetization generated in matter that is exposed to this field (e.g., objects in the magnet bore). The magnetization increases with the field strength and is proportional to the magnetic susceptibility that differs significantly between air, for example around the body and in air-filled cavities like the lung, bones, and biological tissues (Table 2.2.1). Thus, the actual field distribution is not solely defined by the design of the magnet and the adjustment of the magnetic field (e.g., by using the shim coils) but also significantly influenced by the distribution of the magnetic susceptibilities within the bore, i.e., the objects and body in it.

Nowadays, the field homogeneity that can be achieved within the empty bore of the magnet over a typical measurement volume is very high, even for whole-body MR systems. For instance, the relative

TABLE 2.2.1 Magnetic Volume Susceptibilities of Different Materials Relevant In vivo and for Passive Shims

Material	$(\chi - 1)/10^{-6}$ (cm.g.s)
Air	0.03
Bone	−0.9
Water	−0.72
Tissue	−0.73
Bismuth	−13.2
Niobium	237
Zirconium	108
Pyrolytic graphite	−450[1]
	−85[1]

[1] *Perpendicular and parallel to graphite basal plane, respectively.[3]*

peak-to-peak variation (i.e., the relative difference between the maximum and the minimum fields) within a sphere with a diameter of 20 cm is typically about or below 0.03 parts per million (ppm) in state-of-the-art 3 T systems, which corresponds to field deviations of less than ±0.05 µT.

Because the differences between the magnetic susceptibilities of air or bones and tissue (see Table 2.2.1) are an order of magnitude larger (a few tenths ppm), the body is usually a significant source of field inhomogeneities in vivo. Thus, the field in vivo strongly depends on the geometry and orientation of the body part investigated and the distribution of the magnetic susceptibilities within it, which differs considerably between the different body parts and, to some extent, also between individuals, and can vary during the experiment (e.g., due to respiration). The related field deviations can therefore not be considered in the general setup (e.g., in the design of the magnet) but need to be addressed specifically for each examination and individual with a shim adjustment that, in the presence of motion, ideally is updated during the experiment.

2.2.2 FIELD INHOMOGENEITIES IN THE HUMAN SPINAL CORD

Field inhomogeneities in the human spinal cord:

- are mainly caused by the different magnetic susceptibilities of the vertebrae, tissue, vertebral disks, and air (e.g., in the lung)
- can hamper acquisitions of the spinal cord in vivo considerably
- are hard to compensate with the standard shim hardware of whole-body MR systems

Field inhomogeneities often hamper MR acquisitions of the human spinal cord, in particular T_2^*- and diffusion-weighted imaging and MRS. A minor reason for this is the length of the spinal cord, which could require imaging fields of view as large as 400 mm or beyond in the head–feet direction. The homogeneity of the magnetic field in the empty bore for such a large field of view is typically about 4 ppm on standard 3 T MR systems, which already can cause problems in acquisitions sensitive to field inhomogeneities (see Figure 2.2.2). However, more important is the vicinity of the spinal cord to bones, in particular the vertebrae, and air-filled

cavities, notably the lung. The magnetic susceptibilities of bone and, in particular, air differ considerably from those of tissue (see Table 2.2.1) and the vertebral disks, yielding significant field variations in the human spinal cord.

In all spinal cord sections, the alternation of vertebrae and vertebral disks along the spinal cord is a relevant problem. It effectively causes a periodic modulation of the field in the head–feet direction (Figure 2.2.5).[4] Such a modulation within about one or a few centimeters is hard to correct for with standard shim coils (see Section 2.2.3). For about one cycle, i.e., for a few axial slices or within tiny fields of view in the head–feet direction, the shim results achievable may be quite reasonable (see Section 2.2.7). But within a larger dimension, i.e., for typical slice stacks used in functional neuroimaging or for MRS voxels, significant inhomogeneities will remain. For axial acquisitions, the slice positions could be chosen to match either the sections within relatively homogeneous fields (i.e., midvertebrae positions) or positions that have very similar field inhomogeneities (Figure 2.2.5), which is easier to correct for with the standard shim methods. However, for many applications, this is not an option.

In the lower cervical and upper thoracic section of the spinal cord, significant field variations are caused by the lung (Figure 2.2.5). These inhomogeneities occur on a larger scale and, thus, are easier to address with the standard shim coils (see Section 2.2.3), but they are also more variable and much larger in amplitude. Some reduction of these inhomogeneities can be achieved with standard shim methods, but there is still much room for improvements (Figure 2.2.5), inter alia, because the inhomogeneities within the spinal cord depend on the current air volume in the lung (i.e., the respiration state),[88] and

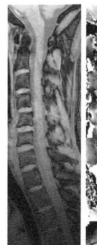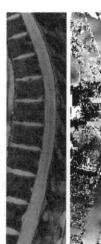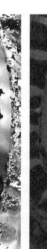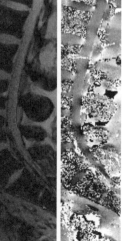

FIGURE 2.2.5 Anatomical reference images and field maps of the cervical, thoracic, and lumbar parts of the spinal cord. The field maps were acquired with a two-echo FLASH sequence and represent the phase difference of the echoes (see Section 2.2.5) without phase unwrapping. The periodic modulation caused by the different susceptibilities of vertebrae and vertebral disks and tissue are visible throughout the cord. Note that the field maps are not corrected for the phase wrap-around (see Section 2.2.5), i.e., black and white in neighboring pixels are likely to reflect very similar fields.

motion of the spinal cord may be relevant (e.g., due to respiration).

Thus, the standard shim methods available on common whole-body MR systems provide only a limited correction of the field inhomogeneities in the spinal cord. For the most affected applications, like BOLD-based functional neuroimaging and MRS, this correction is often not sufficient to obtain reasonable image or spectra quality. But more elaborated techniques, such as a dynamic shim update (see Section 2.2.4) or z-shimming (see Section 2.2.8), could yield a significant improvement.

2.2.3 SHIM HARDWARE

- Shim coils:
  - shim coils generate an additional magnetic field driven by electric currents
  - each coil provides a unique, smooth field shape
  - the electric currents (i.e., the field strength) can be adapted rapidly
  - at least three linear and usually five second-order coils are available around the bore
  - additional, local shim coils have been shown to be beneficial
- Passive shims (dia-, para-, or ferromagnetic materials):
  - only distort the existing magnetic field
  - are located at dedicated positions, preferably close to the target volume
  - can correct for more complex (arbitrarily shaped) field variations
  - their adjustment can be quite time consuming

Hardware used for shimming can be divided into two categories. Shim coils driven by an electric current generate an additional magnetic field ("active shim"; see Section 2.2.3.1) that superimposes the existing magnetic field (e.g., generated by the magnet). Ferromagnetic, paramagnetic, or diamagnetic materials that are placed in the bore of the magnet ("passive shims"; see Section 2.2.3.2) distort the field of the magnetic flux density. Both approaches aim to provide a more homogeneous field in a volume of interest (e.g., around the magnet isocenter or a target volume within the body). However, they differ regarding their flexibility and ability to correct field inhomogeneities. Standard shim coils are somehow limited regarding the field variations that can be compensated, but they can be adjusted flexibly, with an optimized setup being chosen on an acquisition-by-acquisition or even on a slice-by-slice

basis (see Section 2.2.4). Current passive shim devices are less flexible because their adjustment can be quite time consuming (see Section 2.2.4), but they are able to correct more complex field variations.

2.2.3.1 Shim Coils (Active Shim)

Different solutions for shim coils that generate additional magnetic fields have been considered. Commonly available is a set of a few shim coils around the bore, with each of them generating a specific field "pattern". Adjusting the currents of these shim coils appropriately, a reasonable compensation of typical field inhomogeneities can be attained. However, the homogeneity achievable in specific target volumes may be insufficient for some applications. This is why dedicated shim coils have been proposed that are designed to compensate the specific inhomogeneities that typically remain within the target volume. These coils are much smaller and are positioned close to the target ("local shim coils").[5,6] Recently, a promising, more general approach has been presented that involves a fixed array of local coils within the bore around the object.[7,8] It is able to generate complex field variations, like dedicated local coils, but is more flexible, like the standard shim coils, as it is not constrained to a specific target region.

To describe an arbitrary field distribution mathematically, it can be decomposed into a set of basic functions. For the magnetic flux density, a suitable set is based on the so-called spherical harmonics.[9] The individual terms of the decomposition describe unique spatial variations of the field that differ by (1) the power (order) in which the radial coordinate (i.e., the distance from the isocenter) appears in the expressions, and (2) the angular variation. The zeroth-order term corresponds to a homogeneous field, the three first-order terms are linear field variations in three orthogonal directions, and the five second-order terms represent components with a quadratic field variation and more complex angular dependencies (see Figure 2.2.6). Accordingly, any linear or higher-order term appearing in the decomposition describes a deviation from the desired homogeneous field and should be compensated. The linear terms can be corrected easily by the gradient coils using an appropriate constant current offset. But second- and higher-order terms require dedicated shim coils that are designed to provide the desired field distribution (Figure 2.2.6).

Whole-body MR systems with lower field strength (1.5 T) often do not have specific shim coils and are limited to first-order shims. At higher field strength ($\geq$3 T), second-order shim coils are standard in most MR systems (see Figure 2.2.6), and at 7 T or beyond at

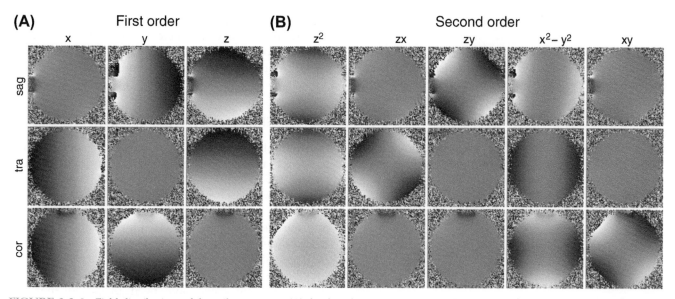

FIGURE 2.2.6 Field distributions of the coils generating (A) the three linear terms (realized by the gradient coils) and (B) the five second-order terms generated by dedicated room-temperature shim coils acquired in a homogeneous, spherical water phantom in three orthogonal planes. Note that the bottleneck of the phantom causes some minor distortions of the field distribution. The field maps represent the phase difference observed in a two-echo FLASH sequence (see Section 2.2.5).

least some third-order coils and sometimes even a few fourth-order coils are available. These coils are usually integrated in the gradient coil unit but have their own power supply. Some vendors also provide superconducting shim coils within the cryostate that are adjusted during the installation of the MR system to optimize the field homogeneity in the empty bore for the specific MR environment ("tune-up shim"). These coils are usually termed "cryo shims", while the standard shim coils are often referred to as "room-temperature shims".

Even with higher-order shim coils, the complex field variations that can be present in a target volume cannot be compensated completely. One option to overcome this limitation is the usage of local shim coils.[5,6] For instance, small coils within the oral cavity can reduce signal losses in T_2^*-weighted functional neuroimaging of the orbitofrontal cortex.[5] For optimum results, local shim coils should be designed to meet the specific needs of the target region. However, with a few coils of different designs that can be positioned and adjusted independently, a quite good compensation can be achieved as has been demonstrated for the human brain.[6] This solution could be adapted for spinal cord applications to reduce larger-scale inhomogeneities (e.g., as caused by the lung).

A promising extension involves a fixed array of small coils that can be controlled independently.[7,8] A setup of 24 coils around the mouse head has been successfully tested on an animal MR system and has been shown to be able to generate a variety of field variations, including third-order terms.[8] Interestingly, it can also provide linear field gradients along any direction, which could

be used to perform the spatial encoding rather than using a dedicated gradient coil. Recently, a first setup for the human head consisting of 48 coils has been developed and has been shown to improve shimming of the human brain at 7 T compared to the standard shim setup involving third-order shim coils.[7] Thus, it seems to be very promising to apply this concept to the human spinal cord because it could also be able to address some of the periodic field variations caused by the vertebrae. However, an issue that needs to be considered is RF coupling of the local shim coils that may distort and reduce the RF field.[6,7]

2.2.3.2 Passive Shim

For passive shimming, ferromagnetic, paramagnetic, or diamagnetic materials are positioned in the bore of the magnet in order improve the field homogeneity in a target region. The simplest realization is to reduce or remove the susceptibility differences that cause the field inhomogeneities, in particular by replacing air in or around the body by a material with a magnetic susceptibility close or equal to that of tissue, such as water[10] (Figure 2.2.7(A)) or a foam of pyrolytic graphite (volume fraction 5%).[11] Regarding the spinal cord, this approach could be applied to reduce effects occurring at the body's surface, but it may interfere with the need to position surface coils as close as possible to the target volume to maximize the signal-to-noise ratio. Furthermore, it is unable to address the usually more pronounced susceptibility differences caused by bones and the air-filled lung.

(A) Passive shimming

Without   With

(B) Static shim adjustment

Tune-up   Adjusted

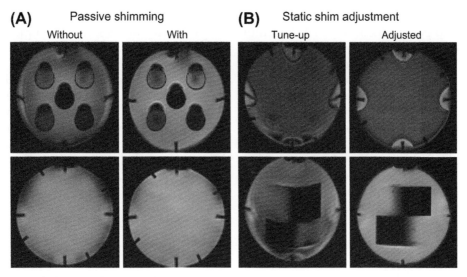

FIGURE 2.2.7 (A) Example for a simple passive-shimming approach in a water phantom acquired with T_2^*-weighted echo-planar imaging. Two different slices close to the bottom of the phantom (top) and about 30 mm apart from the bottom (bottom) are shown, with the phantom alone in the bore where the bottom represents an air–phantom boundary with a considerably difference of magnetic susceptibilities (left), and with a second water phantom attached to the bottom of the first such that no significant difference of magnetic susceptibilities is present (right). The latter setup reduces signal losses and geometric distortions significantly. (B) Examples for the improvements in T_2^*-weighted echo-planar imaging achievable with a static shim involving first- and second-order room-temperature shims. Without an adjustment of the static shim (left), severe geometric distortions and pronounced signal losses occur. These artifacts are considerably ameliorated after an adjustment of the static shim (right).

In a more elaborated approach, dedicated amounts of a shim material with a magnetic susceptibility that differs from that of tissue (see Table 2.2.1) are positioned at different locations (see also Section 2.2.6) within the magnet bore or close to the target volume. To optimize the field homogeneity, the locations and quantities of the material must be carefully chosen (e.g., Refs 12,13) and depend on the susceptibility of the material (see also Section 2.2.6). Due to the variety of locations that are usually available, more complex field corrections can be realized than with standard shim coils (e.g., Ref. 14). To minimize the amount of shim material, only those higher-order field variations are usually corrected for which no room-temperature shim coils are available.

The type of feasible shim materials depends on the specific geometry and application. As a rule of thumb, the larger the distance to the target region is, the higher should be the difference of the material's and the tissue's susceptibilities (see Table 2.2.1). For instance, some vendors use passive shimming materials located around the tunnel to improve the field homogeneity of the empty bore for the specific MR environment as part of the "tune-up shim" during the installation or after major hardware upgrades. In this case, ferromagnetic materials (iron, nickel, cobalt, or alloys of them) are used to attain a significant field distortion in the isocenter ("iron shim").

Several passive shim approaches have been presented that can be adapted to the specific target region investigated. In one variant, ferromagnetic materials have been used to shim the visual cortex of macaque brains.[15] Such materials provide a high efficiency in distorting the field due to their excessive susceptibility and, thus, can provide significant corrections even deeper in the body. But attention must be paid to the considerable force and torque that may act on ferromagnetic materials within the static field. Thus, for adjusting the shim (i.e., the locations of the materials) in humans, either the subject or the shim device may have to be removed from the bore after the measurement of the field distribution for safety reasons. This would require time and a good reproducibility of the subject's or the device's position. However, this approach could provide a good solution to correct typical inhomogeneity patterns that are observed for a target volume independent of the subject. Thus, a fixed passive shim can be set up prior to the examination and used for different subjects.

For an individual, subject- or target-specific shim adjustment, high-susceptibility para- and diamagnetic materials, like graphite, bismuth, niobium, and zirconium (see Table 2.2.1), seem to be more feasible.[3,13,14] They do not create safety issues, but their susceptibility is large enough to cause significant distortions even deeper in the body (e.g., in the human brain), if they are located close to the object. Thus, a subject- or even target-specific shim can easily be realized as has been demonstrated in animals[14] and in the human brain, for example to reduce inhomogeneities in the orbitofrontal and temporal lobes by shim material located in the mouth[3,16] or close to the forehead and ears.[1,13,17] The usage of both dia- and paramagnetic materials (bismuth and zirconium) has been shown to yield better results and outperforms third-order room-temperature shims in the mouse brain at 9.4 T.[14] An adaptation of such approaches to spinal cord applications could be very promising. As long as electrically conducting materials are used, their compatibility with the MR acquisitions must be ensured, for example regarding distortions of the RF field and the induction of eddy currents that could give rise to artifacts and could heat up the material and affect its magnetic susceptibility (i.e., the field correction).

2.2.4 TUNE-UP, STATIC, AND DYNAMIC SHIM

- Tune-up shim:
  - is based on a passive iron shim or cryo shim coils
  - is optimized for the empty bore or a phantom and performed by the manufacturer
- Static shim:
  - involves the adjustment of currents in shim coils and of passive shims
  - is performed for the examination or prior to each measurement
  - is optimized for a specific target volume
- Dynamic shim update:
  - optimized settings are used for each part of the measurement part (e.g., each slice)
  - it is not commonly available on whole-body MR systems; practically limited to shim coils

Several levels of shimming are usually applied to optimize the field homogeneity in the target region. During the installation of an MR system and after major hardware upgrades, the homogeneity of the magnetic field in the empty bore is optimized for the specific MR environment ("tune-up shim"). The setup of the corresponding shim components, the cryo shim coils and the iron shim (see Section 2.2.3), then remains fixed and cannot be adapted by the user. It therefore will not be considered here. The more flexible shim components like the room-temperature shim coils (see Section 2.2.3) can be adapted to correct the field distortions in the body part to investigate that, for example, are induced by the different magnetic susceptibilities of air, bones, and tissue. Usually, this setup is performed specifically for the chosen target volume and is fixed during the acquisition ("static shim"; Section 2.2.4.1), but dynamic

approaches that aim to provide an optimized setup for different subvolumes, for example by updating the shim settings on a slice-by-slice basis, have also been presented ("dynamic shim update"; Section 2.2.4.2). Furthermore, (dynamic) pulse sequence modifications have been used to ameliorate the effects of field inhomogeneities, particularly in T_2^*-weighted acquisitions. Strictly speaking, such techniques should not be considered as "shim" methods because they do not improve the field homogeneity but only aim to compensate the side effects that they have on the signal. Nevertheless, due to their relevance for spinal cord applications, they will be considered in the context of the applications for which they are useful (see Sections 2.2.8 and 2.2.9).

2.2.4.1 Static Shim

The field inhomogeneities in vivo depend on the body's geometry and orientation in the bore and the distribution of bones and air within the body. Thus, a flexible correction of the actual inhomogeneities in the target volume, for example as determined from a field map (see Section 2.2.5), on an acquisition-by-acquisition basis is important.

On standard MR systems, this is realized using the gradient coil (first-order terms) and, if available, the room-temperature shim coils (second- and higher-order terms; see Section 2.2.3.1), but approaches with passive shims have also been proposed (see Section 2.2.3.2). While the room-temperature shim coils are independent of the hardware involved in the MR acquisitions, the gradient coil is also used for the spatial encoding. Thus, the static current offset applied to the gradient coil for shimming may reduce the maximum current available for pulsed gradients on the different axes (i.e., the specified gradient strength usually is not fully usable for pulsed gradients).

With the room-temperature shim coils, a relevant improvement of the field homogeneity can usually be achieved (see Figures 2.2.7(B) and 2.2.9), but higher-order field variations cannot be corrected appropriately. Thus, static, passive shim approaches (see Section 2.2.3.2) have been presented to improve the field homogeneity within the target region. They are suitable for correcting more complex field variations, but their feasibility to improve the homogeneity in the human spinal cord so far has not been demonstrated. Another option is local shim coils or coil arrays (see Section 2.2.3.1), that is, dedicated coils located within the bore close to the target region. So far, such devices are not commonly available but with an appropriately modified geometry could be quite helpful for spinal cord applications.

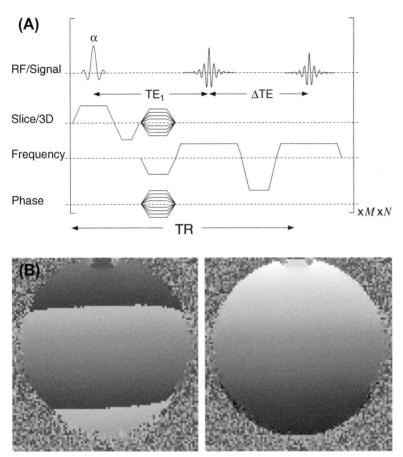

FIGURE 2.2.8 (A) Basic pulse sequence for 3D FLASH imaging with two echoes that could be used for field mapping. (B) Example for phase unwrapping in a water phantom with a linear field gradient (up-down). Due to the large range of field strength in the phantom, the phase wraps around (left), which can be corrected with an unwrapping algorithm (right).

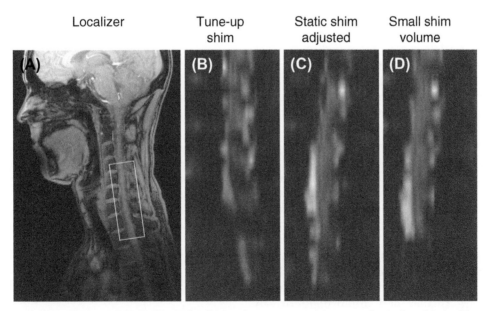

FIGURE 2.2.9 (A) Localizer image; and (B–D) T_2^*-weighted echo-planar images of the cervical spinal cord in healthy volunteers acquired with (B) the tune-up shim (i.e., without a dedicated shim adjustment), (C) an adjustment of the static shim involving first- and second-order room-temperature shims, and (D) a smaller adjustment volume focusing on the upper and central parts of the cord.

2.2.4.2 Dynamic Shim Update

On standard MR systems, the shim currents of the gradient coil and the room-temperature shim coils are adjusted prior to each measurement but are fixed during an acquisition. This means that shim settings should be used that provide a reasonable homogeneity for all parts of the target volume during the experiment. But often, for instance in multislice imaging, only a part of the target volume is covered within a certain period of the acquisition, and a better homogeneity for it could be achieved if a dedicated shim setup could be used. Furthermore, the optimal shim setup may vary during the experiment (e.g., due to respiration or motion). Thus, a dynamic update of the shim settings during the acquisitions would be an attractive option.

Experiments with a dynamic shim update have demonstrated the significant improvement of the field homogeneity that can be obtained in the animal[18] and the human brain,[7,19–25] even if only linear shim terms are considered[19,20,24] but also if standard higher-order terms[18,21–23,25] and shim coil arrays[7] are involved. This holds for imaging and spectroscopy experiments with a temporally constant shim setup for the individual slices or voxels[7,19,20,22–25] and also a shim adapted to the respiratory state that has been shown to reduce signal phase variations in the human brain considerably.[21] While most of these experiments were conducted with home-built hardware, such an update is, in principle, possible on standard whole-body MR systems, at least for the linear terms[24] that are realized by the gradient coil, which is designed and constructed to be switched very rapidly and reliably. However, system access to modify the corresponding current offsets on the fly is often not supported or easy to realize. This also holds for the higher-order coils available on standard MR systems. But their dynamic update is also hampered by the fact that these coils, so far, are not built or intended for rapid current changes; in other words, the hardware may not be feasible to update the currents within the required time of a few milliseconds. Furthermore, significant current changes could cause eddy currents[22,26] that may only decay slowly and can affect the image quality. This means that an eddy current compensation as realized for the gradient coil (e.g., with the so-called preemphasis) may be essential,[18,22,26] in particular as most standard shim coils are unshielded. But there is hope that the severe artifacts that field inhomogeneities can cause at higher static fields trigger the development of a fully dynamic shim update for standard MR systems.

The rapid current update of local shim coils and coil arrays (see Section 2.2.3.1) seems to be easier to realize. First, the coils are smaller and are usually driven by lower voltages and currents. Second, eddy current problems are less relevant because the coils are far away from the cryostate, the major source of eddy currents.

Regarding the human spinal cord, the dynamic shim update is a quite promising technique that can help to overcome substantial limitations of the static shim. For instance, most of the inhomogeneities that are relevant within a single or a few axial slices can be corrected quite well with the room-temperature shim coils that are available on standard MR systems. Only the need to use the same shim setup for the full stack of slices provides a setup that is far from being optimal for most of the slices. Thus, a dynamic update on a slice-by-slice basis could provide a considerable improvement. However, other measurements, e.g., three-dimensional (3D) acquisitions or sagittal acquisitions, could not benefit from a dynamic shim update, because the field variations within each slab or slice are still considerable.

All of the passive shim devices presented so far were static, i.e., the locations of the shim materials were fixed during a measurement. In principle, a dynamic adjustment of the locations during the acquisition should be possible, in particular when using para- or diamagnetic materials (e.g., to provide the best setup for the current slice or consider subject or organ motion). Such a rapid update can be expected to be technically challenging. However, a rapid update is also not as important as for shim coils because passive shims can correct higher-order field variations. Thus, a static setup can already provide a very good solution for the full target volume.

2.2.5 MEASUREMENT OF THE FIELD DISTRIBUTION

Field mapping

- Measurement of the field distribution:
  - is usually based on the phase difference of T_2^*-weighted signals at two different echo times
  - is then sensitive to the ambiguity of the phase (phase wrap-around)
  - the echo times must be chosen to avoid excessive wrap-arounds while providing a sufficient sensitivity
- Localization and pulse sequences:
  - mostly a full 3D data set is acquired, usually with a rapid gradient-echo imaging sequence
  - faster approaches use only a few columnar projection measurements ("MAP shims")

To optimize the field homogeneity, a map of the current field distribution ("field map")[27–30] within the body or the defined target region must be determined. Because the Larmor frequency of the spins depends on the field strength, MRI or MRS can be used to measure such a field map, which does not require extra hardware. But MR acquisitions are prone to artifacts in the presence of field inhomogeneities (see Section 2.2.1) and other experimental imperfections like eddy currents (see Section 2.2.5.3). Such artifacts can yield a distorted field, which must be kept in mind when evaluating field maps (see Section 2.2.7).

In this section, the techniques used to acquire field maps are considered. It will cover the methods used to determine the Larmor frequency (i.e., the field strength) (Section 2.2.5.1), its spatial distribution (Section 2.2.5.2), and the pulse sequences and related artifacts (Section 2.2.5.3). But it should be noted that shimming can also be obtained without a field map but solely based on the signal within the target volume (see Section 2.2.6.1). This option is of particular importance for single-voxel MRS but could also help to improve MRI of small target volumes (see Section 2.2.7).

2.2.5.1 Access to Frequency Information

A reliable but also time-consuming method to determine the spatial distribution of the Larmor frequency is to perform spectroscopic imaging.[27,28,31,32] For each voxel, an MR spectrum is obtained from which the water frequency and, thus, the local field strength can be determined. However, even with fast spectroscopic-imaging techniques, such a field map could take several minutes (e.g., Ref. 33), which often is considered too long for routine usage. Therefore, a much simpler approach was proposed that is based on the phase of a T_2^*-weighted spin echo signal.[30] It deviates from the phase expected for a purely T_2-weighted echo and reflects the field strength. However, this method relies on a perfect and homogeneous RF phase, which is hard to achieve in practice.

Thus, the phase difference method is commonly used where two or more echoes are acquired that exhibit different T_2^* weightings (i.e., echo times) (see Figures 2.2.5, 2.2.6, and 2.2.8(A)).[29] If the field is perfectly homogeneous, all echoes will, ideally, have the same phase. In voxels with a field offset, the corresponding frequency shift introduces a phase difference between the different echoes from which this offset can be estimated. The phase difference and, thus, the sensitivity increase with the echo time difference.

A problem of this approach is the ambiguity of the phase and the wrap-around (or aliasing) that may occur for large echo time differences or pronounced field variations (Figure 2.2.8(B)). With "unwrapping" algorithms,[34-38] the impact of such phase wrapping

can be minimized (see Figure 2.2.8(B)). Such algorithms are based on the assumption that the field variation occurs spatially smooth—that is, that the phase difference shows only minor variations (i.e., no wrapping) within the neighborhood of a voxel that can be met with a sufficiently high spatial resolution and moderate echo time differences. To combine both a high sensitivity (large echo time difference) and a reliable unwrapping (small echo time difference), a range of different echo times can be used. However, in practice, only a few different echo times are usually used, and most standard field-mapping procedures rely on just two echoes (see Figures 2.2.5 and 2.2.6).

A further limitation of the method is that other causes of frequency shifts and phase difference could mimic or mask field inhomogeneities, namely, noise, motion, eddy currents (see Section 2.2.5.3), and chemical shifts. The latter is relevant in vivo because the lipid signal can be significant. Water-selective excitations or fat saturation could be used to eliminate the lipid signal (e.g., Ref. 39), but for this purpose a sufficient field homogeneity is required. Another solution is to use only echo times with a fixed phase relationship of water and lipids.[40] Although the required minimum echo time difference limits the sensitivity, it still seems to be sufficient for typical applications in vivo.[40]

2.2.5.2 Spatial Information

A 3D field map provides the full information about the field distribution. It can depict arbitrary field variations in any target volume and can also be used for more elaborated shim approaches, such as involving local shim coils and passive shims or for a dynamic shim update. Minimum acquisition times are achieved with rapid gradient-echo pulse sequences like FLASH (fast low-angle shot) (see Figure 2.2.8(A); e.g., Refs 39–41) but may last about half a minute or even more. Thus, alternative solutions have been proposed.

They are based on the finding that to determine the field variations that can be corrected with the available shim coils, the full 3D field map is not required but only a minor subset of it, usually a few columnar volumes.[42,43] For instance, to determine the optimum shim settings for a field variation consisting of first- and second-order terms only, only the field distribution along six columnar volumes is needed.[42,43] The most prominent approach is the FASTMAP (fast automatic shimming technique by mapping along projections) technique[42,43] and its enhancements.[44,45] Some extensions that are further optimized, for example for (multiple) thin sections, have also been presented[18,46,47] and, for instance, could be used to provide slice-specific settings for a dynamic shim update (see Section 2.2.4.2).

The localization of the columnar volumes usually is performed with cross-sectional RF excitations (see Section 2.2.5.3).

These approaches are very elegant, but they have two major drawbacks. First, they rely on the assumption that the field variations are not too complex.[47] In cases where higher-order field variations are present, more columns must be acquired to obtain the optimum shim setup,[46] even if these higher-order terms cannot be addressed with the available shim hardware, which increases the acquisition time. Second, a reacquisition of the columns is required if the target volume is changed. This is why full 3D field maps are commonly used for human applications despite their prolonged acquisition time.

2.2.5.3 Pulse Sequences and Artifacts

An important issue is the pulse sequence used for field mapping and its vulnerability to artifacts, in particular eddy currents that can induce (additional) phase shifts that effectively distort the field information. If multiple shots are used for the different echo times, an identical gradient timing relative to the echo could be used, for example by using a nonselective RF pulse for the initial excitation.[42] But commonly, the different echo times are acquired within the same acquisition[41,44] to avoid shot-by-shot phase variations occurring, for instance due to motion. This approach increases the sensitivity to eddy currents and gradient imperfections because more gradient pulses precede the later echo(es) compared to the earlier one(s) (see Figure 2.2.8(A)). Their impact can be reduced by averaging two acquisitions with opposite gradient polarities and using nonequidistant echo times.[48] While an inhomogeneity-related phase effect increases linearly with the echo time, artifacts can be expected to depend mainly on the echo number (e.g. those caused by accumulated gradient imperfections). Thus, for nonequidistant echo times, a fixed phase increment from echo to echo unmasks artifacts.[48]

Regarding the underlying pulse sequence, the most popular is a (multiecho) rapid gradient-echo (FLASH) sequence (e.g., Refs 39–41) (Figure 2.2.8(A); see also Figures 2.2.5 and 2.2.6), in either its two-dimensional or 3D variant. It combines reasonable acquisition times (typically below 1 min for a 3D field map) with high signal efficiency and an overall low sensitivity to imaging artifacts. Faster pulse sequences like echo-planar and spiral imaging have also been proposed (e.g., Refs 49,50) in order to speed up the acquisition, but they suffer from their high sensitivity to imaging artifacts like blurring or geometric distortions in the presence of field inhomogeneities, and are not widely used. However, they can monitor changes of the field inhomogeneity (e.g., due to motion) during an acquisition to apply an appropriate dynamic shim update, as has been demonstrated for MRS in the human brain.[51]

To acquire the columnar volumes required for FAST-MAP and its variants, cross-sectional RF excitations can be used.[42,44] Most commonly, three excitations are used to generate a stimulated echo,[42,44] which, for example, can also be extended to rapid mapping in multiple slices.[18]

2.2.6 SHIM ALGORITHMS

- Signal shim:
  - optimizes the signal amplitude or line width in the target volume
  - does not rely on prior knowledge of the field distribution or the shim coils
- Field map–based shimming:
  - the characteristics of the shim hardware (e.g., coils, passive shims) must be known
  - ideally, hardware constraints (e.g., maximum coil currents) are considered

From the measured field distribution, the optimum shim setup to correct the observed field inhomogeneities must be determined. The basic concepts and potential pitfalls of corresponding algorithms are presented in Section 2.2.6.2. However, first, a signal shim method is covered that is not based on a previously determined field distribution (see Section 2.2.6.1).

2.2.6.1 Signal Shim

The first shim procedures were based on the signal of a cuboidal voxel or of the full object. For a perfectly homogeneous field, the Larmor frequency of all water molecules in the voxel is identical, and their phase coherence is retained for a long time (i.e., no dephasing occurs). This means that (1) the signal decays exponentially and slowly in time (with the transverse relaxation time constant T_2), (2) the time integral of the signal is very large, and (3) its Fourier transformation is very narrow and has a Lorentzian line shape. If the field is inhomogeneous, the Larmor frequencies differ, and the more inhomogeneous the field is, the faster dephasing occurs. As a consequence, (1) the signal decay in time is steeper (and may deviate from an exponential shape), (2) the signal's time integral is reduced, and (3) its Fourier transformation has a broader line width (and may exhibit a non-Lorentzian shape). Thus, changing the shim settings and comparing these signal properties allow one to estimate whether the field homogeneity has been improved or not.

Unfortunately, it is not possible to predict which change of the shim setup may improve the field homogeneity within the voxel. Thus, a simple search for the optimum values is required. It is usually performed interactively by the user by changing the coil currents, evaluating the corresponding variation of the signal, and accepting or rejecting the change until an optimum setting is achieved. With appropriate algorithms (e.g., Ref. 52), the search can be automated, which can be expected to provide reproducible and less user-dependent results.[53]

Despite its somewhat trial-and-error character, this shim procedure is still used, mainly for single-voxel MRS, and could be of interest for targets with small volumes or cross-sectional areas like the spinal cord. However, one should be aware of its limitations (see Section 2.2.7) when applying it.

2.2.6.2 Field Map–Based Shimming

From a field map, the required correction to obtain a homogeneous field can be easily calculated. But an algorithm is needed to determine the optimum shim setup from it, that is, the currents for the different shim coils or the locations and quantities of the passive shim material. This problem can be written as a system of equations that, for example, could be formulated on a voxel-by-voxel basis.

For active shimming with coils, the field provided by all coils is a linear combination of the individual field contributions for each coil for a unit current weighted with an (unknown) individual factor that determines the actual current.[29] In the shim target volume, this combination should be identical to the desired field correction, which yields the individual weighting factors (i.e., coil currents) required.[29] For passive shimming, an equivalent equation can be formulated if fixed locations[14] or setups (e.g., arrangements that correspond to the field decomposition in spherical harmonics[15]) are considered for the shim material. In this case, the solution yields the quantity of the shim material required at each location. If the shim devices have no fixed locations, like for local shim coils or passive shims that can be freely positioned, these locations represent additional degrees of freedom that can be considered.[13]

In principle, the field corrections required by the shim hardware could be determined with simulations or by assuming perfect shim devices, e.g., shim coils that exactly provide the field distribution they were designed for. This is an option for passive shims, but for shim coils it is more reliable to use measured field distributions in order to consider appropriately the deviations occurring in reality.[29]

Because the number of voxels considered usually exceeds the number of shim devices, the system is over-determined. There is usually no perfect solution, for instance because higher-order terms are present for which no coil is available. This means that only an approximation of the desired field correction can be realized, and a criterion or cost function to determine which approximation is considered the best must be defined. Most commonly, the least-squares norm is applied (e.g., Ref. 29), but other options have also been used (e.g., Refs 29,50), for instance the maximum deviation. Usually, the shim setups considered to be optimum are very similar for the different criteria[50]; however, for highly sensitive acquisitions like SSFP, the choice of a suitable criterion may be important.[54]

But the system can also be underdetermined, for example if the number of equations (voxels) is lower than the number of shim devices or due to a degeneracy of the shim coils within the target volume, and no unique solution exists. This could happen for small target volumes or passive shim settings where many locations for shim material may be available. Thus, additional constraints could be introduced into the algorithm, such as choosing the setup with the lowest coil currents or the minimum amount of shim material (e.g., Ref. 55).

The corresponding equations can be solved directly if an appropriate reformulation of the chosen criterion or cost function is possible; otherwise, iterative approaches are used. Even in the absence of noise or artifacts, the latter may end up in a local minimum and not find the optimum shim setup. Furthermore, the problem could be ill conditioned; in other words, a minor variation of the underlying data (e.g., due to noise) could cause a considerably different result. In particular, if the target volume is very small in one direction, even a minor noise influence on the field map could have a major effect on the shim setup chosen. This is why other strategies have been proposed that have an inherently lower sensitivity to noise, for example a regularized algorithm based on a singular value decomposition.[49] Nevertheless, the signal-to-noise ratio of the underlying acquisitions (i.e., the field corrections provided by the coils and the in vivo field map) should be sufficiently high, and the minimum size of the target volume is usually limited.

The optimum shim setup could be beyond the accessible parameter range, e.g., require larger coil currents than feasible or more passive shim material than fits to the dedicated location. Simply clipping these settings to those that can be realized, for instance by using the maximum coil current or amount of material possible, may not provide the best approximation within the accessible parameter range.[56] Thus, more elaborated algorithms consider such constraints and search for the minimum within the accessible parameter range that yields better results.[49,56]

In column-based shim procedures like FASTMAP (see Section 2.2.5.2), a simple polynomial regression for the individual columns is performed from which the optimum shim settings can be calculated analytically.[42,43]

2.2.7 SHIM PRACTICE

- The resolution of standard maps may be too coarse to consider left-right and posterior-anterior field variations in the spinal cord
- Limiting the adjustment volume to the spinal cord can be beneficial
- Iterative runs of the standard shim procedure may improve the results
- If results are insufficient, the start configuration of the shim procedure should be changed
- A manual signal shim could further improve the shim but requires some experience

The standard shim procedure on common whole-body MR systems involves (1) the measurement of a field map in vivo (see Section 2.2.5); (2) the definition of the target volume for which the field homogeneity should be optimized; (3) the calculation of the currents that, if applied to the shim coils available (see Section 2.2.3), provide the best approximation of a homogeneous field within the target region (see Section 2.2.6); and (4) the corresponding adaptation of the static shim currents prior to the measurement (see Section 2.2.4).

The field map (see Section 2.2.5) is usually acquired with a multiecho 3D rapid gradient-echo sequence because it combines a reasonable acquisition time with a low sensitivity to artifacts. From the phase differences observed between the different echoes, typically two with an echo time difference that ensures an identical phase relationship for water and lipids, the field distribution can be estimated. Commonly, the maximum field of view of the system is used for this acquisition to ensure that upon changes of the target volume (e.g., by increasing the number of slices or modifying their position or orientation), no reacquisition of the field map is required. But upon moving the patient table or changing the coil configuration, a reacquisition of the field map is advisable and usually performed automatically. After significant motion, a reacquisition is also recommended but must be triggered by the user. To provide a high signal-to-noise ratio for the field maps and minimize their

acquisition time, a rather coarse spatial resolution of several millimeters is used that can yield acquisition times below 1 min. This spatial resolution is usually sufficient for most applications because excessive phase wrapping is usually still avoided (see Section 2.2.5.1) and the standard shim coils are of lower (e.g. first and second) orders (see Section 2.2.3.1) and provide correction fields that vary slowly in space. However, such a resolution can be too coarse to resolve field variations within the spinal cord in the left-right and posterior-anterior directions. This can limit the value of such a field map and the standard shim procedure based on it for spinal cord applications, and a manual shim adjustment could be helpful (as discussed in this section).

Regarding artifacts of the acquisition that can distort the calculated field map (see Section 2.2.5.3), it should be emphasized that they cannot be unmasked with the performed measurement itself. Consider a perfectly homogeneous field that appears inhomogeneous in the measurements due to artifacts. The shim procedure aims to minimize the observed "inhomogeneities" and will provide a shim setup for which the field map appears homogeneous, i.e., the artifacts of the measurement are "corrected" for. This means that a convergence of the shim procedure during several iterations with an increased field homogeneity measure only proves the reproducibility of the field map measurement. It does not necessarily mean that the field map is correct and the homogeneity really has been improved. This should be kept in mind.

The default target volume, for which the field is optimized, is usually the smallest cuboid that contains the entire measurement volume (e.g., the full fields-of-view of all slices). But the user can flexibly modify its size, position, and orientation and sometimes also the basic shape (e.g., to an ellipsoid) to focus it to a smaller volume of interest. This can improve the homogeneity within this volume considerably at the expense of an increased inhomogeneity in other regions. This holds in particular if the field distribution varies significantly within the measurement volume. Consider, for instance, a small volume of interest that exhibits severe through-slice dephasing, while all other regions in the volume have a quite homogeneous field. A shim setup that corrects the through-slice dephasing will decrease the homogeneity in all other regions, which, if the full volume is evaluated, is not the best approximation of a homogeneous field. This is different if the target volume focuses on the small volume of interest.

For imaging of the spinal cord, the adaptation of the target volume can be an important feature because the spinal cord has a very small cross-section, but a quite large field of view may be required to avoid aliasing. By sacrificing the homogeneity in outer regions that are not of interest, an improvement within the spinal cord could be obtained (see Figure 2.2.9). But it should be kept in mind that (1) usually a minimum size of the target volume is required to ensure that the shim algorithm behaves benignly (see Section 2.2.6.2); and (2) severe inhomogeneities outside of the target volume, which may be induced by optimizing the shim in a small target volume, may cause other adverse effects. For instance, geometric distortions in echo-planar imaging (e.g., stretching in the phase-encoding direction) (cf. Figure 2.2.2) may become excessive and result in aliasing artifacts even for a nominally appropriate field-of-view, or, in single-voxel MRS, the suppression of unwanted signal contributions from outside of the voxel may be insufficient (see Section 2.2.10).

An algorithm (see Section 2.2.6.2) aims to find the currents for the different shim coils available (usually first- and second-order terms) that provide the best homogeneity within the defined target region. It usually yields a good approximation of the optimum settings, but for regions with pronounced inhomogeneities it may just find a local minimum or end up with desired coil currents that exceed the hardware limits. The field homogeneity then may not be sufficient for specific applications like BOLD-based functional neuroimaging.

Thus, in cases of disappointing results, more efforts may be required. An option that sometimes helps is to perform one or two full repetition(s) of the shim procedure, i.e., a reacquisition of the field map and a recalculation of the shim currents. Thereby, it may help to start with a very different shim configuration rather than the result of a previous iteration to increase the chance of leaving or avoiding the local minimum in which the algorithms could be trapped.

In particular for MRS, but also for imaging with small volumes of interest like the spinal cord, a signal shim (see Section 2.2.6.1), often performed by the user interactively, could also be helpful. Thereby, the accumulated signal of the full target volume is considered while changing the currents of the different shim coils. For an increased field homogeneity, the signal decay in time is reduced (i.e., T_2^*), the signal time integral is increased, and its Fourier transformation is narrowed. Thus, it can be estimated whether the homogeneity has been improved or not upon changing a shim current.

Usually, this optimization is conducted on a coil-by-coil basis, starting with the linear terms because they often have the largest impact on the field homogeneity. Two or more iterations should be performed, at least for the linear terms, with decreasing step width. But there are some important issues that must be taken into account. First, it usually is recommended to perform at least one iteration of the standard shim procedure involving a field map prior to the signal shim to start with reasonable values. Second, some waiting time is

needed after changing the shim settings before an evaluation should be performed, because the underlying measurements are usually not performed under fully relaxed conditions but in a dynamic steady state that requires a few seconds to be reestablished for the new settings. As a rule of thumb, at least the first acquisition after changing a coil current should be ignored. Third, the signal measures may not change monotonically with the field homogeneity, in particular far away from the optimum such that it may be required to perform a few steps toward a "worse" signal performance until a major improvement is achieved. Fourth, there is usually an interaction of the shim terms: in general, they are not completely independent. In practice, this means that (1) the optimum setup for a second-order coil may not correspond to the best signal performance unless the corresponding linear coils are readjusted; and (2) after changing one coil current, it may be required to readjust another one to obtain the best shim. Thus, some experience is required to adjust the second-order coils appropriately, and several iterations may be useful that, however, should be terminated with a check of the linear terms. But even if only linear terms are considered, some improvement is usually achievable.

2.2.8 SPECIFIC PROBLEMS AND SOLUTIONS FOR T_2^*-WEIGHTED ACQUISITIONS

T_2^*-Weighted acquisitions

- Problems:
  - signal loss, in particular due to through-slice dephasing
  - geometric distortions and echo time shift in echo-planar imaging
- Solutions:
  - gradient compensation (in the slice direction) and tailored RF excitations can reduce signal losses
  - an echo time shift in echo-planar imaging can be addressed with gradient compensation (in the phase-encoding direction)

T_2^*-weighted acquisitions, such as those used for BOLD-based functional neuroimaging (see Chapter 4.1), are particularly sensitive to field inhomogeneities. This sensitivity is desired to detect changes of the blood oxygenation level (i.e., field inhomogeneities on a microscopic level) but also causes artifacts and signal losses in the presence of macroscopic field inhomogeneities (e.g., due to susceptibility differences) that hamper functional neuroimaging. The standard static shim (see Section 2.2.7) often does not provide a field homogeneity sufficient to avoid such problems, which has been a major motivation to develop and test more elaborated shim techniques.

The main effect of such macroscopic field inhomogeneities is the intravoxel dephasing that can cause significant signal losses, mainly for inhomogeneities in the slice direction (see Section 2.2.1 and Figure 2.2.3), which is a particular problem in the human spinal cord (see Section 2.2.2 and Figure 2.2.10). A simple way to reduce the signal loss is to decrease the voxel size, in particular the slice thickness (e.g., Ref. 57). However, this reduces the signal-to-noise ratio, prolongs the acquisition time, and, in cases of increased in-plane resolution and single-shot pulse sequences like echo-planar imaging, increases the sensitivity to other artifacts like geometric distortions (see Section 2.2.1, Figure 2.2.2, and Chapter 2.1).

Thus, other approaches that are based on modifications of the pulse sequence have been considered to ameliorate the signal dephasing. In particular, two techniques have been used in the past, gradient compensation in the slice direction (the "z-shim"; Section 2.2.8.1) and tailored RF excitations (Section 2.2.8.2), which both provide a compensation at a given echo time. Furthermore, a special issue related to echo-planar imaging is considered in Section 2.2.8.3.

2.2.8.1 Gradient Compensation in the Slice Direction

Gradient compensation of field inhomogeneities,[58–62] applied in the slice direction known as the z-shim, can be considered as a kind of "poor man's" dynamic shim approach. It involves an additional gradient pulse that modulates the Larmor frequencies within the voxel linearly and, thus, manipulates the spins' phases. Ideally, the gradient moment (i.e., the product of its signed amplitude and its duration) is chosen to yield a phase distribution that is inverted compared to the distribution that is caused by the field inhomogeneities and would be present at the echo time without the additional gradient pulse. Thus, the phase distortions induced by the field inhomogeneities and by the additional gradient pulse cancel each other at the echo time, which reduces the signal loss. This can be at the expense of a slightly prolonged echo time due to the time needed for the additional gradient pulse.

A gradient compensation in the slice direction is often sufficient because the signal loss is most pronounced in this direction (see Section 2.2.1 and Figure 2.2.3),[58,60–62] in particular in the human spinal cord. Thus, this section will focus on the z-shim, but the principles presented can easily be adapted to gradient compensation in the phase- and frequency-encoding directions. Indeed, for echo-planar imaging, field inhomogeneities in the phase-encoding direction could also cause a relevant signal decay, which could be ameliorated with gradient compensation as well[59] (see Section 2.2.8.3).

Because the additional gradient pulse provides a linear field variation, effectively only the linear component of the field inhomogeneities can be compensated, i.e., some contributions of the dephasing will remain, and the full signal is not recovered. Furthermore, the best compensation gradient depends on the actual field

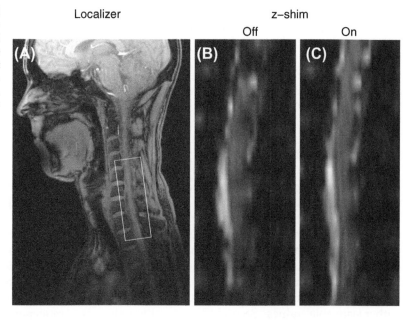

FIGURE 2.2.10 (A) Localizer and (B, C) sagittal views of a stack of axial slices acquired with T_2^*-weighted echo-planar imaging ($1 \times 1 \times 5\,mm^3$, parallel imaging acceleration factor 2, echo time 42 ms) in the cervical spinal cord of a healthy volunteer (B) without and (C) with a single, slice-specific gradient compensation in the slice direction ("z-shim"). With z-shimming, the signal homogeneity along the cord is significantly improved.

inhomogeneity, which may vary between different regions of interest. Thus, different gradient moments must usually be sampled to obtain an optimum signal recovery in all regions, which prolongs the acquisition time and reduces the temporal resolution[58,60,61,63,64] or is at the expense of a reduced signal-to-noise ratio if they are sampled successively in a shot.[62]

To obtain an image that provides the full (compensated) signal intensity for all voxels, the different acquisitions must be combined. A simple approach is a maximum intensity projection that selects the highest pixel intensity of the series on a voxel-by-voxel basis. Unfortunately, the signal-to-noise ratio of such an image effectively corresponds to that of a single acquisition, although multiple acquisitions were performed. With alternative combination schemes that include more or all images (e.g., Ref. 65), such as a sum-of-squares combination of all images[65] or a Fourier transformation over the different acquisitions,[63,64] an improved signal-to-noise ratio can be obtained.

An approach that does not affect the acquisition time or the temporal resolution is to apply a single, slice-specific compensation moment.[66,67] This approach is particularly interesting for axial slices of the spinal cord. In this case, significant through-slice dephasing is present that varies considerably between slices but is very similar within the spinal cord section of a slice. Thus, a good signal recovery for the full spinal cord cross-section within a slice can be achieved[66] (Figure 2.2.10).

To determine the optimum moment for each slice, a field map could be used.[67] However, a high spatial resolution in the head–feet direction is needed with a reasonable signal-to-noise ratio that could require quite long acquisition times. Alternatively, an adjustment measurement could be performed where for each slice, images with different compensation moments are acquired.[66] For each slice, the moment that provides the highest signal amplitude is determined and used in subsequent acquisitions. Thereby, a sufficiently dense sampling of the compensation moments in the adjustment scan is required to hit the optimum or a value close to it.

2.2.8.2 Tailored RF Excitations

Tailored RF excitations are an interesting option because they can compensate the dephasing effect of arbitrary field inhomogeneities. Furthermore, in their most elaborated implementation, they can provide a good signal recovery in multiple regions with different field inhomogeneities simultaneously. Both properties are an improvement compared to the gradient compensation approach (see Section 2.2.8.1).

In the small-tip-angle approximation,[68] the complex RF envelope (magnitude and phase) is the Fourier transformation of the desired, complex excitation profile. If the field distribution along the slice direction is known, the resulting phase distortion present at the chosen echo time can be calculated. Inverting this phase distortion and combining it with a rectangular magnitude profile yields the slice profile required to cancel the inhomogeneity-induced phase distortions. The Fourier transform of this profile yields the envelope of the tailored, slice-selective RF excitation that completely avoids signal losses due to through-slice dephasing.[69,70] It compensates the effect of arbitrary field distributions in the slice direction even if higher-order terms are relevant that cannot be addressed with current shim coils or other techniques like gradient compensation. But, compared to a standard slice-selective RF excitation, it may be required to prolong the RF pulse duration in order to achieve the spatial resolution required to define the through-slice field variation accurately.

In general, several specific RF envelopes are required if the field distribution in the slice direction varies within the target region covered by a slice. Then multiple shots are needed to realize a good signal recovery in all regions, which is similar to the z-shim method (see Section 2.2.8.1). However, for spinal cord applications with axial slices, the variation of the through-slice field within each slice is not that pronounced such that a single, dedicated RF envelope for each slice may provide a good signal recovery in the full cross-section without having a time penalty. This approach is analogous to using a single, slice-specific compensation moment in z-shimming (see Section 2.2.8.2) but is able to correct arbitrary, not only linear, field variations.

To take full advantage of this ability, the through-slice field variations need to be determined with sufficient accuracy. This means that a field map with a high spatial resolution in the slice direction is needed with a sufficiently high signal-to-noise ratio, which may yield quite long acquisition times. As a compromise, an RF excitation that provides a quadratic phase profile could be used.[71] With such a profile, a quite large range of (unknown) field inhomogeneities could be compensated reasonably with a single RF excitation and without a field map or an adjustment scan. In particular, the pronounced signal loss that may occur without compensation or with an inappropriate z-shim can be avoided. However, this is at the expense of an insufficient signal rephasing in regions without through-slice field inhomogeneities, yielding a considerably reduced signal intensity. Thus, this option does not seem to be very attractive for spinal cord applications.

For spinal cord imaging with nonaxial slices, the in-plane variation of the through-slice field inhomogeneities can be expected to be significant, and multidimensional RF excitations[68,72,73] may be required to provide a solution without the need for multiple acquisitions. With 3D-selective RF excitations,[74] full flexibility in the slice direction is achieved such that a region-specific compensation of arbitrary field distributions can be realized.[75] This also includes in-plane field gradients that can hamper single-shot techniques like echo-planar imaging (see Section 2.2.8.3).

A drawback of the multidimensional, tailored RF excitations is their prolonged pulse duration, which may be considerable, in particular for the 3D variant (several tens of milliseconds).[75] While effective echo times can be comparable to standard slice-selective RF excitations if an appropriate trajectory is chosen,[76] the repetition time is significantly increased or multiple shots must be used,[77,78] which hampers their applicability. However, since the advent of parallel transmission techniques,[79] considerable progress has been made to shorten such RF excitations, which finally may lead to rather acceptable RF pulse durations for spinal cord acquisitions.

2.2.8.3 Issues for Echo-Planar Imaging

A problem specific to echo-planar imaging is a shortening or prolongation of the effective echo time, which modulates the BOLD sensitivity.[59] Field inhomogeneities in the phase-encoding direction superimpose the blip gradient pulses that act as a "line feed" to the next k-space line, and amplify or reduce their effect. Thus, the central k-space line may be covered with an "earlier" or "later" echo than expected, which corresponds to a shorter or longer echo time, respectively. This effect is specific to echo-planar imaging because the different echoes are acquired at different echo times. In the worst case, the k-space center may not be covered at all, which results in a severe degradation of the signal intensity and image quality. A simple way to avoid such problems is the application of an additional gradient pulse in the phase-encoding direction that compensates the dephasing effect of the field inhomogeneities and, thus, retains the desired echo time.[59]

Similar to the z-shim (see Section 2.2.8.1), the best compensation may in general require multiple compensation moments to optimize regions that are differently affected by field inhomogeneities.[59] But, again as for z-shim, if a small volume like the spinal cord is targeted with axial slices, a single, slice-specific compensation moment could be sufficient. This may also be helpful because in a stack of parallel slices, not every slice can be expected to be perpendicular to the cord axis which

means that some of the field inhomogeneity present in the longitudinal direction of the spinal cord may have a component in the phase-encoding direction of the slice.

2.2.9 SPECIFIC PROBLEMS AND SOLUTIONS FOR DIFFUSION-WEIGHTED ACQUISITIONS

Diffusion-weighted acquisitions

- Problems:
  - cross-terms of field inhomogeneities with the diffusion-weighted gradient pulses
  - can cause over- or underestimation of diffusion coefficients and distort tensor eigenvectors
- Solutions:
  - the diffusion-weighting preparation can be modified to minimize cross-terms
  - geometrically averaging acquisitions with opposite diffusion-weighting directions reduces cross-term effects

Field inhomogeneities can interfere with the dedicated pulsed gradients applied for diffusion weighting. This interference can modulate the strength or distort the direction of the pulsed diffusion weighting, which could hamper the quantitative determination of diffusion properties and fiber tracking in the spinal cord (see Chapters 3.1 and 3.2).

The diffusion-induced displacement that spins typically exhibit in tissue during an MR experiment is about several tens of micrometers. On this scale, a field inhomogeneity present in a voxel can usually be well approximated by a linear variation that corresponds to a gradient field. This so-called background field gradient also causes a diffusion weighting.[80] In most acquisitions, this effect is very small and can be neglected. However, it could be relevant for the long echo times and the long distance between the RF pulses present in diffusion-weighted acquisitions.[80]

This additional diffusion weighting has two effects (e.g. Ref. 80). First, it causes a signal attenuation that depends on the background field gradients only. Because this attenuation, like the T_2-related signal decay, is present in all acquisitions (with or without pulsed gradients), it is usually not relevant when estimating the diffusion properties. Second, there is an interaction, the so-called cross-term, of the background field gradients with the pulsed gradients that modulates the signal attenuation. It depends on both, the background field gradients and the diffusion weighting, and, thus, is only present if the pulsed gradients are applied.

If this interaction is not taken into account, diffusion coefficients may be under- or overestimated.[80] Furthermore, because the cross-terms depend on the relative orientation of the pulsed and background gradients, the estimation of the diffusion anisotropy may be incorrect[81] and the direction of the eigenvectors could be distorted, which may affect fiber tracking. So far, studies are missing that systematically investigate the influence of such effects in the spinal cord. However, one should be aware of these problems that could be relevant if the field inhomogeneities are pronounced.

Modified time courses of the pulsed diffusion-weighting gradients have been presented that minimize or even fully compensate the cross-terms, independent of the amplitude and direction of the background gradient fields (e.g., Refs 82,83). However, such approaches reduce the diffusion-weighting efficiency (i.e., require longer echo times) and, thus, can reduce the signal-to-noise ratio. Furthermore, such time courses are hard to combine with other demands like eddy current compensation to minimize geometric distortions.

However, if the field variations over the full voxel dimension can be considered to be linear, a simpler solution has been found.[81] By performing a second acquisition with the polarity of all pulsed diffusion-weighting gradients inverted, and averaging the intensities of both acquisitions geometrically, the cross-terms cancel independent of the amplitude and direction of the pulsed diffusion weighting.[81] This approach can also be used to eliminate cross-terms with other pulsed gradients like slice selection and spoiler gradient pulses. It is compatible with any gradient timing and is easy to implement.

2.2.10 SPECIFIC PROBLEMS AND SOLUTIONS FOR MRS

MR Spectroscopy

- Problems:
  - line width broadening
  - insufficient water suppression or spoiling of unwanted signals
- Solutions:
  - choose a voxel position that is less affected by field inhomogeneities
  - use accurate, manual shimming
  - use spatial saturation pulses to minimize signals from outside of the target volume

MRS (see Chapter 5.1) exhibits a high sensitivity to field inhomogeneities. This holds particularly for ^{1}H spectroscopy because the chemical shift differences and couplings are small, i.e., an effectively high-frequency resolution is required, and the amplitude of the metabolite signals is low compared to that of other signals like that of water. Thus, a broadening of the line width and unwanted signal contributions from outside of the target volume can hamper the acquisitions in addition to the side effects that field inhomogeneities have on the localization with slice-selective RF excitations.

The most important effect of field inhomogeneities in MRS is the line width broadening (see Section 2.2.1 and Figure 2.2.4), which, even at inhomogeneity levels that are negligible in most imaging experiments, can degrade the spectrum quality considerably. It hampers the reliable identification and discrimination of the metabolite signals. Furthermore, due to the correspondingly decreased peak-to-noise ratio, the estimation of the metabolite concentrations becomes more unreliable because the uncertainties of the baseline (shape and amplitude) have an increased impact. Other side effects of the line broadening could be an insufficient chemical-shift-selective suppression (e.g., Ref. 84), for example of water or lipids, and a reduced efficiency of spectral editing techniques, which both impair the spectrum quality and analysis.

Second, unwanted signal contributions could occur, particularly in cases of severe field inhomogeneities outside of the target volume, for instance in regions covered by one of the slice-selective RF excitations or close by.[85] These contributions are usually dephased by the spoiler gradient pulses applied. But if the field variations are not small compared to these pulses, some residual signal may remain, in particular if chemical-shift-selective suppression is also degraded or not applied as for lipids.[84] Even if the fraction that effectively is not spoiled is very small, it could be relevant for water and lipids due to (1) their much higher concentration compared to the metabolites and (2) the much larger volume excited by the individual excitations compared to the cross-sectional voxel volume. It should be noted that such artifacts can also be induced by shimming. The optimal shim setup for the spectroscopy voxel can yield considerable field distortions outside that, for example, can degrade the water suppression and cause spurious signal contributions.[84]

Third, as for all localized MR experiments, the slice selection can be affected, yielding not only deviating voxel positions and orientations but also sizes (see Section 2.2.1). This may happen if the amplitudes of the slice selection gradient pulses do not exceed the field variations considerably. Then, the section excited may be shifted, tilted, and narrowed or thickened. However, if the gradient pulse amplitudes are sufficiently large, these effects should cause only minor distortions of the desired cuboidal shape. Furthermore, performing the metabolite quantification on a water reference signal can avoid an over- or underestimation of the concentrations due to a deviating voxel size.

A careful selection of the voxel size and position is a prerequisite to avoid excessive line broadening in the spinal cord.[4,86] For instance, the line width is superior at the C2–C3 level compared to that at the C4–C5 level[86] and is less favorable for voxels spanning several vertebrae.[4] Accurate shimming (see Section 2.2.7) is also of particular importance to minimize or avoid the described inhomogeneity problems. With an elaborated shim procedure, a good field homogeneity is obtained,[86] but a skilled user may achieve a further improvement with an interactive signal shim (see Sections 2.2.6.1 and 2.2.7).

Unspoiled signal contributions from outside of the voxel can be minimized by an appropriate choice of the order in which the three slice-selective RF excitations are applied. Using the slice that is least affected by inhomogeneities for the last excitation—which, for example, can be realized by choosing the appropriate voxel orientation—can yield a significant improvement, as has been demonstrated for the frontal human brain.[87] Spatial saturation pulses with sufficient spoiling can also be used to (further) reduce unwanted signal contributions.[84] Because these saturation pulses are applied prior to the excitation, their spoiler gradient pulses can be increased without prolonging the echo time of the MRS acquisition. Such pulses can also minimize unwanted signal contributions caused by cerebral spinal fluid flow and chemical-shift-displacement artifacts, which due to the small cross-section of the spinal cord can disturb the acquisition.[86]

2.2.11 SUMMARY

Shimming is important for MR experiments of the human spinal cord in order to minimize artifacts like geometric distortions and signal losses and provide sufficient data quality, in particular for BOLD-based functional neuroimaging, diffusion-weighted imaging, and spectroscopy. Unfortunately, the standard shim hardware available on clinical MR systems (see Section 2.2.3) provides only a static shim (see Section 2.2.4) with, typically, up to second-order terms that even after careful adjustment (see Section 2.2.7) often do not yield a satisfactory field homogeneity in the spinal cord. With optimized protocol parameters and acquisitions strategies (see Chapter 2.1), some of the artifacts can be reduced, but they are usually still significant and hamper the experiments.

Work-arounds that can be helpful for specific applications involve modifications or extensions of the pulse sequence, such as adaptation of the pulsed gradient amplitude to avoid geometric distortions or gradient compensation and tailored RF excitations to minimize signal losses in T_2^*-weighted acquisitions. Such approaches can usually be realized at dedicated research sites and require only minimum support by the manufacturer (e.g., to be able to run nonstandard pulse sequences). For tailored RF excitations, the usage of parallel transmission techniques is very helpful to improve their applicability. Such systems are already offered by some manufacturers and are becoming more and more available.

A dynamic shim update (see Section 2.2.4.2) is quite promising, as it can be expected to yield a significant improvement for spinal cord applications, in particular for axial slice orientations. An update of the linear shim terms should be possible with standard pulse sequence programming. An integration of the full functionality, including second- and higher-order terms, into standard MR systems is straightforward and should be feasible for the manufacturers. Due to the severe artifacts that field inhomogeneities can cause at higher static fields, this approach will hopefully be considered in future systems.

More elaborated passive and active shim devices (e.g., local or arrays of shim coils) are very promising solutions, but, so far, it is unlikely that they will become available in the near future. Building one's own devices may be feasible only for cutting-edge research sites with extensive experience in hardware development and may be limited by safety issues and regulations in practice.

Acknowledgments

The author is very grateful to Susann Boretius, Martin Busch, Yasar Goedecke, Martin Koch, Joost Kuijer, Marco Lawrenz, and Petra Pouwels for helpful discussions and to Joachim Graessner (Siemens Healthcare) and Jürgen Bunke (Philips Healthcare) for providing information about the shim techniques of their companies' MR systems.

References

1. Koch KM, Rothman DL, de Graaf RA. Optimization of static magnetic field homogeneity in the human and animal brain in vivo. *Prog Nucl Magn Reson Spectrosc.* 2009;54(2):69–96.

2. Lauterbur PC. Image formation by induced local interactions: examples employing nuclear magnetic resonance. *Nature.* 1973; 242(5394):190–191.

3. Wilson JL, Jenkinson M, Jezzard P. Optimization of static field homogeneity in human brain using diamagnetic passive shims. *Magn Reson Med.* 2002;48(5):906–914.

4. Cooke FJ, Blamire AM, Manners DN, Styles P, Rajagopalan B. Quantitative proton magnetic resonance spectroscopy of the cervical spinal cord. *Magn Reson Med.* 2004;51(6):1122–1128.

5. Hsu J-J, Glover G. Mitigation of susceptibility-induced signal loss in neuroimaging using localized shim coils. *Magn Reson Med.* 2005; 53(2):243–248.

6. Juchem C, Nixon TW, McIntyre S, Rothman DL, de Graaf RA. Magnetic field homogenization of the human prefrontal cortex

with a set of localized electrical coils. *Magn Reson Med.* 2010;63(1): 171–180.

7. Juchem C, Nixon TW, McIntyre S, Boer VO, Rothman DL, de Graaf RA. Dynamic multi-coil shimming of the human brain at 7 T. *J Magn Reson.* 2011;212(2):280–288.

8. Juchem C, Nixon TW, McIntyre S, Rothman DL, de Graaf RA. Magnetic field modelling with a set of individual localized coils. *J Magn Reson.* 2010;204(2):281–289.

9. Roméo F, Hoult DI. Magnet field profiling: analysis and correcting coil design. *Magn Reson Med.* 1984;1(1):44–65.

10. Rosen Y, Bloch BN, Lenkinski RE, Greenman RL, Marquis RP, Rofsky NM. 3 T MR of the prostate: reducing susceptibility gradients by inflating the endorectal coil with a barium sulfate suspension. *Magn Reson Med.* 2007;57(5):898–904.

11. Lee GC, Goodwill PW, Phuong K, et al. Pyrolytic graphite foam: a passive magnetic susceptibility matching material. *J Magn Reson Imaging.* 2010;32(3):684–691.

12. Wilson JL, Jenkinson M, Jezzard P. Protocol to determine the optimal intraoral passive shim for minimisation of susceptibility artifact in human inferior frontal cortex. *Neuroimage.* 2003;19(4): 1802–1811.

13. Yang S, Kim H, Ghim M-O, Lee B-U, Kim D-H. Local in vivo shimming using adaptive passive shim positioning. *Magn Reson Imaging.* 2011;29(3):401–407.

14. Koch KM, Brown PB, Rothman DL, de Graaf RA. Sample-specific diamagnetic and paramagnetic passive shimming. *J Magn Reson.* 2006;182(1):66–74.

15. Juchem C, Muller-Bierl B, Schick F, Logothetis NK, Pfeuffer J. Combined passive and active shimming for in vivo MR spectroscopy at high magnetic fields. *J Magn Reson.* 2006;183(2):278–289.

16. Wilson JL, Jezzard P. Utilization of an intra-oral diamagnetic passive shim in functional MRI of the inferior frontal cortex. *Magn Reson Med.* 2003;50(5):1089–1094.

17. Koch KM, Brown PB, Rothman DL, de Graaf RA. External diamagnetic and paramagnetic shimming of the human brain. *Proc Intl Soc Magn Reson Med.* 2007;15:982.

18. de Graaf RA, Brown PB, McIntyre S, Rothman DL, Nixon TW. Dynamic shimming updating (DSU) for multislice signal acquisition. *Magn Reson Med.* 2003;49(3):409–416.

19. Blamire AM, Rothman DL, Nixon T. Dynamic shim updating: a new approach towards optimized whole brain shimming. *Magn Reson Med.* 1996;36(1):159–165.

20. Ernst T, Hennig J. Double-volume ^{1}H spectroscopy with interleaved acquisitions using tilted gradients. *Magn Reson Med.* 1991; 20(1):27–35.

21. van Gelderen P, de Zwart JA, Starewicz P, Hinks RS, Duyn JH. Real-time shimming to compensate for respiration-induced B_0 fluctuations. *Magn Reson Med.* 2007;57(2):362–368.

22. Koch KM, McIntyre S, Nixon TW, Rothman DL, de Graaf RA. Dynamic shim updating on the human brain. *J Magn Reson.* 2006; 180(2):286–296.

23. Koch KM, Sacolick LI, Nixon TW, McIntyre S, Rothman DL, de Graaf RA. Dynamically shimmed multivoxel ^{1}H magnetic resonance spectroscopy and multislice magnetic resonance spectroscopic imaging of the human brain. *Magn Reson Med.* 2007;57(3):587–591.

24. Morrell G, Spielman D. Dynamic shimming for multi-slice magnetic resonance imaging. *Magn Reson Med.* 1997;38(3):477–483.

25. Sengupta S, Welch EB, Zhao Y, et al. Dynamic B_0 shimming at 7 T. *Magn Reson Imaging.* 2011;29(4):483–496.

26. Sengupta S, Avison MJ, Gore JC, Welch EB. Software compensation of eddy current fields in multislice high order dynamic shimming. *J Magn Reson.* 2011;210(2):218–227.

27. Maudsley AA, Oppelt A, Ganssen A. Rapid measurement of magnetic field distributions using nuclear magnetic resonance. *Siemens Forsch Entwickl Ber.* 1979;8(6):326–331.

28. Maudsley AA, Simon HE, Hilal SK. Magnetic field measurement by NMR imaging. *J Phys E.* 1984;17(3):216–220.

29. Prammer MG, Haselgrove JC, Shinnar M, Leigh JS. A new approach to automatic shimming. *J Magn Reson.* 1988;77(1):40–52.

30. Sekihara K, Matsui S, Kohno H. A new method of measuring static field distribution using modified Fourier NMR imaging. *J Phys E.* 1985;18(3):224–227.

31. Brown TR, Kincaid BM, Ugurbil K. NMR chemical shift imaging in three dimensions. *Proc Natl Acad Sci USA.* 1982;79(11):3523–3526.

32. Maudsley AA, Hilal SK, Perman WH, Simon HE. Spatially resolved high resolution spectroscopy by four-dimensional NMR. *J Magn Reson.* 1983;51(1):147–152.

33. Ericsson A, Weis J, Hemmingsson A, Wikström M, Sperber GO. Measurement of magnetic field variations in the human brain using a 3D-FT multiple gradient echo technique. *Magn Reson Med.* 1995;33(2):171–177.

34. Axel L, Morton D. Correction of phase wrapping in magnetic resonance imaging. *Med Phys.* 1989;16(2):284–287.

35. Jenkinson M. Fast, automated, *N*-dimensional phase-unwrapping algorithm. *Magn Reson Med.* 2003;49(1):193–197.

36. Song SMH, Napel S, Pelc NJ, Glover G. Phase unwrapping of MR phase images using Poisson equation. *IEEE Trans Image Process.* 1995;4(5):667–676.

37. Strand J, Taxt T. Two-dimensional phase unwrapping using robust derivative estimation and adaptive integration. *IEEE Trans Image Process.* 2002;11(10):1192–1200.

38. Ying L, Liang ZP, Munson DC, Koetter R, Frey BJ. Unwrapping of MR phase images using a Markov random field model. *IEEE Trans Med Imaging.* 2006;25(1):128–136.

39. Webb P, Macovski A. Rapid, fully automatic, arbitrary-volume in vivo shimming. *Magn Reson Med.* 1991;20(1):113–122.

40. Schneider E, Glover G. Rapid in vivo proton shimming. *Magn Reson Med.* 1991;18(2):335–347.

41. Kanayama S, Kuhara S, Satoh K. In vivo rapid magnetic field measurement and shimming using single scan differential phase mapping. *Magn Reson Med.* 1996;36(4):637–642.

42. Gruetter R. Automatic, localized in vivo adjustment of all first- and second-order shim coils. *Magn Reson Med.* 1993;29(6):804–811.

43. Gruetter R, Boesch C. Fast noniterative shimming of spatially localised signals. In vivo analysis of the magnetic-field along axis. *J Magn Reson.* 1992;96(2):323–334.

44. Gruetter R, Tkáč I. Field mapping without reference scan using asymmetric echo-planar techniques. *Magn Reson Med.* 2000;43(2): 319–323.

45. Shen J, Rycyna RE, Rothman DL. Improvements on an in vivo automatic shimming method (FASTERMAP). *Magn Reson Med.* 1997;38(5):834–839.

46. Chen Z, Li SS, Yang J, Letizia D, Shen J. Measurement and automatic correction of high-order B_0 inhomogeneity in the rat brain at 11.7 Tesla. *Magn Reson Imaging.* 2004;22(6):835–842.

47. Shen J, Rothman DL, Hetherington HP, Pan JW. Linear projection method for automatic slice shimming. *Magn Reson Med.* 1999;42(6): 1082–1088.

48. Klassen LM, Menon RS. Robust automated shimming technique using arbitrary mapping acquisition parameters (RASTAMAP). *Magn Reson Med.* 2004;51(5):881–887.

49. Kim DH, Adalsteinsson E, Glover GH, Spielman DM. Regularized higher-order in vivo shimming. *Magn Reson Med.* 2002;48(4):715–722.

50. Reese TG, Davis TL, Weisskoff RM. Automated shimming at 1.5 T using echo-planar image frequency maps. *J Magn Reson Imaging.* 1995;5(6):739–745.

51. Hess AT, Tisdall MD, Andronesi OC, Meintjes EM, van der Kouwe AJ. Real-time motion and B_0 corrected single voxel spectroscopy using volumetric navigators. *Magn Reson Med.* 2011;66(2): 314–323.

52. Holz D, Jensen D, Proksa R, Tochtrop M, Vollmann W. Automatic shimming for localized spectroscopy. *Med Phys*. 1988;15(6):898–903.

53. Webb PG, Sailasuta N, Kohler SJ, Raidy T, Moats RA, Hurd RE. Automated single-voxel proton MRS: technical development and multisite verification. *Magn Reson Med*. 1994;31(4):365–373.

54. Lee J, Lustig M, Kim DH, Pauly JM. Improved shim method based on the minimization of the maximum off-resonance frequency for balanced steady-state free precession (bSSFP). *Magn Reson Med*. 2009;61(6):1500–1506.

55. Sánchez H, Liu F, Trakic A, Crozier S. A magnetization mapping approach for passive shim design in MRI. *Conf Proc IEEE Eng Med Biol Soc*. 2006;1:1893–1896.

56. Wen H, Jaffer FA. An in vivo automated shimming method taking into account shim current constraints. *Magn Reson Med*. 1995;34(6):898–904.

57. Merboldt KD, Finsterbusch J, Frahm J. Reducing inhomogeneity artifacts in functional MRI of human brain activation — thin sections vs gradient compensation. *J Magn Reson*. 2000;145(2):184–191.

58. Constable RT. Functional MR imaging using gradient-echo echo-planar imaging in the presence of large static field inhomogeneities. *J Magn Reson Imaging*. 1995;5(6):746–752.

59. Deichmann R, Josephs O, Hutton C, Corfield DR, Turner R. Compensation of susceptibility-induced BOLD sensitivity losses in echo-planar fMRI imaging. *Neuroimage*. 2002;15(1):120–135.

60. Frahm J, Merboldt KD, Hänicke W. Direct FLASH MR imaging of magnetic field inhomogeneities by gradient compensation. *Magn Reson Med*. 1988;6(4):474–480.

61. Glover GH. 3D z-shim method for reduction of susceptibility effects in BOLD fMRI. *Magn Reson Med*. 1999;42(2):290–299.

62. Yang QX, Dardzinski BJ, Li SL, Eslinger PJ, Smith MB. Multigradient echo with susceptibility inhomogeneity compensation (MGESIC): demonstration of fMRI in the olfactory cortex at 3.0 T. *Magn Reson Med*. 1997;37(3):331–335.

63. Yang QX, Wang J, Smith MB, et al. Reduction of magnetic field inhomogeneity artifacts in echo planar imaging with SENSE and GESEPI at high fields. *Magn Reson Med*. 2004;52(6):1418–1423.

64. Yang QX, Williams GD, Demeure RJ, Mosher TJ, Smith MB. Removal of local field gradient artifacts in T$_2^*$-weighted images at high fields by gradient-echo slice excitation profile imaging. *Magn Reson Med*. 1998;39(3):402–409.

65. Constable RT, Spencer DD. Composite image formation in z-shimmed functional MR imaging. *Magn Reson Med*. 1999;42(1):110–117.

66. Finsterbusch J, Eippert F, Büchel C. Single, slice-specific z-shim gradient pulses improve T$_2^*$-weighted imaging of the spinal cord. *Neuroimage*. 2012;59(3):2307–2315.

67. Rick J, Speck O, Maier S, et al. Optimized EPI for FMRI using a slice-dependent template-based gradient compensation method to recover local susceptibility-induced signal loss. *Magn Reson Mater Phys Biol Med*. 2010;23(3):165–176.

68. Pauly J, Nishimura D, Macovski A. A k-space analysis of small-tip-angle excitations. *J Magn Reson*. 1989;81(1):43–56.

69. Chen NK, Wyrwicz AM. Removal of intravoxel dephasing artifact in gradient-echo images using a field-map based RF refocusing technique. *Magn Reson Med*. 1999;42(4):807–812.

70. Glover GH, Lai S. Reduction of susceptibility effects in BOLD fMRI using tailored RF pulses. *Proc Intl Soc Magn Reson Med*. 1998;6:298.

71. Cho ZH, Ro YM. Reduction of susceptibility artifact in gradient-echo imaging. *Magn Reson Med*. 1992;23(1):193–200.

72. Bottomley PA, Hardy CJ. Two-dimensional spatially selective spin inversion and spin-echo refocusing with a single nuclear magnetic resonance pulse. *J Appl Phys*. 1987;62(10):4284–4290.

73. Hardy CJ, Cline HE. Spatial localization in two dimensions using NMR designer pulses. *J Magn Reson*. 1989;82(3):647–654.

74. Pauly JM, Hu BS, Wang SJ, Nishimura DG, Macovski A. A three-dimensional spin-echo or inversion pulse. *Magn Reson Med*. 1993;29(1):2–6.

75. Stenger VA, Boada FE, Noll DC. Three-dimensional tailored RF pulses for reduction of susceptibility artifacts in T$_2^*$-weighted functional MRI. *Magn Reson Med*. 2000;44(4):525–531.

76. Yip CY, Fessler JA, Noll DC. Advanced three-dimensional tailored RF pulse for signal recovery in T$_2^*$-weighted functional magnetic resonance imaging. *Magn Reson Med*. 2006;56(5):1050–1059.

77. Stenger VA, Boada FE, Noll DC. Variable-density spiral 3D tailored RF pulses. *Magn Reson Med*. 2003;50(5):1100–1106.

78. Stenger VA, Giurgi MS, Boada FE, Noll DC. Excitation UNFOLD (XUNFOLD) to improve the temporal resolution of multishot tailored RF pulses. *Magn Reson Med*. 2006;56(3):692–697.

79. Katscher U, Börnert P, Leussler C, van den Brink JS. Transmit SENSE. *Magn Reson Med*. 2003;49(1):144–150.

80. Zhong J, Kennan RP, Gore JC. Effects of susceptibility variations on NMR measurements of diffusion. *J Magn Reson*. 1991;95:267–280.

81. Neeman M, Freyer JP, Sillerud LO. A simple method for obtaining cross-term-free images for diffusion anisotropy studies in NMR microimaging. *Magn Reson Med*. 1991;21(1):138–143.

82. Karlicek RF, Lowe IJ. A modified pulse gradient technique for measuring diffusion in the presence of large background gradients. *J Magn Reson*. 1980;37(1):75–91.

83. Koch MA, Finsterbusch J. Compartment size estimation with double wave vector diffusion-weighted imaging. *Magn Reson Med*. 2008;60(1):90–101.

84. Carlsson Å, Ljungberg M, Starck G, Forssell-Aronsson E. Degraded water suppression in small volume ^{1}H MRS due to localised shimming. *Magn Reson Mater Phys Biol Med*. 2011;24(2):97–107.

85. Moonen CTW, Sobering G, van Zijl PCM, Gillen J, von Kienlin M, Bizzi A. Proton spectroscopic imaging of the human brain. *J Magn Reson*. 1992;98(3):556–575.

86. Henning A, Schär M, Kollias SS, Boesiger P, Dydak U. Quantitative magnetic resonance spectroscopy in the entire human cervical spinal cord and beyond at 3 T. *Magn Reson Med*. 2008;59(6):1250–1258.

87. Ernst T, Chang L. Elimination of artifacts in short echo time H MR spectroscopy of the frontal lobe. *Magn Reson Med*. 1996;36(3):462–468.

88. Verma T, Cohen-Adad J. Effect of Respiration on the B0 Field in the Human Spinal Cord at 3T. *Magn Reson Med*. 2014. http://dx.doi.org/10.1002/mrm.25075.

2.3

Susceptibility Artifacts

Emine U. Saritas[1,2], *Samantha J. Holdsworth*[3], *Roland Bammer*[3]

[1]Department of Bioengineering, University of California, Berkeley, CA, USA

[2]Department of Electrical and Electronics Engineering, Bilkent University, Ankara, Turkey

[3]Center for Quantitative Neuroimaging, Department of Radiology, Stanford University, Stanford, CA, USA

2.3.1 INTRODUCTION: SOURCES OF SUSCEPTIBILITY ARTIFACTS

The uniformity of the B_0 main field in magnetic resonance imaging (MRI) is critical for artifact-free image formation. MRI scanners are manufactured with a stringent requirement of less than one part-per-million (ppm)[a] variation in the B_0 field. However, this 1 ppm theoretical homogeneity easily gets distorted once a subject is placed inside the MRI scanner, mainly due to a 9 ppm magnetic susceptibility difference between air and tissue. The presence of any surgical implants further exacerbates the problem, as different tissue types, air, and metal all interact with and distort the applied magnetic field differently. This interaction is quantified by what is called the magnetic susceptibility of a matter.[1]

The susceptibility variations in tissue on a microscopic scale are in fact the source of many useful contrast mechanisms in MRI, such as blood oxygenation level-dependent (BOLD) functional MRI (fMRI) and diagnosis of cerebral hemorrhage. However, a macroscopic susceptibility variation leads to a global field inhomogeneity, which in turn creates off-resonance induced artifacts in the images. These artifacts manifest as faster T_2^* decay, signal dropouts and pileups, geometric distortions, and incomplete fat suppression. High-field MRI scans especially suffer from susceptibility artifacts, as the absolute size of the field perturbations increases linearly with B_0 field strength. For example, the 9 ppm susceptibility difference between air and tissue corresponds to a 575 Hz field variation at 1.5 T, while it is doubled to a 1150 Hz variation at 3 T. While a global frequency shift can be easily dealt with by

adjusting the center frequency, it is the local field inhomogeneity that perturbs the imaging process.

In vivo MRI of the spinal cord is especially challenging due to susceptibility variations between various tissue types (e.g., vertebrae, muscle, CSF, gray and white matter, fat, air in the lungs and trachea, bowel gas, and surgical implants) that significantly distort the applied magnetic field. As shown by the B_0 field maps of the spine (Figure 2.3.1), the air in the lungs and nasal cavities as well as the curvature in the neck significantly distort the field around the spinal cord. Furthermore, susceptibility differences between vertebral spinous processes and connective tissue create local field inhomogeneities along the spinal cord itself, as seen in Figure 2.3.1(B). Bulk physiologic motion from cardiac and respiratory cycles, CSF pulsation, as well as breathing and swallowing further cause temporal variations of these field inhomogeneities.

This chapter gives an overview of susceptibility artifacts and how they manifest in EPI images of the spinal cord. Methods to alleviate these artifacts will be outlined. Please note that while this chapter mostly presents examples of susceptibility artifacts on sagittal images, axial and coronal orientations are equally affected.

2.3.2 ARTIFACTS IN EPI OF THE SPINAL CORD

Single-shot echo planar imaging (ss-EPI) remains the most frequently used technique for most of the quantitative imaging methods, because it acquires the whole of

---

[a]In MRI, the variations in B_0 field or the differences in resonant frequencies are so small that they are expressed in "parts per million", or ppm. For example, 1 ppm inhomogeneity at 1.5 T corresponds to a 1.5 μT variation in the B_0 field. This field variation would in turn result in a 63.87 Hz off-resonance (i.e., one-millionth of the center frequency of $f_0 = 63.87$ MHz at 1.5 T).

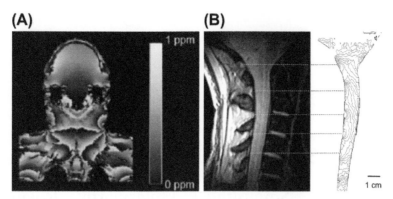

FIGURE 2.3.1 B_0 field maps of the cervical spine, showing over 6 ppm variation in field homogeneity. (A) The coronal view of the cervicothoracic area shows how the lungs and the nasal cavities contribute to field variations. Here, each phase wrap reflects a 1 ppm field change. (B) T_1-weighted sagittal view of the spinal cord and contour plot of the B_0 field map showing local distortions in magnetic field caused by susceptibility differences between vertebral spinous processes and connective tissue. Note how the regions shown with the dashed lines experience high distortion in the EPI image in Figure 2.3.2(C). Contour spacing = 10 Hz at 2 T field, or approximately 0.1 ppm. *Source: (A) from Reference 2; (B) obtained with permission from Ref. 3.*

k-space after a single excitation. This fast imaging capability is especially critical for methods that are sensitive to subject motion (e.g., diffusion-weighted imaging (DWI)) or for methods that require a high temporal resolution (e.g., fMRI).

Although ss-EPI performs relatively well in the brain, the anatomy of the spine as well as the abundance of susceptibility variations make it particularly difficult to produce high-quality ss-EPI images of the spinal cord. The long and narrow anatomy of the spine requires a large field of view (FOV) in the superior-inferior (S/I) direction, and the small cross-sectional size of the spinal cord mandates high-spatial-resolution images. Even in the axial imaging plane, where the spinal cord presents a small region of interest (ROI), the rest of the body dictates a large FOV. Covering a large FOV with high resolution requires long readout durations in EPI, which in turn result in distortions and severe blurring of the images along the phase-encoding (PE) direction. In addition, the long interval between subsequent k-space lines (i.e., echo spacing) causes significant image distortions due to off-resonance effects.

The location-dependent geometric distortion in an EPI image can be expressed as:

$$d_{PE}(r) = \frac{\Delta f(r)\, T_{ESP}\, FOV_{PE}}{N_{int}\, R}. \qquad (2.3.1)$$

Here, $d_{PE}(r)$ is the local displacement of a voxel in the PE direction (i.e., the voxel appears at position $r + d_{PE}(r)$ instead of at r), $\Delta f(r)$ (in Hertz) represents a field inhomogeneity or off-resonance effect observed at position r, and FOV_{PE} is the FOV in the PE direction, T_{ESP} (in seconds) is the time interval between two adjacent echoes during an EPI readout (referred to as the "echo spacing"), N_{int} is the number of interleaves in EPI (e.g., $N_{int} = 1$ for ss-EPI), and R denotes the

acceleration factor for parallel imaging (e.g., $R = 1$ for no acceleration). As seen in Eqn (2.3.1), a large FOV, increased readout duration due to a need for high resolution, and increased susceptibility variations all contribute to geometric distortions in EPI images. For example, a local 6 ppm off-resonance at 3 T, a FOV-$_{PE} = 18$ cm, and $T_{ESP} = 0.5$ ms (all typical numbers in the spine) would cause close to 7 cm local displacement for regular ss-EPI. This level of distortion, as demonstrated in Figure 2.3.2(C), can easily render regular ss-EPI images clinically unusable.

ss-EPI images also exhibit a substantial water–fat misalignment, as the frequency term in Eqn (2.3.1) also applies to chemical shifts. For example, for the aforementioned imaging parameters, the fat image would experience a 4 cm shift in the PE direction with respect to the water image (assuming a chemical shift of 3.5 ppm, i.e., 440 Hz at 3 T). Hence, ss-EPI mandates proper shimming of the ROI, as well as a robust fat suppression or spectrally selective excitation.[4,5] These fat suppression schemes usually take advantage of the chemical shift (i.e., differences in resonant frequencies) between fat and water. Unfortunately, susceptibility variations around the spine can distort the field homogeneity to such an extent that effective fat suppression is often an issue. For example, a local 440 Hz susceptibility-induced off-resonance at 3 T would cause the water signal to be suppressed, instead of the fat signal. Figure 2.3.2(B) demonstrates this phenomenon, where the susceptibility variations around the cervical spine resulted in an incomplete fat suppression (white arrow) and a signal dropout (red arrow).

The position dependency of susceptibility effects causes different regions in the FOV to experience different levels of displacement, further complicating the problem. This nonrigid distortion is typically

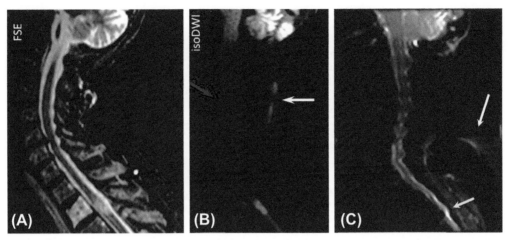

FIGURE 2.3.2   Various manifestations of susceptibility artifacts. (A) T_2-weighted fast spin-echo image showing the anatomy, and (B) corresponding isotropic diffusion-weighted image acquired using interleaved EPI. Susceptibility variations around the spine result in incomplete fat suppression (white arrow) and a signal drop (red arrow). (C) T_2-weighted single-shot EPI of the cervical spine demonstrates high levels of distortion, as well as incomplete fat suppression (white arrow). Local susceptibility differences between vertebral spinous processes and connective tissue, as shown in Figure 2.3.1(B), result in a comb-like appearance of the spine. In the cervicothoracic junction, the signals from the spinal cord and the CSF are piled up, while the neighboring pixels (where CSF was supposed to be) are left devoid of signal (yellow arrow).

observed as signal pileups or dropouts in an EPI image. The cervicothoracic junction in Figure 2.3.2(C) shows one such case, where the signals from the spinal cord and the CSF are piled up, while the neighboring pixels (where CSF was supposed to be) are left devoid of signal (yellow arrow). A less severe manifestation of this susceptibility artifact is the comb-like appearance of the spinal cord in Figure 2.3.2(C), which is caused by the local field inhomogeneities along the spinal cord (see Figure 2.3.1(B)).

2.3.3 METHODS TO REDUCE SUSCEPTIBILITY ARTIFACTS

There are various approaches that can be used to reduce susceptibility artifacts for spinal cord imaging; unfortunately, many of these methods have only been demonstrated in the research arena and are not available on clinical scanners. These approaches target one (or more) of the variables in Eqn (2.3.1), which can be rewritten as:

$$d_{PE}(r) = \frac{\Delta f(r)}{S_k} \qquad (2.3.2)$$

where S_k is the speed of k-space traversal, i.e.,

$$S_k = \frac{\Delta k_{PE}}{\Delta t_{PE}} = \frac{N_{int} R}{FOV_{PE} T_{ESP}} \qquad (2.3.3)$$

Here, Δk_{PE} is the distance between adjacent k-space lines during readout, and Δt_{PE} is the time interval between the echoes from these k-space lines, which is equal to the echo spacing, T_{ESP}.

As seen in Eqn (2.3.2), one can reduce susceptibility artifacts by reducing the *off-resonance effect*, or $\Delta f(r)$. This goal can be achieved to a certain extent by passive or active shimming of the areas of interest (see Section 2.3.3.6 and Chapter 2.2); however, local field inhomogeneities remain unaddressed.

The other (rather more tortuous) method is to *accelerate the traversal of k-space* (i.e., increase S_k) by altering the MRI pulse sequence, as outlined schematically in Figure 2.3.3. A reduction of the *echo spacing* (T_{ESP}) can be achieved by (1) increasing the EPI bandwidth and/or sampling on the gradient ramps of the EPI trajectory, and/or (2) segmenting the k-space trajectory, such as by the readout-segmented EPI approach (a "multishot" method). Interleaved EPI methods speed up the k-space traversal by dividing the k-space into several sections that are each acquired faster but in separate repetition times (TRs).[6–8] A reduction in the *phase-encoding* FOV (FOV$_{PE}$) in spine imaging with standard slice-selective pulses can cause undesired aliasing in the PE direction if the object is larger than FOV$_{PE}$, even after using graphical saturation pulses. Thus, more advanced reduced FOV methods that alter the radiofrequency (RF) pulses or that use outer volume suppression methods have been implemented for the spinal cord.[9–12] Parallel imaging methods provide *acceleration* in k-space by utilizing the complementary spatial encoding information from multiple receiver coil elements to reduce the number of acquired k-space lines.[13–15]

Ideally, a combination of all of these methods could be used; however, each of these techniques presents a rather complicated set of advantages and limitations.

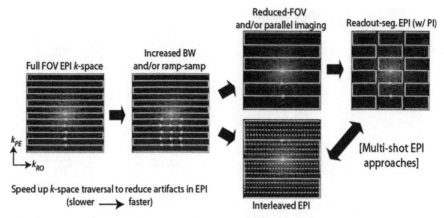

FIGURE 2.3.3   Overview of some of the MRI pulse sequence techniques described in this chapter. To reduce susceptibility artifacts in EPI, we need to speed up k-space traversal (methods are listed in increasing k-space traversal speed, with faster methods on the right). Increased readout bandwidth (BW) and ramp sampling both help decrease the echo spacing between adjacent k-space lines. Reducing the phase-encoding FOV, parallel imaging, and dividing the k-space into interleaves all help to speed up k-space traversal by skipping lines during readout in a single TR. A more advanced multishot method is to segment the k-space along the readout direction to shorten the echo spacing. These methods can be combined to reach a desired level of acceleration.

The remainder of this section discusses various approaches to reduce susceptibility distortions, and their relative advantages and disadvantages.

2.3.3.1 Reduced Echo-Spacing Methods

Susceptibility effects can be alleviated by reducing the echo spacing between adjacent k-space lines during readout in a single TR. For a fixed image resolution, the easiest way to achieve this goal is (1) to increase the readout bandwidth (BW), and/or (2) to acquire data during the gradient ramps (also known as "ramp sampling") in addition to the gradient plateaus. Increasing the bandwidth reduces the signal-to-noise ratio (SNR) due to a shorter readout. However, if a region experiences severe off-resonance effects, the decreased readout duration can actually reduce the dephasing in a voxel, resulting in an *increase* in local signal level. Ramp sampling is an especially important implementation that comes at very little disadvantage, other than the need for 1D-gridding of the data acquired during gradient ramps.

Both ramp sampling and increasing the bandwidth are methods available on most commercial MRI scanners. In some scanners, there is no direct relationship between the echo spacing and the BW, due to hardware limitations (e.g., gradient-switching time). In practice, the user can increase the BW and stop when the echo spacing is at its minimum. Note that although reducing the echo spacing is the easiest way to alleviate susceptibility artifacts, it can fail to provide a significant improvement in image quality, given that the readout bandwidth in an MRI scanner has an upper limit (typically a maximum of ± 250 kHz). The methods described in the remainder of this section usually build on top of

a ramp-sampled, high-bandwidth EPI sequence, and they provide additional ways to speed up k-space traversal in EPI.

2.3.3.2 Reduced Field-of-View Methods

Spinal cord imaging has been shown to benefit from reduced FOV (rFOV) acquisitions that limit the extent of coverage in the phase-encoding direction (i.e., FOV_{PE}). With a much smaller FOV_{PE}, the number of required k-space lines is also reduced (typically between one-half and one-fourth of the full-FOV case), which in turn significantly reduces off-resonance induced artifacts. As expected, the SNR is also reduced by the square root of the FOV_{PE} reduction factor. Although both reduced-FOV and parallel imaging methods reduce the number of acquired k-space lines to achieve high-quality images, they significantly differ in implementation. Parallel imaging methods (see Section 2.3.3.3) take advantage of the orthogonality of coil sensitivities, while the rFOV techniques actively limit the extent of FOV through pulse sequence modifications.

Figure 2.3.4 demonstrates the effectiveness of rFOV techniques, where reducing the FOV_{PE} to one-fourth of its full-FOV value alleviates the distortions in the ss-EPI image of the spinal cord, even in the presence of metallic implants.[16] Recently, a number of rFOV methods have been proposed for high-resolution ss-EPI of the spinal cord. A schematic explanation of some of these methods is given in Figure 2.3.5.

One of these rFOV methods utilizes outer-volume suppression pulses preceding the excitation pulse[10] (shown in Figure 2.3.5(A)). This technique can be implemented by placing suppression bands anterior and/or posterior to the spine. Similar implementations of this

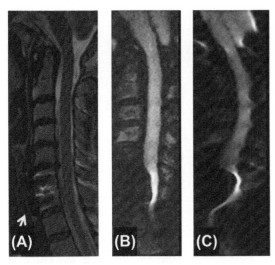

FIGURE 2.3.4 Diffusion-weighted ss-EPI images of the cervical spine of a patient post cervical discectomy and fusion, acquired using a four-channel spine array coil with phase encoding performed in the anterior–posterior direction, and matrix size $= 192 \times 192$. (A) T$_2$-weighted fast spin-echo image is given for anatomical reference. ss-EPI images with (B) a 25% FOV$_{PE}$ (i.e., 18 cm $\times$ 4.5 cm), and (C) full FOV (i.e., 18 cm $\times$ 18 cm). The reduced-FOV image (B) has fourfold reduced distortion when compared to the full-FOV image (C), demonstrating the effectiveness of the reduced-FOV method in alleviating susceptibility-induced distortions. Note that the reduced-FOV method mitigates but does not fully eliminate the metallic artifact associated with the plate between the vertebral bodies. *Source: Figure from Ref. 16.*

method are available on most commercial MRI scanners, and they usually involve graphical prescription of suppression and saturation bands. However, because the suppression efficiency is generally limited, it can lead to partial aliasing artifacts in the PE direction of the images. These artifacts are sometimes difficult to detect, as the aliased signal can resemble noise due to its

attenuated amplitude. Hence, it is imperative to perform phantom tests to assess the level of signal suppression outside the desired FOV$_{PE}$.

Another rFOV technique applies excitation and refocusing RF pulses orthogonally[17] (see Figure 2.3.5(B)), which significantly decreases the SNR of the neighboring slices if interleaved acquisition is performed. This is because the 180° pulse acts as an inversion pulse on the neighboring slice locations. A method called ZOOM-EPI[9] mitigates the SNR loss problem by applying the 180° refocusing pulse at an oblique angle, as shown in Figure 2.3.5(C). This way, the neighboring slices do not experience the refocusing pulse. However, if the neighboring slices are close to each other in space, there can still be a partial cross-saturation of the adjacent slices, resulting in a signal drop along the edges of the FOV in the PE direction. This signal drop can be alleviated by spacing the slices apart (i.e., by placing slice skips) or by extending FOV$_{PE}$. A recent approach called contiguous-slice zonally oblique multislice (CO-ZOOM) mitigates the cross-saturation problem by double refocusing the signal with two 180° pulses applied orthogonally as in Figure 2.3.5(B).[12] However, the resulting prolonged echo time (TE) decreases the signal level.

Instead of utilizing a 1D excitation pulse, 2D spatially selective RF pulses can be used to excite only the ROI for rFOV imaging.[11,18] As shown in Figure 2.3.5(D), because the adjacent slices are not excited, this method is compatible with contiguous multislice imaging without the need for a slice skip. Depending on the implementation, these 2D-RF pulses have excitation profiles periodic in either the phase or the slice direction. A subsequent 180° refocusing pulse can be utilized to refocus only the main lobe of the excitation while preserving the rFOV imaging capabilities,

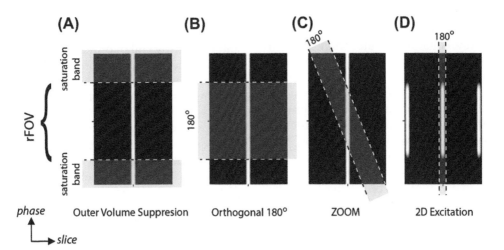

FIGURE 2.3.5 Schematic explanation of various reduced-FOV imaging methods. (A) Outer volume suppression and saturation methods utilize a regular 90° excitation followed by two suppression bands placed anterior and posterior to the region of interest. (B) Regular 90° excitation followed by an orthogonally applied 180° refocusing pulse. The 180° pulse inverts the adjacent slices, reducing the SNR during imaging. (C) ZOOM-EPI method with a tilted 180° refocusing pulse. (D) 2D spatial excitation, followed by a 180° refocusing pulse.

as demonstrated in Figure 2.3.5(D).[11] When the profile is periodic in the slice direction, the fat and water profiles are also shifted in volume in the slice direction. This feature can be exploited by designing a 2D-RF pulse with nonoverlapping fat–water profiles. Then, the subsequent 180° refocusing pulse suppresses the signal from fat without the need for additional fat suppression pulses. However, the periodicity in the slice direction may also restrict the coverage in the slice direction.[11] Likewise, if the excitation profile is periodic in the phase direction, it may place a restriction on the maximum size of the subject. This is because the periodic lobes in the phase direction can otherwise cause aliasing artifacts, as those lobes are now refocused with the 180° pulse.[18] Furthermore, because the 2D-RF pulses tend to have long durations, the slice profiles may be sensitive to off-resonance effects.

Each of these rFOV methods has its own strengths and weaknesses, and the method of choice depends on the application. In the end, they all significantly reduce the susceptibility-induced artifacts in EPI.

2.3.3.3 Parallel Imaging

Parallel imaging helps reduce the effective readout duration by decreasing the number of k-space lines (see Chapter 2.1). Data from multiple channels are then used to fill in the "missing" k-space lines through parallel imaging reconstruction procedures (such as GRAPPA[19]) or unalias reconstructed images (using SENSE[20]). Since a fully sampled k-space data set can be reconstructed from the undersampled k-space acquired in one repetition, parallel imaging–enhanced EPI is relatively robust to motion artifacts.

While parallel imaging is frequently used for distortion reduction in EPI brain scans, its efficacy is limited by both the number of available receiver coils and their geometric arrangement. This is particularly the case for spine array coils, which are often geometrically flat, have poor sensitivity in the anterior–posterior (A/P) direction, and have limited parallel imaging capability in the S/I direction. Figure 2.3.6 compares cervical spine images acquired both with and without parallel imaging performed in the A/P (phase-encoding (PE)) direction. Figure 2.3.6(C) and 2.3.6(D) were acquired with the same scan time as in Figure 2.3.6(B), but with acceleration factors of $R = 2$ and $R = 3$, respectively. While accelerating through k-space results in a two- or threefold reduction in distortion, the overall SNR is reduced for a given scan time. Even though the scan times were adjusted so that the accelerated images had approximately the same number of samples as in the unaccelerated image, one can observe the g-factor noise that obscures the pons region. This is more pronounced for the image with

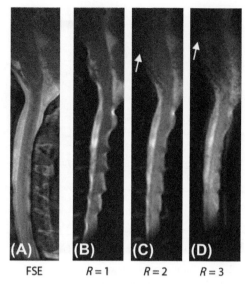

FIGURE 2.3.6 Cervical spine images acquired using a four-channel spine array coil using a matrix size = 192×192 and a FOV = $18\,\text{cm} \times 9\,\text{cm}$ (with PE performed in the A/P direction). (A) T_2-weighted fast spin-echo image is given for anatomical reference. Standard ss-EPI with (B) no acceleration, (C) $R = 2$ giving a twofold reduction in geometric distortion, and (D) $R = 3$ giving a threefold reduction in geometric distortion. All images have the same scan time. Because of the shorter trajectory and g-factor noise present in (C–D), the SNR is reduced overall. Especially the pons area experiences a significant SNR reduction, due to the diminishing coil sensitivity profiles in the A/P direction (white arrow). The decreased image quality with $R = 3$ suggests that $R = 2$ is probably the upper acceleration limit for this spine array coil.

$R = 3$, but it is noticeable even with a modest parallel acceleration factor of $R = 2$. It is for this reason that many studies of the spinal cord utilizing parallel imaging to reduce susceptibility artifacts in EPI only achieve a factor of (or near) 2.[13–15,21] At such small acceleration factors, parallel imaging alone is often not effective in obtaining submillimeter in-plane resolution with adequate image quality.

For cervical scans, one may be inclined to use a head and neck array coil in order to leverage on its improved parallel imaging performance capability. Unfortunately, few conventional head and neck coils have geometric arrangements suitable for high acceleration factors. However, some promising work has been shown with the development of a 32-channel coil that fully covers the brain and cervical spine.[22] Diffusion tensor imaging (DTI) results acquired with this coil are shown in Figure 2.3.7, with noticeable reduction in geometric distortion with increasing acceleration factors (of up to four).

2.3.3.4 Multishot EPI Techniques

As shown in Figure 2.3.3, it is possible to reduce susceptibility artifacts by traversing k-space faster through the use of multishot EPI techniques. The most common

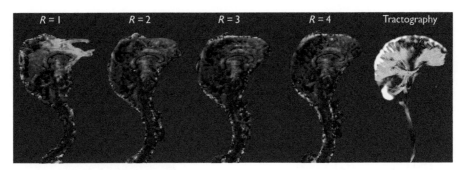

FIGURE 2.3.7 Parallel imaging at various acceleration factors using EPI readout and a 32-channel coil that fully covers the brain and cervical spine.[22] Fractional anisotropy (FA) color maps from this DTI scan show a noticeable reduction in geometric distortion with increasing acceleration factors. GRAPPA reconstruction was utilized for parallel imaging. TR = 14280 ms, echo time (TE) = 80 ms, resolution = $1.7 \times 1.7 \times 1.7$ mm^3, 30 diffusion-encoding directions, b-value = 800 s/mm^2. *Source: Images courtesy of Julien Cohen-Adad.*

multishot EPI technique is called interleaved EPI (IEPI),[23] which is becoming a promising approach in clinical spine DWI acquisitions.[6–8,24–28] With this method, the number of k-space lines per interleaf is reduced by acquiring multiple EPI interleaves in the phase-encoding direction. For example, for $N_{int} = 2$, each interleaf traverses the k-space by skipping every other line. These two interleaves are then combined to form the full k-space data. The disadvantage of the IEPI approach is that motion can occur between the acquisition of different interleaves, which can lead to ghosting artifacts or even result in gaps in k-space (for diffusion-MRI methods after phase correction), leading to aliasing artifacts and residual ghosting in the final image.

Figure 2.3.8 demonstrates that one can acquire anatomically reliable DWI images using IEPI with 11 shots (and 15 echoes per interleaf). According to Eqn

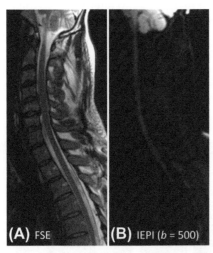

FIGURE 2.3.8 Isotropic diffusion-weighted interleaved EPI sequence showing high geometric fidelity in the spinal cord. (A) T$_2$-weighted fast spin-echo image for anatomical reference, and (B) isotropic diffusion-weighted image acquired using IEPI (15 lines and 11 shots), with b-value = 500 s/mm^2.

(2.3.1), the distortion artifacts can be reduced by a factor that is proportional to the number of interleaves. The shortened readout in IEPI helps to reduce image blurring that is caused by field inhomogeneity and chemical shift. In addition, the flexibility in choice of interleaves in IEPI allows one to use larger acquisition matrices, which enables one to acquire images with higher spatial resolution. With smaller voxel sizes, distortions from intravoxel dephasing can also be mitigated. Multiple signal averages (excitations) can then be used to compensate for the decreased SNR associated with smaller voxels. Some work has coupled the IEPI approach with reduced FOV for DWI, achieving images at a resolution capable of revealing strong diffusional anisotropy in spinal cord white matter.[28]

The trade-off for using a multishot echo planar technique is that the segmentation of k-space not only increases the scan time compared with single-shot EPI but also results in phase error discontinuities from off-resonant spins and random motion-induced phase fluctuations for each interleaf.[29] Phase error discontinuities require echo-time shifting,[29] as well as monitoring and retrospective correction of phase errors by means of navigator echoes.[30,31]

Despite the use of navigators in IEPI, motion remains a difficult problem, particularly for diffusion imaging where significant motion can cause gaps in between the interleaves, resulting in aliasing artifacts. An alternative multishot approach that is less prone to motion is readout-segmented EPI (RS-EPI),[32] which covers k-space with a series of consecutive segments. As in Eqn (2.3.1), in RS-EPI the echo-spacing T_{ESP} is reduced by segmenting the k-space trajectory along the readout dimension. Here, geometric distortion is reduced by an extent that is roughly inversely proportional to the width of the segment. In RS-EPI, each segment acquires a full-FOV (low-resolution) image that is largely motion-free. Thus, correction for motion is required

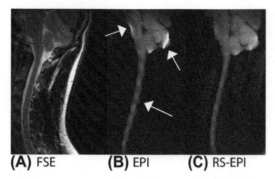

FIGURE 2.3.9 Cervical spine images showing (A) a fast spin-echo for geometric reference, and isotropic diffusion-weighted ($b = 500$ s/mm^2) images acquired at matched resolution (1.5 mm × 1.5 mm × 4 mm) and matched scan time (2:30 min) using (B) EPI (echo spacing = 726 μs) and (C) RS-EPI (effective echo spacing = 316 μs).

only between segments, which can be performed with the use of a navigator image. Any "gaps" in k-space that arise due to this correction are quite benign as demonstrated in DWI neuroimaging.[33] Figure 2.3.9 shows a comparison between EPI and RS-EPI isotropic diffusion-weighted images acquired with the same scan time at a matrix size of 192 × 192. Using 32 × 192 segments in RS-EPI results in a 2.3-fold reduction in distortion. It is possible to further reduce susceptibility artifacts using smaller segment widths, which is analogous to the use of more interleaves in IEPI. However, this comes at a considerable cost in SNR efficiency and greater sensitivity to motion artifacts.

As in reduced-FOV IEPI, it is intuitive to use RS-EPI with reduced-FOV imaging approaches to get the benefits of both methods for reducing distortion. Figure 2.3.10 shows the improvement of image quality in a thoracic DTI scan as one goes from standard (full FOV) EPI, to reduced-FOV ZOOM-EPI, and finally to reduced-FOV ZOOM-RS-EPI.

In addition, equipped with a coil suitable for parallel imaging, one can also benefit from accelerating the RS-EPI trajectory with parallel imaging. As shown in

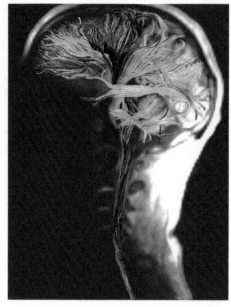

FIGURE 2.3.11 Fiber tractography using parallel imaging combined with RS-EPI. This image was acquired using a 32-channel brain and spine coil,[22] 3 RS-EPI segments, 34 slices, cardiac gating, 2.2 mm isotropic resolution, TR/TE = 15 s/66 ms, matrix = 138 × 104, $R = 3$ (GRAPPA reconstruction), BW = 1510 Hz/pixel, echo spacing = 0.38 ms, twice-refocused pulse, b-value = 800 s/mm^2, 30 diffusion-encoding directions. *Source: Images courtesy of Julien Cohen-Adad.*

Figure 2.3.11, it is possible to achieve high-quality fiber tractography images of the cervical spinal cord and brain with the use of RS-EPI accelerated by a factor of 3.

2.3.3.5 Other (Non-EPI) Techniques

2.3.3.5.1 *Line Scan Imaging*

Line scan imaging is an alternative to the EPI acquisition scheme that has been used for diffusion-weighted MRI in the spinal cord. It consists of sequential single-shot acquisition of PE lines. Line scan imaging is relatively insensitive to B_0-field inhomogeneities, eddy currents, and bulk motion, and can provide rectangular

FIGURE 2.3.10 Comparison between the $b = 0$ s/mm^2 images of a thoracic spine using full FOV EPI (30 × 30 cm, matrix size = 200 × 200), ZOOM-EPI, and ZOOM-RS-EPI (30 × 10 cm, matrix size = 200 × 60 (square pixels)). For ZOOM-RS-EPI, the isotropic DWI (isoDWI, $b = 500$ s/mm^2), fractional anisotropy (FA), and the first eigenvector (color map) are also shown. Note that there is less "disc bulging" into the spinal canal and less blurring on the ZOOM-RS-EPI scans than on the ZOOM-EPI scans.

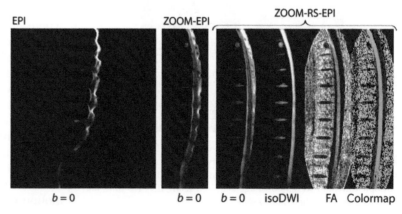

diffusion-weighted images.[34–36] Previous studies have compared single-shot EPI and line scan imaging.[37] It was applied in children,[38] in the human spinal cord,[39–41] and in the spine.[42] However, the trade-off of line scan imaging acquisition schemes is the relatively long acquisition time to image a large volume, and missing k-space lines in the presence of extensive motion.

2.3.3.5.2 Fast Spin-Echo

Rapid acquisition with relaxation enhancement (RARE) is a spin-echo (SE) sequence with refocusing pulses after RF excitation to significantly decrease relaxation time, thus enabling the introduction of more excitation pulses in a given time in comparison to the standard SE sequence. With RARE, the RF refocusing yields signal decay with T_2 rather than T_2^*, making this sequence less sensitive to off-resonance effects and eddy currents.[43] A number of variations of the RARE sequence have been developed, including fast spin-echo (FSE) and turbo spin echo (TSE). Some studies have demonstrated the benefits of FSE for imaging the human spinal cord with DTI.[13,44,45] Although faster than standard SE, this sequence is much slower than EPI.

2.3.3.5.3 Radial and Spiral Acquisition

In contrast to the classical Cartesian k-space filling, radial acquisition is made up of phase lines passing through the center of k-space, while spiral acquisition consists of acquisition in a "spiral" trajectory starting from either the center or periphery of k-space. Hence, in both radial acquisition and spiral acquisition, all readout trajectories are symmetric to the origin of k-space and are equivalent with respect to the reconstruction. This is not the case in conventional Cartesian readout schemes, where a single corrupted data line can degrade the complete image.[46] Due to the high density of data at the center of k-space, the SNR is still acceptable when fewer phase lines are acquired compared to the Cartesian k-space sampling scheme. A disadvantage of radial and spiral acquisition schemes, however, is the potential for streak or "aura" (or swirl) artifacts due to the undersampling of the azimuthal regions in k-space.[47] Instead of single lines, one could acquire blades consisting of several lines, which are then rotated to provide better navigation capabilities.[48,49] This technique is known as periodically rotated overlapping parallel lines with enhanced reconstruction (PROPELLER). A radial EPI technique using this approach has been proposed and yielded very promising results in the abdomen[50] and in the spinal cord.[51] Here, it is important to note that for the EPI-variant of PROPELLER, the readout is along the short axis of the blade to shorten the echo spacing. The radial FSE technique was further improved by using a wider refocusing

slice to decrease B_1-field inhomogeneity effects.[52,53] Additionally, self-navigated, interleaved, variable-density spiral-based DTI acquisition (SNAILS) at high spatial resolutions have recently shown promising results in a cat model of spinal cord injury during free breathing.[54]

2.3.3.6 Decreasing Off-Resonance

In addition to adjusting the imaging parameters, susceptibility artifacts can be reduced by repositioning the subject, reorienting the slice, or applying active- and/or passive-shimming methods. For example, the curvature in the neck creates an abundance of air–tissue interfaces, and the resulting magnetic field inhomogeneity makes fat suppression difficult. To improve the magnetic field homogeneity, the patient's head can be supported by foam pads in order to achieve maximum anteflexion without the patient feeling uncomfortable.[8] In this position, the neck rests nearly flat on the coil, minimizing the volume of air between the spine and the coil. This repositioning makes the subsequent shimming more effective, especially when using surface coils. In kyphotic patients, however, this can be rather difficult to perform. For axial imaging of the spine, instead of repositioning the patient, one can carefully reorient the slices so that they are centered within vertebral bodies.[55] This in turn minimizes the effects of field inhomogeneities from vertebral bodies shown in Figure 2.3.1(B).

Off-resonance artifacts can also be improved by active or passive shimming of the ROI. Of the active-shimming methods, first-order gradient shimming of the ROI is standard in most MRI scanners. These shims only correct for linear variations in the local field. However, spinal cord imaging can significantly benefit from higher order shimming, especially at high field strengths. As seen in Figure 2.3.12(A), both the signal level and the distortion (seen with the curvature of the spine) are improved by applying a second-order shim.

Another way to improve field homogeneity near the air-tissue interface is to fill the air with a material that is susceptibility-matched to tissue to move the inhomogeneities outside the imaging FOV. This is a simple, passive, and direct technique for reducing B_0 inhomogeneities at air-tissue boundaries. For this method to be effective, the susceptibility-matching material needs to be MRI invisible, such that it does not extend the size of the FOV in any direction. These criteria are satisfied by fluids such as perfluorocarbon,[56] barium sulfate-doped water,[57] Kaopectate,[58] and a recently proposed pyrolytic graphite (PG)-doped foam.[59] Figure 2.3.12(A) demonstrates how this PG foam improves the field map around the spine when it is positioned behind the neck.

Although active- and passive-shimming methods can significantly improve the image quality, they both have

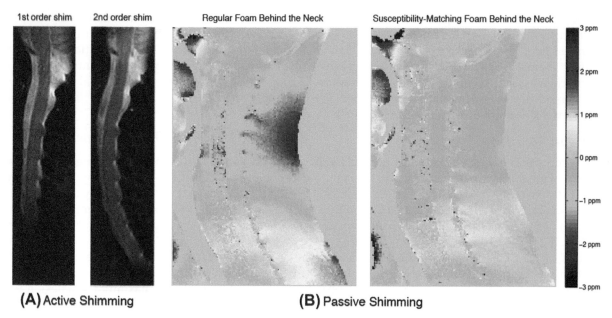

(A) Active Shimming   **(B)** Passive Shimming

FIGURE 2.3.12   Effects of shimming on susceptibility-induced off-resonance. (A) T_2-weighted reduced-FOV ss-EPI images of the spinal cord, acquired at 3 T, with first-order (i.e., linear) shim versus second-order shim. Note the improvement in the signal level and distortion (seen with the curvature of the spine) using higher order shimming. (B) Field maps of the spine acquired with regular foam versus susceptibility-matching foam placed behind the neck. With the susceptibility-matching foam, the air volume in the back of the neck is filled with a material that has the same magnetic susceptibility as that of human tissue. Hence, the field map is significantly improved (*Source: Passive-shimming images courtesy of Gary Lee*). Please see Chapter 2.2 for more information on shimming.

limitations. Active-shimming methods cannot correct for high-spatial-frequency perturbations in the field,[60] because the shim coils are physically too large to generate high-spatial-frequency field patterns deep within a patient.[1] Similarly, passive-shimming methods can only fix the problems where the air–tissue interface is accessible, and they cannot address susceptibility variations due to air in the lungs, trachea, and sinuses. In addition, some of the shimming methods are difficult to apply in clinical settings. Hence, it is best to combine practical shimming methods with acquisition- and reconstruction-based distortion reduction methods, some of which are discussed in Section 2.3.3.7.

2.3.3.7 Distortion Correction Methods

While distortion correction methods have been used for neuroimaging applications for quite some time, there are a few studies that have incorporated and tailored the use of these methods for spinal cord imaging. It is not surprising that these postprocessing methods are not readily available on clinical MRI scanners.

There are a number of "distortion correction" strategies available, including the point spread function (PSF),[61] phase field map method,[62–64] reversed gradient polarity method (RGPM),[65–69] and co-registration methods.[70,71] The first three of these methods must

incorporate extra measurements in the acquisition, and all of these methods require extra postprocessing steps.

In the *phase field map* method, a B_0 field map is acquired for each subject and then used to undistort the accompanying EPI data.[62–64] This method is widely used (e.g., it is implemented in FSL[b], a comprehensive library of analysis tools for fMRI). The standard procedure consists of (1) acquiring two gradient echo images at different TEs, then subtracting the phase data to obtain the phase field map (also see Chapter 2.2); (2) processing it to generate a warping matrix; and (3) applying this warping matrix to EPI series. For regions particularly prone to inhomogeneities (e.g., close to the lungs),[72] phase field maps may exceed 2π, therefore producing "phase wraps". To correct for these phase wraps, one could use automatic algorithms that identify phase discontinuities based on a standard intensity segmentation, and then correct phase errors at wrap interfaces.[73] Acquisition of a more accurate B_0 field map (in comparison with the standard double echo technique) can provide improvement to the phase field map technique in the spinal cord. For example, acquiring more than two echoes could provide a way to unwrap phase maps on a voxel-by-voxel basis.

The *point spread function* (PSF) mapping method uses a separate reference scan that introduces an additional distortion-free dimension in k-space that can be

[b]http://www.fmrib.ox.ac.uk/fsl/fugue/index.html.

Fourier-transformed into the PSF for each voxel. These images provide additional information about distortions in all directions, as well as the intensity distribution for each voxel. By considering the displacement of the PSF, local distortions due to susceptibility and chemical shift effects can be quantified and subsequently corrected. This technique can be combined with other acquisition methods for faster imaging, such as parallel imaging. The PSF method has been shown to reduce artifacts around the intervertebral disks and provide better consistency of fiber tractography compared with uncorrected images.[74] However, a disadvantage of this approach is that the correction is performed in k-space, which can be problematic for diffusion MRI data due to the large phase shifts introduced by diffusion encoding.[75]

The RGPM or "blip-up blip-down" method uses an additional EPI volume acquired with the same FOV and matrix, but using a reversed PE direction (i.e., it is rotated 180°). Reversing the PE results in a sign reversal of $\Delta f(r)$ in Eqn (2.3.1). As a result, images acquired with reversed gradients exhibit distortions in the opposite direction. Using images acquired with both the positive and the negative phase gradients, geometric and intensity correction fields are estimated and subsequently applied to EPI data sets. In DTI, the same deformation field can be applied to all diffusion-weighted data after motion correction. Since this method does not involve extensive calibration measurements like in the case of the PSF mapping method, nor does it rely on measured field maps, it is relatively practical to use with minimal scan time increase. Figure 2.3.13 shows EPI images acquired with opposite PE gradients, with subsequent

correction using the phase map estimated from the difference between these two images.

For *co-registration methods*, geometric distortion is corrected using nonlinear registration procedures, by warping distorted EPI images onto a corresponding undistorted (anatomical) reference image, so that their global shape would tend to be similar to their theoretical undistorted one.[71] The reference image is typically a T_2-weighted FSE sequence, acquired with the same FOV as the EPI image. The method consists of (1) manually segmenting the ROI to optimize the registration procedure, (2) normalizing intensity histograms for both EPI and FSE images, and (3) estimating a slice-dependent nonrigid deformation field constrained in the PE direction. This method is advantageous because no additional volume acquisition is required, except a reference image without distortion, which is incidentally generally acquired by default in standard protocols. However, the task of eliminating distortions in this way can be difficult, as the contrast between the reference and EPI image is often quite different, and the transformation has considerably more degrees of freedom than a simple rigid-body transform.[75] This method has been shown in fMRI brain data to provide improved matching between anatomical and functional MRI data; however, it does not fully remove the geometrical distortions since it does not rely on an accurate measure of these distortions.[71]

In all of the methods discussed here, intensity errors can also be corrected using the geometric displacement map. For example, if two voxels are stretched, the intensity in each voxel will be reduced. Similarly, if two voxels are squeezed, their intensity will be increased. Intensity correction will therefore multiply each distortion-corrected voxel by a correcting factor to compensate for intensity error. It should be noted that while voxels that are stretched due to distortion can be restored, the spatial details of the voxels that are bunched up cannot be recovered (these voxels will only be spread across a voxel range after correction). Note that the fidelity of all distortion correction methods relies on a reasonable image quality. That is, if the underlying image is overly distorted, the methods result in an inaccurate measurement of the displacement field and in lost anatomical information.

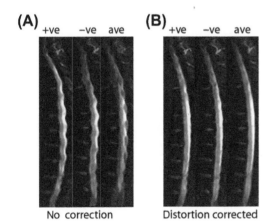

FIGURE 2.3.13 Distortion correction using the reversed gradient polarity method (RGPM). (A) T_2-weighted images of the thoracic spine acquired with a positive (+ve) and negative (−ve) phase-encoding gradient, and the average of the two images (ave). (B) Distortion-corrected images produced by using the displacement map calculated from the +ve and −ve images. A substantial improvement of image quality can be seen, particularly when the +ve and −ve images are averaged.

2.3.4 COMPARISON OF METHODS TO REDUCE SUSCEPTIBILITY ARTIFACTS

A basic summary of the methods that reduce susceptibility artifacts in EPI, and their relative advantages and disadvantages, are given in Box 2.3.1. To demonstrate the improvements in susceptibility artifacts achieved

BOX 2.3.1

BASIC SUMMARY OF METHODS THAT REDUCE SUSCEPTIBILITY ARTIFACTS IN EPI, AND THEIR RELATIVE ADVANTAGES AND DISADVANTAGES

Method	Target Parameter	Pros	Cons	Difficulty (*Easiest and ***Hardest)
Increased BW	T_{ESP}	• Simple and effective	• Limited by gradient and BW specs	*Available on most scanners
Ramp sampling	T_{ESP}	• Simple • Improved signal-to-noise ratio (SNR)	• Provides minor improvement	*Available on most scanners
Reduced FOV	FOV_{PE}	• Significant reduction in distortion level • A variety of methods to choose from	• May require modifications to RF pulses • May reduce SNR and/or affect slice coverage (depending on method of choice)	**Available on some scanners
Parallel imaging	R	• Can be combined with other methods (e.g., with reduced-FOV methods)	• Requires suitable phased-array coils—typically allows only $R \leq 2$ in A/P direction in spine • May cause spatially correlated noise	**
Interleaved EPI (IEPI)	N_{int}	• Flexibility to choose number of interleaves based on desired distortion reduction	• Increased temporal footprint • Increased scan time • Prone to motion between interleaves • May require navigator echoes and tailored reconstruction	***
Readout-segmented (RS)-EPI	T_{ESP}	*Compared with IEPI* • More effective motion correction • In DWI, much improved data consistency and fewer "gaps" in k-space	• Increased temporal footprint • Prone to motion between segments—requires tailored reconstruction for motion correction and gridding *Compared with IEPI* • Inefficient use of gradients reduce SNR • Reduction in distortion through selection of segment width limited	***
Shimming	$\Delta f(r)$	• Also improves signal level and fat suppression	• Only fixes large-scale off-resonance effects	**Available on most scanners
Distortion correction methods (postprocessing)		• Effective in correcting residual distortions • Data used for distortion correction can be used to boost SNR (for RGPM)	• Requires additional postprocessing • Increases scan time (for most approaches) • Not effective if original images are overly distorted	***

Note that compared with standard EPI, all of these approaches (excluding ramp sampling, shimming, and distortion correction) to varying degrees come at a reduced SNR efficiency.

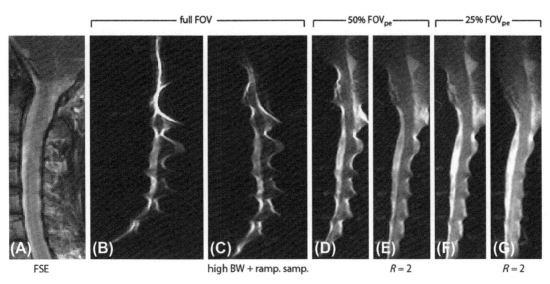

FIGURE 2.3.14 Comparison of some of the acquisition-based methods to reduce susceptibility artifacts. T_2-weighted EPI images of the cervical spine were acquired with a high in-plane resolution of 0.94 mm × 0.94 mm (corresponding to a 192 × 192 matrix size for full-FOV images), using a four-channel spine array coil at 3 T. The scan time was kept constant for all methods. (A) Fast spin echo (FSE) image showing anatomical reference. (B–C) Full FOV (18 cm × 18 cm) images, where (B) is acquired without ramp sampling, and (C) with ramp sampling and higher bandwidth (BW). Although these two simple changes help reduce the geometric distortion (see the difference in the curvature of the spine between (B) and (C)), the image quality is still not good. Reducing the FOV, on the other hand, significantly helps with the image quality. (D–E) 50% FOV_{PE} (i.e., 18 cm × 9 cm) images; and (F–G) 25% FOV_{PE} (i.e., 18 cm × 4.5 cm) images. Note that (E) and (B) also incorporate a parallel acceleration factor (R) of 2, with (G) displaying the best overall image quality among the compared images. While (E) and (F) have roughly the same geometric distortion properties, (E) shows some parallel imaging–induced noise in the pons.

via some of the methods presented in this chapter, in vivo T_2-weighted EPI of the cervical spinal cord was performed on a healthy subject, with the results shown in Figure 2.3.14. An FSE image is included for anatomical reference. The regular (i.e., "full-FOV") EPI images exhibit very high levels of distortion. The spinal cord has a comb-like appearance due to susceptibility differences between the cord, CSF, and vertebral bodies. The cord appears to have an unnatural convex curvature, instead of its concave shape as given in the anatomical reference in Figure 2.3.14(A). These artifacts are only slightly alleviated by ramp sampling at a higher BW. Reducing the FOV, however, significantly helps with the distortions and signal dropouts. A combination of reduced-FOV imaging and parallel imaging achieves the best overall image quality in this comparison. Further improvements in image quality can be achieved via the distortion correction methods mentioned in Section 2.3.3.7.

Combining distortion correction techniques with acquisition-based methods can further improve the quality of resulting images. Figure 2.3.15 shows such an example where thoracic spine images were produced using a combination of three of the methods mentioned in this chapter: reduced FOV imaging, the RS-EPI trajectory, and RGPM distortion correction. The combination of these methods (Figure 2.3.15(D)) provides an image that anatomically closely matches the undistorted FSE image (Figure 2.3.15(A)).

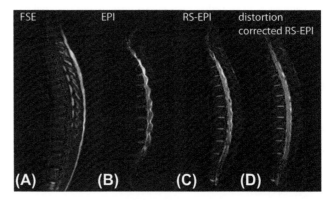

FIGURE 2.3.15 T_2-weighted thoracic spine images showing a comparison between (B) EPI and (C) readout-segmented (RS)-EPI. In (D), the RS-EPI image has been distortion corrected with the use of a $b = 0$ image acquired with a negative phase-encoding gradient, helping to remove some of the residual distortion inherent in the RS-EPI trajectory. In (A), an undistorted FSE image is shown for anatomic reference.

2.3.5 CONCLUSION

The susceptibility variations around the spine cause significant distortions in EPI images, making it difficult to obtain quantitative images of the spinal cord. Luckily, there is an arsenal of techniques that can be used to provide high-quality quantitative spine images. These techniques, some of which are described in this chapter, can be further improved with the advent of advanced spine-array and head and neck coils that can achieve high acceleration factors. Combining postprocessing distortion correction techniques (such as RGPM correction) with acquisition-based methods (such as rFOV imaging, RS-EPI, and parallel imaging), one may be able to "come close" to providing distortion-free spinal cord EPI-based images that are robust to motion.

References

1. Schenck JF. The role of magnetic susceptibility in magnetic resonance imaging: MRI magnetic compatibility of the first and second kinds. *Med Phys.* 1996;23(6):815–850.
2. Bammer R, Fazekas F. Diffusion imaging of the human spinal cord and the vertebral column. *Top Magn Reson Imaging.* 2003;14(6):461–476.
3. Cooke FJ, et al. Quantitative proton magnetic resonance spectroscopy of the cervical spinal cord. *Magn Reson Med.* 2004;51(6):1122–1128.
4. Fischer H, Ladebec R. Echo-planar imaging image artifacts. In: Schmitt F, Stehling MK, Turner R, eds. *Echo-Planar Imaging: Theory, Technique and Application.* Berlin: Springer-Verlag; 1998:179–200.
5. Delfaut EM, et al. Fat suppression in MR imaging: techniques and pitfalls. *Radiographics.* 1999;19(2):373–382.
6. Bammer R, et al. Diffusion-weighted MR imaging of the spinal cord. *AJNR Am J Neuroradiol.* 2000;21(3):587–591.
7. Ries M, et al. Diffusion tensor MRI of the spinal cord. *Magn Reson Med.* 2000;44(6):884–892.
8. Bammer R, et al. Diffusion-weighted imaging of the spinal cord: interleaved echo-planar imaging is superior to fast spin-echo. *J Magn Reson Imaging.* 2002;15(4):364–373.
9. Wheeler-Kingshott CAM, et al. Investigating cervical spinal cord structure using axial diffusion tensor imaging. *NeuroImage.* 2002;16(1):93–102.
10. Wilm BJ, et al. Reduced field-of-view MRI using outer volume suppression for spinal cord diffusion imaging. *Magn Reson Med.* 2007;57(3):625–630.
11. Saritas EU, et al. DWI of the spinal cord with reduced FOV single-shot EPI. *Magn Reson Med.* 2008;60(2):468–473.
12. Dowell NG, et al. Contiguous-slice zonally oblique multislice (CO-ZOOM) diffusion tensor imaging: examples of in vivo spinal cord and optic nerve applications. *J Magn Reson Imaging.* 2009;29(2):454–460.
13. Tsuchiya K, et al. Diffusion-weighted MRI of the cervical spinal cord using a single-shot fast spin-echo technique: findings in normal subjects and in myelomalacia. *Neuroradiology.* 2003;45(2):90–94.
14. Tsuchiya K, Fujikawa A, Suzuki Y. Diffusion tractography of the cervical spinal cord by using parallel imaging. *AJNR Am J Neuroradiol.* 2005;26(2):398–400.
15. Cercignani M, et al. Sensitivity-encoded diffusion tensor MR imaging of the cervical cord. *AJNR Am J Neuroradiol.* 2003;24(6):1254–1256.
16. Zaharchuk G, et al. Reduced field-of-view diffusion jmaging of the human spinal cord: comparison with conventional single-shot echo-planar imaging. *AJNR Am J Neuroradiol.* 2011;32(5):813–820.
17. Jeong EK, et al. High-resolution DTI with 2D interleaved multislice reduced FOV single-shot diffusion-weighted EPI (2D ss-rFOV-DWEPI). *Magn Reson Med.* 2005;54(6):1575–1579.
18. Finsterbusch J. High-resolution diffusion tensor imaging with inner field-of-view EPI. *AJNR Am J Neuroradiol.* 2009;29(4):987–993.
19. Griswold MA, et al. Generalized autocalibrating partially parallel acquisitions (GRAPPA). *Magn Reson Med.* 2002;47(6):1202–1210.
20. Pruessmann KP, et al. SENSE: sensitivity encoding for fast MRI. *Magn Reson Med.* 1999;42(5):952–962.
21. Maieron M, et al. Functional responses in the human spinal cord during willed motor actions: evidence for side- and rate-dependent activity. *J Neurosci.* 2007;27(15):4182–4190.
22. Cohen-Adad J, et al. 32-Channel RF coil optimized for brain and cervical spinal cord at 3 T. *Magn Reson Med.* 2011;66(4):1198–1208.
23. Mckinnon GC. Ultrafast interleaved gradient-echo-planar imaging on a standard scanner. *Magn Reson Med.* 1993;30(5):609–616.
24. Thurnher MM, Bammer R. Diffusion-weighted MR imaging (DWI) in spinal cord ischemia. *Neuroradiology.* 2006;48(11):795–801.
25. Plank C, et al. Diffusion-weighted MR imaging (DWI) in the evaluation of epidural spinal lesions. *Neuroradiology.* 2007;49(12):977–985.
26. Demir A, et al. Diffusion-weighted MR imaging with apparent diffusion coefficient and apparent diffusion tensor maps in cervical spondylotic myelopathy. *Radiology.* 2003;229(1):37–43.
27. Summers P, et al. A preliminary study of the effects of trigger timing on diffusion tensor imaging of the human spinal cord. *AJNR Am J Neuroradiol.* 2006;27(9):1952–1961.
28. Holder CA, et al. Diffusion-weighted MR imaging of the normal human spinal cord in vivo. *AJNR Am J Neuroradiol.* 2000;21(10):1799–1806.
29. Feinberg DA, Oshio K. Phase errors in multishot echo-planar imaging. *Magn Reson Med.* 1994;32(4):535–539.
30. Decrespigny AJ, et al. Navigated diffusion imaging of normal and ischemic human brain. *Magn Reson Med.* 1995;33(5):720–728.
31. Butts K, et al. Diffusion-weighted interleaved echo-planar imaging with a pair of orthogonal navigator echoes. *Magn Reson Med.* 1996;35(5):763–770.
32. Porter DA, Heidemann RM. High resolution diffusion-weighted imaging using readout-segmented echo-planar imaging, parallel imaging and a two-dimensional navigator-based reacquisition. *Magn Reson Med.* 2009;62(2):468–475.
33. Holdsworth SJ, et al. Robust GRAPPA-accelerated diffusion-weighted readout-segmented (RS)-EPI. *Magn Reson Med.* 2009;62(6):1629–1640.
34. Gudbjartsson H, et al. Line scan diffusion imaging. *Magn Reson Med.* 1996;36(4):509–519.
35. Finsterbusch J, Frahm J. Diffusion-weighted single-shot line scan imaging of the human brain. *Magn Reson Med.* 1999;42(4):772–778.
36. Finsterbusch J, Frahm J. Diffusion tensor mapping of the human brain using single-shot line scan imaging. *J Magn Reson Imaging.* 2000;12(3):388–394.
37. Kubicki M, et al. Comparison of single-shot echo-planar and line scan protocols for diffusion tensor imaging. *Acad Radiol.* 2004;11(2):224–232.
38. Robertson RL, et al. MR line-scan diffusion imaging of the spinal cord in children. *AJNR Am J Neuroradiol.* 2000;21(7):1344–1348.
39. Maier SE. Examination of spinal cord tissue architecture with magnetic resonance diffusion tensor imaging. *Neurotherapeutics.* 2007;4(3):453–459.
40. Maier SE, Mamata H. Diffusion tensor imaging of the spinal cord. *Ann N Y Acad Sci.* 2005;1064:50–60.
41. Mamata H, et al. Collateral nerve fibers in human spinal cord: visualization with magnetic resonance diffusion tensor imaging. *NeuroImage.* 2006;31(1):24–30.
42. Bammer R, et al. Line scan diffusion imaging of the spine. *AJNR Am J Neuroradiol.* 2003;24(1):5–12.
43. Hennig J, Nauerth A, Friedburg H. RARE imaging: a fast imaging method for clinical MR. *Magn Reson Med.* 1986;3(6):823–833.
44. Xu D, et al. Single-shot fast spin-echo diffusion tensor imaging of the brain and spine with head and phased array coils at 1.5 T and 3.0 T. *Magn Reson Imaging.* 2004;22(6):751–759.

45. Sarlls JE, et al. Isotropic diffusion weighting in radial fast spin-echo magnetic resonance imaging. *Magn Reson Med.* 2005; 53(6):1347–1354.

46. Dietrich O, et al. Diffusion-weighted imaging of the spine using radial k-space trajectories. *Magma.* 2001;12(1):23–31.

47. Bernstein M, King K, Zhou X. Handbook of MRI Pulse Sequences. In: E.A. Press, ed. Elsevier Academic Press; 2004, 1040.

48. Pipe JG. Motion correction with PROPELLER MRI: application to head motion and free-breathing cardiac imaging. *Magn Reson Med.* 1999;42(5):963–969.

49. Pipe JG, Zwart N. Turboprop: improved PROPELLER imaging. *Magn Reson Med.* 2006;55(2):380–385.

50. Deng J, Omary RA, Larson AC. Multishot diffusion-weighted SPLICE PROPELLER MRI of the abdomen. *Magn Reson Med.* 2008;59(5):947–953.

51. Wang FN, et al. PROPELLER EPI: an MRI technique suitable for diffusion tensor imaging at high field strength with reduced geometric distortions. *Magn Reson Med.* 2005;54(5):1232–1240.

52. Sarlls J, Pierpaoli C. High-resolution diffusion tensor imaging at 3T with radial-FSE. *Proceedings of the 16th Annual Meeting of ISMRM.* Toronto, Canada; 2008.

53. Sarlls JE, Pierpaoli C. Diffusion-weighted radial fast spin-echo for high-resolution diffusion tensor imaging at 3T. *Magn Reson Med.* 2008;60(2):270–276.

54. Ellingson BM, Sulaiman O, Kurpad SN. High-resolution in vivo diffusion tensor imaging of the injured cat spinal cord using self-navigated, interleaved, variable-density spiral acquisition (SNAILS-DTI). *Magn Reson Imaging.* 2010;28(9):1353–1360.

55. Cohen-Adad J, et al. BOLD signal responses to controlled hypercapnia in human spinal cord. *NeuroImage.* 2010;50(3):1074–1084.

56. Eilenberg SS, Tartar VM, Mattrey RF. Reducing magnetic-susceptibility differences using liquid fluorocarbon pads (Sat Pad(Tm))—results with spectral presaturation of fat. *Artif Cells Blood Substitutes Immobilization Biotechnol.* 1994;22(4):1477–1483.

57. Rosen Y, et al. 3T MR of the prostate: reducing susceptibility gradients by inflating the endorectal coil with a barium sulfate suspension. *Magn Reson Med.* 2007;57(5):898–904.

58. Mitchell DG, et al. Comparison of Kaopectate with barium for negative and positive enteric contrast at MR imaging. *Radiology.* 1991;181(2):475–480.

59. Lee GC, et al. Pyrolytic graphite foam: a passive magnetic susceptibility matching material. *J Magn Reson Imaging.* 2010;32(3): 684–691.

60. Schneider E, Glover G. Rapid in vivo proton shimming. *Magn Reson Med.* 1991;18(2):335–347.

61. Robson MD, Gore JC, Constable RT. Measurement of the point spread function in MRI using constant time imaging. *Magn Reson Med.* 1997;38(5):733–740.

62. Jezzard P, Balaban RS. Correction for geometric distortion in echo-planar images from B-0 field variations. *Magn Reson Med.* 1995;34(1):65–73.

63. Cusack R, Brett M, Osswald K. An evaluation of the use of magnetic field maps to undistort echo-planar images. *NeuroImage.* 2003;18(1):127–142.

64. Reber PJ, et al. Correction of off resonance-related distortion in echo-planar imaging using EPI-based field maps. *Magn Reson Med.* 1998;39(2):328–330.

65. Chang H, Fitzpatrick JM. A technique for accurate magnetic-resonance-imaging in the presence of field inhomogeneities. *IEEE Trans Med Imaging.* 1992;11(3):319–329.

66. Andersson JLR, Skare S, Ashburner J. How to correct susceptibility distortions in spin-echo echo-planar images: application to diffusion tensor imaging. *NeuroImage.* 2003;20(2):870–888.

67. Skare S, Andersson JLR. Correction of MR image distortions induced by metallic objects using a 3D cubic B-spline basis set: application to stereotactic surgical planning. *Magn Reson Med.* 2005;54(1):169–181.

68. Kannengiesser SAR, Wang Y, Haacke EM. Geometric distortion correction in gradient-echo imaging by use of dynamic time warping. *Magn Reson Med.* 1999;42(3):585–590.

69. Bowtell RMD, Commandre MJ, Glover PM. Correction of geometric distortions in echo planar images. *Proceedings of the 2nd Annual Meeting of ISMRM.* San Francisco, CA; 1994.

70. Ardekani S, Sinha U. Geometric distortion correction of high-resolution 3 T diffusion tensor brain images. *Magn Reson Med.* 2005;54(5):1163–1171.

71. Villain N, et al. A simple way to improve anatomical mapping of functional brain imaging. *J Neuroimaging.* 2010;20(4):324–333.

72. Cohen-Adad J, Lundell H, Rossignol S. Distortion correction in spinal cord DTI: what's the best approach? *Proceedings of the 17th Scientific Meeting of ISMRM.* Honolulu, HI, USA; 2009:3178.

73. Jenkinson M. Fast, automated, N-dimensional phase-unwrapping algorithm. *Magn Reson Med.* 2003;49(1):193–197.

74. Lundell H, et al. Fast diffusion tensor imaging and tractography of the whole cervical spinal cord using point spread function corrected echo planar imaging. *Magn Reson Med.* 2013;69(1): 144–149.

75. Andersson JSS, Skare ST. Image distortion and its correction in diffusion MRI. In: J DK, ed. *Diffusion MRI: Theory, Methods, and Applications.* Oxford University Press; 2010:285–302.

Ultra-High Field Spinal Cord Imaging

Seth A. Smith[1,2], Richard D. Dortch[1,2],
Robert L. Barry[1,2], John C. Gore[1,2]

[1]Radiology and Radiological Sciences, Vanderbilt University Medical Center, Nashville, TN USA [2]Vanderbilt University
Institute of Imaging Science, Vanderbilt University, Nashville, TN USA

2.4.1 BACKGROUND

2.4.1.1 Importance of High Field

In the early 1980s, magnetic resonance imaging (MRI) was introduced into clinical practice and has subsequently undergone technical advancements that have resulted in improvements in image quality. For nearly 20 years, 1.5 T has been the most common field strength in use for clinical MRI of the human spinal cord. In fact, according to current European Union regulations, scanners operating at field strengths of 3 T or higher are considered research scanners. Recently, higher field strength MRI has shown that greater information may be obtained from the spinal cord with higher spatial resolution. As a result, many groups have adopted MRI scanners operating at 3 T for routine use and neuroscience research applications. Continuing this trend to higher fields, scanners operating at 7 T (or even higher) have recently been introduced into research. Currently, there are approximately 40+ human MRI scanners worldwide operating at these "ultra-high" fields. To date, most of the work at 7 T has focused on studies of the brain. However, it is likely that higher field strengths will also provide significant new opportunities for smaller structures of the human body, in particular the spinal cord and associated nerves.

The motivation for higher field strength is supported by the fact that each increase in field strength in the past has led to substantial improvements in image quality, anatomical detail, spectral fidelity, and in some cases new information about tissue composition, metabolism, pathology, and organ system function. However, each major increase in field strength has

also introduced new technical challenges that have required creative scientific and engineering solutions to realize the full potential that can be achieved. MRI image quality is constrained by the ratio of the available signal to the noise, the random, unavoidable image perturbations that make the detection of small signal differences challenging. The magnitude of the raw MRI signal increases with the square of the field strength, while the noise mostly scales linearly with the field strength; thus, the available SNR increases linearly. In principle, the greater than twofold higher SNR afforded at 7 T compared to 3 T can be used for higher spatial resolution, more rapid scan times, or to detect subtle tissue differences that may not be appreciated at lower field. In addition, some intrinsic tissue properties are field dependent and can contribute more significantly to image contrast at higher field strengths. For example, variations in tissue magnetic susceptibility—often dominated by blood oxygenation/volume and tissue iron concentration—give rise to MRI signal changes that increase dramatically at high field. The former of these is the so-called blood oxygenation level-dependent (BOLD) effect; therefore, ultra-high field affords the ability to detect BOLD signal changes with greater sensitivity. Additionally, the spectral separation of metabolite resonances increases with field strength. As a result, spectroscopic imaging and chemical exchange saturation transfer (CEST) techniques at ultra-high field can offer better-resolved spectra and potentially greater spectral information than is available at lower field strength.

While the impact of 7 T on brain imaging has been reported at length in recent literature, applications to the spinal cord at 7 T have been limited. The goal of this chapter is to describe some of the early experiences with 7 T imaging of the spinal cord, provide an outline of the current challenges and proposed solutions, and attempt to see into the future of what 7 T MRI may offer for spinal cord imaging.

2.4.1.2 Challenges/Solutions at High Field

All major advances in magnet field strength have provided challenges as well as opportunities. Here we discuss the following topics: specific absorption rate (SAR), transmit field (B_1) inhomogeneities, and static field (B_0) inhomogeneities/susceptibility artifacts.

2.4.1.2.1 Specific Absorption Rate

The standard relative measure of power deposition, SAR, scales with the product of B_0^2 and the root-mean-squared B_1; thus, the pulse sequence SAR increases approximately fivefold with an increase from 3 to 7 T. To address this concern, it is often necessary to modify sequences that require high peak RF power, or rapid readout schemes that make use of multiple, high amplitude refocusing pulses (e.g., fast spin echo). Thus, to reduce SAR, either the repetition time (TR) or the applied RF pulses must be lengthened. In cases where this is not possible because of scan time limitations, alternative acquisition strategies should be considered. Thus, SAR places a limit on the sequences that can be used "out of the box" at 7 T. Indeed, the majority of standard clinical sequences employed at lower field strengths for anatomical spinal cord imaging (e.g., short tau inversion recovery [STIR], T_1- and T_2-weighted fast spin echoes, and fat-saturation preparation) are, in many cases, not practical for high field application.

2.4.1.2.2 Static Field Inhomogeneity and Susceptibility

Rapid changes in B_0 arising from tissue interfaces with different magnetic susceptibility (e.g., tissue and air) can significantly affect image quality in the spinal cord at ultra-high field. For certain acquisitions (e.g., echo planar imaging, EPI), these susceptibility effects can result in significant geometric distortions and transverse magnetization dephasing, or signal "drop-out," that scale with field strength. For example, artifacts shown in Chapter 2.3 would be even more exacerbated at 7 T, as the amount of distortion is proportional to B_0. For the spinal cord in particular, susceptibility-related artifacts can arise from a number of structures (susceptibility mismatch between the vertebral bodies and surrounding tissue/cerebrospinal fluid or between the bony structures and the disc space), and can be time varying (cardiac pulsation, respiration). Thus, the spinal cord experiences a combination of global, slowly spatially varying perturbations in B_0, local variation along the extent of the cord,[1] and a rapidly time-evolving component. An example of a typical axial

7 T B_0 map at the level of C3 is shown in Figure 2.4.1(A) with a resolution-matched anatomical image showing the location of the spinal cord (arrow).

Given the small diameter of the cord, correcting the B_0 homogeneity within the axial plane may require sophisticated image-based shimming techniques with second- and/or third-order shimming. Thus, high field scanners need to be equipped with higher order shims that are not commonly implemented at lower fields in order to perform robust spinal cord imaging. For larger volumes along the rostral-caudal extent of the cord, more sophisticated approaches may be required (e.g., dynamic shimming[2,3] for multislice acquisitions) due to the highly nonlinear nature of these perturbations. There are, however, available approaches that can mitigate many of the effects of the static field variations of the cord at lower field (see Chapter 2.2), though additional work is needed to evaluate their effectiveness at 7 T.

Perhaps a larger issue is that B_0 can dynamically change due to motion (e.g., CSF pulsation, swallowing, and breathing)[4] such that changes in the thorax can affect the uniformity of B_0 elsewhere. For example, a previous 7 T study of the brain[5] found up to a 5 Hz variation (peak-to-peak) in B_0 in the brain over the course of the respiratory cycle, and it was noted that this effect increased moving from anterior to posterior regions. Raj et al.,[6] noted similar effects that increased from the superior to inferior portions of the brain. Recently, it was shown that temporal variations in B_0 are even larger in the spinal cord due to its relative proximity to the throat and lungs.[88] Fast, single-shot readouts (e.g., EPI) might be considered to reduce some of the effects of these temporal variations on image quality; however, these sequences typically suffer from a lower spatial resolution than is required for many applications. As a result, multishot sequences, which are much more sensitive to temporal variations in B_0, are often required. As such, one must either (1) remove the dynamic variations prospectively and/or (2) estimate them and correct for their effects retrospectively prior to reconstruction.[7] The former can be achieved via respiratory and/or cardiac gating or triggering[8] or via breath-held sequences. The latter can be achieved via navigated sequences[9] that measure and correct for the temporal variation in B_0 in the spinal cord. Prior to investigating each of these techniques, a thorough characterization of the spatiotemporal variation in B_0 in the spinal cord, along with identification of the sources and of these variations at 7 T, is needed.

2.4.1.2.3 Transmit Field Inhomogeneity

Sequences that rely on B_1 uniformity are further compromised when operating at 7 T, where the RF pulse wavelength becomes smaller than the dimensions of the body to be imaged. At 300 MHz (7 T) and above, standing wave and "near-field" phenomena[10] give rise to

FIGURE 2.4.1 Anatomical and field maps of the cervical spinal cord at the level of C3. *Panel (A)*: B_0 Field map (in Hz). Calculated using a gradient echo with $\Delta TE = 0.5$ ms. *Panel (B)*: B_1 field map (reported as a fraction of the nominal flip angle) calculated using a gradient echo with a TR extension of 100 ms and a flip angle $= 60°$.

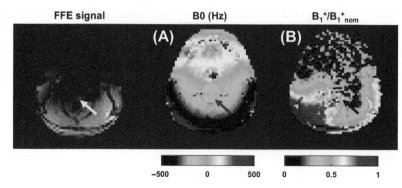

large variations in the transmit RF field. Multichannel transmit systems,[11] advanced RF pulse designs (e.g., SPOKES pulse,[12] optimized adiabatic pulses,[13] composite pulses[13,14]), and high-dielectric materials[15,16] have all been employed to improve the transmit field homogeneity. While these approaches have not been demonstrated in practical applications, each is expected to improve the B_1 uniformity in the cord. Additional work is needed to evaluate which approaches are best suited for spinal cord imaging at higher field strengths. In instances where one is interested in only small axial volumes such as the spinal cord (~ 1.5 cm in cross-sectional size), it should be noted that some of these approaches may be less valuable or necessary as the transmit field varies slowly relative to the diameter of the spinal cord. An example of this can be seen in Figure 2.4.1(B). Note that while B_1 is relatively homogeneous across the diameter of the cord, it is approximately 50% of the nominal prescribed value based on assuming the field is uniform everywhere. Therefore, attention must be paid to calibrating the RF power properly, which is not straightforward for certain coil designs (e.g., surface coils), and may be a larger issue than absolute B_1 uniformity in the cord. Fortunately, there are a number of B_1 mapping techniques (e.g.,[17,18]), which can be used to calibrate the RF power, and from this the appropriate RF power and pulse design can be derived.

2.4.2 ANATOMICAL MRI

As has been pointed out in earlier chapters, the spinal cord is a somatotopically organized structure. Therefore, the higher-resolution imaging afforded at 7 T provides the opportunity to better assess the precise locations of lesions in the cord and relate these to specific neurological dysfunction. Histopathologically, studies have shown spinal cord GM may contain lesions that are related to neurological dysfunction,[19,20] and at higher resolutions it may be possible to visualize such lesions. Also, it may be possible to assess the health of the nerve roots, which convey information to and from the spinal cord. Damage to the nerve roots can mimic the deleterious neurological effects arising from spinal cord lesions.[21] In conditions like spinal cord trauma, degenerative disc disease, or bony malformations, the nerve roots may be involved to a greater degree than the spinal cord itself. Finally, segmentation of the spinal cord may be related to the clinical presentation in multiple sclerosis.[22,23] In previous studies, the focus has been on the C2-C3 junction and the cross-sectional area (CSA) is measured.[24,25] Even with this coarse measure, the relationship between atrophy and neurological dysfunction may be appreciated. Even at 3 T, segmentation of GM and WM[26] has shown promise and at 7 T the reliability of atrophy measurements may be significantly increased.

Generally speaking, a clinical spinal cord imaging study at lower field strength incorporates T_1-weighted, T_2-weighted, short-tau inversion recovery (STIR), and fluid attenuated inversion recovery (FLAIR) sequences, though other methods may also be used and tailored to the pathology of interest. Currently, there are a limited

---

PROS AND CONS OF ULTRA-HIGH FIELD MRI

Pros

- Increased SNR → can achieve higher spatial resolution or reduced scan time
- Increased spectral resolution → MRS, CEST
- Increased sensitivity to tissue susceptibility → fMRI, delineating tissue microstructure
- Prolonged T_1 → MT, CEST

Cons

- Increased power deposition → SAR
- B_1 inhomogeneity → inconsistent and/or reduced flip angles (variable contrast, reduced SNR)
- B_0 inhomogeneity → Susceptibility artifacts, signal voids in GRE imaging, periodic signal fluctuation
- Decreased T_2 and T_2^* → spectral line broadening, lower SNR in DWI
- Decreased shimming effectiveness
- Cost/Site requirements

number of reports on spinal cord anatomical imaging at 7 T.[27] In Sigmund et al.,[27] the authors demonstrated the impact of the higher SNR at 7 T over lower field strength, which they used to obtain higher spatial resolution. Specifically, they focused their attention on T_2^*-weighted imaging with short echo times. From their presentation, subtle structures are well visualized within the cord.

Other examples of 7 T anatomical MRI are given in Figure 2.4.2, which shows that a nominal resolution of 0.3 mm in-plane can be readily achieved (Figure 2.4.2(A)) using a conventional gradient echo sequence (all scanning details given at the end of the chapter). Note the greater detail seen of the gray matter in the lateral and dorsal horns. No longer is the butterfly-shaped gray matter simply a thin H-shaped structure in the body of the cord, but at this resolution, fine details of the lateral and ventro-lateral gray matter horns can be appreciated. In Figure 2.4.2(F–G) a 1D phase navigator has been applied to each of five echoes and the first three echoes have been averaged to increase the contrast from the CSF, GM, and WM. In addition to the improved contrast within the cord, the spinal cord nerve roots can be visualized within the surrounding CSF using this technique.

The increased SNR at high field can also be used to reduce acquisition times with resolutions comparable to conventional anatomical imaging at lower field strength. In Figure 2.4.2(B–C), axial T_2^*- and T_1-weighted gradient echo acquisitions are shown at resolutions typical of 3 T MRI in the spinal cord ($0.8 \times 0.8 \times 4$ mm^3) and obtained in less than 8 min. In concordance with the fact that T_1 values for WM and GM are similar at lower field strengths,[28] T_1-weighted imaging of the spinal cord at 7 T shows little contrast between WM and GM (Figure 2.4.2(C)), especially when compared with the T_2^*-weighted acquisition (Figure 2.4.2(B)). Similar T_2^*-weighted images of the cervical spinal cord in a patient with multiple sclerosis are given in Figure 2.4.2(D–E). Note the dorsal column lesion in panel D (arrow), and the bilateral tissue signal aberrations in the lateral columns in panel E (arrow).

To date, there have been no publications regarding spinal cord FLAIR or STIR at 7 T. Performing FLAIR imaging at 7 T is problematic due to the requirement of a uniform inversion RF pulse over the entire structure of interest, which for the brain is challenging, yet possible[13,14] with tailored inversion and refocusing pulses, and alternative readout parameters. Recently, Zwanenburg and Visser[29,30] proposed a high resolution 3D FLAIR for the brain. They showed that a T_2 preparation prior to inversion aided in enhancing the contrast between tissue types while minimizing T_1 contrast. The T_2 preparation consisted of a 90° pulse followed by a pulse train of adiabatic 180° pulses and a final 90° flip-back pulse. While not currently in use, this type of acquisition paradigm may prove to be equally beneficial for imaging inflammation

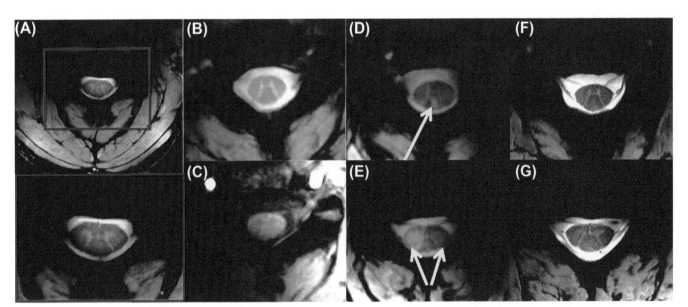

FIGURE 2.4.2   Anatomical gradient echo images of the cervical spinal cord at 7 T. *Panel (A)*: 2D gradient echo, FOV = $180 \times 180 \times 5$ mm^3, resolution = $0.3 \times 0.3 \times 5$ mm^3, TR/TE/α = 31 ms/15 ms/25°, SENSE × 2, scan time = 1 min/slice. *Panel (B–C)*: 2D multi-echo gradient echo, FOV = $198 \times 178 \times 3$ mm^3, resolution = $0.37 \times 0.37 \times 3$ mm^3, TR/TE = 514 ms/(7.83, 15, 22.21, 29.43) ms, SENSE = 2, phase stabilization applied, scan time = 4:24. Note: image shows average of the first three echo times. *Panel (D)*: multislice gradient echo, FOV = $180 \times 180 \times 60$ mm^3, resolution = $0.6 \times 0.6 \times 4$ mm^3, TR/TE/α = 221 ms/9.1 ms/25°, SENSE × 2, scan time = 3:45. *Panel (E)*: 3D gradient echo, FOV = $180 \times 180 \times 60$ mm^3, resolution = $0.6 \times 0.6 \times 4$ mm^3, TR/TE/α = 50 ms/4.4 ms/100°, SENSE × 2, scan time = 4:20. *Panel (F–G)*: multislice gradient echo, FOV = $180 \times 180 \times 60$ mm^3, resolution = $0.6 \times 0.6 \times 4$ mm^3, TR/TE/a = 221 ms/9.1 ms/25, GRAPPA × 2, scan time = 3:45. *Source: Figure F,G courtesy Dr Cohen-Adad, A.A. Martinos Center, Boston, Massachusetts.*

in the spinal cord, and a similar preparation phase could easily be adopted for both FLAIR and STIR imaging.

Some preliminary reports demonstrated the benefits of 7 T for characterizing the pathological spinal cord in ALS[31] and spinal cord injury.[32] In the latter study, the high spatial resolution (300 micron in-plane) enabled the clear delineation of signal abnormality likely due to Wallerian degeneration of ascending dorsal column.

2.4.3 QUANTITATIVE MRI

2.4.3.1 Relaxometry

Relationships between relaxation parameters and microanatomical features such as myelination[33] and iron content[34] have previously been investigated with the goal of developing quantitative imaging biomarkers of disease. Unfortunately, while relaxation parameters are sensitive to overall tissue composition, they are not necessarily specific to a given microanatomical feature. There are, however, exceptions to this general rule. For example, Whittall and Mackay[35] have shown that multicomponent characterization of white matter T_2 allows for the separation of the bulk signal into two components: (1) a short-T_2 from water residing between myelin bilayers and (2) a long-T_2 from water residing within and between axons. More recently, a relationship between the size of the short-T_2 and myelin content in the spinal cord[36] has been shown, indicating that more specific information about myelination may be available via multicomponent relaxation measurements. It should be noted, however, that such measurements at 7 T are difficult because these sequences invoke high SAR and rely on the use of multiple refocusing pulses that are nonuniform at higher field.

In addition to providing information on tissue composition, NMR relaxation measurements at ultra-high field are essential for sequence optimization (e.g., optimization of white matter/gray matter contrast in T_1-weighted scans). It is well known that T_1 increases while T_2 and T_2^* decrease with increasing magnetic field strength. Thus, sequences that are optimized for spinal cord imaging at clinical field strengths yield suboptimal results at ultra-high field.

2.4.3.1.1 Spin–Spin Relaxation (T_2)

Spin echo sequences are most commonly used to measure T_2. The spin echo signal $S(\text{TE})$ is given by:

$$S(\text{TE}) = S_0 e^{\frac{-\text{TE}}{T_2}} + v, \qquad (2.4.1)$$

where S_0 is the equilibrium signal (related to proton density, instrument factors, and T_1-weighting if present), v reflects noise, and TE is the echo time. In the ideal case, estimates of T_2 and S_0 can be obtained via nonlinear

regression of images at different TE values to Eqn (2.4.1); however, variations in B_0 and B_1 can affect these estimates.

The spin echo signal is maximized when the refocusing pulse is a uniform $180°$ over the entire structure of interest; therefore, spin echo sequences are exquisitely sensitive to B_1 homogeneity. If one spin echo is acquired per TR, variations in the effective flip angle simply result in a reduction in the observed signal amplitude. For T_2 measurements, this reduction factor can then be folded into S_0 (Eqn (2.4.1)), and the estimate of T_2 remains accurate. Often, however, multiple spin echoes are acquired per TR to more efficiently sample the T_2 decay curve. For multiple echo sequences, variations of this effective flip angle can result in signal contributions from non-spin echo pathways (e.g., stimulated echoes that evolve according to T_1) that cannot be accounted for by this simple model. In such cases, contributions from non-spin echo pathways must be minimized. At lower field strengths, composite (e.g., $90_x 180_y 90_x$)[37] pulses are often used in concert with crusher gradients to minimize these non-spin-echo signal contributions. At 7 T, more robust pulses will likely need to be developed to account for B_1 inhomogeneity,[14] especially when imaging over the rostral-caudal volume of the spinal cord in which we would expect a simultaneous variation in B_0. It should be noted that such pulse designs often require high amplitude pulses; therefore, considerations of SAR are required when developing robust refocusing pulses for high field applications. In summary, T_2 estimation at high field is challenging, but there remain several options that warrant investigation.

2.4.3.1.2 Effective Spin–Spin Relaxation (T_2^*)

Spoiled gradient echo sequences, both single and multi-echo, are most commonly used to quantify T_2^*. In this case, the observed signal equation can be expressed as:

$$S(\text{TE}) = S_0 e^{\frac{-\text{TE}}{T_2^*}} + v. \qquad (2.4.2)$$

Again, in the ideal case, one can estimate T_2^* via nonlinear regression of gradient echo images at different TE values to Eqn (2.4.2). In reality, the signal from gradient echo sequences is also sensitive to spatial variations in B_0, or background field gradients. Thus, in the presence of a background field gradient, the signal equation must be altered to include an additional term $f_{\Delta\phi}$ that accounts for background-gradient-induced signal loss:

$$S(\text{TE}) = S_0 e^{\frac{-\text{TE}}{T_2^*}} f_{\Delta\phi}(\text{TE}) + v. \qquad (2.4.3)$$

To accurately quantify T_2^* in the presence of a significant background field gradient, one has two options: (1) account for the effect by including $f_{\Delta\phi}$ as a free parameter in the regression model[38] or (2) correct for the effect as described following.

The most straightforward way to remove background field gradients is by appropriate shimming. A number of automated techniques are available in order to optimize shim values (see Chapter 2.2). Even with advanced shimming methods, complete removal of susceptibility-induced background field gradients is often not possible, as they tend to be highly nonlinear and time varying. As a result, additional techniques are likely to be needed in order to accurately quantify T_2^* in the spinal cord at ultra-high field. There are a number of sequence-based prospective approaches for minimizing the effect of background gradients on the observed signal. For example, RF pulses[39] and/or additional slice refocus gradients (so-called "z-shimming")[40] can be designed with phase profiles that are the inverse of the profile generated by the background gradients themselves. Although promising, the TE-dependence (i.e., different corrections are needed for images acquired at different TE values) of these sequence-based approaches makes them difficult to implement for the measurement of T_2^*. Therefore, direct estimation of background gradients from an acquired B_0 map (from which an estimate of $f_{\Delta\phi}$ can be obtained[41]) is often recommended. In summary, there are viable options for measuring T_2^* in the spinal cord at ultra-high field, but an accurate estimate of the effect of background field gradients on the observed signal is necessary.

2.4.3.1.3 Spin-Lattice Relaxation (T_1)

T_1 can be estimated via saturation recovery (SR), inversion recovery (IR), or multi-flip angle echo (MFA) approaches. Generally speaking, SR and IR can be prohibitively long. In contrast, MFA sequences can be acquired with a short TR (because they are not delay dependent), allowing for a much more rapid T_1 estimation. Unfortunately, MFA estimates of T_1 can be biased in the presence of magnetization transfer (MT).[42] As a result, we limit the following discussion to SR and IR approaches.

The measurement of T_1 relies on knowing the state of the longitudinal magnetization at the beginning of the delay period (TR for SR, TI for IR), which depends upon knowing the effective flip angle of the excitation or inversion RF pulse. As previously mentioned, there are RF pulse designs that can mitigate the effect of B_0 and B_1 variations on the effective flip angle. At ultra-high field, however, some uncertainty in the effective flip angle can remain even when such pulses are used. In this case, the signal equation must be modified. For an SR sequence, the signal as a function of delay time (TD) is:

$$S(TD) = S_0\left[1 - (1-\cos\theta)e^{\frac{-TD}{T_1}}\right] + v. \qquad (2.4.4)$$

For a spin echo acquisition, TD = TR−TE is the time from the center of the spin echo to the next excitation pulse and θ is the effective flip angle; for a gradient echo acquisition with a 90° excitation pulse, TD = TR. Thus, the parameters T_1, θ, and S_0 can be estimated via nonlinear regression of images acquired at different TR values to Eqn (2.4.3). Similarly, the signal for the IR sequence can be expressed as:

$$S(TI, TD) = S_0\left[1 - (1-\cos\theta)e^{\frac{-TI}{T_1}} + e^{\frac{-TD}{T_1}}\right] + v. \qquad (2.4.5)$$

and T_1, θ, and S_0 are estimated in the same manner. For the IR sequence, TD accounts for the recovery of magnetization from a point of saturation following excitation to the next inversion pulse. For spin echo sequences, this is approximately the time from the center of the last spin echo to the next inversion pulse. For a gradient echo sequence with a perfect 90° excitation, this is the time from excitation pulse to the next inversion pulse. However, for a gradient echo sequence with smaller excitation flip angles, there is not a point at which $M_z \approx 0$ after the excitation. In this case, one has two options: (1) increase TR to ensure full recovery prior to the inversion pulse (if TR > $5T_1$, the TD term can be ignored in Eqn (2.4.4)) or (2) apply RF pulses after the readout to saturate M_z. An example of the latter is described in the following section in which an extension of the IR approach has been employed to investigate quantitative MT mapping at ultra-high field strengths.

2.4.3.2 Magnetization Transfer

In addition to protons associated with free water, there are protons associated with immobile macromolecules in tissue.[43] Conventional imaging sequences cannot capture signals from these macromolecular protons since their T_2s are extremely short (<<1 ms). These macromolecular protons can, however, be indirectly detected by exploiting their interactions with the free water pool via chemical exchange and/or dipole–dipole interactions (referred to as magnetization transfer, MT).[44] Greater detail of the MT effect, acquisition methods, and impact on spinal cord imaging can be found in Chapter 3.4.

With respect to high field imaging, previous work has shown that MT saturation (and MTR contrast) increases with field strength due to the prolongation of T_1. Unfortunately, because the MTR is also sensitive to RF power,[45] these gains are typically lost by the increased SAR limitations at 7 T. Thus, for a given RF power, a longer TR is typically required to remain within SAR limitations, and T_1 elongation alone may be insufficient to provide the same MT effect that could be achieved at lower fields.[45] These issues are further exacerbated by the large B_1 variations encountered at higher fields, which result in spatial variation in MTR that may not be related to the underlying tissue composition but rather to field inhomogeneity. This effect can be mitigated via B_1 mapping and correction schemes[46–48] or via so-called quantitative MT (qMT) approaches (see Chapter 3.4), which typically involves collecting a series of MT-weighted images with different MT pulse offsets and/or powers and fitting the data to one of many models. Unfortunately, this is an even higher power deposition method, thus SAR limitations for saturation-based qMT measurements at ultra-high field can be prohibitive.

In an alternative approach, Dortch et al.[49] have proposed a low-SAR inversion recovery-based method to perform high-resolution qMT imaging at 7 T. This method, referred to as selective inversion recovery (SIR) qMT imaging, is based upon measuring the biexponential recovery of the free water pool in the presence of MT after an on-resonance inversion pulse. The SIR qMT sequence (Figure 2.4.3(A)) is similar to the inversion recovery sequence used to measure T_1 with two modifications. First, short inversion times (≈ 10 ms or less) are sampled in order to capture the fast-recovering component of the biexponential curve, which has been shown to be related to MT. Second, a T_2-selective inversion pulse is applied. This is achieved

via a low-power inversion pulse, whose duration is much longer than the T_2 of the macromolecular pool and much shorter than the T_2 of the free water pool. Ideally, this pulse inverts the free pool magnetization with minimal saturation of the macromolecular pool. Thus, this pulse maximizes the disparity between the two pools and, in turn, the sensitivity of the signal to MT.

Previous work has shown the feasibility of applying SIR qMT in the brain at 7 T[49]; and here we demonstrate the feasibility of applying the same technique in the spinal cord. To correct for the effect of B_1 and B_0 on the inversion pulse, a composite inversion pulse has been employed.[49] To acquire these data efficiently and to remain within SAR limitations, a low flip angle turbo field echo sequence (similar to an MPRAGE[50] sequence) was employed for the readout. This readout also allows for single-shot data to be acquired, thus minimizing the impact of motion on the data. Because this is a low flip angle gradient echo approach, a long TR would typically need to be employed to ensure full recovery of magnetization prior to each inversion pulse, resulting in prohibitively long scan times. To get around this issue, we have designed[49] a train of RF pulses to saturate both pools following the TFE readout, allowing for the reduction in TR without biasing the estimated qMT parameters. Sample data and estimates of the macromolecular-to-free pool size ratio (PSR) in the spinal cord using this approach is shown in Figure 2.4.3(B). Details of the acquisition paradigm are given in the Figure legend.

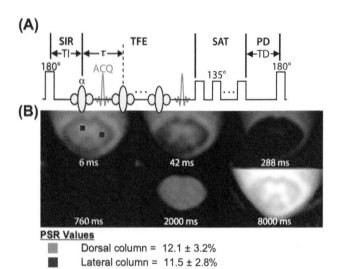

FIGURE 2.4.3   *Panel (A)*: SIR pulse sequence with a low flip angle turbo field echo readout (TFE). The TFE readout is followed by a train of RF pulses designed to saturate (SAT) both pools and a predelay (PD) period to allow for partial z-magnetization recovery. Legend: TI = inversion time, TD = predelay, τ = TFE pulse spacing, α = excitation pulse flip angle, and ACQ = acquisition. *Panel (B)*: SIR images (6 of 14 TIs shown) from a slice at C3; and ROIs for the dorsal column (green), the lateral column (red), and gray matter (blue). Also given are the mean ± SD PSR values across four healthy volunteers for each of these ROIs. Note the slightly elevated PSR values in white matter tracts relative to gray matter. *Acquisition parameters*: 3D SIR sequence with a flow-compensated TFE readout: FOV = $180 \times 180 \times 50$ mm³, resolution = $1 \times 1 \times 5$ mm³, TI = 6–8000 m (14 log-spaced values), TD = 2.5 s, TFE factor = 180, τ/TE = 5.7/3.6 ms, $\alpha = 15°$, total imaging time ∼15 min.

2.4.3.3 Chemical Exchange Saturation Transfer

While all imaging sequences benefit from the increased SNR afforded at higher field strengths, spectroscopic techniques also benefit from the increase in spectral dispersion and longer T_1 at high fields. In this section, we focus on the impact of field strength on CEST and how it can be used in the spinal cord.

CEST imaging can be thought of as a spectrally selective MT experiment[51] and has been shown to report on the biochemical composition of tissues.[52–60] Contrary to general MT, the CEST effect is driven by direct chemical exchange of chemically shifted, labile protons (hydroxyl, amide, amine, and sulfhydryl moieties).[58] Specifically, labile protons with a relatively slow exchange rate and sufficient chemical shift from water can be saturated by spectrally selective RF irradiation. Note that unlike general MT applications, which rely on large B_1 pulses, CEST relies on lower power, narrower bandwidth irradiation. As a result, SAR limitations are often not encountered with CEST imaging as they are for MT imaging. Additionally, the increased spectral separation at high field has led investigators to increasingly lean on 7 T for CEST applications (e.g., amide protons,[53,61,62] glutamate,[63] and myoinositol protons[52]).

CEST preparations are most commonly performed by applying a single, spectrally selective pulse or pulse train[53,56,61] prior to an imaging readout. By acquiring a series of images over a range of CEST pulse offset frequencies ($\Delta\omega$) and normalizing to an acquisition without RF irradiation, a so-called CEST z-spectrum[64] for each voxel can be obtained. For more details on CEST experiments, see to Chapter 3.4. To perform high quality CEST measurements in the spinal cord, we face three main challenges: (1) B_0 field inhomogeneities and fluctuations, (2) B_1 inconsistencies/inhomogeneities, and (3) resolution. While these concerns are similar to those when imaging the spinal cord at any field strength and with any technique, the specific impacts to the CEST experiment at high field are outlined here.

2.4.3.3.1 B_0 Inhomogeneity and Fluctuations

In general, static field inhomogeneities can be corrected by appropriately shifting the z-spectrum such that the minimum of the CEST spectra for each voxel is set to $\Delta\omega = 0$. While there are methods to do this,[65,66] B_0 fluctuation due to respiration, swallowing, and cardiac pulsation are more difficult to correct. That is, at ultra-high field, these effects can change the local field sufficiently during the preparation, or acquisition, resulting in a time-dependent variation in the frequency offset. In principle, gating strategies can be employed; however, it is imperative that the TR remains constant for CEST when steady state acquisitions are used. Therefore, navigated approaches may be more ideal and should be investigated.

2.4.3.3.2 B_1 Inconsistencies/Inhomogeneities

CEST imaging also relies on confidence that the power of the RF irradiation is constant across space and time. At higher field strengths, B_1 inhomogeneities result in reduced saturation efficiency and consistency. That is, the resonance of interest may not be saturated sufficiently or consistently, thus the observed CEST effect can be either noisy or even nonexistent. It should be pointed out, however, that the choice of CEST sequence (pulsed, pulse-train, or continuous wave) and the shape of the CEST irradiation pulse(s) will have an effect on the impact of field inhomogeneities, and tailored RF waveforms (c.f. Selective Inversion Recovery in Section 2.4.3.2) may provide a more consistent irradiation profile at ultra-high field. Nevertheless, it has been suggested that the acquisition of a B_1 map[67] prior to the CEST experiment can provide a "scaling factor" for the RF irradiation, which may provide at least a first-order correction for inefficient B_1. Additionally, with the advent of multichannel transmit systems, the fidelity of the transmit fields can be greatly improved.

2.4.3.3.3 Resolution

CEST compared to conventional MR acquisitions is a low SNR method. As a result, large voxel sizes (e.g., $2 \times 2 \times 3$ mm^3) are often obtained in combination with multiple averaged acquisitions. The latter of these can result in prohibitively long scan times, especially in cases where the entire z-spectrum is sampled. Thus, the need for higher resolution in the spinal cord has further prompted the development of CEST at 7 T. Recently, Jones et al. have developed a CEST approach in which the CEST saturation is interleaved with a steady state acquisition,[53] which shows promise in increasing the speed with which CEST spectra can be obtained. Faster CEST acquisitions will allow for higher resolution (with more averages) to be obtained and open the door for higher resolution spinal cord acquisitions.

2.4.3.3.4 Sample Data

In spite of these limitations, CEST data can be obtained in the spinal cord at 7 T. Figure 2.4.4 shows a CEST data set in the cervical spinal cord of a healthy volunteer at 7 T. Scan parameters can be found in the Figure legend. Figure 2.4.4(A) shows a montage of the spinal cord when the RF irradiation frequency offset is varied. Note that near resonance the tissue signal is nearly completely saturated. Figure 2.4.4(B) shows the CEST z-spectra for WM (black dots) and GM (gray dots), a fit to a single Lorentzian (solid lines) and the resulting deviation of the data from the Lorentzian fit (dashed). Lastly, Figure 2.4.4(C) shows the map of the amide proton transfer (APT) effect ($\Delta\omega = 3.5$ ppm). Note that in Figure 2.4.4(B) it is difficult to accurately visualize the amide peak in the CEST spectra potentially due to pulse duration, spoiling, and lipid contamination, and underpins the shortcomings of the acquisition and analysis method. Thus, there is a need for optimization for each anatomy. Nevertheless, development of optimized CEST preparation, readout schemes, and appropriate shimming CEST should be considered feasible for spinal cord imaging at 7 T.

2.4.3.4 Diffusion-Weighted/Diffusion Tensor Imaging

The higher SNR afforded at 7 T may be particularly advantageous for diffusion tensor imaging (DTI). Specifically, DTI at 7 T can utilize this increase in SNR for increased spatial resolution, reduced acquisition time, and/or increased diffusion weighting—this may allow for more accurate fractional anisotropy (FA),

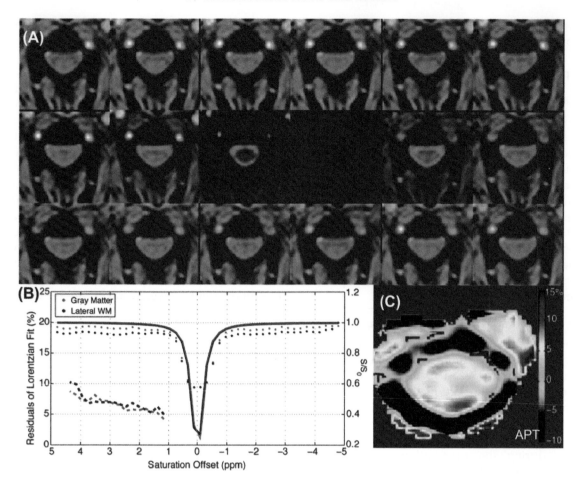

FIGURE 2.4.4 Chemical exchange saturation transfer (CEST) acquisition *(Panel (A))*, calculated spectra from gray and lateral column white matter *(Panel (B))* and a calculated amide proton transfer (APT) image *(Panel (C))*. *Acquisition parameters*: 3D gradient echo with turbo field echo readout (TFE factor = 63), FOV = $180 \times 180 \times 40$ mm^3, resolution = $1.5 \times 1.5 \times 5$ mm^3, TR/TE/α = 4.8 ms/3 ms/25°, SENSE = 2. RF irradiation was performed with 25 Gaussian pulses (1 µT, 25 ms, 80% duty cycle) leading to a pulse train of 500 ms. Offset frequency range was −5 to 5 ppm with 0.2 ppm spacing (48 offset frequencies). Total scan time = 10 min.

mean diffusivity (MD), and fiber tracking. However, there are many confounding issues at high field that may nullify the benefits of improved SNR.[68] Specifically deleterious for DTI is a reduction in T_2 (from approximately 77 ms at 3 T to 50 ms at 7 T[69]). The resulting faster signal decay cancels some of the gains in SNR and results in increased image blurring from the single-shot EPI readouts that are typically used. Stronger susceptibility-induced B_0 inhomogeneities near tissue-air or tissue-bone can also cause significant image distortion. In the spinal cord, this is further exacerbated by the complicated motions surrounding the spinal cord, which corrupt DTI data when large motion-sensitive diffusion gradients are applied. Conventional, lower field DTI experiments use single-shot EPI, which at 7 T, is particularly challenging, especially in the spinal cord. One very promising alternative is to use multishot EPI with parallel imaging techniques (see Chapter 2.3).

Currently, high spatial-resolution diffusion-weighted images and corresponding tensor-derived information have been presented using multishot EPI approaches for in vivo human brain at 7 T,[70,71] but to date, no spinal cord DTI at 7 T has appeared in the literature. Even with the promising advancements in high field DTI of the brain, there remain significant challenges to adopt these for spinal cord imaging.

2.4.4 BOLD FUNCTIONAL MRI

Functional MRI (fMRI) has rapidly expanded since its emergence two decades ago, and it is estimated that more than a dozen fMRI articles are published daily. It is well established as the single most powerful method available for detecting changes in neural activity in vivo, albeit indirectly by detection of changes in the BOLD signal.

Functional MRI of the spinal cord is still an emerging field (details of the different methodologies can be found in Chapters 4.1 and 4.2), and the two orders of magnitude fewer publications on spinal cord fMRI (compared to brain fMRI) can potentially be attributed to two main reasons. First, the functional organization of the spinal cord is complex and layer specific,[72] relatively underexplored, and it remains unclear whether the spinal cord exhibits functional connectivity akin to the brain's resting-state networks. Secondly, and perhaps most significantly, are the technical hindrances to spinal cord fMRI. At 1.5 T and even 3 T, temporal SNR and BOLD contrast limit the spatial resolution and sensitivity to the BOLD effect, so large voxels and/or thicker slices are typically necessary. The higher SNR and much greater BOLD contrast from 7 T fMRI have already shown significant advantages over lower field studies of the brain for detecting activation at high spatial resolution for a wide range of

applications. For example, recent work in the brain has shown a dramatic improvement in the sensitivity and spatial specificity of BOLD activation at the laminar scale using submillimeter resolution.[73] However, questions remain regarding the impact of higher field strengths on spinal cord fMRI experiments.

Nearly all fMRI (both brain and spinal cord) at lower fields make use of multislice single-shot sequences such as EPI and FSE. EPI sequences are largely limited to coarse spatial resolution (typically $\sim 30\,\mathrm{mm}^3$ voxels at 3 T) and are artifact ridden in areas where there are multiple tissue interfaces and B_0 field inhomogeneities. At 7 T, single-shot EPI is penalized to an even greater degree due to shorter T_2^* and significant field inhomogeneities. For FSE sequences, robustness is intimately linked to the fidelity of the refocusing pulses and is also limited to coarse resolution since long FSE echo trains result in a T_2-blurring effect.

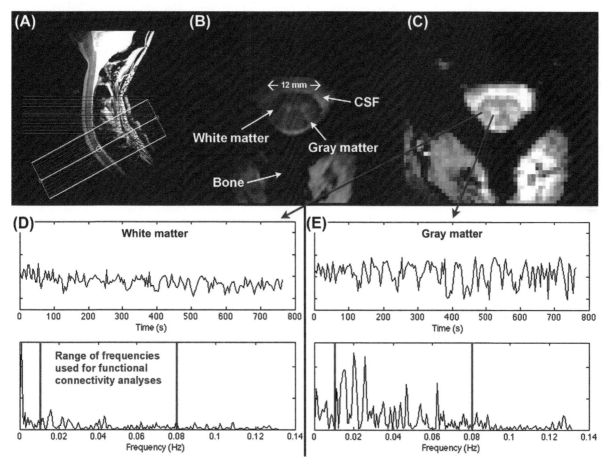

FIGURE 2.4.5 *Panel (A)*: mid-sagittal slice from a healthy volunteer showing the complete cervical spinal cord and slice placement for data shown in Panels (B–E). Due to the natural curve in the spinal cord, two stacks were necessary for data acquisition. *Panel (B)*: T_2^*-weighted anatomical image of the spinal cord at C4 acquired with $0.6 \times 0.6 \times 4\,\mathrm{mm}^3$ voxels (15 slices acquired in 3 min 48 s). *Panel (C)*: a high-resolution axial functional-weighted image at approximately the same level as in Panel (B). This sequence acquired 24 slices ($1 \times 1 \times 4\,\mathrm{mm}^3$) voxels every 3.81 s. The only preprocessing step applied to these functional data was a manual de-spiking filter to suppress volumes with obvious swallowing-related artifacts. *Panel (D)*: time series (*top*) for a single white matter voxel identified in *Panel (C)* and the corresponding power spectrum density (PSD) (*bottom*). The PSD reveals no significant power in the range of frequencies typically associated with resting state functional connectivity. *Panel (E)*: time series (*top*) for a single gray matter voxel identified in Panel (C) and its PSD (*bottom*). Most of the power in this gray matter voxel lies in the 0.01–0.08 Hz frequency range associated with functional connectivity in the brain.

Recent literature on the brain points toward the utilization of underexplored, alternative 3D-imaging strategies that can provide similar sensitivity to BOLD effects but offer high spatial or temporal resolution, reduced T_2^* blurring, and diminished geometric distortions.[74] Because these scans may be slower than their single-shot counterparts, the ability at higher field to make use of increased acceleration factor and/or short TRs is essential. For example, a recent 7 T study in the brain demonstrated that functional volumes can be acquired with high temporal resolution (1 s) at finer spatial resolutions ($\sim$2–4 mm^3) using more than threefold k-space undersampling.[75]

Such approaches may afford an opportunity to study spinal cord functionality in detail at much higher resolution at 7 T. It can be seen that the 3D-gradient echo BOLD-weighted acquisition in Figure 2.4.5(C) is devoid of many of the artifacts that we are accustomed to seeing in single-shot methods even at lower field strengths. Additionally, there is growing interest in the resting state activity of tissues of the central nervous system and Figure 2.4.5(D–E) show two panels of the resting state fluctuations (top panels) and resulting power spectra (bottom panels) derived from voxels in the WM (left) and GM (right). While these data are preliminary, they demonstrate the plausibility of performing resting-state fMRI in the spinal cord at 7 T. Additional data will need to be obtained to discern whether or not these novel fMRI sequences can be employed in the spinal cord with sufficient sensitivity to detect task-related BOLD changes.

2.4.5 MAGNETIC RESONANCE SPECTROSCOPY

Magnetic resonance spectroscopy and spectroscopic imaging (MRS/MRSI) have extensively characterized metabolic composition and change associated with neurological disease in the brain[76,77] and spinal cord.[78] Three main metabolites have drawn the most attention in MRS/MRSI of the CNS: (1) N-acetyl aspartate (NAA), (2) total choline (Cho), and (3) total creatine (Cr)—these are primarily sensitive to axonal integrity, demyelination/gliosis, and overall metabolic activity, respectively. Other metabolites/neurochemicals such as γ-aminobutyric acid (GABA),[79–82] glutamate/glutamine,[83,84] myoinositol,[85] etc., have recently become more accessible due to advanced editing sequences, higher SNR receiver coils, and more sophisticated pulses.

While MRS/MRSI face significant challenges in the spinal cord, some excellent reports have proven the necessity to push forward spectroscopic applications in the spinal cord. At lower field strengths, the primary challenges for performing MRS/MRSI in the spinal cord are (1) the need for higher SNR, (2) the impact of spatially (and temporally) varying B_0 and B_1 fields, and (3) the need for higher spectral resolution to resolve the metabolites of interest. At lower field, most commonly, single voxel MRS is utilized (with[1] and without[86] water suppression) over a voxel size of $\sim$2 cm^3. To gain sufficient SNR, a high number of acquisitions are obtained compared to the brain, which can in some cases make spectroscopic scans prohibitive for routine clinical use. At higher fields, the quasi-linear relationship between the SNR and field strength may offer the opportunity for either much more rapid acquisitions (at the same resolution), or perhaps better, higher resolution acquisitions from which it may be possible to begin to study individual structures within the spinal cord. Additionally, as has been shown in the brain,[87] the increase in spectral resolution at higher field may allow metabolites that are challenging to visualize at lower field may become more straightforward to image in the cord.

It should be noted, however, that higher field strength does pose some significant hurdles compared to lower field. Primarily, the increased sensitivity to susceptibility requires a carefully designed shimming routine. Additionally, because of the proximity of the spinal cord to the heart and lungs, at higher field there will likely be a greater temporally varying field to consider.

Nevertheless, the possibility of greater SNR and spectral resolution coupled with the growing need to understand the metabolic profile of healthy and diseased spinal cords will likely result in a growth of spinal cord MRS/MRSI over the next years.

2.4.6 CONCLUDING REMARKS

7 T MRI has recently become an active area of research and of exploratory application. The possibility of increased resolution and/or acquisition speed resulting from the increased available SNR has opened up the door for a more detailed examination of the spinal cord. The increased spectral dispersion may allow for high resolution CEST and advanced MR spectroscopy to be performed. Lastly, the sensitivity to susceptibility, which increases at higher field, may also serve to augment fMRI of the spinal cord. However, there are significant challenges that are faced at higher field (field inhomogeneity, power deposition, shorter T_2/T_2^*, increased susceptibility effects). Fortunately, there are solutions to overcome these impediments that are appearing in the literature at a rapid pace. While in its infancy for spinal cord imaging, ultra-high field may lead to many more exciting opportunities for novel contrasts to be explored in health and disease.

References

1. Henning A, Schar M, Kollias SS, Boesiger P, Dydak U. Quantitative magnetic resonance spectroscopy in the entire human cervical spinal cord and beyond at 3T. *Magn Reson Med*. 2008;59(6): 1250–1258.

2. Sengupta S, Avison MJ, Gore JC, Brian Welch E. Software compensation of eddy current fields in multislice high order dynamic shimming. *J Magn Reson*; 210(2): 218–227.

3. Sengupta S, Welch EB, Zhao Y, et al. Dynamic B0 shimming at 7 T. *Magn Reson Imaging*; 29(4): 483–496.

4. Mikulis DJ, Wood ML, Zerdoner OA, Poncelet BP. Oscillatory motion of the normal cervical spinal cord. *Radiology*. 1994;192(1): 117–121.

5. Van de Moortele PF, Pfeuffer J, Glover GH, Ugurbil K, Hu X. Respiration-induced B_0 fluctuations and their spatial distribution in the human brain at 7 Tesla. *Magn Reson Med*. 2002;47(5):888–895.

6. Raj D, Anderson AW, Gore JC. Respiratory effects in human functional magnetic resonance imaging due to bulk susceptibility changes. *Phys Med Biol*. 2001;46(12):3331–3340.

7. Figley CR, Stroman PW. Development and validation of retrospective spinal cord motion time-course estimates (RESPITE) for spin-echo spinal fMRI: Improved sensitivity and specificity by means of a motion-compensating general linear model analysis. *NeuroImage*. 2009;44(2):421–427.

8. Spuentrup E, Buecker A, Koelker C, Guenther RW, Stuber M. Respiratory motion artifact suppression in diffusion-weighted MR imaging of the spine. *Eur Radiol*. 2003;13(2):330–336.

9. Jeong HK, Gore JC, Anderson AW. High-resolution human diffusion tensor imaging using 2-D navigated multishot SENSE EPI at 7 T. *Magn Reson Med*.

10. Van de Moortele PF, Akgun C, Adriany G, et al. B(1) destructive interferences and spatial phase patterns at 7 T with a head transceiver array coil. *Magn Reson Med*. 2005;54(6):1503–1518.

11. Katscher U, Bornert P, Leussler C, van den Brink JS. Transmit SENSE. *Magn Reson Med*. 2003;49(1):144–150.

12. Jankiewicz M, Zeng H, Moore JE, et al. Practical considerations for the design of sparse-spokes pulses. *J Magn Reson*. 2010;203(2): 294–304.

13. Moore J, Jankiewicz M, Zeng H, Anderson AW, Gore JC. Composite RF pulses for B1+-insensitive volume excitation at 7 Tesla. *J Magn Reson*; 205(1): 50–62.

14. Moore J, Jankiewicz M, Anderson AW, Gore JC. Evaluation of non-selective refocusing pulses for 7 T MRI. *J Magn Reson*; 214(1): 212–220.

15. de Heer P, Brink WM, Kooij BJ, Webb AG. Increasing signal homogeneity and image quality in abdominal imaging at 3 T with very high permittivity materials. *Magn Reson Med*; 68(4): 1317–1324.

16. Teeuwisse WM, Brink WM, Webb AG. Quantitative assessment of the effects of high-permittivity pads in 7 Tesla MRI of the brain. *Magn Reson Med*; 67(5):1285–1293.

17. Sacolick LI, Wiesinger F, Hancu I, Vogel MW. B1 mapping by Bloch-Siegert shift. *Magn Reson Med*. 2010;63(5):1315–1322.

18. Yarnykh VL. Actual flip-angle imaging in the pulsed steady state: a method for rapid three-dimensional mapping of the transmitted radiofrequency field. *Magn Reson Med*. 2007;57(1):192–200.

19. Cohen AB, Neema M, Arora A, et al. The relationships among MRI-defined spinal cord involvement, brain involvement, and disability in multiple sclerosis. *J Neuroimaging*; 22(2): 122–128.

20. Poloni G, Minagar A, Haacke EM, Zivadinov R. Recent developments in imaging of multiple sclerosis. *Neurologist*; 17(4): 185–204.

21. Kachramanoglou C, De Vita E, Thomas DL, et al. Metabolic changes in the spinal cord after brachial plexus root re-implantation. *Neurorehabil Neural Repair*. 2013;27(2):118–124.

22. Coulon O, Hickman SJ, Parker GJ, Barker GJ, Miller DH, Arridge SR. Quantification of spinal cord atrophy from magnetic resonance images via a B-spline active surface model. *Magn Reson Med*. 2002;47(6):1176–1185.

23. Horsfield MA, Sala S, Neema M, et al. Rapid semi-automatic segmentation of the spinal cord from magnetic resonance images: application in multiple sclerosis. *NeuroImage*; 50(2): 446–455.

24. Filippi M, Rocca MA, De Stefano N, et al. Magnetic resonance techniques in multiple sclerosis: the present and the future. *Arch Neurol*; 68(12): 1514–1520.

25. Rocca MA, Horsfield MA, Sala S, et al. A multicenter assessment of cervical cord atrophy among MS clinical phenotypes. *Neurology*; 76(24):2096–2102.

26. Yiannakas MC, Kearney H, Samson RS, et al. Feasibility of grey matter and white matter segmentation of the upper cervical cord in vivo: a pilot study with application to magnetisation transfer measurements. *Neuroimage*; 63(3): 1054–1059.

27. Sigmund EE, Suero GA, Hu C, et al. High-resolution human cervical spinal cord imaging at 7 T. *NMR Biomed*; 25(7): 891–899.

28. Smith SA, Edden RA, Farrell JA, Barker PB, Van Zijl PC. Measurement of T1 and T2 in the cervical spinal cord at 3 Tesla. *Magn Reson Med*. 2008;60(1):213–219.

29. Visser F, Zwanenburg JJ, Hoogduin JM, Luijten PR. High-resolution magnetization-prepared 3D-FLAIR imaging at 7.0 Tesla. *Magn Reson Med*; 64(1): 194–202.

30. Zwanenburg JJ, Hendrikse J, Visser F, Takahara T, Luijten PR. Fluid attenuated inversion recovery (FLAIR) MRI at 7.0 Tesla: comparison with 1.5 and 3.0 Tesla. *Eur Radiol*; 20(4): 915–922.

31. Cohen-Adad J, Zhao W, Keil B, et al. 7-T MRI of the spinal cord can detect lateral corticospinal tract abnormality in amyotrophic lateral sclerosis. *Muscle Nerve*. 2013;47(5):760–762.

32. Cohen-Adad J, Zhao W, Wald LL, Oaklander AL. 7T MRI of spinal cord injury. *Neurology*. 2012;79(22):2217.

33. Kolind SH, Laule C, Vavasour IM, et al. Complementary information from multi-exponential T2 relaxation and diffusion tensor imaging reveals differences between multiple sclerosis lesions. *NeuroImage*. 2008;40(1):77–85.

34. Haacke EM, Chengb NYC, House MJ, et al. Imaging iron stores in the brain using magnetic resonance imaging. *Magn Reson Imaging*. 2005;23(1):1–25.

35. MacKay A, Whittall K, Adler J, Li D, Paty D, Graeb D. In vivo visualization of myelin water in brain by magnetic resonance. *Magn Reson Med*. 1994;31(6):673–677.

36. Minty EP, Bjarnason TA, Laule C, Mackay AL. Myelin water measurement in the spinal cord. *Magn Reson Med*. 2009;61(4): 883–892.

37. Levitt M, Freeman R. Compensation for pulse imperfections in NMR spin-echo experiments. *J Magn Reson*. 1981;43:65–80.

38. Fernandez-Seara MA, Wehrli FW. Postprocessing technique to correct for background gradients in image-based R2* measurements. *Magn Reson Med*. 2000;44(3):358–366.

39. Nk Chen, Wyrwicz AM. Removal of intravoxel dephasing artifact in gradient-echo images using a field-map based RF refocusing technique. *Magn Reson Med*. 1999;42(4):807–812.

40. Truong TK, Chakeres DW, Scharre DW, Beversdorf DQ, Schmalbrock P. Blipped multi gradient-echo slice excitation profile imaging (bmGESEPI) for fast T2* measurements with macroscopic B_0 inhomogeneity compensation. *Magn Reson Med*. 2006;55(6): 1390–1395.

41. Dortch RD, Does MD. Temporal DeltaB0 and relaxation in the rat heart. *Magn Reson Med*. 2007;58(5):939–946.

42. Ou X, Gochberg DF. MT effects and T1 quantification in single-slice spoiled gradient echo imaging. *Magn Reson Med*. 2008; 59(4):835–845.

43. Henkelman RM, Stanisz GJ, Graham SJ. Magnetization transfer in MRI: a review. *NMR Biomed.* 2001;14(2):57–64.

44. Wolff SD, Balaban RS. Magnetization transfer contrast (MTC) and tissue water proton relaxation in vivo. *Magn Reson Med.* 1989;10(1):135–144.

45. Smith SA, Farrell JA, Jones CK, Reich DS, Calabresi PA, van Zijl PC. Pulsed magnetization transfer imaging with body coil transmission at 3 Tesla: feasibility and application. *Magn Reson Med.* 2006;56(4):866–875.

46. Ropele S, Filippi M, Valsasina P, et al. Assessment and correction of B1-induced errors in magnetization transfer ratio measurements. *Magn Reson Med.* 2005;53(1):134–140.

47. Samson RS, Wheeler-Kingshott CA, Symms MR, Tozer DJ, Tofts PS. A simple correction for B1 field errors in magnetization transfer ratio measurements. *Magn Reson Imaging.* 2006;24(3):255–263.

48. Volz S, Noth U, Rotarska-Jagiela A, Deichmann R. A fast B1-mapping method for the correction and normalization of magnetization transfer ratio maps at 3 T. *Neuroimage*; 49(4):3015–3026.

49. Dortch RD, Moore J, Li K, et al. Quantitative magnetization transfer imaging of human brain at 7 T. *NeuroImage.* 2012.

50. Mugler 3rd JP, Brookeman JR. Three-dimensional magnetization-prepared rapid gradient-echo imaging (3D MP RAGE). *Magn Reson Med.* 1990;15(1):152–157.

51. Ward KM, Aletras AH, Balaban RS. A new class of contrast agents for MRI based on proton chemical exchange dependent saturation transfer (CEST). *J Magn Reson.* 2000;143(1):79–87.

52. Haris M, Cai K, Singh A, Hariharan H, Reddy R. In vivo mapping of brain myo-inositol. *NeuroImage*; 54(3): 2079–2085.

53. Jones CK, Polders D, Hua J, et al. In vivo three-dimensional whole-brain pulsed steady-state chemical exchange saturation transfer at 7 T. *Magn Reson Med*; 67(6): 1579–1589.

54. Jones CK, Schlosser MJ, van Zijl PC, Pomper MG, Golay X, Zhou J. Amide proton transfer imaging of human brain tumors at 3T. *Magn Reson Med.* 2006;56(3):585–592.

55. Kogan F, Singh A, Cai K, Haris M, Hariharan H, Reddy R. Investigation of chemical exchange at intermediate exchange rates using a combination of chemical exchange saturation transfer (CEST) and spin-locking methods (CESTrho). *Magn Reson Med.* 2012;68(1):107–119.

56. Sun PZ, Sorensen AG. Imaging pH using the chemical exchange saturation transfer (CEST) MRI: correction of concomitant RF irradiation effects to quantify CEST MRI for chemical exchange rate and pH. *Magn Reson Med.* 2008;60(2):390–397.

57. van Zijl PC, Jones CK, Ren J, Malloy CR, Sherry AD. MRI detection of glycogen in vivo by using chemical exchange saturation transfer imaging (glycoCEST). *Proc Natl Acad Sci USA.* 2007;104(11):4359–4364.

58. van Zijl PC, Yadav NN. Chemical exchange saturation transfer (CEST): what is in a name and what isn't? *Magn Reson Med*; 65(4):927–948.

59. Zhou J, Payen JF, Wilson DA, Traystman RJ, van Zijl PC. Using the amide proton signals of intracellular proteins and peptides to detect pH effects in MRI. *Nat Med.* 2003;9(8):1085–1090.

60. Zhu H, Jones CK, van Zijl PC, Barker PB, Zhou J. Fast 3D chemical exchange saturation transfer (CEST) imaging of the human brain. *Magn Reson Med*; 64(3): 638–644.

61. Dula AN, Asche EM, Landman BA, et al. Development of chemical exchange saturation transfer at 7 T. *Magn Reson Med*; 66(3): 831–838.

62. Mougin OE, Coxon RC, Pitiot A, Gowland PA. Magnetization transfer phenomenon in the human brain at 7 T. *NeuroImage.* 2010;49(1):272–281.

63. Cai K, Haris M, Singh A, et al. Magnetic resonance imaging of glutamate. *Nat Med*; 18(2): 302–306.

64. Bryant RG. The dynamics of water-protein interactions. *Annu Rev Biophys Biomol Struct.* 1996;25:29–53.

65. Kim M, Gillen J, Landman BA, Zhou J, van Zijl PC. Water saturation shift referencing (WASSR) for chemical exchange saturation transfer (CEST) experiments. *Magn Reson Med.* 2009;61(6):1441–1450.

66. Zhou J, Blakeley JO, Hua J, et al. Practical data acquisition method for human brain tumor amide proton transfer (APT) imaging. *Magn Reson Med.* 2008;60(4):842–849.

67. Singh A, Cai K, Haris M, Hariharan H, Reddy R. On B(1) inhomogeneity correction of in vivo human brain glutamate chemical exchange saturation transfer contrast at 7 T. *Magn Reson Med.* 2013;69(3):818–824.

68. Speck O, Zhong K. *Diffusion Tensor Imaging at 7T: Expectations vs. Reality Check.* 2009. Honolulu. p. 1462.

69. Polders DL, Leemans A, Hendrikse J, Donahue MJ, Luijten PR, Hoogduin JM. Signal to noise ratio and uncertainty in diffusion tensor imaging at 1.5, 3.0, and 7.0 Tesla. *J Magn Reson Imaging*; 33(6): 1456–1463.

70. Heidemann RM, Porter DA, Anwander A. Diffusion imaging in humans at 7 T using readout-segmented EPI and GRAPPA. *Magn Reson Med.* 2010;64(1):9–14.

71. Jeong HK, Anderson AW, Gore JC. Multi-Shot SENSE DWI at 7T. In: *Proceedings of the 18th Annual Meeting of ISMRM.* Stockholm; 2010: 1616.

72. Kandel E, Schwartz JH, Jessell TM. *Principles of Neural Science.* McGraw-Hill Companies; 2000.

73. Polimeni JR, Fischl B, Greve DN, Wald LL. Laminar analysis of 7 T BOLD using an imposed spatial activation pattern in human V1. *NeuroImage*; 52(4): 1334–1346.

74. Barry RL, Strother SC, Gatenby JC, Gore JC. Data-driven optimization and evaluation of 2D EPI and 3D PRESTO for BOLD fMRI at 7 Tesla: I. Focal coverage. *NeuroImage*; 55(3): 1034–1043.

75. Newton AT, Rogers BP, Gore JC, Morgan VL. Improving measurement of functional connectivity through decreasing partial volume effects at 7 T. *NeuroImage*; 59(3): 2511–2517.

76. Ross B, Kreis R, Ernst T. Clinical tools for the 90s: magnetic resonance spectroscopy and metabolite imaging. *Eur J Radiol.* 1992;14(2):128–140.

77. Van Zijl PC, Barker PB. Magnetic resonance spectroscopy and spectroscopic imaging for the study of brain metabolism. *Ann N Y Acad Sci.* 1997;820:75–96.

78. Ciccarelli O, Wheeler-Kingshott CA, McLean MA, et al. Spinal cord spectroscopy and diffusion-based tractography to assess acute disability in multiple sclerosis. *Brain.* 2007;130(Pt 8):2220–2231.

79. Edden RA, Barker PB. Spatial effects in the detection of gamma-aminobutyric acid: improved sensitivity at high fields using inner volume saturation. *Magn Reson Med.* 2007;58(6):1276–1282.

80. Edden RA, Puts NA, Barker PB. Macromolecule-suppressed GABA-edited magnetic resonance spectroscopy at 3T. *Magn Reson Med*; 68(3): 657–661.

81. Waddell KW, Avison MJ, Joers JM, Gore JC. A practical guide to robust detection of GABA in human brain by J-difference spectroscopy at 3 T using a standard volume coil. *Magn Reson Imaging.* 2007;25(7):1032–1038.

82. Zhu H, Edden RA, Ouwerkerk R, Barker PB. High resolution spectroscopic imaging of GABA at 3 Tesla. *Magn Reson Med*; 65(3): 603–609.

83. Gu M, Zahr NM, Spielman DM, Sullivan EV, Pfefferbaum A, Mayer D. Quantification of glutamate and glutamine using constant-time point-resolved spectroscopy at 3 T. *NMR Biomed.*

84. Henry ME, Lauriat TL, Shanahan M, Renshaw PF, Jensen JE. Accuracy and stability of measuring GABA, glutamate, and glutamine by proton magnetic resonance spectroscopy: a phantom study at 4 Tesla. *J Magn Reson*; 208(2): 210–218.

85. Ciccarelli O, Toosy AT, De Stefano N, Wheeler-Kingshott CA, Miller DH, Thompson AJ. Assessing neuronal metabolism in vivo by modeling imaging measures. *J Neurosci*; 30(45): 15030–15033.

86. Hock A, Macmillan EL, Fuchs A, et al. Non-water-suppressed proton MR spectroscopy improves spectral quality in the human spinal cord. *Magn Reson Med*. 2013;69(5):1253–1260.

87. Fuchs A, Luttje M, Boesiger P, Henning A. SPECIAL semi-LASER with lipid artifact compensation for (1) H MRS at 7 T. *Magn Reson Med*. 2013;69(3):603–612.

88. Verma T, Cohen-Adad J. Effect of Respiration on the B0 Field in the Human Spinal Cord at 3T, *Magn Reson Med*. 2014. http://dx.doi.org/10.1002/mrm.25075.

PART III

IMAGING SPINAL CORD STRUCTURE

Diffusion-Weighted Imaging of the Spinal Cord

Benjamin M. Ellingson[1], Julien Cohen-Adad[2]

[1]Department of Radiological Sciences, David Geffen School of Medicine, University of California-Los Angeles, Los Angeles, CA, USA [2]Institute of Biomedical Engineering, Polytechnique Montreal; Functional Neuroimaging Unit, CRIUGM, Université de Montréal, Montreal, QC, Canada

3.1.1 PRINCIPLES OF DIFFUSION-WEIGHTED MAGNETIC RESONANCE IMAGING

3.1.1.1 Basic Concept of Diffusion Weighting

Water molecules in tissue undergo Brownian motion, which means that molecules are not perfectly static over time but experience random microscopic displacements due to thermal agitation. This effect can be characterized by a diffusion coefficient. Compared to free water, where this effect is equal whatever the direction of observation is (i.e., it is isotropic), in tissue the molecular displacement is restricted and hindered[a] by the tissue structures (i.e., it is anisotropic), where it is faster along certain directions and slower along others. This is a very important consideration for the discussion of water diffusion measurements in tissue using magnetic resonance imaging (MRI), as it will become clearer later on in this chapter.

MRI is inherently sensitive to the movement of water molecules in tissue because in MRI a spatial position is characterized by its own phase and frequency that are encoded during the experiment. On average, at a voxel size level of a few millimeter cube, the thermal motion of water molecules is negligible but can be encoded by sensitizing the MRI acquisition to the average displacement taking place during a certain time.

To aid in understanding diffusion-weighted MR images of the spinal cord, it may be helpful to explore the basic physical principles of the diffusion process in general terms. Traditionally, the net movement of a substance (e.g., spins or protons in the nuclear magnetic resonance (NMR) experiment, or generically "water protons" in the NMR experiment and throughout this chapter) can be characterized by a diffusion coefficient (D), a variable relating the concentration gradient to the rate of transfer of water molecules through a unit of area.[1] The flux of water in one direction is related to the diffusion coefficient by Fick's first law of diffusion:

$$F = -D\frac{\partial C}{\partial r} \tag{3.1.1}$$

where F is the mass flux (mass/time), D is the diffusion coefficient (area/time), C is the concentration of water protons (mass/volume), and r is the length coordinate. If we assume the system is in steady state (i.e., no net water protons added or subtracted from the system), Fick's first and second law of diffusion can be combined to form the second-order wave equation for diffusion:

$$\frac{\partial C(r,t)}{\partial t} = D\frac{\partial^2 C(r,t)}{\partial r^2} \tag{3.1.2}$$

where $C(r,t)$ denotes the concentration of water protons as a function of both distance, r, and time, t.

In the diffusion-weighted MRI experiment, no real or significant measurable "concentration gradients" of water protons exist (i.e., "zero-flux"). Thus, any "concentration gradients" in the diffusion MRI experiment must be thought of in terms of the concentration of "tagged" water protons, such as is performed in

---

[a]Hindered diffusion refers to the diffusion of water with a Gaussian displacement pattern, such as in the extracellular space. Restricted diffusion refers to the diffusion of water in restricted geometries, yielding a non-Gaussian pattern of displacement, and is found in the intracellular space bounded for example by axonal or dendritic membranes.

123

diffusion tracer experiments. In any sense, if no physical concentration gradients are assumed in this condition, we must describe the concentration of water protons in terms of the probability of their displacement across both space and time, $P(r_0|r, t)$, where r_0 is the initial position of the water protons. Assuming the probability displacement function follows a Gaussian distribution, which is the simple solution using random walks, Einstein's equation for mean displacement applies,[1,2]

$$\langle r - r_0 \rangle = \sqrt{6Dt} \qquad (3.1.3)$$

and it results in the solution:

$$P(r_0|r, t) = \frac{1}{\sqrt{(4\pi Dt)^2}} e^{-\frac{(r-r_0)^2}{4Dt}} \qquad (3.1.4)$$

The application of this Gaussian probability distribution of water protons to the Bloch equations is the basis of conventional diffusion-weighted MRI.

3.1.1.2 Bloch Equations with Diffusion Terms

The time-evolving magnetization density in an NMR experiment can be defined by the Bloch equations (including relaxation terms):

$$\frac{\mathrm{d}\overrightarrow{\mathbf{M}}(t)}{\mathrm{d}t} = \mathrm{j}\gamma\overrightarrow{\mathbf{M}}(t) \times \overrightarrow{\mathbf{B}} + \frac{(M_z(0) - M_z(t))\cdot\widehat{\mathbf{k}}}{T_1}$$
$$- \frac{M_x(t)\widehat{\mathbf{i}} + M_y(t)\widehat{\mathbf{j}}}{T_2} \qquad (3.1.5)$$

where $\overrightarrow{\mathbf{M}}(t)$ is the magnetization density vector at time t, $M_z(0)$ is the initial longitudinal magnetization, $M_z(t)$ is the longitudinal magnetization at time t, $M_x(t)$ is the transverse component of the magnetization density vector in the x-orientation at time t, $M_y(t)$ is the transverse component of the magnetization density vector in the y-orientation at time t, γ is the gyromagnetic ratio for protons ($\gamma = 42.58\,\mathrm{MHz/T}$), $\overrightarrow{\mathbf{B}}$ is the external magnetic field vector, T_1 is the spin–lattice relaxation rate, T_2 is the spin–spin relaxation rate, j is the imaginary number $\mathrm{j} = \sqrt{-1}$, and $\widehat{\mathbf{i}}$, $\widehat{\mathbf{j}}$, and $\widehat{\mathbf{k}}$ denote unit vectors in the x, y, and z orientation.

In 1956, Torrey described the Bloch equations in terms of self-diffusion of an NMR species (e.g., water protons) having a diffusion coefficient, D.[3] By applying an arbitrary time-dependent linear magnetic field gradient, $\overrightarrow{\mathbf{g}}(t)$, we are able to describe the magnetization density vector as:

$$\frac{\mathrm{d}\overrightarrow{\mathbf{M}}(t)}{\mathrm{d}t} = \mathrm{j}\gamma\overrightarrow{\mathbf{M}}(t) \times \overrightarrow{\mathbf{g}}(t) + \frac{(M_z(0) - M_z(t))\cdot\widehat{\mathbf{k}}}{T_1}$$
$$- \frac{M_x(t)\widehat{\mathbf{i}} + M_y(t)\widehat{\mathbf{j}}}{T_2} + D\nabla^2\overrightarrow{\mathbf{M}}(t) \qquad (3.1.6)$$

which has the solution:

$$\overrightarrow{\mathbf{M}}(t) = \overrightarrow{\mathbf{M}}(0)\cdot\left(1 - \exp\left\{-\frac{t}{T_1}\right\}\right)\cdot\exp\left\{-\frac{t}{T_2}\right\}\cdot$$
$$\exp\left\{-D\gamma^2\int_0^t\left[\left(\int_0^{t''}\overrightarrow{\mathbf{g}}(t')\mathrm{d}t'\right)^2\right]\mathrm{d}t''\right\} \qquad (3.1.7)$$

This solution can be rewritten in generic terms as:

$$\overrightarrow{\mathbf{M}}(t) = \overbrace{\overrightarrow{\mathbf{M}}(0)}^{\substack{\text{Initial}\\\text{Magnetization}}} \cdot \overbrace{\left(1 - e^{-\frac{t}{T_1}}\right)}^{\substack{\text{Spin–Lattice}\\\text{Relaxation}}} \cdot \overbrace{e^{-\frac{t}{T_2}}}^{\substack{\text{Spin–Spin}\\\text{Relaxation}}} \cdot \overbrace{e^{-b\cdot D}}^{\substack{\text{Diffusion}\\\text{Weighting}}} \qquad (3.1.8)$$

where b, generally referred to as the "b-value", represents the level of diffusion weighting (or attenuation) observed in the resulting magnetization as a function of diffusion "encoding" experimental parameters defined as:

$$b = \gamma^2\int_0^t\left[\left(\int_0^{t''}\overrightarrow{\mathbf{g}}(t')\mathrm{d}t'\right)^2\right]\mathrm{d}t'' \qquad (3.1.9)$$

For example, using a *gradient recalled echo (GRE)* experiment, the total magnetization at echo time TE at steady-state for a repetition time TR is:

$$\overrightarrow{\mathbf{M}}(\mathrm{TE}, \mathrm{TR}) = \overrightarrow{\mathbf{M}}(0)\cdot\left(1 - \exp\left\{-\frac{\mathrm{TR}}{T_1}\right\}\right)\cdot\exp\left\{-\frac{\mathrm{TE}}{T_2}\right\}\cdot$$
$$\exp\left\{-D\gamma^2\int_0^{\mathrm{TE}}\left[\int_0^{t''}\overrightarrow{\mathbf{g}}(t')\mathrm{d}t'\right]^2\mathrm{d}t''\right\} \qquad (3.1.10)$$

Alternatively, using a *spin-echo (SE)* experiment, the total magnetization at echo time TE at steady-state for a repetition time TR is:

$$\overrightarrow{\mathbf{M}}(\mathrm{TE}, \mathrm{TR}) = \overrightarrow{\mathbf{M}}(0)\cdot\left(1 - \exp\left\{-\frac{\mathrm{TR}}{T_1}\right\}\right)\cdot\exp\left\{-\frac{\mathrm{TE}}{T_2}\right\}$$
$$\cdot\exp\left\{-D\gamma^2\left[\int_0^{\mathrm{TE}/2}\left[\left(\int_0^{t''}\overrightarrow{\mathbf{g}}(t')\mathrm{d}t'\right)^2\right]\mathrm{d}t''\right.\right.$$
$$- 4\cdot\int_0^{\mathrm{TE}/2}\left[\left(\int_0^{t''}\overrightarrow{\mathbf{g}}(t')\mathrm{d}t'\right)^2\right]\mathrm{d}t''$$
$$\cdot\int_{\mathrm{TE}/2}^{\mathrm{TE}}\left[\left(\int_0^{t''}\overrightarrow{\mathbf{g}}(t')\mathrm{d}t'\right)^2\right]\mathrm{d}t''$$
$$\left.\left.+ 4\cdot\int_{\mathrm{TE}/2}^{\mathrm{TE}}\left[\left(\int_0^{t''}\overrightarrow{\mathbf{g}}(t')\mathrm{d}t'\right)^2\right]\mathrm{d}t''\right]\right\} \qquad (3.1.11)$$

Note that while both of these experiments result in dramatically different dependencies of diffusion-related signal attenuation on the gradient waveforms, both sequences can be expressed in terms of $e^{-b \cdot D}$, differing only in their expression for b.

The simplest method of employing diffusion sensitivity is through the use of bipolar diffusion sensitizing gradients to the GRE experiment (in a single direction), as illustrated in Figure 3.1.1(A). Here, G reflects the gradient amplitude and δ reflects the duration of each bipolar gradient pulse. Using Eqn (3.1.9), we see the expression for the b-value as a function of the diffusion-encoding scheme is:

$$b = \frac{2}{3}\gamma^2 G^2 \delta^3 \tag{3.1.12}$$

Similarly, a monopolar pulse of similar amplitude and duration results in the same expression for b-value for the SE case (Figure 3.1.1(B)). This also can be extended to n-refocusing pulses in the SE experiment (Figure 3.1.1(C)), resulting in an expression for b-value of:

$$b = \frac{\gamma^2 G^2 \delta}{3n^2} \tag{3.1.13}$$

In 1965, Stejskal and Tanner introduced the most commonly employed diffusion-encoding scheme called *pulsed gradient spin-echo (PGSE)* encoding.[4] In contrast to previous diffusion MR experiments, the PGSE experiment involves a *diffusion time* (also called mixing time), Δ, in addition to the encoding time, δ (Figure 3.1.1(D)).

$$b = \gamma^2 G^2 \delta^2 \left(\Delta - \frac{\delta}{3} \right) \tag{3.1.14}$$

Note that a *stimulated echo acquisition mode (STEAM)*, which replaces the π-refocusing pulse by two

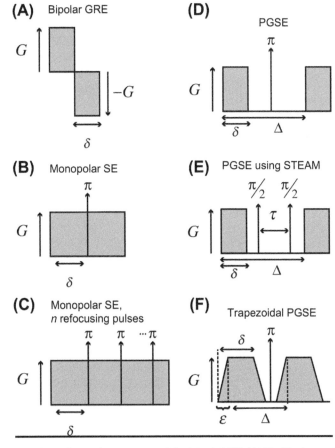

FIGURE 3.1.1 Common gradient encoding schemes for measuring diffusivity in MRI. (A) The bipolar gradient recalled echo (GRE) dephases the spins in the first monopolar lobe, then refocuses the spins in the second, opposite, monopolar lobe. (B) A monopolar spin-echo (SE) sequence performs similarly to the bipolar GRE sequence, but uses a p-refocusing pulse to refocus the spins. (C) The monopolar SE sequence can be extended to "n" refocusing pulses, leading to a higher level of diffusion weighting. (D) The pulsed-gradient spin-echo (PGSE) experiment first proposed by Stejskal and Tanner, where a diffusion time Δ is introduced between dephasing and rephrasing diffusion sensitizing gradient pulses. (E) In stimulated echo acquisition mode (STEAM), the π-refocusing pulse is replaced by two $\pi/2$ pulses in order to store the magnetization vector along the longitudinal axis, resulting in T_1 decay instead of T_2/T_2^* decay and allowing for longer diffusion times because $T_1 \gg T_2/T_2^*$. (F) Using trapezoidal gradient waveforms in the PGSE experiment better estimates the physical gradients used for PGSE by adjusting for maximum gradient slew rate.

$\pi/2$-pulses separated by a length of time t, should be used to probe long diffusion times, since the phase encoded spins can be stored within the longitudinal orientation instead of transverse plane, making them subject to T_1 decay and minimal T_2-related signal attenuation (Figure 3.1.1(E)). Taking into consideration limitations on gradient slew rates, the use of trapezoidal diffusion-encoding gradients (Figure 3.1.1(F)) allows for an accurate real-world approximation to the rectangular gradients proposed in the PGSE experiments, with a b-value of:

$$b = \gamma^2 G^2 \left[\delta^2 \left(\Delta - \frac{1}{3}\delta \right) + \frac{\varepsilon^3}{30} - \frac{\delta \cdot \varepsilon^2}{6} \right] \quad (3.1.15)$$

where G/ε is the gradient slew rate, which is typically assumed to be the maximum for a specific system. It is important to point out that the imaging gradients themselves, during readout of the image, contribute to diffusion weighting and should be included in the calculations of b for an exact solution of the equation.

3.1.1.3 The Apparent Diffusion Coefficient

Although the diffusion MR experiment can provide an *estimate* for the physical diffusion coefficient in an image voxel using the magnetic field gradients, the measured diffusion coefficient in MRI is often referred to as an *apparent diffusion coefficient*, or *ADC*, because it reflects the average diffusion coefficient in a voxel, affected by many biophysical factors and experimental setup.

Estimation of the diffusion coefficient in fast-moving liquids will typically be underestimated in highly tortuous environments due to the relatively long diffusion times (milliseconds) used in conventional MR experiments. These relatively long diffusion times are a direct reflection of magnetic field gradient hardware limitations, primarily in terms of slew rate. For example, consider a single water molecule diffusing through a relatively tortuous environment with a fixed diffusion time, Δ (Figure 3.1.2, *top row*). If this water molecule is diffusing relative slowly and the spacing between barriers is sufficiently large compared to the ensemble average distance traveled by the diffusing water molecule during this diffusion time ($\langle r - r_0 \rangle < r_{\text{boundaries}}$), then the actual diffusion coefficient will be accurately represented by the measured, apparent, diffusion coefficient with MRI (ADC$\cong D$) (Figure 3.1.2(A)). Alternatively, if the water molecule is diffusing relatively quickly such that the spacing between barriers is smaller than the *actual* distance traveled by diffusion water molecule during the diffusion time of the experiment ($l_{\text{actual}} > r_{\text{boundaries}}$), then the diffusion coefficient will

not be accurately represented by the measured, or apparent, diffusion coefficient detected by MRI (ADC $< D$) (Figure 3.1.2(B)). In this case, the apparent diffusion coefficient, ADC, is related to the actual diffusion coefficient, D, by the square of the *tortuosity* of the environment, θ^2:[5–7]

$$\text{ADC} = \frac{D}{\theta^2} \quad (3.1.16)$$

Tortuosity is a variable relating the actual total distance the water molecule travels during the diffusion time to the shortest distance between the start and end points of the water molecule's path.

$$\theta = \frac{l_{\text{actual}}}{\langle r - r_0 \rangle} \quad (3.1.17)$$

The current example assumes a constant diffusion time; however, the same situation arises when *different* diffusion times are used within the same tissue architecture (Figure 3.1.2, *bottom row*). Specifically, if short diffusion times are employed then minimal diffusion restriction is observed (ADC$\cong D$) (Figure 3.1.2(C)), whereas if longer diffusion times are used then the diffusion coefficient will again *not* be accurately represented by the apparent diffusion coefficient (ADC $< D$) (Figure 3.1.2(D)).

The physical diffusion coefficient of water molecules can also be influenced by kinematic viscosity and temperature of the environment, as illustrated by the Einstein–Stokes equations[8]:

$$D = \frac{RT}{6\pi N v r} \quad (3.1.18)$$

Here, R is the universal gas constant, T is the absolute temperature, N is Avogadro's number, v is the kinematic viscosity, and r is the approximate radius of the water molecule. As this equation suggests, the measured diffusion coefficient is proportional to temperature and inversely proportional to viscosity. This relationship is particularly important when interpreting spinal cord diffusion MR measurements during pathological conditions, where changes in tissue viscosity can occur as a result of axonal or myelin degeneration, necrosis, or inflammatory cell infiltration. Additionally, acute spinal cord injury above the T6 spinal level can result in changes in core body temperature from neurogenic shock,[9,10] which may potentially confound diffusivity measurements.

Also, the ADC will depend on the direction of the applied diffusion gradients due to the complex tissue microstructure that can have different coherences. For example, measuring the ADC along a fiber bundle or across it, using the same diffusion time can give very different results.

Constant diffusion time,
different boundary spacing

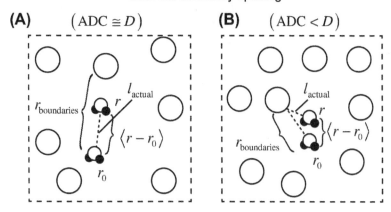

Constant boundary spacing,
different diffusion time

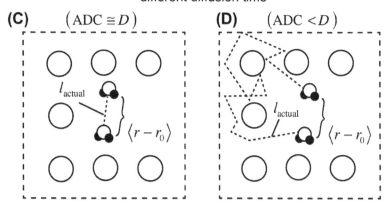

FIGURE 3.1.2 Differences between apparent diffusion coefficient (ADC) and physical diffusion coefficient (D). (A) For a constant diffusion time, physical diffusion coefficient is equal to ADC when the distance between boundaries, $r_{boundaries}$, is sufficiently larger than the diffusion distance, $\langle r - r_0 \rangle$. (B) For the same diffusion time, the diffusion MRI experiment underestimates the physical diffusion coefficient when the distance between boundaries is less than the diffusion distance (i.e., tortuosity of the environment). (C) For a fixed tissue environment with the same boundaries, the diffusion experiment with a short diffusion time will result in better estimation of the physical diffusion coefficient due to lack of restricted diffusion. (D) For the same environment, a long diffusion time (as is typically employed clinically) results in underestimation of the physical diffusion coefficient due to tortuosity and diffusion restriction.

KEY CONCEPTS IN DIFFUSION-WEIGHTED IMAGING

b-value   Parameter that sets the amplitude of the diffusion weighting. Typical values range between 500 and 3000 s/mm^2

q-space   3-dimensional space that represents the amplitude (b-value) and directions of all diffusion-encoding gradients. It is set by the user before each diffusion-weighted (DW) acquisition

Shell   refers to the q-space sampling distribution on a sphere with constant radius (constant q). For example, diffusion tensor imaging (DTI) and Q-Ball utilize single-shell sampling

3.1.2 MODELING THE DIFFUSION PROPERTIES

Several reconstruction methods exist for diffusion weighted imaging (DWI) such as DTI, Q-Ball Imaging (QBI), persistent angular structure MRI (PASMRI), and diffusion spectrum imaging (DSI). This section will review some of the most popular reconstruction methods. Good reviews on reconstruction methods are in Refs 11,12. Note that the type of reconstruction is strongly tightened to the acquisition parameters (notably q-space sampling), therefore the reconstruction method has to be carefully chosen before setting up the imaging protocol. Figure 3.1.3 summarizes the different techniques with the recommended q-space sampling and protocol length.

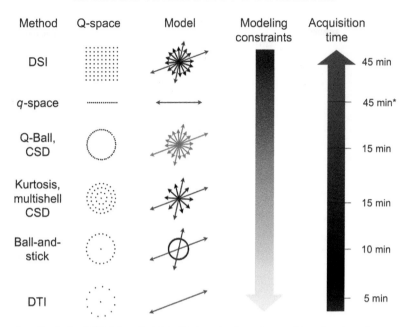

FIGURE 3.1.3   Summary of methods for DWI. Note that this list is not exhaustive and is only given for general overview of the existing methods. The first column lists the name of the techniques, the second column shows the typical *q*-space sampling, the third column shows the information obtained from the diffusion profile: if color coded, information about the amount of diffusion is known. DSI technique enables to obtain the full probability density function (PDF), i.e., orientation and magnitude of water diffusion, however is extremely time consuming (typical acquisition >45 min). Q-space imaging provides the PDF in one direction, although with higher *q*-range and finer sampling compared to DSI. (*) Note that *q*-space imaging is typically performed on systems equipped with strong gradients to be able to acquire very high *b*-values (>10,000 s/mm^2). QBI provides the diffusion orientation distribution function (dODF). Similarly, constrained spherical deconvolution (CSD) gives access to the fiber orientation distribution function (fODF). Q-Ball and CSD lose the information on the magnitude of water diffusion. QBI, particularly CSD, are therefore well suited for tractography. Kurtosis imaging contains quantitative information about the non-Gaussian diffusion profile (especially useful at high *b*-values, where restricted diffusion is better depicted). Ball-and-stick model provides the orientation and magnitude for up to *N* anisotropic compartments. DTI is the simplest model but is also the quickest to acquire.

3.1.2.1 Diffusion Tensor Imaging

A "diffusion tensor" is a 3×3 matrix useful in describing the diffusion characteristics of anisotropic media, where diffusion rates vary with respect to orientation. Diffusion tensor magnetic resonance images are calculated from data obtained from DWIs, but measured in six or more noncollinear diffusion-encoding directions. Specifically, the diffusion sensitizing gradients are applied using combinations of the three imaging gradients (slice select, phase encode, and frequency encode; or alternatively the *z*, *y*, and *x* directions), sampling the diffusion weighting along various orientations, one at a time. From these multiple DWI measurements, regression or nonlinear techniques can be used to estimate the 3×3 tensor field that describes the preferred magnitude and orientation of the self-diffusion properties of water (Figure 3.1.4(A)). The diffusion tensor, **D**, is positive and symmetric, therefore it only has six unique values (i.e., $D_{xy} = D_{yx}$, $D_{xz} = D_{zx}$ and $D_{yz} = D_{zy}$). As a result, DWI data must be obtained in a minimum of six sensitizing directions to determine the tensor values. However, it is usually recommended to acquire at least 20 directions to obtain a robust and accurate estimate of the diffusion tensor.[13]

$$\mathbf{D} = \begin{bmatrix} D_{xx} & D_{yx} & D_{zx} \\ D_{xy} & D_{yy} & D_{zy} \\ D_{xz} & D_{yz} & D_{zz} \end{bmatrix} \qquad (3.1.19)$$

The preferred diffusion magnitude and direction are found from decomposition of the *eigenvalues* and *eigenvectors* for the diffusion tensor (**D**) in each image voxel. The eigenvalues (λ) are represented by a diagonal matrix, as shown in Figure 3.1.4(B). To each one of the three eigenvalues is associated an eigenvector ($\boldsymbol{\varepsilon}$), i.e., a unitary vector indicating the direction of the diffusion process. The eigenvalues are also ordered so that λ_1 is the principal eigenvalue representing the diffusivity along $\boldsymbol{\varepsilon}_1$. Popular DTI metrics are derived from these eigenvalues, such as the fractional anisotropy (*FA*), axial diffusivity (AD) and radial diffusivity (RD), defined in the "Diffusion Tensor indices" box. Because diffusion of water in spinal cord white matter is more anisotropic than gray matter, anisotropy indices are often useful for identifying spinal gray and white matter. The mean diffusivity (MD) is defined as the average of the three eigenvalues.

(A)

$$
\begin{bmatrix}
D_{xx} & D_{yx} & D_{zx} \\
D_{xy} & D_{yy} & D_{zy} \\
D_{xz} & D_{yz} & D_{zz}
\end{bmatrix}
$$

(B)

$$
\begin{bmatrix}
\lambda_3 & 0 & 0 \\
0 & \lambda_2 & 0 \\
0 & 0 & \lambda_1
\end{bmatrix}
$$

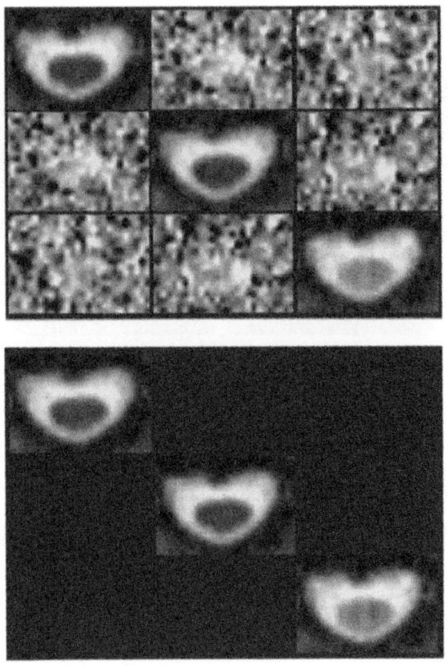

FIGURE 3.1.4 The diffusion tensor and eigenvalues. (A) A fully constructed 3×3 diffusion tensor of the human cervical spinal cord. (B) The resulting eigenvalues from the diffusion tensor. Images were collected using a custom two-dimensional radiofrequency excitation pulse and a reduced field-of-view readout scheme with $b = 500 \, s/mm^2$ and six directions.

DIFFUSION TENSOR INDICES

Fractional Anisotropy:

$$
FA = \sqrt{\frac{3}{2}} \, \frac{\sqrt{(\lambda_1 - \langle D \rangle)^2 + (\lambda_3 - \langle D \rangle)^2 + (\lambda_3 - \langle D \rangle)^2}}{\sqrt{\lambda_1^2 + \lambda_2^2 + \lambda_3^2}}
$$

Mean Diffusivity

$$
MD = \frac{(\lambda_1 + \lambda_2 + \lambda_3)}{3}
$$

Axial Diffusivity:

$$
AD = \lambda_\parallel = \lambda_1
$$

Radial Diffusivity:

$$
RD = \lambda_\perp = \frac{(\lambda_2 + \lambda_3)}{2}
$$

3.1.2.2 Ball-and-Stick Model

Introduced in Ref. 14, the ball-and-stick model is a partial volume model, where the diffusion-weighted MR signal is split into several anisotropic components (each one representing a fiber orientation) and a single isotropic component. This model can be fitted to DWI data (similar sampling scheme as for DTI). This model is notably implemented in BedPostX available in FSL (http://fsl.fmrib.ox.ac.uk/fsl/fslwiki/FDT) and in camino (http://www.camino.org.uk).

3.1.2.3 High Angular Resolution Diffusion Imaging

Diffusion tensors quantify mean diffusion within the space of a voxel, on the order of millimeters, providing only an average quantification of the microscopic diffusion process. The result is integration of diffusion characteristics for every axon localized in each voxel. If axons were homogeneously aligned within an image voxel, the first eigenvector of the tensor would accurately approximate their direction.[15] However, the tensor model is not capable of resolving multiple fiber orientations within the same voxel.[16,17] Although the use of the second eigenvector has been proposed as a means of resolving crossing fibers in spinal cord,[18,19] there are major limitations imposed by the tensor model. For example, the three eigenvectors are, by definition, orthogonal. Thus, when the primary direction is defined by the first eigenvector—longitudinal fibers in the case of the spinal cord—the second eigenvector is limited in terms of degrees of freedom since its direction is necessarily on the plane orthogonal to longitudinal fibers. In the presence of nonorthogonal fiber crossings, the typical process of orthogonal decomposition of the tensor becomes less efficient.[11]

To overcome this issue, model-free approaches have been proposed to measure the microscopic diffusion properties without constraining its representation. These methods are collectively known as diffusion spectrum imaging[20] and have already demonstrated benefits for imaging the brain.[21] However, long acquisition times are required to adequately sample q-space and retrieve the three-dimensional diffusion profile. To reduce acquisition times, sampling of q-space in a single direction has been proposed,[22] allowing the distinction of diffusion

FIGURE 3.1.5 Fiber orientations estimated using DT, QBI, and PAS of an axial
slice at the cervical enlargement overlaid on
FA (DT) and GFA (QBI and PAS); note the diagonal orientation of the spinal cord. Ventral
roots and terminating fibers from the corticospinal tract are marked with green and white
ellipses, respectively. *Source: Reproduced with
permission from Lundell et al.*[35]

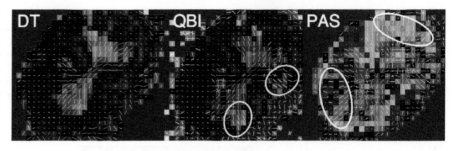

properties of various types of axons.[23,24] Q-space techniques for the spinal cord will be discussed in Chapter
3.2. Another approach is to sample the *q*-space restricted
to a single sphere. This method is known as high angular
resolution diffusion imaging (HARDI). Some popular
HARDI reconstructions methods include QBI,[17,25,26]
deconvolution techniques,[27–30] diffusion orientation
transform[31] and persistent angular structure.[12] Note
that HARDI data can always be used to fit the diffusion
tensor model to it too.

HARDI was successfully applied in the ex vivo
spinal cord of rats,[32] cats,[33] and monkey.[34] Results
demonstrated that HARDI is able to retrieve crossing
fiber information, where the DTI approach was constrained to a unique diffusion direction. The retrieval
of longitudinal, commissural, and dorsoventral fibers
was notably demonstrated.[33] Berens et al. demonstrated
particular diffusion properties in the dorsal horn of spinal cord injured rats, such as increased diffusivity in the
plane orthogonal to dorsoventral tracts (Figure 3.1.5).

3.1.2.4 Diffusion Kurtosis Imaging

The diffusional kurtosis is a quantitative measure of the
degree to which the diffusion displacement probability
distribution deviates from a Gaussian form.[36,37] As such,
diffusion kurtosis imaging (DKI) may provide new
markers of pathological processes in the white matter.[38]
A spinal cord study showed that kurtosis imaging is sensitive to axonal and myelin damage in a rat model of axotomy.[39] Acquisition of kurtosis imaging can be done by
sampling *q*-space with multishells (e.g., 5 shells) varying
from 200 to 3000 s/mm^2. For a comprehensive explanation of the diffusion kurtosis, see Chapter 3.2.

3.1.3 DATA ACQUISITION

Various pulse sequences are available for DW-MRI of
the spinal cord. The most commonly used is echo
planar imaging (EPI) because it is fast and produces
high signal-to-noise ratio (SNR). However, due to the
sensitivity of EPI readout to susceptibility artifacts,
strategies can and should be employed, such as multishot EPI, parallel imaging, and reduced field-of-view

techniques. See Chapter 2.3 for an overview of strategies and non-EPI pulse sequences that can be used. In
the following sections, we will mostly assume
EPI-based acquisition.

3.1.3.1 Eddy Currents and Twice-Refocused Pulse

Eddy currents are electric currents induced in the
gradient coils by the presence of large-varying diffusion-encoding gradients. When eddy currents decay
slowly, a residual magnetic field gradient remains present during the EPI readout, causing distortion of the
image such as translation, scaling, and shearing.
The pattern of distortion depends on the direction of
the diffusion-encoding gradient. One consequence of
eddy current distortions is that the calculated DTI metrics will become blurred. It is, however, possible to correct eddy current distortions using standard packages
(e.g., FSL eddy_correct or topup). For a comprehensive
view of the manifestation of eddy current distortions,
see Chapter 2.2 (Figure 2.2.2(C)–(E)).

A twice-refocused pulse sequence has been introduced in Ref. 40 and aims at minimizing eddy currents. The sequence adds a second refocusing pulse
in order to cancel out eddy currents. It is implemented
in most scanners and is widely used by the DW community. One downside of the twice-refocused scheme,
however, is that it imposes a longer TE. Consequently,
the SNR is reduced, given that $SNR \propto e^{-TE/T_2}$.
Although this is not a problem in typical brain acquisitions where SNR is not a strong constraint, in the
case of spinal cord DTI this may become an issue.
Indeed, spatial resolution in spinal cord DTI is typically limited by the available SNR. Modern gradients
have eddy current compensation systems built into
them, so might offer satisfactory performance in terms
of the generated eddy current; it is encouraged to try
running DTI sequences in the spinal cord with the
standard single refocusing pulse. Of course, data quality needs to be assessed by visually inspecting DW
data in the form of a movie. Overlaying a grid on
the movie helps to assess the presence of eddy current
distortions.

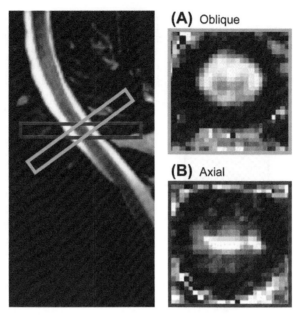

FIGURE 3.1.6 Slice orientation influence on image quality. (A) Oblique FA images of the spinal cord such that the cord is perpendicular to the R-C axis. (B) Straight axial FA images (i.e., orthogonal to the main magnetic field B_0) show significant partial volume effects, particularly when the spinal cord is not perpendicular to the prescribed image plane. Note that the poor quality of the image on panel B can also partly be related to B_0 inhomogeneity due to the proximity of the imaging plane to the intervertebral disk. It is important to note that although the oblique slice is also subject to B_0 inhomogeneity, the impact on the image is different because the bulk susceptibility profile at the disk interface has a particular orientation, and the interplay between this orientation and the orientation of the slice will impact the amount of susceptibility artifact. Images were acquired with a 1.5 T MR scanner using a single-shot, twice-refocused, SE DW-EPI sequence, $b = 1000$ s/mm^2, 25 directions, and a slice thickness of 5 mm.

3.1.3.2 Slice Orientation

In human spinal cord acquisitions, subjects are usually positioned head-first supine. There are two main strategies for slice orientation. The first one consists of acquiring thick slices perpendicular to the rostro-caudal (R-C) axis with high in-plane resolution (Figure 3.1.6(A)), taking advantage of the gross symmetry of the cord along the R-C axis.[41–61] The main advantage is to obtain high in-plane spatial resolution and quantify the integrity of specific spinal tracts (e.g., corticospinal tracts (CST), fasciculus gracilis). Note that this oblique orientation is preferred to a *straight* axial acquisition because less partial volume artifacts are present through plane (Figure 3.1.6(B)). Note that elongated voxels result in more averaging of the diffusion signal in one specific direction, therefore biasing estimation of DTI metrics.

The second strategy consists of acquiring sagittal slices, usually using isotropic voxels.[62–71] The latter approach offers the benefits of extensive spinal coverage using only a few slices. Moreover, isotropic voxels enable the exploration of the anatomical structure of the white matter without bias.[72,73] Some studies used sagittal acquisition with large slice thickness (~5 mm) to gain SNR (see Chapter 2.3), but large partial volume effect exists between the spinal cord and the surrounding CSF, as well as between the white and the gray matter tissue, rendering it difficult to quantitatively assess specific white matter tracts.

3.1.3.3 Spatial Resolution and SNR

Spatial resolution is set by the voxel size, i.e., in-plane resolution and slice thickness. SNR is proportional to the square root of the voxel size. DTI acquisition in the spinal cord is highly constrained by the SNR. While typical acquisitions in the brain are done at $3 \times 3 \times 3$ mm^3 resolution, spinal cord acquisitions are done at about $1 \times 1 \times 5$ mm^3 (for axial orientation). This gives a voxel size of 27 mm^3 in the brain and 5 mm^3 in the spinal cord, so SNR is typically more than five times lower than in regular brain acquisitions. Moreover, good coil sensitivity is more difficult to achieve compared to the brain (see Chapter 2.1), which further decreases the SNR in typical spinal cord acquisitions.

Differences in spatial resolution and slice thickness can result in significant differences in image quality and DTI measurements between brain and spinal cord or between different spinal cord protocols. For example, errors in the estimated indices are highly correlated with the available SNR. Figure 3.1.7 demonstrates the effects of slice thickness on SNR (as measured using the technique suggested by Kaufmann et al.[74]) and variability in ADC measurement.

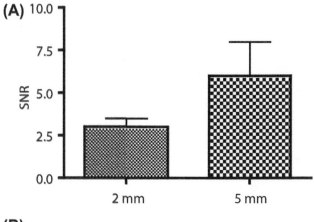

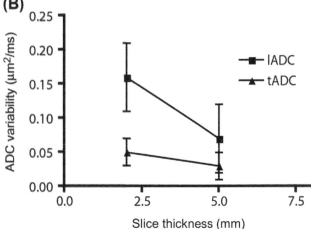

FIGURE 3.1.7   Effects of slice thickness on SNR and ADC variability. (A) T_2-weighted image SNR across multiple slices in $n = 10$ volunteers at 2 mm and 5 mm slice thickness. (B) Longitudinal and transverse ADC measurement variability in the same subjects showing decreased variability with increased slice thickness. Images were acquired with a 1.5 T MR scanner using a single-shot, twice-refocused, SE DW-EPI sequence, $b = 1000$ s/mm^2, and 25 directions. Error bars reflect standard deviation across population.

To compensate for poor SNR, it is encouraged to either increase the number of averages (SNR $\propto \sqrt{N_{averages}}$) or to increase the number of diffusion-encoding directions.

3.1.3.4 Angular Resolution: b-Value and Number of Directions

Angular resolution in DW-MRI is dictated by the b-value and by the number of directions in which magnetic gradients are applied to get the DW signal (q-space sampling). At high b-values the signal is more attenuated yielding low SNR data.[75] Hence, a compromise should be found between the angular resolution and the SNR required to get interpretable data.

There is an ongoing debate as to whether increasing the number of directions over a certain threshold yields significant benefits for diffusion modeling.[13,76–78] An article by Landman et al. suggests increasing the

number of directions rather than the number of averaging.[79] A study based on Monte Carlo simulations showed that optimal DTI reconstruction is made possible when using 20–30 directions for gradient encoding.[13] Additionally, the q-space sampling scheme also has an impact on the estimation of the diffusion tensor.[80] For spinal cord imaging, many studies pointed out the axial symmetry of the cord as an argument for imaging with a reduced number of directions.[81,82] However, the computed ADC along or across the fibers is biased for regions where axons curve or change direction, namely in some complex anatomical projections of nerve roots or following spinal cord injury (SCI). Furthermore, as mentioned in Ref. 55, these acquisitions are dependent on subject positioning within the scanner, so that the cord axis is aligned with the longitudinal gradient. When only a small section of the cord is imaged, this may be possible. However, for ADC along a specific direction, e.g., z, quantification along a larger extent of the cord, the curvature may induce a bias in the proton signal attenuation where longitudinal fibers are no longer aligned with the gradient. To prevent this, Madi et al. used an icosahedral scheme up to 42 gradient directions and showed the benefit of high angular resolved gradient directions. In the case of model-free approaches, however, as many directions as possible are needed to robustly reconstruct the orientation distribution function (ODF).[83,84] However, there is a trade-off with acquisition duration. To minimize this trade-off, researchers try to measure the diffusion profile using nonhomogeneous sampling of the q-space. They notably claim that when a particular orientation of fiber bundles is assumed, it becomes beneficial to record more DW data in the plane orthogonal to those fibers. Recent studies proposed methods to estimate the diffusion profile online,[84] enabling the dynamic adaptation of q-space sampling using a data-driven loop (Figure 3.1.8).[85]

3.1.3.5 Cardiac Gating

Significant motion of the spinal cord has been reported in the R-C[86] and in the antero-posterior (A-P) direction[66,87,88] along with CSF pulsation. This motion modifies the ADC in specific directions, thus biasing FA quantifications along the cord. Cord motion could arise from two distinct phenomena. The first one is related to the dilation of arteries following cardiac systole, as observed in the brain.[89] The second source of motion may be related to CSF pulsation. After cardiac systole, increase of cerebral blood volume causes a compression of the subarachnoid space, yielding abrupt CSF flow in the spinal region.[90,91] During the diastole, CSF flows back to supraspinal regions at relatively high velocity.[92] Hence, it has been suggested that data should be acquired at a certain phase of the cardiac rhythm where cord motion is minimal.[86]

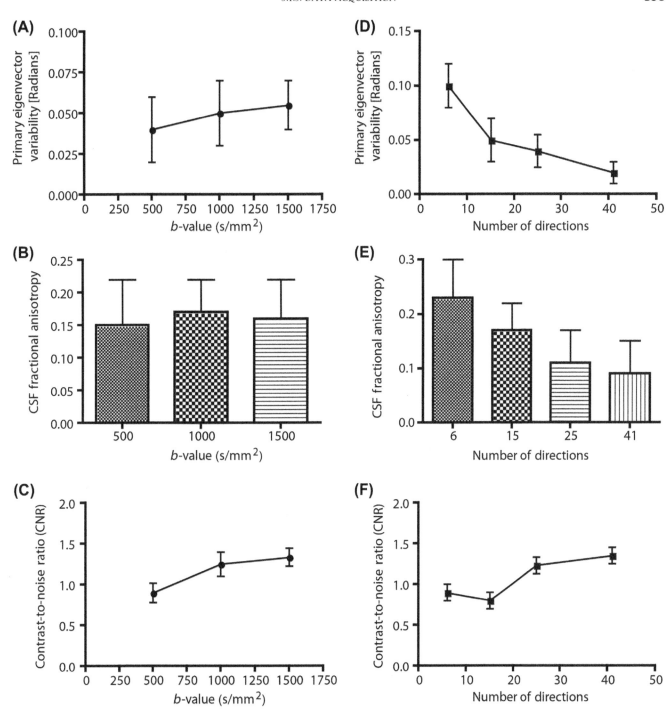

FIGURE 3.1.8 Influence of *b*-value and number of directions on primary eigenvector orientation, FA in the CSF, and contrast-to-noise ratio (CNR) between gray and white matter in FA images. (A) The variability in primary eigenvector orientation was calculated for each patient with respect to the mean vector orientation for that patient. This measurement was then repeated across subjects. This panel shows the mean of variance in primary eigenvector orientation (error bars reflect standard deviation across population). Primary eigenvector variability is relatively constant across *b*-values when the number of directions is held constant. (B) CSF fractional anisotropy is also relatively constant across *b*-values if the number of directions is held constant. (C) CNR between gray and white matter increases with increasing *b*-values. (D) Primary eigenvector variability decreases with increasing number of diffusion sensitizing directions. (E) CSF fractional anisotropy decreases with increasing number of directions. (F) CNR between gray and white matter on FA images increases slightly with increasing number of directions. Images were acquired in 10 healthy volunteers with a 1.5 T MR scanner using a single-shot, twice-refocused, SE DW-EPI sequence.

3.1.3.6 Respiratory Gating

Similarly to cardiac pulsations, motion due to respiration can significantly further degrades image quality.[69,93] Respiratory gating has been used successfully to limit respiration-related motion artifacts.[44,55,94,95] More advanced methods rely on the acquisition of expiration and inspiration phases to reduce motion occurring between phase encoding lines, thus allowing faster acquisition.[69] Additionally to moving structures, respiration could have another negative impact related to susceptibility effects. When imaging the thoracic region, air volume in the lungs regularly changes, its volume causing variations in local B_0-field homogeneity. This can cause susceptibility effects such as time-varying geometric distortions in the phase-encoding direction as shown in the brain[96–98] and spinal cord.[181] This effect is even more notable at ultra high field but can already be encountered at 3 T. To circumvent this issue, dynamic shimming has been proposed[99] and has shown encouraging results in the brain at 7 T.[100]

3.1.4 DATA PROCESSING

3.1.4.1 Motion Correction

This step consists of realigning all DW dataset acquired in one subject over the course of several minutes, during which the subject may have moved. Typically for the brain, most methods consist in registering each DW image to a single target, which could be the $b = 0$ image or the average of the DW images. Registration is typically done by estimating an affine transformation matrix (three rotations and three translations). Given that head motion is rigid (i.e., nondeformable structure) and that DW images of the brain usually contain >100,000 voxels, this procedure is usually robust and accurate. Unfortunately this does not hold for the spinal cord because (1) many fewer voxels are contained in the spinal cord, therefore estimating a transformation matrix might be less robust; (2) motion is usually nonrigid due to the segmental structure of the spine associated with swallowing, neck readjustment, and B_0-variations inducing nonrigid image distortion close to the thoracic area. Several techniques can help optimize motion correction procedure for the spinal cord.

In case of axial acquisition, it may help to correct each slice independently, to notably account for the nonrigid motion of structures across slices.[101,102] Indeed, there could be more motion in slices close to the lungs due to the respiration, which induces variations in the B_0 field (and therefore time-dependent translation of the image in the phase-encoding direction). Slice-by-slice motion correction is achieved by first splitting the data along the Z direction, then estimating transformation matrix for each slice using three degrees of freedom,

and then concatenating back each slice to recover the whole volume. The implementation could be achieved using scripts (e.g., shell or Matlab) that are combined with freely available packages such as FSL (FLIRT), SPM, or AFNI (AIR). An example of a slice-wise algorithm is presented in Chapter 4.1. The existing motion correction software usually allows to set the degree of freedom and to choose the target image. As for the target image, it is possible to use either the mean DW image or the $b = 0$ image, although the former ensures more robust correction of DW images, due to similar contrast. Note that if you wish to perform several registration steps (e.g., intrasubject then intersubject), it is recommended to output the transformation matrix at each step, then apply the transformation only once to avoid multiple interpolations, which can add smoothing or interpolation errors in the data. In some cases it is also desired to crop the area outside the spinal region (e.g., crop out the muscles surrounding the spine) in order to optimize the accuracy of the registration of the spinal cord. One limitation of this method is that depending on the orientation of the diffusion-encoding gradient, the signal from the spinal cord can be very attenuated. In that case, registration to the target image can be unreliable. To address this issue, it is possible to compute the mean signal in a region of interest encompassing the spinal cord and then set an arbitrary threshold. If the mean signal passes the threshold, the image is corrected. If not, the registration matrix calculated at the previous instance is used.

If DWI acquisition is done in the sagittal plane, volume-based motion correction is more appropriate. However, given the likely presence of nonrigid motion (notably A-P motion that is more important close to the thoracic region), it might be appropriate to perform nonrigid transformations.

Note that after correcting for motion, it is recommended to apply the same correction to the b-matrix.[103]

3.1.4.2 Distortion Correction (Susceptibility Artifacts)

In addition to optimizing acquisition methods with respect to susceptibility artifacts, it is possible to correct distortions during data processing. Given that off-resonance effects are negligible in the frequency-encoding direction due to the fast sampling of RF echoes, one can make the assumption that reconstructed images show susceptibility distortions in the phase encoding direction only. To correct for these distortions in the image domain, various strategies use nonlinear registration algorithms constrained in one direction. The reader is referred to Chapter 2.3, where the most commonly used techniques are described: phase field

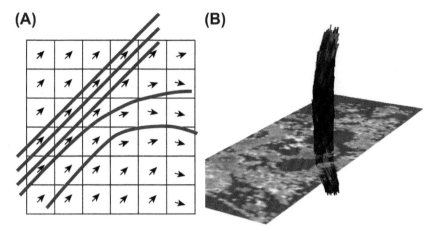

FIGURE 3.1.9 Diffusion tensor tractography. (A) Relationship between artificial white matter tracts (red lines) and primary eigenvector orientation (black arrows). (B) DTI tractography of the cervical spinal cord performed for a neurologically intact participant. DTI data was collected using a custom two-dimensional radiofrequency excitation pulse and a reduced field-of-view readout scheme with $b = 500\,\text{s}/\text{mm}^2$ and six directions. Blue color of tracts = rostral–caudal orientation. Slice shown is FA image.

map, reversed gradient polarity method, point spread function, and co-registration. In most methods, a deformation field is estimated and can be applied to all DW data after they have been motion-corrected. Ideally, the deformation field is multiplied to the motion correction transformation matrix, and the resulting transformation matrix is applied only once to the data.

3.1.5 TRACTOGRAPHY

Fiber tracking or *tractography* uses information from DWI data to obtain a 3D representation of fiber architecture in the white matter. Tractography incorporates information from the diffusion tensor or from the ODF (see HARDI techniques) by linking neighboring voxels having similar maximum diffusion direction, creating *pseudo*-axonal tracts that can be used to visualize microstructural orientation (Figure 3.1.9).

Although used predominantly in the brain, diffusion tractography can also be applied to spinal cord DTI. Application of tractography in the spinal cord has demonstrated the feasibility of retrieving major longitudinal pathways and axon bundles oriented in the R-C direction[43,94,104–108] along with spinal nerves.[109] An important motivation for tracking specific pathways in the spinal cord is the ability to obtain quantitative measurements along those pathways, to correlate the integrity of specific tracts with the severity of functional deficits.[43,82] To successfully perform these measurements, white and gray matter in the spinal cord must be segmented accurately, despite the limited spatial resolution in the axial plane. For this purpose, methods based on fuzzy-logic technique have been suggested to automatically and efficiently segment white and gray matter on DTI maps.[110]

Various tractography methods have been developed, leveraging differences in computational time, tract orientation accuracy, and other criteria. The main difference between tractography methods involves the

technique in which artificial tracts utilize adjacent information to plan their next trajectory.[111] For example, two of the most common approaches to tractography include the streamlines tracking technique (STT) and the tensor deflection technique (TEND). STT primarily utilizes information from the largest eigenvector (i.e., the eigenvector corresponding to the largest eigenvalue) to create tracts,[112,113] whereas TEND deflects the incoming eigenvector by the diffusion tensor orientation, resulting in a smoother approximation.[114,115] A probabilistic approach to tractography has also been developed for use in quantification of common white matter tract orientations in the brain.[116,117] Using this approach, the ADC is first measured in a large number of directions, every image voxel is considered a seed point for tract growth, and the most probable tract orientations are calculated. Probabilistic tractography also has the advantage of allowing for better flexibility in the quantification of white matter directionality, potentially limiting the number of false negatives.[118]

Several implementations exist and are freely available as software package such as MedINRIA, TrackVis, DTIstudio, and Camino.

One has to be very careful when interpreting results from tractography. Firstly, reconstructed fiber bundles do not represent real axonal tracts but merely traces the path where water diffusion shows some sort of coherence.[72,119] For instance, false negatives could be induced by the presence of crossing fibers, which would artificially decrease the FA and stop the tracking procedure. Inversely, false positives could be induced by fibrous structures such as scar tissue in which water diffusion also has anisotropic properties.[120] It is also important to point out that it is not possible to distinguish anterograde from retrograde conduction pathways using tractography (i.e., descending or ascending pathways in the cord).

To illustrate the need for caution in tractography, Figure 3.1.10 shows an example of tractography

FIGURE 3.1.10 Tractography in a healthy subject. Acquisition was performed using the standard EPI sequence with the following parameters: sagittal orientation, TR/TE = 4000/86 ms, 1.8×1.8 mm^2 in-plane resolution, 1.8 mm slice thickness, $R = 2$ acceleration. The left panel shows tractography performed on the raw data. The right panel shows tractography performed on the same dataset, after distortion correction using the reversed-gradient method. A false apparent interruption of the tracts can be observed on the data hampered by susceptibility distortions.

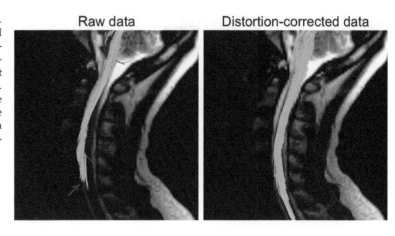

Raw data   Distortion-corrected data

performed in a healthy subject, before and after correcting for susceptibility artifacts, which as we have seen in previous chapters can induce strong image distortions. On the raw data, a false apparent interruption of the tracts is clearly observed and can be misinterpreted as an interruption of white matter tracts.[121] This result highlights that careful interpretation of tractography data is strongly encouraged, especially in the spinal cord where susceptibility artifacts can be prominent. Moreover, these limitations provide an incentive to perform region of interest (ROI)-based analysis of DTI metrics, in place of metrics such as "fiber counts", which is highly sensitive to artifacts. However, if the user is knowledgeable about data acquisition parameters and performs a careful assessment of the raw data before tractography, it may still be possible to use tractography with confidence on the results.

3.1.6 QUANTIFY DWI METRICS IN THE SPINAL CORD

Firstly, what are the metrics that need to be considered? Popular metrics arise from the diffusion tensor and include FA, MD, and axial and radial diffusivities.

However, other metrics could also be quantified depending on the reconstruction method. For example, if DKI is employed, the mean kurtosis could be calculated and used as a potential marker for white matter pathology.

Once DWI data are preprocessed and metrics calculated, one may want to quantify those metrics in the spinal cord in order to test the presence of white matter abnormalities under certain pathologies. Two popular methods exist and are summarized in Figure 3.1.11. Note that a third method exist, which consists in registering the spinal cord to a template and then quantify metrics using a template-based white matter atlas. However, this method is still at its infancy therefore we will not cover it here.

3.1.6.1 Tractography-Based Quantification

This approach consists of reconstructing the underlying fiber bundles via tractography algorithms. Once reconstructed, DTI metrics can be quantified within the tracts (i.e., within the voxels that include the tracts).[122] It is possible to predefine seed points in various regions of the spinal cord and then quantify metrics in specific segments of the spinal cord.[106,123]

FIGURE 3.1.11 Two popular methods to quantify DTI metrics within the spinal cord. The tractography-based method is less subject dependent and more automatic, whereas the ROI-based method is more accurate and less prone to tractography errors.

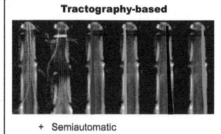

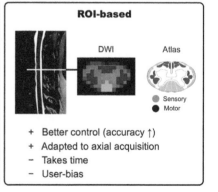

Tractography-based

+ Semiautomatic
− Partial volume effect (accuracy ↓)
− Not applicable with gapped slices
− Susceptibility distortions

ROI-based

DWI   Atlas

● Sensory
● Motor

+ Better control (accuracy ↑)
+ Adapted to axial acquisition
− Takes time
− User-bias

Pros: (1) this method can be relatively fast as tractography is a semiautomatic procedure; (2) it has relatively low user bias. *Cons*: (1) requires data acquired for optimized tractography, typically sagittal orientation with isotropic voxels. This precludes axial acquisition with a large gap between slices. This usually results in a trade-off for in-plane (i.e., axial) resolution. (2) substantial inaccuracies can occur as a result of partial volume effects caused by tracts that don't keep following a specific spinal pathway. This can occur due to the nonlongitudinal branches across spinal segments and in the gray matter area. (3) Residual susceptibility distortions can cause degradation/interruption of the reconstructed fiber bundles.[121] (4) Pathological conditions can decrease anisotropy in spinal pathways, which can cause degradation/interruption of the reconstructed fiber bundles and therefore bias the study.[124]

3.1.6.2 ROI-Based Quantification

Alternatively, it is possible to manually draw ROIs by selecting voxels in various segments of the spinal cord to probe the integrity of specific tracts. For instance, ROI in the dorsal segment includes ascending sensory columns, and ROI in the dorsolateral segment includes the corticospinal tracts. As an alternative to manual drawing, fuzzy-logic methods can be employed.[110] ROI-based methods have notably been employed in Refs 106,125–129. To minimize user bias in the definition of the ROI, i.e., circularity induced by defining ROIs based on DTI metrics, ROIs should be defined on the mean $b = 0$ or diffusion-weighted image. Defining the ROI on a completely different image with a different contrast (e.g., high-res structural) is possible but requires accurate registration due to the potential mismatch between DW data and anatomical data caused by subject motion and susceptibility distortions. *Pros*: (1) more accurate and "forces" the user to assess the quality of the ROI; (2) can be performed on axial acquisitions with large gaps providing high in-plane resolution, hence well-defined spinal segments; *Cons*: (1) user-bias; (2) time-consuming.

3.1.7 DIFFUSION CHARACTERISTICS OF THE NEUROLOGICALLY INTACT SPINAL CORD

Water diffusivity in the CNS is anisotropic, in which diffusion occurs preferentially in a particular direction. Diffusion anisotropy is attributed to cylindrical symmetry of intra- and extracellular structures within the spinal cord, which allows for diffusion coefficients to be reduced to transverse (D_t or tADC) and longitudinal (D_l or lADC) components.[130–134] Although collection of *only* transverse and longitudinal components has the added benefit of reducing scan time significantly, making ADC measurements in only the transverse and longitudinal orientations tends to overestimate low ADCs and underestimate high ADCs due to slight misalignment of the spinal cord with the main field orientation.[134] Most notably, transverse diffusion is restricted by the axon membrane, myelin sheath, neurofilaments, and microtubules. Variations in the properties of these barriers, along with intra- and extracellular volume, are the basis for interpreting the status of the spinal cord using DTI.

The contribution of cellular barriers to diffusion depends largely on membrane permeability and axon size. Ford et al.[135] used numerical simulations and an animal model to demonstrate dependence of membrane permeability and axon diameter on measurements of tADC, suggesting little contribution of membrane permeability on tADC in large diameter axons and dominance of membrane permeability on tADC when examining small caliber axons. More complex numerical simulations involving various axon geometries have also been performed with similar results.[136,137]

Histological data from animal models further supports the conclusions from numerical simulations, verifying that tADC depends primarily on axon size. Schwartz et al.[138] showed a significant correlation between cellular morphometric parameters and ADCs using combined histological analyses and high resolution ex vivo DTI. This study confirmed the results of numerical simulations, showing that tADCs are reduced for axons with a smaller diameter, including axons both with and without myelin. These results were also

> **PROCESSING PIPELINE FOR DIFFUSION-WEIGHTED MRI OF THE SPINAL CORD**
>
> - Motion correction: for axial acquisition, usually split the data in Z and perform slice-by-slice realignment
> - Distortion correction: corrects for susceptibility-induced distortions
> - Estimate metrics using the desired model. For example, if DTI, calculate FA, radial diffusivity (RD), axial diffusivity (AD), and MD
> - Make ROI: Using tractography or manual segmentation of spinal cord regions, or using recent template-based approaches.
> - Compute metrics within ROI

replicated in live excised lamprey spinal cords at high magnetic field strengths.[131] lADC has shown to be inversely correlated with both neurofilament and microtubule density as demonstrated in the rat optic nerve.[139] This inverse relationship between lADC and microtubule or neurofilament density may be interpreted as a reduced local viscosity provided by neurofilaments and microtubules, since they run parallel to axon orientation.

Extracellular morphology also contributes to diffusion characteristics within the CNS. If the total volume of the spinal cord does not change, an increase in extracellular volume fraction will result in an increase in the observed ADC due to the significantly higher ADC within the extracellular compartment compared to the intracellular compartment. Alternatively, if axons are tightly packed or if the extracellular matrix has a high degree of fibrosis or collagen infiltration, the ADC is lower. In the rat cervical spinal cord, regions with larger axonal spacing and extracellular volume fraction have larger transverse and longitudinal ADCs, and, conversely, a higher axon density has been shown to result in smaller transverse and longitudinal ADCs.[138] In the human spinal cord, lADC typically ranges from 1.0×10^{-3} to $2.3 \times 10^{-3}\,\text{mm}^2/\text{s}$ and tADC typically ranges from 0.1×10^{-3} to $1.0 \times 10^{-3}\,\text{mm}^2/\text{s}$. The observed range in ADCs is highly dependent on the specific microstructure of the tissue under investigation, but also depends on pulse sequence parameters such as diffusion time (Δ-value) and echo time (TE). Despite differences in pulse sequences, if signal attenuation is plotted versus the degree of diffusion weighting (i.e., b-value) for the human studies, it produces a mean ADC in the human cervical spinal cord of approximately $1 \times 10^{-3}\,\text{mm}^2/\text{s}$.[140,141]

3.1.8 DIFFUSION CHARACTERISTICS FOLLOWING SPINAL CORD TRAUMA

Trauma to the spinal cord, and changes occurring during healing, result in alterations of tissue microstructure that are measurable via diffusion MRI. DTI has the potential to noninvasively provide information about the location and severity of an injury that might prove useful in the diagnosis and prognosis of a spinal injury. Further, DTI measures could be used as an indicator of neural degeneration and healing. Because of the changes in tissue structure during inflammation and healing, DTI measures are likely to depend on the stage of injury, varying from the acute to chronic stages. Note that DTI can and has been successfully applied to other diseases such as multiple sclerosis, amyotrophic lateral sclerosis and tumors. However given that these are already well covered by Chapter 1.1, we will only focus on the application of DTI to traumatic spinal cord injury.

3.1.8.1 Acute SCI

In the acute stages of SCI, direct mechanical injury as well as more indirect modalities, including hypoxia, ischemia, hemorrhage, and edema, contribute to diffusion changes that can be detected using DTI. Mechanical disruption of neural tissue structure results in immediate death of cells in the region of the insult. The stretching and tearing of large axons results in damage to axonal membranes and an increase in membrane permeability.[142] This cell death and disruption of the cell membrane is reflected by an increased ADC in animal studies[143,144] and in numerical simulations of diffusivity changes associated with injury.[135,145] The increase in diffusivity may be as high as a double the baseline diffusion measurements.[144] Immediately following compressive or impact-induced spinal trauma, blood flow to the injury site is restricted, resulting in ischemia.[146–148] Exploration of ischemia in the CNS via DWI has indicated a significant decrease in the ADCs following transient induced ischemia ($\sim 1\,\text{h}$) in the mouse optic nerve.[149] Sagiuchi et al.,[150] Bammer et al.,[151] Mamata et al.,[152] and Küker et al.[153] all report a decrease in the measured ADC in the early onset of spinal stroke, indicative of the ischemic events following infarction. Bammer et al.[151] and Demir et al.[154] documented a decrease in the ADC within the center of the spinal cord in patients with cervical spondylotic myelopathy, which was thought to occur due to vascular compromise. Although the precise mechanisms responsible for changes in the diffusion characteristics following acute ischemia are still speculative, it is believed that a shift in water from the high ADC extracellular compartment to the low ADC extracellular compartment during ischemia causes the decrease in the observed ADC. Currently, DTI is being used routinely in the clinical assessment of ischemic and hypoxic injuries in the CNS. The earliest DTI-sensitive morphological changes after spinal insult occur as hemorrhages in the central gray matter adjacent to the central canal. These hemorrhages spread radially from the central canal, primarily affecting the anterior horns and neighboring white matter regions around the injury epicenter[155,156] and then extend in the rostral and caudal directions.[157]

Edema also occurs in the first moments of traumatic SCI primarily resulting from mechanical disruption of axon cell membranes, damage to local blood vessels and electrolytic imbalances.[158,159] This damage to cell membranes would be expected to contribute to the increase in the transverse component of the ADC observed in acute SCI.[143,144] As a result, axons are spaced further apart and water molecules can diffuse larger distances before barriers are encountered. In addition to an increase in transverse diffusion, DTI in acute spinal trauma often exhibits a decrease in lADC, resulting in an overall decrease in diffusion anisotropy in the lesion sites during the period of severe edema and hemorrhage.[143] This decrease in the lADC has been largely attributed to metabolic dysfunction as opposed to specific changes in axon morphology.[160]

3.1.8.2 Subacute SCI

Following the initial response to spinal trauma there is infiltration of inflammatory cells from both the CNS and periphery. In human SCI, astrocytes begin to line the edge of the lesion within the first week and make up the cavity boundary seen in chronic SCI. In addition to the activation of cells originating in the CNS, inflammatory cells also infiltrate the spinal cord in the subacute stages of injury, primarily consisting of polymorphonuclear granulocytes and macrophages[158]; however, there is evidence that Schwann cells, meningeal cells, and fibroblasts also invade the spinal cord,[161] although it is unclear if they affect diffusion characteristics of the injured spinal cord because their relative size and influence on degeneration is limited.

It is unclear how these reactive cell types influence diffusion measurements in the injured spinal cord. Reactive cells, such as glia, produce collagenous scar tissue that is expected to have a relatively high impact on tissue diffusivity. Schwartz et al.[120] demonstrated that glial scar orientation can even be identified through the use of DTI tractography. Consequently, DTI eigenvector orientations show sensitivity to glial cell orientations, although only if they are in sufficient numbers to significantly affect the overall orientation of the particular voxel microstructure. Thus, in the subacute stage of SCI, astrocytes may only have an influence on DTI measurements close to the injury epicenter or in relatively close proximity to the forming lesion cavity. The influx of high numbers of astrocytes, microglia, and macrophages is also predicted to decrease the extracellular volume, which could decrease the overall ADC, counteracting the initial increase associated with edema.

Degeneration of axons following injury, termed Wallerian degeneration,[162] contributes to changes in diffusivity even at locations distant from the injury site. Axon degeneration first manifests as disintegration of the myelin sheath and cytoskeletal proteins including microtubules and neurofilaments. If the distal portion of the axon is not reconnected in a functional pathway, it may eventually die, resulting in complete anterograde degeneration. The proximal ends of the damaged axons produce a retraction bulb, effectively cleaving off the leaking axoplasm.

During the degeneration process, tADC is typically elevated above baseline levels.[82,144] The primary explanation for the increase in tADC lies in the tissue structural changes that occur during degeneration along with direct effects on the intra- and extracellular space. Anterograde degeneration results in rapid degeneration of both the axonal membrane and myelin sheath, decreasing the number and extent of transverse diffusion boundaries. This is expected to contribute to a higher transverse diffusion coefficient. Retrograde degeneration also shows a similar, but slightly larger, increase in tADC in experimental animal models.[144] This significant increase in tADC is most likely due to axon swelling and the subsequent increase in intracellular space.[158]

Gray matter undergoes multiple morphological changes that have been implicated in neurological symptoms, such as spasticity[163] and chronic pain,[164] and may also contribute to alterations in DTI measurements. For example, the rat motoneuron undergoes morphological changes after injury consisting of a significant decrease in the number of dendrites and significant increase in the length of the remaining dendrites.[163] In a mouse model of spinal injury, similar morphological changes in spinal neurons have been reported; in addition, an enlargement of the soma during the subacute stages can also occur.[165] The typical diffusion characteristics of gray matter have not been thoroughly examined after SCI, although baseline measurements of the uninjured spinal cord have been documented.[166] Gray matter is typically less anisotropic than white matter, and, therefore, gray matter has a lower FA,[166,167] although the rostral–caudal orientation of cellular structures in the spinal cord gray matter results in a higher FA than brain gray matter.[145,151,168] The eigenvectors of spinal gray matter show similar rostral–caudal dominance; eigenvectors in voxels with low eigenvalues show orientations that may follow microstructures and the predominant soma orientation.[134] Given the sensitivity of diffusion to gray matter microstructures, it is conceivable that large changes in soma morphology following SCI may influence diffusion measurements. Although not documented in the current literature, an increase in overall ADC and a decrease in diffusion anisotropy are likely in spinal gray matter in the acute and subacute stages of injury due to the increase in soma size and decrease in the number of dendritic projections.

3.1.8.3 Chronic SCI

The late phase of SCI, defined months to years after the initial injury, shows that differences in tissue morphology in chronic injury likely impact DTI measurements. Although most of the degenerative processes are stabilized by the chronic stage, there is evidence to suggest degeneration even long after the injury. For

FIGURE 3.1.12 Suggested DWI acquisition in axial orientation. The yellow box represents the slice positioning. The red slabs represent the saturation bands that achieve outer volume suppression (to avoid aliasing). The green box represents the area where shim coefficients are estimated.

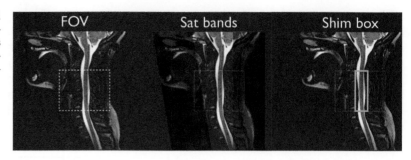

example, progressive demyelination can occur even during chronic injury.[169–171] Remyelination, if it occurs, results in significantly decreased myelin sheath thickness,[169,172–174] resulting in an altered white matter structure in chronic injury. Preferential loss of large diameter axons also occurs in chronic injury,[173] resulting in predominantly small, unmyelinated axons in damaged axonal tracts. Further, extensive longitudinal spreading of lesions following spinal cord injury has also been documented,[175] resulting in drastic and widespread changes in the spinal cord morphology including cystic formation and necrosis. Finally, significant atrophy of the spinal cord also occurs in late stages of spinal cord injury causing the remaining axons to be compressed and tightly packed, as illustrated in Figure 3.1.6(E). These structural changes are all expected to contribute to differences in water diffusivity in chronic injury.

Diffusion characteristics in chronic injury have not been thoroughly explored, however preliminary evidence of gross morphological changes and atrophy have been illustrated using DTI in the human spinal cord.[101,176–179] These studies demonstrate significant changes in diffusion distributions in chronic injury, indicative of expected changes in the spinal cord microstructure. Specifically, the white matter tADCs are lower than uninjured controls and demonstrate a kurtosis (or flattening) of the diffusion distribution. Because tADC is dependent on axon diameter,[135] a shift in the mean transverse diffusion may correspond to preferential loss of larger diameter axons. Kurtosis in the distribution is consistent with a greater heterogeneity of the white matter tissue. Results from these studies support the use of DTI for monitoring the status of the spinal cord after injury, though more research is needed to document the progression of changes in diffusion characteristics and to verify the precise morphological changes responsible for differences in diffusivity.

3.1.9 RECIPES FOR IMPLEMENTATION OF CLINICAL DIFFUSION IMAGING OF THE SPINAL CORD

The following protocols use the EPI sequence with reduced-FOV (field-of-view) combined with saturation bands and can be used with most clinical scanners. Please note that these protocols are only given as example and could not possibility be applicable to all scanners. You will have to adapt some of the parameters that are constrained by your MRI system, such as the bandwidth, TE, etc. Also, you should test the efficiency of the saturation bands in suppressing aliasing using first a phantom of similar volume as the neck or the body, depending on the spinal cord region that you intend to scan. If your system has more advanced reduced FOV techniques, such as the ZOOM or the 2D-RF selective excitation technique, you should use them.

Parameters	Protocol 1	Protocol 2	Comments
GEOMETRY			
Slice orientation	Axial	Sagittal	For axial, be perpendicular to the cord.
FOV (mm)	128 × 64	200 × 100	
Matrix	128 × 64	100 × 50	Fewer distortions with fewer phase lines.
Slice thickness (mm)	5	2	
Acceleration[b]	2	2	GRAPPA (Siemens), SENSE (Philips), ARC (GE).
N slices	10	12	
Slice order	Interleave	Interleave	

[b]Be aware that acceleration is only possible if there is enough coil coverage in the phase encoding direction. With the typical neck coil (anterior and posterior elements), there is enough coverage for acceleration of 2. However, for thoracic or lumbar imaging, there is usually only a spine array matrix posteriorly, therefore not enough coil element if phase-encoding direction is A-P. In that case, acceleration may not be advised.

Parameters	Protocol 1	Protocol 2	Comments
Packages/Group	1–2	1	For axial orientation, if the cord is too curved it is possible to divide the blocks into multiple blocks, each having a different orientation to maximize orthogonality with the cord. See Ref. 180.
Nex/Average	3	3	
PE direction	A/P	A/P	
BW/Pixel	~1000 Hz	~1000 Hz	Set to minimize echo spacing and hence susceptibility distortions.
CONTRAST			
TR	~2 s	~2 s	Cardiac gated
TE	minimum	minimum	
Trigger delay	150 ms	150 ms	See Summers et al.[86]
Partial Fourier	6/8	6/8	Helps to reduce the TE (hence gain SNR), however may be subject to more artifacts.
Shimming	Manual	Manual	Manually set the shim box
Fat suppression	SPAIR	SPAIR	
Saturation bands	1 or 2	1	To prevent aliasing artifacts. Sat bands should be placed anteriorly and posteriorly to the spine (see Figure 3.1.12)
DIFFUSION			
b-value (s/mm^2)	800	800	Stejskal–Tanner (single refocusing)
# Directions	30	30	
Number of *b* = 0	5 (at the beginning)	5 (at the beginning)	Non-diff weighted
Dynamic stabilization	On	On	Readjusting center frequency
Total scan time	**~5 min**	**~5 min**	3:30 min without cardiac gating.

References

1. Crank J. *The Mathematics of Diffusion.* New York: Oxford University Press Inc.; 1975, 494.
2. Einstein A. *Investigations on the Theory of Brownian Movement.* New York: Dover; 1956.
3. Torrey HC. Bloch equations with diffusion terms. *Phys Rev.* 1956; 104(3):563–565.
4. Stejskal EO, Tanner JE. Spin diffusion measurements: spin echoes in the presence of a time-dependent field gradient. *J Chem Phys.* 1965;42(1):288–292.
5. Hrabe J, Hrabetova S, Segeth K. A model of effective diffusion and tortuosity in the extracellular space of the brain. *Biophys J.* 2004;87(3):1606–1617.
6. Nicholson C. Diffusion and related transport mechanisms in brain tissue. *Rep Prog Phys.* 2001;64(7):815–884.
7. Nicholson C, Phillips JM. Ion diffusion modified by tortuosity and volume fraction in the extracellular microenvironment of the rat cerebellum. *J Physiol.* 1981;321:225–257.
8. Kawasaki K. Kinetic equations and time correlation functions of critical fluctuations. *Ann Phys.* 1970;61(8):1–56.
9. Laird AS, Carrive P, Waite PM. Cardiovascular and temperature changes in spinal cord injured rats at rest and during autonomic dysreflexia. *J Physiol.* 2006;577(Pt 2):539–548.
10. Dumont RJ, Okonkwo DO, Verma S, et al. Acute spinal cord injury, part I: pathophysiologic mechanisms. *Clin Neuropharmacol.* 2001;24(5):254–264.
11. Hagmann P, Jonasson L, Maeder P, Thiran JP, Wedeen VJ, Meuli R. Understanding diffusion MR imaging techniques: from scalar diffusion-weighted imaging to diffusion tensor imaging and beyond. *Radiographics.* 2006;26(suppl 1):S205–S223.
12. Alexander DC. Multiple-fiber reconstruction algorithms for diffusion MRI. *Ann N Y Acad Sci.* 2005;1064:113–133.
13. Jones DK. The effect of gradient sampling schemes on measures derived from diffusion tensor MRI: a Monte Carlo study. *Magn Reson Med.* 2004;51(4):807–815.
14. Behrens TE, et al. Probabilistic diffusion tractography with multiple fibre orientations: what can we gain? *Neuroimage.* 2007; 34(1):144–155.
15. Lazar M, Alexander AL. An error analysis of white matter tractography methods: synthetic diffusion tensor field simulations. *Neuroimage.* 2003;20(2):1140–1153.
16. Tuch DS, Reese TG, Wiegell MR, Makris N, Belliveau JW, Wedeen VJ. High angular resolution diffusion imaging reveals intravoxel white matter fiber heterogeneity. *Magn Reson Med.* 2002;48(4):577–582.
17. Campbell JS, Siddiqi K, Rymar VV, Sadikot AF, Pike GB. Flow-based fiber tracking with diffusion tensor and q-ball data: validation and comparison to principal diffusion direction techniques. *Neuroimage.* 2005;27(4):725–736.
18. Mamata H, De Girolami U, Hoge WS, Jolesz FA, Maier SE. Collateral nerve fibers in human spinal cord: visualization with magnetic resonance diffusion tensor imaging. *Neuroimage.* 2006;31(1):24–30.
19. Maier SE, Mamata H. Diffusion tensor imaging of the spinal cord. *Ann N Y Acad Sci.* 2005;1064:50–60.
20. Wedeen VJ, Hagmann P, Tseng WY, Reese TG, Weisskoff RM. Mapping complex tissue architecture with diffusion spectrum magnetic resonance imaging. *Magn Reson Med.* 2005;54(6): 1377–1386.
21. Schmahmann JD, Pandya DN, Wang R, et al. Association fibre pathways of the brain: parallel observations from diffusion spectrum imaging and autoradiography. *Brain.* 2007;130(pt 3): 630–653.
22. Callaghan PT, Eccles CD, Xia Y. NMR microscopy of dynamic displacements: k-space and q-space imaging. *J Phys E Sci Instrum.* 1988;21(8):820–822.
23. Assaf Y, Mayk A, Cohen Y. Displacement imaging of spinal cord using q-space diffusion-weighted MRI. *Magn Reson Med.* 2000; 44(5):713–722.
24. Ong HH, Wright AC, Wehrli SL, et al. Indirect measurement of regional axon diameter in excised mouse spinal cord with q-space imaging: simulation and experimental studies. *Neuroimage.* 2008; 40(4):1619–1632.
25. Tuch DS. Q-ball imaging. *Magn Reson Med.* 2004;52(6):1358–1372.
26. Zhan W, Yang Y. How accurately can the diffusion profiles indicate multiple fiber orientations? A study on general fiber crossings in diffusion MRI. *J Magn Reson.* 2006;183(2):193–202.

27. Tournier JD, Calamante F, Gadian DG, Connelly A. Direct estimation of the fiber orientation density function from diffusion-weighted MRI data using spherical deconvolution. *Neuroimage*. 2004;23(3):1176–1185.

28. Descoteaux M, Deriche R, Knösche TR, Anwander A. Deterministic and probabilistic tractography based on complex fibre orientation distributions. *IEEE Trans Med Imaging*. 2009;28(2):269–286.

29. Dell'Acqua F, Rizzo G, Scifo P, Clarke RA, Scotti G, Fazio F. A model-based deconvolution approach to solve fiber crossing in diffusion-weighted MR imaging. *IEEE Trans Biomed Eng*. 2007; 54(3):462–472.

30. Anderson AW, Ding Z. Sub-voxel measurement of fiber orientation using high angular resolution diffusion tensor imaging. In: *Proceedings of the 10th Annual Meeting of ISMRM*. Honolulu, USA; 2002:440.

31. Ozarslan E, Shepherd TM, Vemuri BC, Blackband SJ, Mareci TH. Resolution of complex tissue microarchitecture using the diffusion orientation transform (DOT). *Neuroimage*. 2006;31(3): 1086–1103.

32. Berens SA. *Use of MRI to Study Excitotoxic Spinal Cord Injury*. Florida, USA: University of Florida; 2006.

33. Cohen-Adad J, Descoteaux M, Rossignol S, Hoge RD, Deriche R, Benali H. Detection of multiple pathways in the spinal cord using q-ball imaging. *Neuroimage*. 2008;42(2):739–749.

34. Lundell H, Nielsen JB, Ptito M, Dyrby TB. Distribution of collateral fibers in the monkey cervical spinal cord detected with diffusion-weighted magnetic resonance imaging. *Neuroimage*. 2011;56(3):923–929.

35. Lundell H, et al. Crossing fibers in lateral white matter of the cervical spinal cord detected with diffusion MRI in monkey postmortem. In: *Proceedings of the 17th Annual Meeting of ISMRM*. Honolulu, USA; 2009:1497.

36. Hui ES, Cheung MM, Qi L, Wu EX. Towards better MR characterization of neural tissues using directional diffusion kurtosis analysis. *Neuroimage*. 2008;42(1):122–134.

37. Jensen JH, Helpern JA, Ramani A, Lu H, Kaczynski K. Diffusional kurtosis imaging: the quantification of non-gaussian water diffusion by means of magnetic resonance imaging. *Magn Reson Med*. 2005;53(6):1432–1440.

38. Cheung MM, et al. Does diffusion kurtosis imaging lead to better neural tissue characterization? A rodent brain maturation study. *Neuroimage*. 2009;45(2):386–392.

39. Farrell JAD, et al. q-space and conventional diffusion imaging of axon and myelin damage in the rat spinal cord after axotomy. *Magn Reson Med*. 2010;63(5):1323–1335.

40. Reese TG, Heid O, Weisskoff RM, Wedeen VJ. Reduction of eddy-current-induced distortion in diffusion MRI using a twice-refocused spin echo. *Magn Reson Med*. 2003;49(1):177–182.

41. Elshafiey I, Bilgen M, He R, Narayana PA. In vivo diffusion tensor imaging of rat spinal cord at 7 T. *Magn Reson Imaging*. 2002;20(3):243–247.

42. Holder CA, Muthupillai R, Mukundan S, Eastwood JD, Hudgins PA. Diffusion-weighted MR imaging of the normal human spinal cord in vivo. *AJNR Am J Neuroradiol*. 2000;21(10): 1799–1806.

43. Gullapalli J, Krejza J, Schwartz ED. In vivo DTI evaluation of white matter tracts in rat spinal cord. *J Magn Reson Imaging*. 2006; 24(1):231–234.

44. Kim JH, Loy DN, Liang HF, Trinkaus K, Schmidt RE, Song SK. Noninvasive diffusion tensor imaging of evolving white matter pathology in a mouse model of acute spinal cord injury. *Magn Reson Med*. 2007;58(2):253–260.

45. Nevo U, Hauben E, Yoles E, et al. Diffusion anisotropy MRI for quantitative assessment of recovery in injured rat spinal cord. *Magn Reson Med*. 2001;45(1):1–9.

46. Ohgiya Y, Oka M, Hiwatashi A, et al. Diffusion tensor MR imaging of the cervical spinal cord in patients with multiple sclerosis. *Eur Radiol*. 2007;17(10):2499–2504.

47. Schwartz ED, Yezierski RP, Pattany PM, Quencer RM, Weaver RG. Diffusion-weighted MR imaging in a rat model of syringomyelia after excitotoxic spinal cord injury. *AJNR Am J Neuroradiol*. 1999;20(8):1422–1428.

48. Tsuchiya K, Fujikawa A, Suzuki Y. Diffusion tractography of the cervical spinal cord by using parallel imaging. *AJNR Am J Neuroradiol*. 2005;26(2):398–400.

49. Brooks JC, Beckmann CF, Miller KL, et al. Physiological noise modelling for spinal functional magnetic resonance imaging studies. *NeuroImage*. 2008;39(2):680–692.

50. Backes WH, Mess WH, Wilmink JT. Functional MR imaging of the cervical spinal cord by use of median nerve stimulation and fist clenching. *AJNR Am J Neuroradiol*. 2001;22(10):1854–1859.

51. Endo T, Spenger C, Westman E, et al. Reorganization of sensory processing below the level of spinal cord injury as revealed by fMRI. *Exp Neurol*. 2008;209(1):155–160.

52. Govers N, Beghin J, Van Goethem JW, et al. Functional MRI of the cervical spinal cord on 1.5 T with fingertapping: to what extent is it feasible? *Neuroradiol*. 2007;49(1):73–81.

53. Kornelsen J, Stroman PW. fMRI of the lumbar spinal cord during a lower limb motor task. *Magn Reson Med*. 2004;52(2):411–414.

54. Lilja J, Endo T, Hofstetter C, et al. Blood oxygenation level-dependent visualization of synaptic relay stations of sensory pathways along the neuroaxis in response to graded sensory stimulation of a limb. *J Neurosci*. 2006;26(23):6330–6336.

55. Madi S, Hasan KM, Narayana PA. Diffusion tensor imaging of in vivo and excised rat spinal cord at 7 T with an icosahedral encoding scheme. *Magn Reson Med*. 2005;53(1):118–125.

56. Maieron M, Iannetti GD, Bodurka J, Tracey I, Bandettini PA, Porro CA. Functional responses in the human spinal cord during willed motor actions: evidence for side- and rate-dependent activity. *J Neurosci*. 2007;27(15):4182–4190.

57. Moffitt MA, Dale BM, Duerk JL, Grill WM. Functional magnetic resonance imaging of the human lumbar spinal cord. *J Magn Reson Imaging*. 2005;21(5):527–535.

58. Stroman PW, Krause V, Malisza KL, Frankenstein UN, Tomanek B. Characterization of contrast changes in functional MRI of the human spinal cord at 1.5 T. *Magn Reson Imaging*. 2001;19(6):833–838.

59. Yoshizawa T, Nose T, Moore GJ, Sillerud LO. Functional magnetic resonance imaging of motor activation in the human cervical spinal cord. *NeuroImage*. 1996;4(3 pt 1):174–182.

60. Ng MC, Wu EX, Lau HF, Hu Y, Lam EY, Luk KD. Cervical spinal cord BOLD fMRI study: modulation of functional activation by dexterity of dominant and non-dominant hands. *Neuroimage*. 2008;39(2):825–831.

61. Wilm BJ, Gamper U, Henning A, Pruessmann KP, Kollias SS, Boesiger P. Diffusion-weighted imaging of the entire spinal cord. *NMR Biomed*. 2009;22(2):174–181.

62. Stroman PW, Kornelsen J, Lawrence J. An improved method for spinal functional MRI with large volume coverage of the spinal cord. *J Magn Reson Imaging*. 2005;21(5):520–526.

63. Bammer R, Augustin M, Prokesch RW, Stollberger R, Fazekas F. Diffusion-weighted imaging of the spinal cord: interleaved echo-planar imaging is superior to fast spin-echo. *J Magn Reson Imaging*. 2002;15(4):364–373.

64. Cercignani M, Horsfield MA, Agosta F, Filippi M. Sensitivity-encoded diffusion tensor MR imaging of the cervical cord. *AJNR Am J Neuroradiol*. 2003;24(6):1254–1256.

65. Jeong EK, Kim SE, Guo J, Kholmovski EG, Parker DL. High-resolution DTI with 2D interleaved multislice reduced FOV single-shot diffusion-weighted EPI (2D ss-rFOV-DWEPI). *Magn Reson Med*. 2005;54(6):1575–1579.

66. Kharbanda HS, Alsop DC, Anderson AW, Filardo G, Hackney DB. Effects of cord motion on diffusion imaging of the spinal cord. *Magn Reson Med.* 2006;56(2):334–339.

67. Murphy BP, Zientara GP, Huppi PS, et al. Line scan diffusion tensor MRI of the cervical spinal cord in preterm infants. *J Magn Reson Imaging.* 2001;13(6):949–953.

68. Shen H, Tang Y, Huang L, et al. Applications of diffusion-weighted MRI in thoracic spinal cord injury without radiographic abnormality. *Int Orthop.* 2007;31(3):375–383.

69. Spuentrup E, Buecker A, Koelker C, Guenther RW, Stuber M. Respiratory motion artifact suppression in diffusion-weighted MR imaging of the spine. *Eur Radiol.* 2003;13(2):330–336.

70. Thurnher MM, Bammer R. Diffusion-weighted MR imaging (DWI) in spinal cord ischemia. *Neuroradiology.* 2006;48(11):795–801.

71. Tsuchiya K, Katase S, Fujikawa A, Hachiya J, Kanazawa H, Yodo K. Diffusion-weighted MRI of the cervical spinal cord using a single-shot fast spin-echo technique: findings in normal subjects and in myelomalacia. *Neuroradiol.* 2003;45(2):90–94.

72. Basser PJ, Pajevic S, Pierpaoli C, Duda J, Aldroubi A. In vivo fiber tractography using DT-MRI data. *Magn Reson Med.* 2000;44(4):625–632.

73. Jones DK, Williams SC, Gasston D, Horsfield MA, Simmons A, Howard R. Isotropic resolution diffusion tensor imaging with whole brain acquisition in a clinically acceptable time. *Hum Brain Mapp.* 2002;15(4):216–230.

74. Kaufman L, Kramer DM, Crooks LE, Ortendahl DA. Measuring signal-to-noise ratios in MR imaging. *Radiology.* 1989;173(1):265–267.

75. Ronen I, Ugurbil K, Kim DS. How does DWI correlate with white matter structures? *Magn Reson Med.* 2005;54(2):317–323.

76. Lee JW, Kim JH, Kang HS, et al. Optimization of acquisition parameters of diffusion-tensor magnetic resonance imaging in the spinal cord. *Invest Radiol.* 2006;41(7):553–559.

77. Ni H, Kavcic V, Zhu T, Ekholm S, Zhong J. Effects of number of diffusion gradient directions on derived diffusion tensor imaging indices in human brain. *AJNR Am J Neuroradiol.* 2006;27(8):1776–1781.

78. Hosey T, Williams G, Ansorge R. Inference of multiple fiber orientations in high angular resolution diffusion imaging. *Magn Reson Med.* 2005;54(6):1480–1489.

79. Landman BA, Farrell JA, Jones CK, Smith SA, Prince JL, Mori S. Effects of diffusion weighting schemes on the reproducibility of DTI-derived fractional anisotropy, mean diffusivity, and principal eigenvector measurements at 1.5T. *Neuroimage.* 2007;36(4):1123–1138.

80. Papadakis NG, Xing D, Huang CL, Hall LD, Carpenter TA. A comparative study of acquisition schemes for diffusion tensor imaging using MRI. *J Magn Reson.* 1999;137(1):67–82.

81. Gulani V, Iwamoto GA, Jiang H, Shimony JS, Webb AG, Lauterbur PC. A multiple echo pulse sequence for diffusion tensor imaging and its application in excised rat spinal cords. *Magn Reson Med.* 1997;38(6):868–873.

82. Schwartz ED, Chin CL, Shumsky JS, et al. Apparent diffusion coefficients in spinal cord transplants and surrounding white matter correlate with degree of axonal dieback after injury in rats. *AJNR Am J Neuroradiol.* 2005;26(1):7–18.

83. Perrin M, Poupon C, Rieul B, et al. Validation of q-ball imaging with a diffusion fibre-crossing phantom on a clinical scanner. *Philos Trans R Soc London.* 2005;360(1457):881–891.

84. Poupon C, Poupon F, Roche A, Cointepas Y, Dubois J, Mangin JF. Real-time MR diffusion tensor and Q-ball imaging using Kalman filtering. *Conf Med Image Comput Comput Assist Interv.* 2007;10(pt 1):27–35.

85. Peng H, Arfanakis K. Diffusion tensor encoding schemes optimized for white matter fibers with selected orientations. *Magn Reson Imaging.* 2007;25(2):147–153.

86. Summers P, Staempfli P, Jaermann T, Kwiecinski S, Kollias S. A preliminary study of the effects of trigger timing on diffusion tensor imaging of the human spinal cord. *AJNR Am J Neuroradiol.* 2006;27(9):1952–1961.

87. Figley CR, Stroman PW. Investigation of human cervical and upper thoracic spinal cord motion: implications for imaging spinal cord structure and function. *Magn Reson Med.* 2007;58(1):185–189.

88. Figley CR, Yau D, Stroman PW. Attenuation of lower-thoracic, lumbar, and sacral spinal cord motion: implications for imaging human spinal cord structure and function. *AJNR Am J Neuroradiol.* 2008;29:1450–1454.

89. Dagli MS, Ingeholm JE, Haxby JV. Localization of cardiac-induced signal change in fMRI. *Neuroimage.* 1999;9(4):407–415.

90. Alperin N, Vikingstad EM, Gomez-Anson B, Levin DN. Hemodynamically independent analysis of cerebrospinal fluid and brain motion observed with dynamic phase contrast MRI. *Magn Reson Med.* 1996;35(5):741–754.

91. Du Boulay G, O'Connell J, Currie J, Bostick T, Verity P. Further investigations on pulsatile movements in the cerebrospinal fluid pathways. *Acta Radiol Diagn (Stockh).* 1972;13(0):496–523.

92. Henry-Feugeas MC, Idy-Peretti I, Blanchet B, Hassine D, Zannoli G, Schouman-Claeys E. Temporal and spatial assessment of normal cerebrospinal fluid dynamics with MR imaging. *Magn Reson Imaging.* 1993;11(8):1107–1118.

93. Cai J, Sheng K, Sheehan JP, Benedict SH, Larner JM, Read PW. Evaluation of thoracic spinal cord motion using dynamic MRI. *Radiother Oncol.* 2007;84(3):279–282.

94. Fenyes DA, Narayana PA. In vivo diffusion characteristics of rat spinal cord. *Magn Reson Imaging.* 1999;17(5):717–722.

95. Loy DN, Kim JH, Xie M, Schmidt RE, Trinkaus K, Song SK. Diffusion tensor imaging predicts hyperacute spinal cord injury severity. *J Neurotrauma.* 2007;24(6):979–990.

96. Van de Moortele PF, Pfeuffer J, Glover GH, Ugurbil K, Hu X. Respiration-induced B0 fluctuations and their spatial distribution in the human brain at 7 Tesla. *Magn Reson Med.* 2002;47(5):888–895.

97. Raj D, Anderson AW, Gore JC. Respiratory effects in human functional magnetic resonance imaging due to bulk susceptibility changes. *Phys Med Biol.* 2001;46(12):3331–3340.

98. Brosch JR, Talavage TM, Ulmer JL, Nyenhuis JA. Simulation of human respiration in fMRI with a mechanical model. *IEEE Trans Biomed Eng.* 2002;49(7):700–707.

99. van Gelderen P, de Zwart JA, Starewicz P, Hinks RS, Duyn JH. Real-time shimming to compensate for respiration-induced B0 fluctuations. *Magn Reson Med.* 2007;57(2):362–368.

100. Duyn JH, van Gelderen P, Li TQ, de Zwart JA, Koretsky AP, Fukunaga M. High-field MRI of brain cortical substructure based on signal phase. *Proc Natl Acad Sci U S A.* 2007;104(28):11796–11801.

101. Cohen-Adad J, El Mendili M-M, Lehéricy S, et al. Demyelination and degeneration in the injured human spinal cord detected with diffusion and magnetization transfer MRI. *Neuroimage.* 2011;55(3):1024–1033.

102. Smith SA, Jones CK, Gifford A, et al. Reproducibility of tract-specific magnetization transfer and diffusion tensor imaging in the cervical spinal cord at 3 tesla. *NMR Biomed.* 2010;23(2):207–217.

103. Leemans A, Jones DK. The B-matrix must be rotated when correcting for subject motion in DTI data. *Magn Reson Med.* 2009;61(6):1336–1349.

104. Maier SE. Examination of spinal cord tissue architecture with magnetic resonance diffusion tensor imaging. *Neurotherapeutics.* 2007;4(3):453–459.

105. Wheeler-Kingshott CA, Hickman SJ, Parker GJ, et al. Investigating cervical spinal cord structure using axial diffusion tensor imaging. *Neuroimage*. 2002;16(1):93–102.

106. Ciccarelli O, Wheeler-Kingshott CA, McLean MA, et al. Spinal cord spectroscopy and diffusion-based tractography to assess acute disability in multiple sclerosis. *Brain*. 2007;130(8):2220–2231.

107. Bilgen M, Al-Hafez B, Berman NE, Festoff BW. Magnetic resonance imaging of mouse spinal cord. *Magn Reson Med*. 2005;54(5):1226–1231.

108. Ellingson BM, Ulmer JL, Schmit BD. Optimal diffusion tensor indices for imaging the human spinal cord. *Biomed Sci Instrum*. 2007;43:128–133.

109. Benner T, van der Kouwe A, Sorensen A, et al. Fiber Tracking of cervical spinal cord and nerves. In: *Proceedings 16th Scientific Meeting, International Society for Magnetic Resonance in Medicine*. Toronto, Canada; 2008. p. 846.

110. Ellingson BM, Ulmer JL, Schmit BD. Gray and white matter delineation in the human spinal cord using diffusion tensor imaging and fuzzy logic. *Acad Radiol*. 2007;14(7):847–858.

111. Mori S, van Zijl PC. Fiber tracking: principles and strategies – a technical review. *NMR Biomed*. 2002;15(7–8):468–480.

112. Basser PJ, Pajevic S, Pierpaoli C, Duda JT, Aldroubi A. In vivo tractography using DT-MRI data. *Magn Reson Med*. 2000;39(4):625–632.

113. Mori S, Crain BJ, Chacko VP, van Zijl PC. Three-dimensional tracking of axonal projections in the brain by magnetic resonance imaging. *Ann Neurol*. 1999;45(2):265–269.

114. Weinstein DM, Kindlmann GL, Lundberg EC. Tensorlines: advection-diffusion based propagation through diffusion tensor fields. In: *IEEE Visualization Proceedings*. 1999. San Francisco.

115. Lazar M, Weinstein D, Hasan K, Alexander AL. Axon tractography with tensorlines. *Proc Intl Soc Mag Reson Med*. 2000;8:482.

116. Mori S, Kaufmann WE, Davatzikos C, et al. Imaging cortical association tracts in human brain. *Magn Reson Imaging*. 2002;47(2):215–223.

117. Mori S, Davatzikos C, Xu D, et al. A probabilistic map approach for the analysis of DTI-based fiber tracking and its application to white matter injuries. *Proc Intl Soc Mag Reson Med*. 2001;9:1522.

118. Behrens TE, Woolrich MW, Jenkinson M, et al. Characterization and propagation of uncertainty in diffusion-weighted MR imaging. *Magn Reson Med*. 2003;50(5):1077–1088.

119. Johansen-Berg H, Behrens TE. Just pretty pictures? What diffusion tractography can add in clinical neuroscience. *Curr Opin Neurol*. 2006;19(4):379–385.

120. Schwartz ED, Duda J, Shumsky JS, Cooper ET, Gee J. Spinal cord diffusion tensor imaging and fiber tracking can identify white matter tract disruption and glial scar orientation following lateral funiculotomy. *J Neurotrauma*. 2005;22(12):1388–1398.

121. Cohen-Adad J, Lundell J, Rossignol S. Distortion correction in spinal cord DTI: What's the best approach? *Proceedings of the 17th Annual Meeting of ISMRM*. Honolulu, USA; 2009:3178.

122. Van Hecke W, Leemans A, Sijbers J, Vandervliet E, Van Goethem J, Parizel PM. A tracking-based diffusion tensor imaging segmentation method for the detection of diffusion-related changes of the cervical spinal cord with aging. *J Magn Reson Imaging*. 2008;27(5):978–991.

123. Cohen-Adad J, Leblond H, Delivet-Mongrain H, Martinez M, Benali H, Rossignol S. Wallerian degeneration after spinal cord lesions in cats detected with diffusion tensor imaging. *Neuroimage*. 2011;57(3):1068–1076.

124. Mohamed FB, Hunter LN, Barakat N, et al. Diffusion tensor imaging of the pediatric spinal cord at 1.5T: preliminary results. *AJNR Am J Neuroradiol*. 2011;32(2):339–345.

125. Onu M, Gervai P, Cohen-Adad J, et al. Human cervical spinal cord funiculi: investigation with magnetic resonance diffusion tensor imaging. *J Magn Reson Imaging*. 2010;31(4):829–837.

126. Cohen-Adad J, Benali H, Hoge RD, Rossignol S. In vivo DTI of the healthy and injured cat spinal cord at high spatial and angular resolution. *Neuroimage*. 2008;40(2):685–697.

127. Klawiter EC, Schmidt RE, Trinkaus K, et al. Radial Diffusivity Predicts Demyelination in ex-vivo Multiple Sclerosis Spinal Cords. *Neuroimage*. 2011;55(4):1454–1460.

128. Lindberg PG, Feydy A, Maier MA. White matter organization in cervical spinal cord relates differently to age and control of grip force in healthy subjects. *J Neurosci*. 2010;30(11):4102–4109.

129. Qian W, Chan Q, Mak H, et al. Quantitative assessment of the cervical spinal cord damage in neuromyelitis optica using diffusion tensor imaging at 3 Tesla. *J Magn Reson Imaging*. 2011;33(6):1312–1320.

130. Pattany PM, Puckett WR, Klose KJ, et al. High-resolution diffusion-weighted MR of fresh and fixed cat spinal cords: Evaluation of diffusion coefficients and anisotropy. *AJNR Am J Neuroradiol*. 1997;18(6):1049–1056.

131. Takahashi M, Hackney DB, Zhang G, et al. Magnetic resonance microimaging of intraaxonal water diffusion in live excised lamprey spinal cord. *Proc Nat Acad Sci USA*. 2002;99(25):16192–16196.

132. Franconi F, Lemaire L, Marescaux L, Jallet P, Le Jeune JJ. In vivo quantitative microimaging of rat spinal cord at 7T. *Magn Reson Med*. 2000;44(6):893–898.

133. Schwartz ED, Cooper ET, Chin CL, Wehrli S, Tessler A, Hackney DB. Ex vivo evaluation of ADC values within spinal cord white matter tracts. *AJNR Am J Neuroradiol*. 2005;26(2):390–397.

134. Inglis BA, Yang L, Wirth 3rd ED, Plant D, Mareci TH. Diffusion anisotropy in excised normal rat spinal cord measured by NMR microscopy. *Magn Reson Imaging*. 1997;15(4):441–450.

135. Ford JC, Hackney DB. Numerical model for calculations of apparent diffusion coefficient (ADC) in permeable cylinders – comparison with measured ADC in spinal cord white matter. *Magn Reson Med*. 1997;37(3):387–394.

136. Hwang SN, Chin CL, Wehrli FW, Hackney DB. An image-based finite difference model for simulating restricted diffusion. *Magn Reson Med*. 2003;50(2):373–382.

137. Stanisz G, Szafer A, Wright GA, Henkelman RM. An analytical model of restricted diffusion in bovine optic nerve. *Magn Reson Med*. 1997;37(1):103–111.

138. Schwartz ED, Cooper ET, Fan Y, et al. MRI diffusion coefficients in spinal cord correlate with axon morphometry. *Neuroreport*. 2005;16(1):73–76.

139. Kinoshita Y, Ohnishi A, Kohshi K, Yokota A. Apparent diffusion coefficient on rat brain and nerves intoxicated with methylmercury. *Environ Res*. 1999;80(4):348–354.

140. Ellingson BM, Ulmer JL, Kurpad SN, Schmit BD. Diffusion tensor MR imaging of the neurologically intact human spinal cord. *AJNR Am J Neuroradiol*. 2008;29(7):1279–1284.

141. Ellingson BM, Schmit BD, Ulmer JL, Kurpad SN. Diffusion tensor magnetic resonance imaging in spinal cord injury. *Concepts Magn Reson Part A*. 2008;32A(3):219–237.

142. Shi R, Pryor JD. Pathological changes of isolated spinal cord axons in response to mechanical stretch. *Neuroscience*. 2002;110(4):765–777.

143. Ford JC, Hackney DB, Alsop DC, et al. MRI characterization of diffusion coefficients in a rat spinal cord injury model. *Magn Reson Med*. 1994;31(5):488–494.

144. Deo AA, Grill RJ, Hasan K, Narayana PA. In vivo serial diffusion tensor imaging of experimental spinal cord injury. *J Neurosci Res*. 2006;83(5):801–810.

145. Ford JC, Hackney DB, Lavi E, Phillips M, Patel U. Dependence of apparent diffusion coefficients on axonal spacing, membrane permeability, and diffusion time in spinal cord white matter. *J Magn Reson Imaging.* 1998;8(4):775–782.

146. Ducker TB, Saleman M, Perot PL, Balentine D. Experimental spinal cord trauma. I. Correlation of blood flow, tissue oxygen, and neurologic status in the dog. *Surg Neurol.* 1978;10(1):60–63.

147. Holtz A, Nystrom B, Gerdin B. Spinal cord blood flow measured by ^{14}C-iodoantipyrine autoradiography during and after graded spinal cord compression in rats. *Surg Neurol.* 1989;31(5):350–360.

148. Rivlin AS, Tator CH. Regional spinal cord blood flow in rats after severe cord trauma. *J Neurosurg.* 1978;49(6):470–477.

149. Sun S, Liang H, Le T, Armstrong RC, Cross AH, Song S. Differential sensitivity of in vivo and ex vivo diffusion tensor imaging to evolving optic nerve injury in mice with retinal ischemia. *Neuroimage.* 2006;32(3):1195–1204.

150. Sagiuchi T, Iida H, Tachibana S, Kusumi M, Kan S, Fujii K. Diffusion-weighted MRI in anterior spinal artery stroke of the cervical spinal cord. *J Comput Assist Tomogr.* 2003;27(3):410–414.

151. Bammer R, Fazekas F, Augustin M, et al. Diffusion-weighted MR imaging of the spinal cord. *AJNR Am J Neuroradiol.* 2000;21(3): 587–591.

152. Mamata H, Jolesz FA, Maier SE. Apparent diffusion coefficient and fractional anisotropy in spinal cord: age and cervical spondylosis-related changes. *J Magn Reson Imaging.* 2005;22(1): 38–43.

153. Kuker W, Weller M, Klose U, Krapf H, Dichgans J, Nagele T. Diffusion-weighted MRI of spinal cord infarction–high resolution imaging and time course of diffusion abnormality. *J Neurol.* 2004; 251(7):818–824.

154. Demir A, Ries M, Moonen CT, et al. Diffusion-weighted MR imaging with apparent diffusion coefficient and apparent diffusion tensor maps in cervical spondylotic myelopathy. *Radiology.* 2003;229(1):37–43.

155. Sandler AN, Tator CH. Review of the effect of spinal cord trauma on the vessels and blood flow in the spinal cord. *J Neurosurg.* 1976;45(6):638–646.

156. Wagner Jr FC, Dohrmann GJ, Bucy PC. Histopathology of transitory traumatic paraplegia in the monkey. *J Neurosurg.* 1971; 35(2):272–276.

157. Hagg T, Oudega M. Degenerative and spontaneous regenerative processes after spinal cord injury. *J Neurotrauma.* 2006;23(3):264–280.

158. Balentine JD. Pathology of experimental spinal cord trauma. *Lab Invest.* 1978;39(3):236–253.

159. Mautes AE, Weinzierl MR, Donovan F, Noble LJ. Vascular events after spinal cord injury: contribution to secondary pathogenesis. *Phys Ther.* 2000;80(7):673–687.

160. Schwartz ED, Hackney DB. Diffusion-weighted MRI and the evaluation of spinal cord axonal integrity following injury and treatment. *Exp Neurol.* 2003;184(2):570–589.

161. Blakemore WF. Remyelination by Schwann cells of axons demyelinated by intraspinal injection of 6-aminonicotinamide in the rat. *J Neurocytol.* 1975;4(6):745–757.

162. Waller A. Experiments on the section of glossopharyngeal and hypoglossal nerves of the frog and observation of the alternatives produced thereby in the structure of their primitive fibres. *Philos Trans R Soc Lond B Biol Sci.* 1850;140:423.

163. Kitzman P. Alterations in axial motoneuron morphology in the spinal cord injured spastic cat. *Exp Neurol.* 2005;192(1):100–108.

164. Finnerup NB, Gyldensted C, Nielsen E, Kristensen AD, Bach FW, Jensen TS. MRI in chronic spinal cord injury patients with and without central pain. *Neurology.* 2003;61(11):1569–1575.

165. Uchida K, Baba H, Maezawa Y, Furukawa S, Furukawa N, Imura S. Histological investigation of spinal cord lesions in the spinal hyperostotic mouse (twy/twy): morphological changes in anterior horn cells and immunoreactivity to neurotropic factors. *J Neurol.* 1998;245(12):781–793.

166. Ellingson BM, Ulmer JL, Kurpad SN, Schmit BD. Diffusion tensor magnetic resonance imaging of the neurologically intact human spinal cord. *AJNR Am J Neuroradiol.* 2008;29(7):1279–1284.

167. Ford JC, Hackney DB, Joseph PM, et al. A method for in vivo high resolution MRI of rat spinal cord injury. *Magn Reson Med.* 1994;31(2):218–223.

168. Fraidakis M, Klason T, Cheng H, Olson L, Spenger C. High resolution MRI of intact and transected rat spinal cord. *Exp Neurol.* 1998;153(2):299–312.

169. Totoiu MO, Keirstead HS. Spinal cord injury is accompanied by chronic progressive demyelination. *J Comp Neurol.* 2005;486(4): 373–383.

170. Waxman SG. Demyelination in spinal cord injury. *J Neurol Sci.* 1989;91(1–2):1–14.

171. Bunge RP, Pucket WR, Becerra JL, Marcillo A, Quencer RM. Observation on the pathology of human spinal cord injury. A review and classification of 22 new cases with details from a case of chronic cord compression with extensive focal demyelination. *Adv Neurol.* 1993;59:75–89.

172. Blakemore WF. Pattern of remyelination in the CNS. *Nature.* 1974; 249(457):577–578.

173. Blight AR, Decrescito V. Morphometric analysis of experimental spinal cord injury in the cat: the relation of injury intensity to survival of myelinated axons. *Neuroscience.* 1986;19(1):321–341.

174. Harrison BM, McDonald WI. Remyelination after transient experimental compression of the spinal cord. *Ann Neurol.* 1977; 1(6):542–551.

175. Ito T, Oyanagi K, Wakabayashi K, Ikuta F. Traumatic spinal cord injury: a neuropathological study on the longitudinal spreading of the lesions. *Acta Neuropathol (Berl).* 1997;93(1): 13–18.

176. Ellingson BM, Ulmer JL, Kurpad SN, Schmit BD. Diffusion tensor MR imaging in chronic spinal cord injury. *AJNR Am J Neuroradiol.* 2008;29(10):1976–1982.

177. Ellingson BM, Prost RW, Ulmer JL, Schmit BD. Morphology and morphometry in chronic spinal cord injury assessed using diffusion tensor imaging and fuzzy logic. *Conf Proc IEEE Eng Med Biol Soc.* 2006;1(1):1885–1888.

178. Ellingson BM, Ulmer JL, Schmit BD. A new technique for imaging the human spinal cord in vivo. *Biomed Sci Instrum.* 2006;42: 255–260.

179. Ellingson BM, Ulmer JL, Schmit BD. Morphology and morphometry of human chronic spinal cord injury using diffusion tensor imaging and fuzzy logic. *Ann Biomed Eng.* 2008;36(2): 224–236.

180. Xu J, Shimony JS, Klawiter EC, et al. Improved in vivo diffusion tensor imaging of human cervical spinal cord. *Neuroimage.* 2013; 67:64–76.

181. Verma T, Cohen-Adad J. Effect of Respiration on the B0 Field in the Human Spinal Cord at 3T. *Magn Reson Med.* 2013 (in press). http://dx.doi.org/10.1002/mrm.25075.

Q-Space Imaging: A Model-Free Approach

Torben Schneider, Claudia A.M Wheeler-Kingshott

NMR Research Unit, Department of Neuroinflammation, Queen Square MS Centre, UCL Institute of Neurology,
University College London, London, UK

In Chapter 3.1, the diffusion of water molecules was described according to the diffusion tensor model, which assumes a Gaussian probability of displacement associated to the diffusion of water molecules. This assumption is true in free systems, but it is also applied for water in complex biological structures. In this chapter, the q-space theory is explored as a model free from assumptions, and we discuss its limitations and its translation to in vivo applications to the spinal cord. One of the main advantages of q-space imaging (QSI) is that it allows probing of tissue microstructures with higher fidelity than diffusion tensor imaging (DTI) because of its sensitivity to restriction and hindrance.

All concepts relative to DTI are discussed in Chapter 3.1, and it is assumed that the user is familiar with magnetic resonance imaging (MRI) diffusion experiments.

3.2.1 Q-SPACE THEORY

Nonparametric approaches (e.g., those based on q-space theory)[1] do not model the displacement probability explicitly and therefore give a more accurate representation of the diffusion mechanism in complex biological tissue. The notion that structural information is obtainable through the study of q-space has been pioneered by Refs 2 and 3. The following derivation forms the basis of q-space analysis, where $P(r|r', t)$ is the conditional displacement probability of water (i.e., expressing the probability of a water molecule diffusing from position r to r' over the time period t). In a pulsed gradient spin echo (PGSE) diffusion experiment (see Chapter 3.1 for details), if the diffusion gradient pulse duration δ is negligible compared to the diffusion time Δ ($\delta \ll \Delta$), any motion of water molecules during the diffusion gradient time can be neglected. In this short gradient pulse (SGP) regime, the normalized echo attenuation S for a specific PGSE experiment can be

expressed as the integral over all water molecules of the net phase shift of each molecule caused by the diffusion gradient vector g and diffusion gradient duration δ, weighted by the probability of its movement from r to r' during diffusion time Δ (also called the mixing time). Thus:

$$S(g, \delta, \Delta) = \iint P(r)P(r|r', \Delta)\exp[-i \cdot \gamma \delta g \cdot (r' - r)]\mathrm{d}r'\mathrm{d}r,$$

(3.2.1)

with γ being the gyromagnetic ratio for the nucleus under observation (e.g., the proton ^{1}H).

In a typical diffusion MRI experiment, the spatial dimension of the prescribed voxel is several magnitudes bigger than the length scale of diffusion motion. Hence, it is useful to consider the average displacement probability density function (dPDF) $P'(R, t)$ (often referred to as the "average propagator"[4]), describing the ensemble average probability of a particle moving the distance R during diffusion time t independent of starting position r within the voxel, which is defined as:

$$P'(R, t) = \int P(r)P(r|r + R, t)\mathrm{d}r.$$

(3.2.2)

Combining Eqns (3.2.1) and (3.2.2), the signal attenuation can be expressed as:

$$S(g, \delta, \Delta) = \int P'(R, \Delta)\exp[-i \cdot \gamma \delta g \cdot R]\mathrm{d}R.$$

(3.2.3)

Furthermore, by introducing the q-value $q = (2\pi)^{-1}\gamma\delta g$ and rewriting Eqn (3.2.3) as:

$$S(q, \Delta) = \int P'(R, \Delta)\exp[i2\pi q \cdot R]\mathrm{d}R,$$

it is evident that there is a simple Fourier relationship between the observed signal $S(q, \Delta)$ and the average displacement probability $P'(R,t)$. This Fourier relationship can be exploited to infer the average displacement probability of diffusing water at a certain diffusion time within a sample without the need to impose any constraints on characteristics of the probability distribution itself.

> The displacement *PDF* or *diffusion propagator* is the average probability of a particle moving a certain distance during a given diffusion time. The PDF is calculated by measuring the signal attenuation at various gradient amplitudes (g).

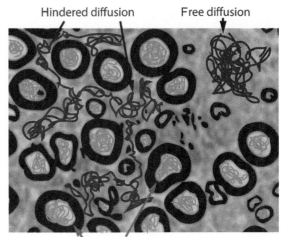

FIGURE 3.2.1 Cartoon of diffusion paths in the presence of different tissue environments. Restricted diffusion (shown in green): the molecule's motion is constrained within a confined space (e.g., within in the intra-axonal spaces). Hindered diffusion (shown in red): the free motion of water molecules is hindered by the dense packing of axons (e.g., within the extra-axonal space). Free diffusion (shown in blue): pure Brownian motion in the absence of barriers.

3.2.2 FREE, HINDERED, AND RESTRICTED DIFFUSION

Diffusion in nervous tissue can deviate significantly from simple Gaussian behavior in the presence of cell membranes and structures that hinder or restrict the diffusion of water molecules.[5]

In the simplest case, the change in signal attenuation due to molecule–barrier interaction can be interpreted as a change in the apparent diffusion coefficient (ADC), while assuming that the displacement probability distribution remains Gaussian. This simple interpretation also forms the basis for DTI (see Chapter 3.1 for details) and has shown great sensitivity to pathological changes that affect this interaction. However, measuring ADC or the more popular rotationally invariant DTI indices lacks specificity. By employing the q-space analysis, instead, it is possible to infer the shape and size of the molecular surrounding environment.

In the absence of any interacting barriers, free diffusion (or unrestricted diffusion) describes the pure Brownian motion of water (i.e., molecules diffusing freely in all directions). As described in Chapter 3.1, in the case of free diffusion in all three dimensions, the average displacement probability takes the form of a simple Gaussian distribution and Einstein's equation for the mean displacement R applies:

$$R = \sqrt{6D\Delta}. \tag{3.2.4}$$

In other words, in a free diffusing medium, the mean displacement has a simple dependency on the diffusion time Δ and the diffusivity D of the medium.

In reality, free diffusion is rarely encountered in a biological tissue sample. Instead, the presence of restricting barriers, such as cell walls, membranes, or myelin, impedes the motion of the water molecules and alters the displacement probability. In this case, the diffusion displacement probability not only is influenced by the diffusivity of the medium but also, more importantly, informs about the characteristics of the surrounding environment on the scale of the mean displacement R.

The observed effects on the diffusion MR signal can be quite diverse, depending on the type and location of barriers within the sample. It is helpful to further distinguish between restricted and hindered diffusion (see Figure 3.2.1 for illustration). Restricted diffusion is observed if the movement of water molecules is confined to closed spaces, e.g., inside impermeable cell walls. Those molecules experience restricted diffusion in that the molecules cannot displace farther than the confines of the cell. In hindered diffusion, the movement of molecules is impeded, although it is not confined within a limited space. Hindered diffusion best describes water motion in the space that is between densely packed cells or axons with semipermeable membranes and surrounded by myelin sheaths.

> * *Free diffusion* Water molecules move freely in all directions of space, following a Gaussian distribution
> * *Restricted diffusion* Water molecules are confined in closed spaces, such as the intra-axonal space
> * *Hindered diffusion* Water molecules are constrained within extra-axonal spaces

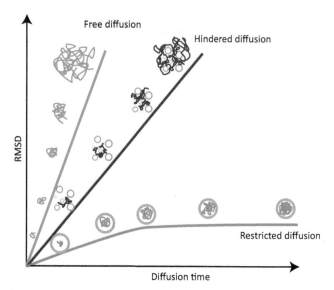

FIGURE 3.2.2   Illustration of the behavior of molecule displacement in the long diffusion time limit. For free diffusion (blue), the linear relationship between the squared mean molecule displacement and diffusion time is governed by Einstein's equation. The squared mean displacement in hindered diffusion (red) also increases monotonously with diffusion time, albeit at a lower rate than in free diffusion. In restricted diffusion (green), the possible displacement of each molecule is limited by the size of the confining space and therefore ultimately reaches a plateau for long diffusion times.

3.2.2.1 Restricted Diffusion and the Long Diffusion Time Limit

Figure 3.2.2 illustrates the expected relationship between diffusion time and the root mean square displacement ($\text{RMSD} = \sqrt{\langle R^2 \rangle}$) in hindered and restricted diffusion. According to Einstein's equation (Eqn 3.2.4), free diffusion shows a linear relationship between diffusion time and RMSD. In the hindered-diffusion scenario, the RMSD is reduced compared to free diffusion, but it is still approximately linear with distance. In the restricted diffusion scenario, the RMSD is limited by the confinement of the restricting compartment. From Figure 3.2.2, it also becomes clear that the observed motion pattern of restricted diffusion has a strong dependency on the diffusion time. Consider the simple case of water

molecules exclusively diffusing within an impermeable compartment of size a. For short diffusion times $\Delta \ll a^2/D$, the motion pattern is very similar to free diffusion, as most molecules have not yet explored the confines of the compartment. With increasing diffusion time, more diffusing molecules will exhibit a behavior influenced by the boundaries of the compartment. Finally, at long diffusion times $\Delta \gg a^2/D$, most molecules explore the extent of the confining geometry, and the mean displacement converges to the upper limit of the confining dimension a.

In the long diffusion time limit, all molecules have fully experienced the confining space; the conditional displacement probability (Eqn (3.2.1)) becomes independent of starting position and therefore is equivalent to the molecular density function $\rho(r)$ of the confining space. Furthermore, in the long diffusion time limit, the average displacement probability P' (Eqn (3.2.2)) also reduces to the autocorrelation function of $\rho(r)$:

$$P'(R, t \rightarrow \infty) = \int \rho(r)\rho(r + R)\mathrm{d}r \qquad (3.2.5)$$

In simple geometries, this autocorrelation relationship can be directly exploited to estimate the size of the confining space.

3.2.3 Q-SPACE IMAGING

The combination of q-space analysis with MRI methods is called q-space imaging (QSI).[1,6] QSI provides the full displacement probability profile in each voxel of the imaged volume. However, visualization and quantification of the full displacement profile in each voxel are usually impracticable. Instead, it is more common to derive parameters from the dPDF (see Section 3.2.1) that summarize the features of the displacement profile. The most widely used parameters are zero displacement probability (P_0), full width of half maximum (FWHM), and kurtosis (K). The QSI analysis steps and the significance of the P_0, FWHM, and K parameter maps are outlined in Figure 3.2.4.

Ideal gradient   Short gradient   Long gradient
pulse   pulse   pulse

- - - -   Diffusion trajectories during
          Diffusion gradient pulses

——— Diffusion trajectory between
          gradient pulses

⊗ "Centre of mass" location of
          diffusion trajectory

FIGURE 3.2.3   Illustration of the center of mass effect caused by a finite gradient pulse duration. In the ideal case (left), no motion occurs during the diffusion-encoding gradients. In the short gradient pulse case (middle), only a small amount of motion occurs during the diffusion-encoding gradients, which is negligible in view of the displacement encoded during the diffusion time. In the long gradient pulse case (right), the molecules already explore a significant portion of the confining space during the encoding gradient, and thus the observed displacement during the diffusion time is artifactually smaller.

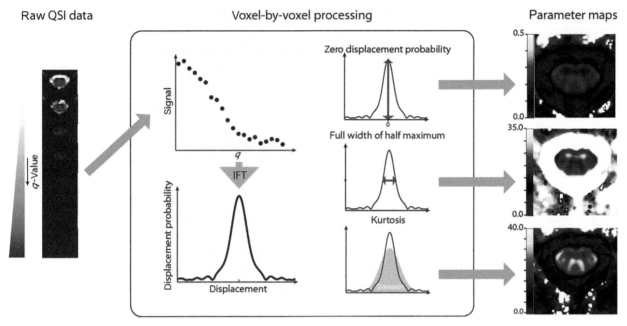

FIGURE 3.2.4   Outline of a QSI-processing pipeline and resulting parameter maps. Left panel: Example of DWI-weighted images (g applied perpendicular to fibers) with a linearly increasing q-value. Middle panel: The inverse fast Fourier transform of the q-space data points is performed on a voxel-by-voxel basis. Right panel: Example maps of P_0, FWHM, and K in a healthy volunteer.

The P_0 and FWHM parameters describe the height and width of the displacement profile (dPDF). Generally, a high P_0 and low FWHM can be interpreted as indicators of a more hindered diffusion; low P_0 and wide FWHM are related to more free or less hindered diffusion (Figure 3.2.4). The FWHM is of particular theoretical interest as it is directly related to the size of the restricted compartment in simple geometries via the autocorrelation function[2,7] described in Eqn (3.2.5). Some studies report the RMSD as described in the equation instead of the FWHM,[2] and suggest the conversion between FWHM and RMSD as:

$$RMSD = 1.443 \ FWHM.$$

However, the equality is true only if the diffusion profile is truly Gaussian.

The kurtosis parameter (here defined as the excess kurtosis[8]) describes how much a distribution differs from the normal distribution. Kurtosis is defined as the standardized fourth central moment of a distribution minus 3 (to make the kurtosis of the normal distribution equal to zero). For a finite sample of n data points, the kurtosis K is computed as:

$$K = \frac{\frac{1}{n}\sum_{i=1}^{n}(x_i - x')^4}{\left(\frac{1}{n}\sum_{i=1}^{n}(x_i - x')^2\right)^2} - 3$$

with x' being the sample mean. A high kurtosis distribution has a narrower peak and a long, fat tail compared to a normal distribution. A low kurtosis distribution has a more rounded peak and a shorter, thinner tail. In the

context of diffusion analysis, the kurtosis parameter can be used to quantify how much the dPDF differs from a Gaussian displacement distribution.[9] High K values can therefore be interpreted as an indicator of restricted diffusion in a sample. The kurtosis parameter can also be directly estimated from a subset of q-space measurements as described in Chapter 3.1.

3.2.4 LIMITATIONS OF QSI

QSI parameters measured in nervous tissue are often interpreted as a direct indicator of axonal architecture, such as the mean axon diameter. Early studies have demonstrated that q-space analysis can indeed provide exact estimates of the geometry in simple samples (e.g., yeast cells[2] or blood cells[7]). However, experiments on real nervous tissue have shown that the interpretation of q-space parameters in axonal tissue is more complicated.[6,10–12] Assaf and Cohen[10] were the first to demonstrate that the displacement profile of nervous tissue can be expressed as a combination of at least two compartments exhibiting hindered and restricted diffusion. A recent study of QSI in the in vivo human brain by Nilsson et al.[13] confirmed that the FWHM perpendicular to white matter fibers did not change with diffusion time, which is an indication of restricted diffusion across the white matter bundles. In contrast, the parallel FWHM increased linearly with the square root of diffusion time, which suggests hindered diffusion, as expected from theory (Figure 3.2.1). The two compartments are often attributed to intracellular (IC) and extracellular (EC) water, although there is an ongoing debate over the interpretation of these results (see e.g., Refs 14 and 15).

Since q-space analysis provides the average displacement probability over the whole voxel, the q-space measurement is affected by both IC and EC compartments as well as by the amount of exchange between the two. As a result, the dPDF may be broader than the actual size of the confining space would suggest, due to the addition of displacements from hindered diffusion in the EC compartments. Other factors, such as the distribution of sizes and the variety of shapes of cells and membranes in tissue, further complicate the interpretation of q-space parameters to infer the real axon diameter distributions.

3.2.4.1 Effect of Gradient Pulse Width and Maximum q

Unlike modern nuclear magnetic resonance (NMR) spectrometers and preclinical small-bore scanners, most clinical MRI systems are equipped with only limited maximal gradient strength (usually 40–60 mT/m). On these systems, the necessary high q-values for q-space analysis cannot be achieved without prolonged diffusion gradient pulse durations. Mitra and Halperin[16] showed that the effective molecule displacement, measured with a finite diffusion pulse δ, is equivalent to the distance between the center of mass and the molecule trajectories occurring while the diffusion gradients are applied. If the SGP condition $\delta \ll \Delta$ is fulfilled, the observed distance between the center of mass and the trajectories is approximately the same as the true displacement of the molecule. However, if δ is long, molecule movement will occur during the diffusion gradient pulses, and only the displacement between the centers of mass will be observed. As illustrated in Figure 3.2.3, in the case of restricted diffusion, an increase in gradient pulse duration will cause the underestimation of the true displacement.

When implementing QSI protocols on a clinical scanner, one has to be aware of the effect of the finite gradient pulse duration and its implications. Usually, clinical studies of QSI have to violate the SGP condition to achieve sufficiently high q-values. As expected from the center of mass effect, this causes an artifactual reduction of displacement. This has been confirmed in simulation[17,18] and various experimental studies in phantoms,[19,20] excised tissue,[21,22] and even in vivo human scans.[13] As a consequence, the estimated displacement profile has to be interpreted with caution as it will not reflect the true displacement in the tissue. This effect also makes it impossible to compare results between studies under different experimental conditions if the SGP is violated.

The SGP violation is a fundamental problem in q-space analysis and can be avoided only with an increase of the maximum gradient strength. As an additional advantage of stronger gradients, echo-planar imaging (EPI) read-outs can be shortened, thereby decreasing the echo time, yielding gains in SNR, and reducing susceptibility distortions.

Some experimental scanners are equipped with gradient systems capable of generating up to 300 mT/m (Human Connectome Project, Harvard/MGH-UCLA, Boston, MA, USA) and demonstrated promising results for q-space axon diameter measurements in the human corpus callosum in vivo.[23] However, those dedicated systems are designed for a specific research project, and the general availability of these strong whole-body gradients in the future is doubtful due to their high costs. Economic feasibility aside, the use of higher gradient strengths and shorter pulse widths also increases the risk of peripheral nerve stimulation (PNS)[24] and might cause more discomfort for the subjects. There is also a safety issue that limits the gradients' duty cycle when requiring high amplitudes to be reached in short times. In fact, there are restrictions on the dB/dt rate of change that is considered safe because a changing magnetic field can induce electrical currents that can harm the subject. As a consequence, this in turn may constrain the adoption of such systems for clinical scanners.

Gradient insert coils offer a practical alternative to achieve higher gradient strength. These coils can be designed for a specific region of interest in the body. Their smaller size allows larger amplitudes and makes stronger gradients more practical to implement. They also reduce the risk of PNS for the subject due to their reduced length and reduced cross-sectional area (only the head is exposed).

Few dedicated gradient coils have been developed for different clinical 3 T and 7 T scanners.[25,26] To date, human neuroimaging applications have focused on the brain. However, some of these existing designs already cover the (upper) cervical cord or might be adapted easily to cover the upper cord segments. However, it should be noted that these insert gradients suffer from important nonlinearities outside the very center of the gradient; therefore, they would be suboptimal when the imaging region is located at the extremity of the gradients. Aside from image distortions (which could be corrected using distortion field maps estimated from the specifications of the gradients), diffusion-encoding gradients would also suffer from gradient nonlinearities and should be accounted for in q-space experiments. Novel open gradient designs (e.g., Ref. 27) offer potential advantages for DWI in the lower cord segments.

The gain from improved gradient strength is immense for q-space analysis (and diffusion imaging in general) and few other subdisciplines of MRI (e.g., all fast imaging methods such as fMRI due to better EPI performance). Wide commercial availability is hampered by the fact that improved gradient performance has little effect on the quality of routine MRI scans. As a result, the commercial interest in offering better gradient systems or gradient inserts is low.

3.2.5 ACQUISITION OF QSI DATA IN THE SPINAL CORD

In theory, q-space analysis can provide the diffusion displacement profile in any arbitrary direction, similarly to diffusion spectrum imaging (see Chapter 3.1). However, accurate estimation of the dDPF requires a large number of q-samples along a single gradient direction (typically, between 16 and 32 samples in one direction are acquired). In practice, this limits the number of directions that can be investigated in vivo within a clinically acceptable time.

To reduce the number of q-space directions sampled, q-space samples are typically only applied perpendicular to the fibers where the restriction effect is most pronounced and occasionally also parallel to the fiber orientation where the effect of restriction is least apparent.[6,11,19,28–30]

While in general the alignment of the gradients with respect to the underlying tissue fiber organization is difficult to achieve in complex systems such as the brain, one can take advantage of the homogeneous organization of spinal cord white matter. Under the assumption that the majority of white matter tracts in the spinal cord align in longitudinal directions, diffusion will therefore be most restricted perpendicular to the long axis of the cord and most hindered (least restricted) parallel to it. The small number of collateral fibers is usually neglected, although Lundell et al.[31] have demonstrated recently that those fibers might be detectable by diffusion-weighted imaging. Table 3.2.1 shows an example of a QSI protocol. In this protocol, QSI data are acquired perpendicular and parallel to the longitudinal axis.

A major confounding factor in clinical QSI is the presence of noise in the images. The noise distribution in MR magnitude images is known to be Rician distributed.[34] Also note that when using phased-array coils, the noise distribution of the magnitude images becomes more complex (see Chapter 2.1). As a consequence, the MR signal exhibits a nonzero bias when SNR is low. This becomes a problem for high q-weighted encodings because of their inherently low SNR. At very large q-values, the true signal and the persistent noise floor become indistinguishable. As a result, the level of the nonzero noise floor effectively determines the resolution of the displacement probability. In a simulation

TABLE 3.2.1 Imaging and Diffusion Parameters for a QSI Protocol

Imaging Parameters		Q-Space Parameters		
FOV	64×64 mm^2	δ	14 ms	*31 steps*
Matrix size	64×64	Δ	75 ms	
Slice thickness	5 mm			
Voxel size	$1 \times 1 \times 5$ mm^3	G	0 mT/m	
TE	Minimum (130 ms)		2 mT/m	
			...	
TR	5000 ms		60 mT/m	
			62 mT/m	
Signal averages	1			
Number of slices	10			

Each acquired in three directions
Two orthogonal acquisitions perpendicular to the long axis of the SC
One acquisition parallel to the long axis of the SC

Adapted from Refs 32 and 33.

study by Lätt et al.,[17] the effect of the signal-to-noise-floor ratio (SNFR) on q-space measurements was demonstrated. The results showed that at least SNFR > 10 is required to achieve enough q-space resolutions to distinguish even relatively large compartments of size 15–25 μm.

The spin-echo EPI (SE-EPI) diffusion acquisition is by far the most commonly used sequence for QSI. In SE-EPI, the SNR (and SNFR) are governed by the T2 decay of the tissue. The choice of the diffusion time Δ has the biggest influence on the echo time (TE). As discussed in this chapter, the diffusion time Δ has to be long enough to allow spins sufficient time to encounter barriers to diffusion. Users therefore have to ensure that the chosen diffusion time of the experiment is long enough to see the effects of restricted diffusion. In the proposed protocol, we chose a diffusion time of 75 ms, which, for values of $D = 1$–2 μm^2/ms (typically found in in vivo nervous tissue), corresponds to a mean displacement of 20–30 μm and thus is several magnitudes bigger than the average axon diameter expected in the spinal cord (1–2 μm).[35] In view of the required long diffusion times and hence long echo times, it is advisable to use a combination of partial Fourier sampling and phased-array coils to reduce the length of the echo train, and use small field-of-view imaging techniques (e.g., Refs 36–38) to increase SNR and reduce susceptibility distortions in the QSI data.

Stimulated echo (STE) sequences are an alternative to achieve long diffusion times with shorter TE instead of the conventional SE (see figure in Chapter 3.1). STE acquisitions are much less affected by the short T2 decay, and SNR is dominated by the T1 decay signal of the tissue. However, STE sequences come with an inherent 50% SNR penalty, which makes them inferior to SE sequences in the shorter diffusion time range.

3.2.6 DATA PROCESSING

Even modern whole-body scanner gradients are not sufficient for achieving the high q-values needed to resolve the compartment sizes usually found in spinal cord white matter (1–2 μm). There are two possible approaches to increase the spatial resolution of the displacement profile: extrapolation of the signal in q-space (before Fourier transformation of the signal) or interpolation in displacement space (after Fourier transformation of the signal).

Cohen and Assaf[39] recommend zero filling the acquired data for larger q values (i.e., when the signal decays toward the noise floor at large q values). In cases where the signal is not fully decayed, zero filling will introduce discontinuities in q-space, which result in truncation artifacts (side lobes) after Fourier transformation. In these cases, model-driven data extrapolation seems to be the better choice. Cohen and Assaf[39] suggest using a biexponential model to extrapolate QSI data, as it produces a good fit to the data.[32,40] However, data-fitting methods always introduce some degree of model dependence, and the "model-free" q-space results must be interpreted with that in mind.

Alternatively, the dPDF can be interpolated directly in displacement space. Most commonly, simple linear interpolation is used to increase the resolution of the original dPDF. Other methods such as b-spline interpolation have the additional benefit of producing smoother dPDFs and offer more realistic distribution curves. While the former methods assume no particular shape of the dPDF, other methods impose a priori knowledge to explain the dPDF. Assaf and Cohen[10] fitted a bi-Gaussian model to explain the displacement profile and attributed the two displacement profiles to the IC and EC compartments. Ong and Wehrli[41] used a similar mixture model but replaced one of the Gaussian PDFs with a more complex expression that restricted diffusion within circular pores with gamma-distributed diameters. They showed that the axon radius distributions they calculated in different tracts of the rat spinal cord agreed with diameter distributions measured from histology. These approaches violate the model-free nature of the q-space analysis. Instead, they can be seen as a hybrid between q-space analysis and geometric tissue models (as in Chapter 3.3).

3.2.7 CURRENT IN VIVO SPINAL CORD APPLICATION OF QSI

Despite the challenges of q-space acquisition, the promise of parameters reflecting tissue microstructure more closely than the model-driven DTI indices has promoted attempts to set up protocols for assessing pathology in the spinal cord in humans in vivo. The search for new indices that can be affected by pathology with higher specificity or sensitivity to microstructural changes is ongoing and aided by the advent of better technology.

The most thorough study presented to date, performing q-space imaging of the spinal cord in vivo in patients, is by Farrell et al.,[32] where they compared q-space-derived parameters with more conventional quantitative measurements of tissue integrity. In fact, in this pilot work, they acquired magnetization transfer (MT) images and reconstructed MT cerebrospinal fluid (MTCSF) maps (see Chapter 3.4) as well as DW images with DW gradients along two orthogonal directions in the cross-sectional plane of the cervical spinal cord. All reported findings are relative to the in-plane diffusion properties of water molecules in spinal cord tissue as no measurements were performed along the main axis of the spinal cord. The acquisition protocol for the DW part of the exam consisted of 31 linearly spaced q-values from 0 to 414 per cm, for a maximum $b = 4685$ s/mm^2 (see Chapter 3.1 for the definition of b). Comparisons of mean ADC values with RMSD and P_0 values between patients with multiple sclerosis (MS) and healthy subjects as well as between lesional tissue and normal-appearing white matter (NAWM) showed that RMSD and P_0 have the potential to be sensitive to disease in a complementary and possibly more sensitive way than ADC or MTCSF. In Figure 3.2.5, the comparison of RMSD, P_0, ADC, MTCSF, and MTR is shown for different slices and for four different subjects, including a healthy control, a relapsing remitting MS (RRMS) patient, and two secondary progressive MS (SPMS) patients. While the ADC and MT-based measurements are often within the healthy subjects' range, it is clear that both RMSD and P_0 are departing from the healthy subject's range in several cases along the cervical cord, demonstrating a potentially greater sensitivity to pathology.

In different papers, Hori et al. presented q-space data of patients with spinal cord damage, including neurinomas, myeloma, and syringohydromyelia,[42] and a cohort of 50 subjects with spinal cord compression.[43] These studies acquired DW data with a very quick suboptimal protocol for six or 12 q-factors along, respectively, three

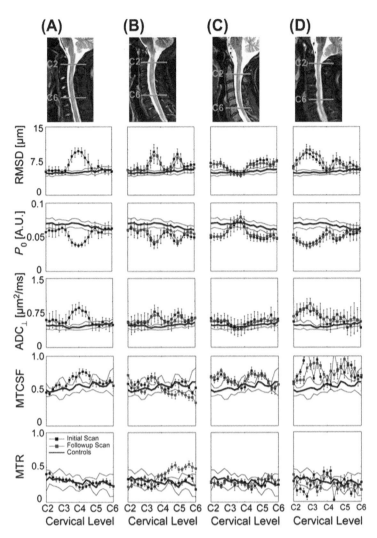

FIGURE 3.2.5 Mean displacement (RMSD), maximum probability of zero displacement P_0, mean diffusion ADC, magnetization transfer ratio (MTR), and MTCSF in a region placed over the dorsal column white matter in (A) a 25-year-old male subject with RRMS, (B) a 31-year-old female subject with RRMS, (C) a 43-year-old female with SPMS, and (D) a 41-year-old male with SPMS. The solid black lines are indicating the mean ± one standard deviation of healthy volunteers for each measurement. In blue are the results along the cervical spinal cord for each subject. In red, measurements were performed again at a second visit, 2–4 months after the initial scan. Interestingly, RMSD and P_0 seems to reveal abnormal values, especially in (C), where the other measured quantities (MTR, MTCSF, ADC) are within the normal range, suggesting that potentially these q-space indices may be more sensitive to pathological changes. *Source: Reproduced from Ref. 32.*

or six non-collinear DW directions. Thy reported their findings by averaging results along DW directions sampled across or along the spinal cord. Both of these studies do not report results in healthy subjects. In spinal cord compression, the RMSD value seemed to be increased in patients with greater compression, although no correlation with clinical scores was reported. This increase in RMSD was also accompanied by a reduction in FA and an increase in the mean ADC.

Further studies in larger cohorts are needed to confirm the place of q-space in clinical applications. Clearly, excised animal work has shown the sensitivity of q-space parameters to tissue microstructure (e.g., Refs 6 and 41; see also Chapter 3.3) and its change in consequence of an insult such as, for example, that generated by spinal cord axotomy[44] and by hemi-crush injury.[45] The sensitivity to myelin structure was also shown in myelin-deficient spinal cord rats, where RMSD was found to be increased in the abnormal spinal cords compared to healthy tissue.[46]

Several publications in excised samples but also in humans in vivo have reported the tendency of the DW signal behavior to depart from a multiexponential decay, which normally characterizes healthy white matter tissue, and to approximate a monoexponential decay in severely damaged areas. Comparison of absolute q-space metrics between studies performed on different scanners, under different circumstances, and using different protocols is strongly not recommended. Given the dependency of the decay on the diffusion time, it is imperative that q-space studies in humans using scanners with limited hardware capabilities and limited scan time must be performed with well-balanced cohorts of patients and healthy controls.

3.2.8 CONCLUSION

In conclusion, in view of the several technical and experimental difficulties, QSI parameters should be interpreted as relative markers rather than absolute measures of microstructural features such as *mean axonal diameter*. However, several studies have shown that *q*-space analysis does add valuable information about the structural organization in nervous tissue and can increase the sensitivity to various pathological conditions.[28,32,47]

Some evidence already exists to support the use of QSI as a complement to DTI studies. Further work will need to prove the sensitivity and specificity of QSI to underlying mechanisms of damage and repair in pathological conditions.[48]

References

1. Callaghan P. *Principles of Nuclear Magnetic Resonance Microscopy.* Clarendon Press; 1991.

2. Cory DG, Garroway AN. Measurement of translational displacement probabilities by NMR: an indicator of compartmentation. *Magn Reson Med.* 1990;14(3):435–444.

3. Callaghan PT, Coy A, MacGowan D, Packer KJ, Zelaya FO. Diffraction-like effects in NMR diffusion studies of fluids in porous solids. *Nature.* 1991;351(6326):467–469. http://dx.doi.org/10.1038/351467a0.

4. Kärger J, Heink W. The propagator representation of molecular transport in microporous crystallites. *J Magn Reson.* 1983;51(1):1–7, 1969.

5. Bihan DL. Molecular diffusion, tissue microdynamics and microstructure. *NMR Biomed.* 1995;8(7):375–386.

6. Assaf Y, Mayk A, Cohen Y. Displacement imaging of spinal cord using *q*-space diffusion-weighted MRI. *Magn Reson Med.* 2000; 44(5):713–722.

7. Kuchel PW, Coy A, Stilbs P. NMR "diffusion-diffraction" of water revealing alignment of erythrocytes in a magnetic field and their dimensions and membrane transport characteristics. *Magn Reson Med.* 1997;37(5):637–643.

8. Kenney JF, Keeping ES. *Mathematics of Statistics.* Van Nostrand; 1957.

9. Jensen JH, Helpern JA. MRI quantification of non-Gaussian water diffusion by kurtosis analysis. *NMR Biomed.* 2010;23(7): 698–710.

10. Assaf Y, Cohen Y. Assignment of the water slow-diffusing component in the central nervous system using *q*-space diffusion MRS: implications for fiber tract imaging. *Magn Reson Med.* 2000;43(2):191–199.

11. Bar-Shir A, Cohen Y. High *b*-value *q*-space diffusion MRS of nerves: structural information and comparison with histological evidence. *NMR Biomed.* 2008;21(2):165–174.

12. King MD, Houseman J, Roussel SA, Van Bruggen N, Williams SR, Gadian DG. *q*-Space imaging of the brain. *Magn Reson Med.* 1994; 32(6):707–713.

13. Nilsson M, Lätt J, Nordh E, Wirestam R, Ståhlberg F, Brockstedt S. On the effects of a varied diffusion time in vivo: is the diffusion in white matter restricted? *Magn Reson Imaging.* 2009;27(2):176–187.

14. Kiselev VG, Il'yasov KA. Is the "biexponential diffusion" biexponential? *Magn Res Med.* 2007;57(3):464–469.

15. Mulkern RV, Haker SJ, Maier SE. On high b diffusion imaging in the human brain: ruminations and experimental insights. *Magn Reson Imaging.* 2009;27(8):1151–1162.

16. Mitra PP, Halperin BI. Effects of finite gradient-pulse widths in pulsed-field-gradient diffusion measurements. *J Magn Reson Ser A.* 1995;113(1):94–101.

17. Lätt J, Nilsson M, Malmborg C, et al. Accuracy of *q*-space related parameters in MRI: simulations and phantom measurements. *IEEE Trans Med Imaging.* 2007;26(11):1437–1447.

18. Linse P, Soderman O. The validity of the short-gradient-pulse approximation in NMR studies of restricted diffusion: simulations of molecules diffusing between planes, in cylinders and spheres. *J Magn Reson Ser A.* 1995;116(1):77–86.

19. Avram L, Assaf Y, Cohen Y. The effect of rotational angle and experimental parameters on the diffraction patterns and micro-structural information obtained from *q*-space diffusion NMR: implication for diffusion in white matter fibers. *J Magn Reson.* 2004;169(1):30–38.

20. Lätt J, Nilsson M, Rydhög A, Wirestam R, Ståhlberg F, Brockstedt S. Effects of restricted diffusion in a biological phantom: a *q*-space diffusion MRI study of asparagus stems at a 3T clinical scanner. *Magn Reson Mater Phys, Biol Med.* 2007;20(4):213–222.

21. Bar-Shir A, Avram L, Ozarslan E, Basser PJ, Cohen Y. The effect of the diffusion time and pulse gradient duration ratio on the diffraction pattern and the structural information estimated from *q*-space diffusion MR: experiments and simulations. *J Magn Reson.* 2008;194(2):230–236.

22. Malmborg C, Sjöbeck M, Brockstedt S, Englund E, Söderman O, Topgaard D. Mapping the intracellular fraction of water by varying the gradient pulse length in *q*-space diffusion MRI. *J Magn Reson.* 2006;180(2):280–285.

23. Mcnab JA, Witzel T, Bhat H, et al. In vivo human brain measurements of axon diameter distributions in the corpus callosum using 300 MT/m maximum gradient strengths. In: *Proceedings Intl Soc Mag Reson Med.* 2012: 680.

24. Ham C, Engels J, Van de Wiel G, Machielsen A. Peripheral nerve stimulation during MRI: effects of high gradient amplitudes and switching rates. *J Magn Reson Imaging.* 1997;7(5):933–937.

25. Cohen-Adad J, McNab JA, Benner T, et al. Improving High-Resolution Q-Ball Imaging with a Head Insert Gradient: Bootstrap and SNR Analysis. In: *Proceedings Intl Soc Mag Reson Med.* 2011.

26. Mayer D, Zahr NM, Adalsteinsson E, Rutt B, Sullivan EV, Pfefferbaum A. In vivo fiber tracking in the rat brain on a clinical 3T MRI system using a high strength insert gradient coil. *NeuroImage.* 2007;35(3):1077–1085.

27. Feldman RE, Scholl TJ, Alford JK, Handler WB, Harris CT, Chronik BA. Results for diffusion-weighted imaging with a fourth-channel gradient insert. *Magn Reson Med.* 2011;66(6): 1798–1808.

28. Assaf Y, Ben-Bashat D, Chapman J, et al. High b-value *q*-space analyzed diffusion-weighted MRI: application to multiple sclerosis. *Magn Reson Med.* 2002;47(1):115–126.

29. King MD, Houseman J, Gadian DG, Connelly A. Localized *q*-space imaging of the mouse brain. *Magn Reson Med.* 1997;38:930–937.

30. Lätt J, Nilsson M, Wirestam R, et al. In vivo visualization of displacement-distribution-derived parameters in *q*-space imaging. *Magn Reson Imaging.* 2008;26:77–87.

31. Lundell H, Nielsen JB, Ptito M, Dyrby TB. Distribution of collateral fibers in the monkey cervical spinal cord detected with diffusion-weighted magnetic resonance imaging. *NeuroImage.* 2011;56:923–929.

32. Farrell JAD, Smith SA, Gordon-Lipkin EM, Reich DS, Calabresi PA, van Zijl PCM. High b-value *q*-space diffusion-weighted MRI of the human cervical spinal cord in vivo: feasibility and application to multiple sclerosis. *Magn Reson Med.* 2008;59(5):1079–1089.

33. Schneider T, Ciccarelli O, Kachramanoglou C, Thomas D, Wheeler-Kingshott C. Reliability of tract-specific *q*-space imaging metrics in healthy spinal cord. In: *Proc Intl Soc Mag Reson Med: 680.* Melbourne; 2011.

34. Gudbjartsson H, Patz S. The Rician distribution of noisy MRI data. *Magn Reson Med*. 1995;34(6):910–914.

35. Golabchi FN, Brooks DH, Hoge WS, De Girolami U, Maier SE. Pixel-based comparison of spinal cord MR diffusion anisotropy with axon packing parameters. *Magn Reson Med*. 2010;63(6):1510–1519.

36. Saritas EU, Cunningham CH, Lee JH, Han ET, Nishimura DG. DWI of the spinal cord with reduced FOV single-shot EPI. *Magn Reson Med*. 2008;60(2):468–473.

37. Wheeler-Kingshott CAM, Hickman SJ, Parker GJM, et al. Investigating cervical spinal cord structure using axial diffusion tensor imaging. *NeuroImage*. 2002;16(1):93–102.

38. Wilm BJ, Svensson J, Henning A, Pruessmann KP, Boesiger P, Kollias SS. Reduced field-of-view MRI using outer volume suppression for spinal cord diffusion imaging. *Magn Reson Med*. 2007; 57(3):625–630.

39. Cohen Y, Assaf Y. High b-value q-space analyzed diffusion-weighted MRS and MRI in neuronal tissues—a technical review. *NMR Biomed*. 2002;15(7–8):516–542.

40. Nossin-Manor R, Duvdevani R, Cohen Y. Effect of experimental parameters on high b-value q-space MR images of excised rat spinal cord. *Magn Reson Med*. 2005;54(1):96–104.

41. Ong HH, Wehrli FW. Quantifying axon diameter and intra-cellular volume fraction in excised mouse spinal cord with q-space imaging. *NeuroImage*. 2010;51(4):1360–1366.

42. Hori M, Motosug U, Fatima Z, Ishigame K, Araki T. Mean displacement map of spine and spinal cord disorders using high b-value q-space imaging-feasibility study. *Acta Radiol*. 2011;52(10): 1155–1158.

43. Hori M, Fukunaga I, Masutani Y, et al. New diffusion metrics for spondylotic myelopathy at an early clinical stage. *Eur Radiol*. 2012; 22(8):1797–1802.

44. Farrell JA, Zhang J, Jones MV, et al. q-Space and conventional diffusion imaging of axon and myelin damage in the rat spinal cord after axotomy. *Magn Reson Med*. 2010;63(5): 1323–1335.

45. Nossin-Manor R, Duvdevani R, Cohen Y. Spatial and temporal damage evolution after hemi-crush injury in rat spinal cord obtained by high b-value q-space diffusion magnetic resonance imaging. *J Neurotrauma*. 2007;24(3):481–491.

46. Biton IE, Duncan ID, Cohen Y. q-Space diffusion of myelin-deficient spinal cords. *Magn Reson Med*. 2007;58(2): 993–1000.

47. Assaf Y, Mayzel-Oreg O, Gigi A, et al. High b value q-space-analyzed diffusion MRI in vascular dementia: a preliminary study. *J Neurol Sci*. 2002;203–204:235–239.

48. Toga AW, Clark KA, Thompson PM, Shattuck DW, Van Horn JD. Mapping the human connectome. *Neurosurgery*. 2012; 71(1):1–5.

Advanced Methods to Study White Matter Microstructure

Yaniv Assaf[1], Daniel C. Alexander[2]

[1]Department of Neurobiology, George S. Wise Faculty of Life Sciences, Tel Aviv University, Tel Aviv, Israel [2]Centre for Medical Image Computing, Department of Computer Science, University College London, London, United Kingdom

3.3.1 INTRODUCTION: DIFFUSION IMAGING AND TISSUE MICROSTRUCTURE

Diffusion imaging and particularly diffusion tensor imaging (DTI)[1] have become standard tools for assessment of white matter in the brain. Although somewhat more technically challenging to implement in the spinal cord, these methods are now also commonplace in studies of the spinal cord.[2–5]

DTI provides two unique pieces of information over any preceding method. First, it provides an estimate of the dominant orientation of local fibers in each image voxel.[1,6,7] That information is the foundation of tractography and structural connectivity mapping in the brain. In the spinal cord fiber orientation information is less useful, since the fiber structure is simpler and generally predicted quite easily, but disruptions to that structure may still be important in injury or disease.

The second key information from DTI is a set of orientationally invariant indices, e.g., fractional anisotropy (FA) and mean diffusivity (MD)[7,8] that provide crude, but useful, markers of microstructural integrity. These quantitative parameters have been used widely in the brain, spinal cord, and peripheral nervous system, as well as a range of other organs and tissue types. For a full description of DTI theory and application to the spinal cord, see Chapter 3.1.

In recent years, some drawbacks in both these unique aspects of DTI have become increasingly evident. The DT model provides only a single fiber orientation in each image voxel and fails in areas of heterogenous white matter such as fiber crossings.[9,10] Crossing fibers are less widespread in the spinal cord, where the white

matter is more regularly ordered, but crossings and other complex fiber configurations do occur. Moreover, the simple DTI microstructure indices lack specificity. White matter contains several cellular components (cells, axons, myelin), each with its own dimensions, density, and other properties that affect water mobility. Simple parameters such as the FA or MD provide only a very crude description of the complex environment that summarizes many different effects.[11–13] The recent trend in diffusion imaging has been to develop more sophisticated models that enable estimation of these different components individually to provide more specific information on the geometry and physiology of white matter tissue.[11,14–19] This chapter summarizes the state of the art for studying white matter through diffusion and speculates on their potential in the spinal cord.

3.3.2 ADVANCED METHODS FOR STUDYING WHITE MATTER

As the *b*-value increases, the DT model rapidly becomes inadequate to explain diffusion measurements from white matter. Significant departures occur even at $b = 1000 \text{ s/mm}^2$ in vivo.[9,10,20,21] These departures indicate a non-monoexponential decay of the signal arising from complex diffusion processes in multiple compartments. The existence of non-Gaussian diffusion in neuronal tissue has motivated over the last decade several innovations in data acquisition and analysis to capture and exploit the extra information in the signal to estimate more useful tissue features. These methods divide into two groups: (1) model based and (2) model free. While all approaches assume some kind of underlying signal model, the classification refers to the use (or not) of a biophysical model with parameters reflecting specific tissue properties. For a detailed treatment of the model-free methods, see Chapter 3.2.

3.3.2.1 Model-Free Techniques

The simplest model-free approach is q-space imaging (QSI),[22,23] often referred to in 3D as diffusion spectrum imaging (DSI).[24] For an extensive treatment of q-space theory and applications, see also Chapter 3.2. This kind of analysis relies on the very basic signal model in which the diffusion-weighted signal is the Fourier transform of the diffusion propagator.[11,22,25,26] By varying the length, strength, and orientation of the gradient pulses in the diffusion imaging acquisition sequence, we can sample the signal at various wavevectors. QSI and DSI work by acquiring a set of measurements typically with wavevectors in a grid configuration and inverting the Fourier transform to obtain a discrete representation of the diffusion propagator.

Several parameters can be extracted from such analysis. If measured along a particular direction, the displacement distribution function can be characterized by its width (mean displacement $<D>$) and height (probability for zero displacement P_0).[11] These parameters were found to be extremely useful for characterization of the human brain and excised spinal cords (see section 3.3.3 following).[11,13,27] If the QSI experiment is done in 3D, as in DSI, the analysis provides the diffusion orientation density function (ODF) by projecting the propagator onto a sphere via a radial integration.[24,28] This ODF has peaks in each of potentially many different fiber directions, so provides a better basis for tractography than DTI.

For tractography alone, DSI is uneconomical in terms of acquisition time, and various other methods try to estimate the diffusion ODF and related functions from more economical high angular resolution diffusion imaging (HARDI) acquisition; see[28] for a review. Q-ball imaging[29–33] uses the Funk–Radon transform as an approximate mapping from HARDI data to the diffusion ODF. PAS-MRI[34] estimates a diffusion ODF with greater sensitivity to fiber orientations. Spherical deconvolution techniques[30,35–38] combine the model-based techniques described in the next section with a model-free description of the ODF to obtain a fiber ODF. See Ref. 28 for an explanation and comparison of these various ideas.

Hybrid diffusion imaging (HYDI)[39] provides a framework to estimate all of the common DSI parameters, including $<D>$, P_0, and the diffusion ODF, from multishell HARDI data, which is more economical than full DSI. Diffusion kurtosis imaging[40] (see also Chapters 3.1 and 3.2) uses multishell HARDI and estimates an additional parameter, the diffusion kurtosis tensor, which characterizes the departure from the Gaussian model used in DTI.

All these parameters are useful markers of tissue integrity that often provide complementary information to the basic DTI indices. However, they remain nonspecific and difficult to associate with specific features of the tissue microstructure.

3.3.2.2 Model-Based Techniques

The model-based approaches include several frameworks with increasing complexity of the model. The most basic model includes a multiexponential decay function,[20,21] anomalous diffusion,[41] or a stretched exponential function.[42,43] Such models can adequately characterize the deviation from Gaussian diffusion, such as the non-Gaussian diffusion that stems from restricted diffusion, in a similar way to model-free techniques like diffusion kurtosis. A biophysical interpretation can be attached to some parameters; for example, associating a separate tissue compartment to each exponential component provides an estimate of the orientation and volume fraction of each compartment.

More directly, biophysical models employ a geometric description of the tissue compartments and exploit restricted diffusion as a window on the geometry. These models are built from assumptions on the diffusion properties of water in different compartments of the tissue. For example, Stanisz et al.[17] proposed a model with three compartments: axonal, glial, and extracellular space. The axons are elongated ellipsoids, and the glia are spherical. Each has a semipermeable membrane and unique volume fractions and internal diffusivity. The composite hindered and restricted model of diffusion (CHARMED)[15,44] assumes that the diffusion within axons is restricted perpendicular to the axons, while elsewhere (cells, extra cellular matrix, and parallel to the axons) it is hindered or free. The minimal model of white matter diffusion (MMWMD)[14,45] combines elements of both CHARMED and Stanisz's model in an attempt to identify the simplest model that explains diffusion data from white matter. Zhang et al.,[19] following the earlier work of Jespersen et al. and Kaden et al.,[46–48] extend the MMWMD to include fiber orientation dispersion, which is another significant influence on the signal. Panagiotaki et al.[49] define a taxonomy of models for diffusion in white matter, which relates all those mentioned herein within a broader framework of compartment models and performs a statistical comparison of their ability to explain measured signals.

From such models parameters such as the axonal density, diameter distribution, and intra/extra cellular diffusivity can be estimated and mapped.[50,51] The models also extend to include other parameters such as cell permeability and shape. However, the modeling process rapidly becomes complex and the number of parameters increases rapidly rendering estimation ill posed if signal-to-noise ratio is not sufficient (as is likely in high b-value diffusion imaging). Despite that, successful demonstrations and systems are now in the literature. For example, the restricted diffusion volume fraction (axonal density) maps from CHARMED analysis were found to be extremely useful and sensitive in the brain and provide an alternative to FA that relates more specifically to axon density.[15] The Neurite Orientation Dispersion and Density Imaging (NODDI) technique[52] extends the set of specific parameters to include indices of fiber orientation dispersion and CSF volume fraction, thus separating the three key parameters that influence FA in brain imaging.

AxCaliber,[50,53,54] an application of CHARMED, models, aside from axonal density, can also estimate the axon diameter distribution. The model assumes that this distribution has a gamma function shape. Based on a multi diffusion time experiment where in each diffusion time a different population of axons will experience restricted diffusion, the estimation of the gamma function becomes feasible. This method was demonstrated on the rat corpus callosum and on excised spinal cord (see following).

The ActiveAx technique[14] uses the MMWMD together with an optimized multishell HARDI acquisition protocol to map an axon diameter index over the brain. The simple model and optimized experiment design enable the technique to be orientationally invariant. Thus, unlike earlier techniques,[17,50] which require the fiber to have known and fixed orientation, ActiveAx provides indices for fibers in all orientations from a single acquisition. However, the index provided is less quantitative than the AxCaliber axon diameter distribution because it provides only a single summary statistic of the full distribution. In theory, the axon diameter index reflects the average axon diameter weighted by axon volume,[14] although there are some departures from this complicated interpretation.[45] Nevertheless, in fixed monkey brains using data from a 4.7 T high field scanner with 140 mT/m[14] and 300 mT/m,[45] the technique provides maps that reflect what we expect from histology. In vivo human results[14] are noisier, but an ROI analysis also reflects the expected trends. As an alternative to ActiveAx, Barazany et al.[54] suggested an extension of AxCaliber into 3D to allow estimation of the full axon diameter distribution function for any orientated fiber system.

While current axon diameter estimation techniques[14,17,50] show good results in experimental animal

systems with high gradients available, on human systems they largely remain scientific demonstrations rather than tools for large-scale studies; the human data sets in Alexander et al.[14] took over 1 h to acquire. Further work is required to realize the potential of these techniques for human studies. Modeling advances, such as those described in Panagiotaki et al.[49] and Zhang et al.[19] make incremental but significant improvements. Greater advances are likely to come from improvements in data acquisition to increase sensitivity to the specific parameters of interest. For example, oscillating gradients[55,56] and generalized waveforms[57,58] can provide orders of magnitude more sensitivity to small axon diameters. Exploitation of such pulse sequences potentially offers much greater sensitivity and practical axon diameter mapping techniques for human studies in the near future.

In the spinal cord, the orientational invariance of ActiveAx is less of an advantage than in the brain because of the simpler orientational structure of the cord. However, the model and experiment design optimization that underpin the technique also provide advantages when the orientation is known; Schneider et al.[59] demonstrate this in the corpus callosum, and that extension is directly applicable to the spinal cord.[60] Measures of orientation dispersion from NODDI are likely to find use in the spinal cord as well as the brain both for studying the intersections of peripheral nerves with the cord, where orientation dispersion can be significant, and for pinpointing different kinds of pathology more precisely. The benefits of alternative pulse sequences are equally applicable in the spinal cord and will help provide more precise information in more manageable acquisition times as these techniques develop.

3.3.3 APPLICATIONS IN SPINAL CORD

- QSI in the spinal cord (see also Chapter 3.2)

    QSI is a model-free approach that can characterize diffusion MRI signal measured at a wide range of b value.[11,13] Being a model-free framework, the extracted parameters also have a vague meaning. From the displacement distribution function two parameters are extracted: the mean displacement ($<D>$) and the probability for zero displacement (P_0). Although these two parameters are not particularly specific to any diffusing component in the tissue, it is assumed that if the experiments are done at sufficient high b values ($>10,000$ s/mm^2) and exactly perpendicular to the fibers, these two parameters ($<D>$ and P_0) represent mostly restricted diffusion. Some support for this assumption comes from experiments on excised optic nerve where it was shown the $<D>$ does not change when increasing the diffusion time indicating restricted diffusion (probably within the axons).[20,25]

This method was applied first on two studies in the spinal cord: (1) a development study[11]; (2) a degeneration study.[61]

In the development experiment, excised spinal cords of rats at different ages (from postnatal day 3 to adulthood) were scanned with QSI protocol. It was shown that the $<D>$ reduces with age while the P_0 increases, indicating increase in restricted diffusion with age (probably due to myelination) (Figure 3.3.1).[11] While this observation accompanies FA changes with age (increase with myelination) it seems that changes in $<D>$ are much more dramatic and span over a much broader range of values increasing the sensitivity of this parameter.

In the degeneration study, an animal model of white matter degeneration (following exposure to hypertension and diabetes) was used. In that model severe pathology in the white matter was observed (following histology), including demyelination, redundant myelin, and cytoplasm filled balloons between split myelin layers.[61] This was manifested by reduction both in $<D>$ and P_0 (Figure 3.3.2). As in the development study, although there was also reduction in the anisotropy index, the QSI parameters were much more sensitive and the magnitude of effect was much larger.

Additional experiments on neurodegeneration included exploring the spinal cord of the porcine exposed to a model of multiple sclerosis (MS) (experimental autoimmune encephemyelitis).[62] In this

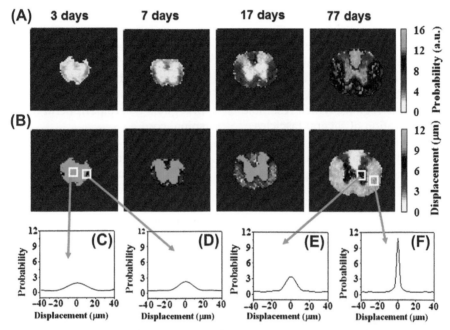

FIGURE 3.3.1 QSI applied to a development study in the ex vivo rat spinal cord. (A): Mean displacement $<D>$. (B): Probability of zero displacement P_0. The $<D>$ reduces with age while the P_0 increases, indicating increase in restricted diffusion with age (probably due to myelination).

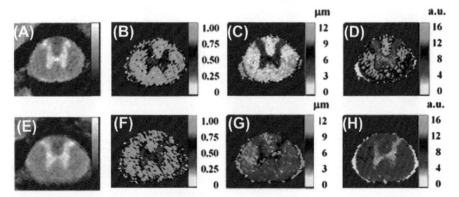

FIGURE 3.3.2 QSI applied to a study of white matter degeneration in the rat spinal cord. Top row: control rat. Bottom row: stroke prone spontaneous hypertensive rat. (A, E): T1-weighted MR image; (B, F): low b value diffusion anisotropy index (σ) image; (C, G): high b value q-space displacement image $<D>$; and (d, h) high b value q-space probability image P_0.

study high correspondence was observed between histological measures of demyelination and gliosis and QSI parameters. As in the previous studies, the high sensitivity of QSI over DTI was also demonstrated.

- AxCaliber in the spinal cord

  AxCaliber allows the estimation of the axon diameter distribution on each voxel.[50,53] This method was implemented on an excised porcine spinal cord with the purpose of segmenting the spinal cord based on its axon diameter properties.[50] Within the white matter of the spinal cord run several fascicles transmitting information to and from the brain. This information can be related to motor or sensory functions and within the sensory subdivision is made sensitive to pain, temperature, and other types of sensation. Each pathway (e.g., pain) passes through specific regions within the spinal cord and is characterized by a unique axon distribution. For example, the fibers that transmit pain are characterized by very small axons. AxCaliber analysis, combined with cluster analysis of the gamma function parameters, was able to segment the spinal cord into several regions, which resemble the known anatomical location of several fascicles (Figure 3.3.3). This experiment indicated that (1) AxCaliber is feasible in the spinal cord, and (2) it can be used to characterize the physiological properties of different regions within the spinal cord (since the axon diameter is linearly correlated with conduction velocity).

- ActiveAx in the spinal cord

  Schneider et al.[60] demonstrate ActiveAx in a fixed monkey spinal cord, which shows good consistency of axon density and diameter indices in laterally corresponding regions and along the length of specific pathways; see Figure 3.3.4. It also shows contrast in axon density and diameter among different pathways. The full ActiveAx protocol originally designed for the brain where fibers exist with all possible orientations is somewhat excessive in the spinal cord, where the dominant fiber orientation is inferior-superior. Schneider's work[59,60] uses the experiment design optimization that underpins ActiveAx to construct a different protocol designed for fibers with known orientation. Simulation experiments show that when the fiber orientation is known, we can achieve similar parameter estimation accuracy with around half the measurements by exploiting that knowledge rather than assuming arbitrary fiber orientation. Further work is required to evaluate and exploit this promising work, although care must be taken even in the spinal cord that fiber orientation adheres to the assumption, as complex fiber architectures can appear in regions where peripheral nerves branch out of the spinal cord.[63]

- NODDI in the spinal cord is showing promise in preliminary work. For example, Grussu et al.[64] show that changes in white matter in MS appear primarily in the neurite density maps rather than orientation dispersion index, which DTI analysis cannot distinguish.

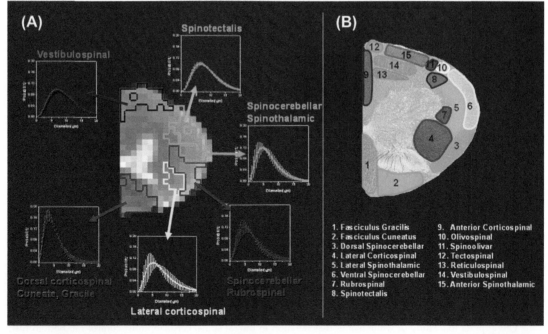

FIGURE 3.3.3 AxCaliber results in an excised porcine spinal cord. (A): Axon diameter distribution as measured with MRI. (B): Parcellation of white matter tracts from an atlas.

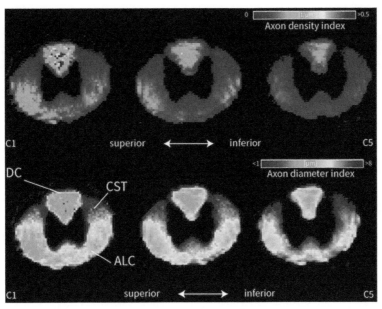

FIGURE 3.3.4 Axial slice of upper cervical cord showing axon density in μm^{-2} (top) and axon diameter in μm (bottom) in the corticospinal tracts (CST), anterolateral column (ALC) and dorsal column (DC).

BOX 3.3.1

COMPARISON BETWEEN METHODS

DTI	Basser Biop. J.[1]	Simple, stable, useful phenomenological indices.	No direct biophysical interpretation of parameters.
CHARMED	Assaf MRM[15]	Separates axon density and orientation distribution.	No axon diameter estimate.
AxCaliber	Assaf MRM[12]	Measurements of axon diameter distribution.	Not currently viable on live human subjects. Fiber orientation known and specified beforehand.
ActiveAx	Alexander *NeuroImage*[14]	Orientationally invariant axon diameter and density indices.	Single summary parameter for axon diameter. Demonstration of weak sensitivity on live human subjects.
NODDI	Zhang *NeuroImage*[52]	Separates three white matter parameters confounded in FA: Neurite density, orientation dispersion, and CSF partial volume. Clinically viable with 10–20 min acquisition protocol.	No axon diameter estimate.

3.3.4 SUMMARY

Diffusion MRI, and particularly DTI, has already become a powerful tool to study spinal cord pathophysiology. However, in this chapter we reviewed alternative approaches to study the diffusion properties of the tissue giving a glance into its microstructure (see summary in Box 3.3.1). Those methods, although more complicated (both experimentally and in analysis) seem to provide invaluable information on the tissue that might boost the information extracted on the spinal cord. Future research should explore the added value of these methods and their applicability in clinical conditions.

References

1. Basser PJ, Mattiello J, LeBihan D. MR diffusion tensor spectroscopy and imaging. *Biophys J.* 1994;66:259–267.
2. Bosma R, Stroman PW. Diffusion tensor imaging in the human spinal cord: development, limitations, and clinical applications. *Crit Rev Biomed Eng.* 2012;40:1–20.
3. Clark CA, Werring DJ. Diffusion tensor imaging in spinal cord: methods and applications—a review. *NMR Biomed.* 2002;15: 578–586.
4. Fujiyoshi K, Konomi T, Yamada M, et al. Diffusion tensor imaging and tractography of the spinal cord: From experimental studies to clinical application. *Exp Neurol.* 2012.
5. Thurnher MM, Law M. Diffusion-weighted imaging, diffusion-tensor imaging, and fiber tractography of the spinal cord. *Magn Reson Imaging Clin N Am.* 2009;17:225–244.
6. Basser PJ, Pajevic S, Pierpaoli C, Duda J, Aldroubi A. In vivo fiber tractography using DT-MRI data. *Magn Reson Med.* 2000;44: 625–632.
7. Pierpaoli C, Jezzard P, Basser PJ, Barnett A, Di Chiro G. Diffusion tensor MR imaging of the human brain. *Radiology.* 1996;201: 637–648.
8. Pierpaoli C, Basser PJ. Toward a quantitative assessment of diffusion anisotropy. *Magn Reson Med.* 1996;36:893–906.
9. Alexander AL, Hasan KM, Lazar M, Tsuruda JS, Parker DL. Analysis of partial volume effects in diffusion-tensor MRI. *Magn Reson Med.* 2001;45:770–780.
10. Alexander DC, Barker GJ, Arridge SR. Detection and modeling of non-Gaussian apparent diffusion coefficient profiles in human brain data. *Magn Reson Med.* 2002;48:331–340.
11. Assaf Y, Mayk A, Cohen Y. Displacement imaging of spinal cord using q-space diffusion-weighted MRI. *Magn Reson Med.* 2000;44: 713–722.
12. Assaf Y, Pasternak O. Diffusion tensor imaging (DTI)-based white matter mapping in brain research: a review. *J Mol Neurosci.* 2008; 34:51–61.
13. Cohen Y, Assaf Y. High b-value q-space analyzed diffusion-weighted MRS and MRI in neuronal tissues – a technical review. *NMR Biomed.* 2002;15:516–542.
14. Alexander DC, Hubbard PL, Hall MG, et al. Orientationally invariant indices of axon diameter and density from diffusion MRI. *NeuroImage.* 2010;52:1374–1389.
15. Assaf Y, Basser PJ. Composite hindered and restricted model of diffusion (CHARMED) MR imaging of the human brain. *NeuroImage.* 2005;27:48–58.
16. Assaf Y, Blumenfeld T, Levin G, Yovel Y, Basser PJ. AxCaliber—A method to measure the axon diameter distribution and density in neuronal tissues. *Proc Intl Soc Magn Reson Med.* 2006;14:637.
17. Stanisz GJ, Szafer A, Wright GA, Henkelman RM. An analytical model of restricted diffusion in bovine optic nerve. *Magn Reson Med.* 1997;37:103–111.
18. Zhang H, Barazany D, Assaf Y, Lundell HM, Alexander DC, Dyrby T. A comparative study of axon diameter imaging techniques using diffusion MRI. *Proc Intl Soc Magn Reson Med.* 2011.
19. Zhang H, Hubbard PL, Parker GJ, Alexander DC. Axon diameter mapping in the presence of orientation dispersion with diffusion MRI. *NeuroImage.* 2011;56:1301–1315.
20. Assaf Y, Cohen Y. Non-mono-exponential attenuation of water and N-acetyl aspartate signals due to diffusion in brain tissue. *J Magn Reson.* 1998;131:69–85.
21. Niendorf T, Dijkhuizen RM, Norris DG, van Lookeren Campagne M, Nicolay K. Biexponential diffusion attenuation in various states of brain tissue: implications for diffusion-weighted imaging. *Magn Reson Med.* 1996;36:847–857.
22. Callaghan PT, Coy A, Macgowan D, Packer KJ, Zelaya FO. Diffraction-like effects in NMR diffusion studies of fluids in porous solids. *Nature.* 1991;351:467–469.
23. Cory DG, Garroway AN. Measurement of translational displacement probabilities by NMR—an indicator of compartmentation. *Magn Reson Med.* 1990;14:435–444.
24. Wedeen VJ, Hagmann P, Tseng WY, Reese TG, Weisskoff RM. Mapping complex tissue architecture with diffusion spectrum magnetic resonance imaging. *Magn Reson Med.* 2005;54:1377–1386.
25. Assaf Y, Cohen Y. Assignment of the water slow-diffusing component in the central nervous system using q-space diffusion MRS: implications for fiber tract imaging. *Magn Reson Med.* 2000;43:191–199.
26. King MD, Houseman J, Roussel SA, van Bruggen N, Williams SR, Gadian DG. q-Space imaging of the brain. *Magn Reson Med.* 1994; 32:707–713.
27. Assaf Y, Ben-Bashat D, Chapman J, et al. High b-value q-space analyzed diffusion-weighted MRI: application to multiple sclerosis. *Magn Reson Med.* 2002;47:115–126.
28. Seunarine KK, Alexander DC. Multiple fibers: beyond the diffusion tensor. In: Johansen-Berg H, Behrens TE, eds. *Diffusion MRI: From Quantitative Measurement to In Vivo Neuroanatomy.* Academic Press; 2009:56–74.
29. Aganj I, Lenglet C, Sapiro G, Yacoub E, Ugurbil K, Harel N. Reconstruction of the orientation distribution function in single- and multiple-shell q-ball imaging within constant solid angle. *Magn Reson Med.* 2010;64:554–566.
30. Anderson AW. Measurement of fiber orientation distributions using high angular resolution diffusion imaging. *Magn Reson Med.* 2005;54:1194–1206.
31. Descoteaux M, Angelino E, Fitzgibbons S, Deriche R. Regularized, fast, and robust analytical Q-ball imaging. *Magn Reson Med.* 2007; 58:497–510.
32. Hess CP, Mukherjee P, Han ET, Xu D, Vigneron DB. Q-ball reconstruction of multimodal fiber orientations using the spherical harmonic basis. *Magn Reson Med.* 2006;56:104–117.
33. Tuch DS. Q-ball imaging. *Magn Reson Med.* 2004;52:1358–1372.
34. Jansons KM, Alexander DC. Persistent angular structure: new insights from diffusion MRI data. Dummy version. *Inf Process Med Imaging.* 2003;18:672–683.
35. Alexander DC. Maximum entropy spherical deconvolution for diffusion MRI. *Inf Process Med Imaging.* 2005;19:76–87.
36. Dell'Acqua F, Rizzo G, Scifo P, Clarke RA, Scotti G, Fazio F. A model-based deconvolution approach to solve fiber crossing in diffusion-weighted MR imaging. *IEEE Trans Biomed Eng.* 2007;54: 462–472.
37. Sakaie KE, Lowe MJ. An objective method for regularization of fiber orientation distributions derived from diffusion-weighted MRI. *NeuroImage.* 2007;34:169–176.
38. Tournier JD, Calamante F, Gadian DG, Connelly A. Direct estimation of the fiber orientation density function from diffusion-weighted MRI data using spherical deconvolution. *NeuroImage.* 2004;23:1176–1185.
39. Wu YC, Alexander AL. Hybrid diffusion imaging. *NeuroImage.* 2007;36:617–629.
40. Jensen JH, Helpern JA, Ramani A, Lu H, Kaczynski K. Diffusional kurtosis imaging: the quantification of non-Gaussian water diffusion by means of magnetic resonance imaging. *Magn Reson Med.* 2005;53:1432–1440.
41. Hall MG, Alexander DC. *MICCAI Workshop on Computational Diffusion MRI.* 2008. New York: 9–18.
42. De Santis S, Gabrielli A, Bozzali M, Maraviglia B, Macaluso E, Capuani S. Anisotropic anomalous diffusion assessed in the human brain by scalar invariant indices. *Magn Reson Med.* 2011;65:1043–1052.

43. Hall MG, Barrick TR. From diffusion-weighted MRI to anomalous diffusion imaging. *Magn Reson Med.* 2008;59:447–455.

44. Assaf Y, Freidlin RZ, Rohde GK, Basser PJ. New modeling and experimental framework to characterize hindered and restricted water diffusion in brain white matter. *Magn Reson Med.* 2004;52: 965–978.

45. Dyrby TB, Sogaard LV, Hall MG, Ptito M, Alexander DC. Contrast and stability of the axon diameter index from microstructure imaging with diffusion MRI. *Magn Reson Med.* 2012.

46. Jespersen SN, Bjarkam CR, Nyengaard JR, et al. Neurite density from magnetic resonance diffusion measurements at ultrahigh field: comparison with light microscopy and electron microscopy. *NeuroImage.* 2010;49:205–216.

47. Jespersen SN, Kroenke CD, Ostergaard L, Ackerman JJ, Yablonskiy DA. Modeling dendrite density from magnetic resonance diffusion measurements. *NeuroImage.* 2007;34:1473–1486.

48. Kaden E, Knosche TR, Anwander A. Parametric spherical deconvolution: inferring anatomical connectivity using diffusion MR imaging. *NeuroImage.* 2007;37:474–488.

49. Panagiotaki E, Schneider T, Siow B, Hall MG, Lythgoe MF, Alexander DC. Compartment models of the diffusion MR signal in brain white matter: a taxonomy and comparison. *NeuroImage.* 2012;59:2241–2254.

50. Assaf Y, Blumenfeld-Katzir T, Yovel Y, Basser PJ. AxCaliber: a method for measuring axon diameter distribution from diffusion MRI. *Magn Reson Med.* 2008;59:1347–1354.

51. Barazany D, Basser PJ, Assaf Y. In-vivo measurement of the axon diameter distribution in the rat's corpus callosum. *Proc Intl Soc Magn Reson Med.* 2008;16.

52. Zhang H, Schneider T, Wheeler-Kingshott CA, Alexander DC. NODDI: practical in vivo neurite orientation dispersion and density imaging of the human brain. *NeuroImage.* 2012;64: 1000–1016.

53. Barazany D, Basser PJ, Assaf Y. In vivo measurement of axon diameter distribution in the corpus callosum of rat brain. *Brain.* 2009;132:1210–1220.

54. Barazany D, Jones D, Assaf Y. AxCaliber 3D. *Proc Intl Soc Magn Reson Med.* 2011;19:76.

55. Callaghan PT. *Principles of Nuclear Magnetic Resonance Microscopy.* Oxford: Clarendon Press; 1991. New York: Oxford University Press.

56. Does MD, Parsons EC, Gore JC. Oscillating gradient measurements of water diffusion in normal and globally ischemic rat brain. *Magn Reson Med.* 2003;49:206–215.

57. Drobnjak I, Siow B, Alexander DC. Optimizing gradient waveforms for microstructure sensitivity in diffusion-weighted MR. *J Magn Reson.* 2010;206:41–51.

58. Siow B, Drobnjak I, Lythgoe MF, Alexander DC. Optimised gradient waveform spin-echo sequence for diffusion weighted MR in a microstructure phantom. *Proc Intl Soc Magn Reson Med.* 2011.

59. Schneider T, Wheeler-Kingshott CA, Alexander DC. In-vivo estimates of axonal characteristics using optimized diffusion MRI protocols for single fibre orientation. *MICCAI.* 2010:183–190.

60. Schneider T, Lundell H, Dyrby TB, Alexander DC, Wheeler-Kingshott CA. Optimized diffusion MRI protocols for estimating axon diameter with known fibre orientation. *Proc Intl Soc Magn Reson Med.* 2010;1561.

61. Assaf Y, Mayk A, Eliash S, Speiser Z, Cohen Y. Hypertension and neuronal degeneration in excised rat spinal cord studied by high-b value q-space diffusion magnetic resonance imaging. *Exp Neurol.* 2003;184:726–736.

62. Biton IE, Duncan ID, Cohen Y. High b-value q-space diffusion MRI in myelin-deficient rat spinal cords. *Magn Reson Imaging.* 2006;24:161–166.

63. Lundell H, Nielsen JB, Ptito M, Dyrby TB. Distribution of collateral fibers in the monkey cervical spinal cord detected with diffusion-weighted magnetic resonance imaging. *NeuroImage.* 2011;56:923–929.

64. Grussu F, Schneider T, Hugh KHZ, et al. Towards spinal cord microstructure mapping with the neurite orientation dispersion and density imaging. *Proc Intl Soc Magn Reson Med.* 2013; 21:2095.

3.4

Magnetization Transfer

Mina Kim[1], Mara Cercignani[2]

[1]Department of Diagnostic Radiology, University of Hong Kong, Hong Kong, China
[2]Clinical Imaging Science Centre, Brighton and Sussex Medical School, University of Sussex, Falmer, East Sussex, UK

Magnetization transfer (MT), first demonstrated in vivo by Wolff and Balaban,[1] is a contrast mechanism based on the exchange of magnetization occurring between groups of spins characterized by different molecular environments. MT produces a source of contrast alternative to T_1 and T_2, which has become widely used in clinical imaging to improve the suppression of static tissue in MR angiography and to increase lesion visibility on conventional MRI when gadolinium-based contrast agents are used. As the MT effect reflects the relative density of macromolecules such as proteins and lipids, it has been associated with myelin content in white matter (WM) of the brain and of the spinal cord. In the attempt to measure myelination, several approaches to quantify the MT effect have thus been proposed. This chapter will review some of the basic theory of MT, the modeling, and the application to spinal cord imaging. It will also present some of the most recent developments, including chemical exchange saturation transfer (CEST).

3.4.1 THE MT PHENOMENON AND ITS RELATIONSHIP TO MYELIN

The simplest model of MT identifies two compartments (or "pools") of protons: those in free water ("liquid" or "free" pool) and those bound to macromolecules ("macromolecular" or "semisolid" pool). The former pool is the main contributor to the MRI signal, while the latter one is assumed to be MRI invisible due to its extremely short T_2 ($\sim 10^{-5}$ s). Nevertheless, macromolecular protons are characterized by a broader absorption line shape than the liquid ones, which makes them sensitive to off-resonance irradiation (Figure 3.4.1).

Selective saturation of the macromolecular pool can thus be achieved by applying radio-frequency (RF) energy several kilohertz off resonance from the Larmor frequency. At the field strength typical of clinical scanners (1–3 T), the natural line width of free water is of the order of few tens of Hz; therefore, the direct saturation of the liquid pool by off-resonance irradiation is minimal.

Nevertheless, as an exchange of magnetization occurs between the two pools via cross-relaxation and chemical exchange, this selective saturation is transferred to the liquid pool, and hence results in an attenuation of the MRI signal.

As a consequence, MT is able to probe indirectly macromolecules such as proteins and lipids. Myelin is a lipid–protein structure (its dry mass is approximately 70–80% lipids and 20–30% proteins) wrapped around axons in both the central (CNS) and the peripheral nervous system (PNS). In the CNS (including the spinal cord), myelin is primarily found in the WM, although it is present in smaller quantities also in the gray matter (GM). The main purpose of myelin is to act as an insulator, thus increasing the speed of action potential transmission. The ability to measure myelin in vivo would have very important consequences, as myelin is the primary target of demyelinating diseases (such as multiple sclerosis, MS), but it is also believed to be involved in degenerative processes secondary to neuronal or axonal damage. Additionally, processes of myelination during neurodevelopment are believed to be responsible for a number of psychiatric disorders.[2] MT imaging, together with diffusion-weighted imaging (Chapter 3.1), q-space imaging (Chapters 3.2 and 3.3), and short T_2 mapping (Chapter 3.5) are among the most promising MR techniques for the assessment of myelin.

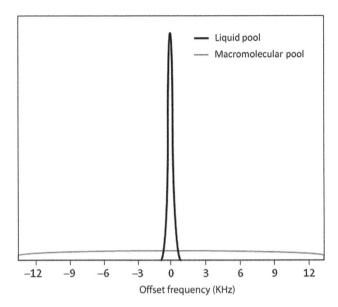

FIGURE 3.4.1 Schematic representation of the absorption line shapes of the liquid (black) and macromolecular pool (gray). The narrow line width of the liquid protons makes them relatively insensitive to off-resonance irradiation at frequencies larger than 1 kHz.

MAGNETIZATION TRANSFER MEASURES

- *MT-weighted*—Magnetization transfer affects the contrast of the image, but it is not quantitative
- *MTR (MT ratio)*—Semiquantitative measure reflecting the amount of bound protons and calculated from two images
- *MTCSF*—MT-weighted scan normalized to the CSF signal. Only one image needed, but results dependent on T_1/T_2
- *qMT*—quantitative MT technique that models the signal change with two pools (bound and free). Parameters determined from it include the exchange rate (RM_0^B), the macromolecular pool ratio (F), and the T_2 of the bound pool (T_2^B). Long scan times are associated with this measure because it needs several data points to fit the model to the data
- *CEST*—Selective irradiation of labile proton pools resonating at frequencies other than water

3.4.2 MT CONTRAST AND MTR

MT saturation results in a suppression of the MRI signal that is proportional to the amount of macromolecules in a given tissue. For this reason MT contrast has been used from the start to suppress unwanted signal.

For example, in MR angiography, the signal contrast between the blood and other tissue can always be enhanced by using MT (which does not affect blood) to further suppress the background tissue signal.[3] With a similar purpose MT imaging can be applied to spinal cord imaging to improve contrast and sharpness between spinal cord and cerebrospinal fluid (CSF) and to increase the conspicuity of focal lesions.[4]

In this chapter, however, we focus on the quantitative applications of the technique.

The simplest approach to quantify the degree of signal loss in an MT-saturated experiment is to express it as the MT ratio (MTR). The MTR is computed as the percentage difference of two images, one acquired with off-resonance saturation (M_S) and one without (M_0):

$$MTR = \frac{M_0 - M_S}{M_0} \times 100. \quad (3.4.1)$$

This simple operation can be computed on a voxel-by-voxel basis to obtain an MTR map, typically expressed as percentage units (pu), although in some cases is expressed as a fraction. As discussed in the previous section, some evidence suggests that molecules associated with myelin dominate the MT exchange process in WM and that MTR increases with myelin content. MTR was shown to be sensitive to subtle damage in the normal-appearing WM of patients with demyelinating diseases, such as multiple sclerosis.[5]

The MTR became very popular as an approach to characterize WM disease and was soon extended to imaging of the cord.[6] An example of MTR *map* of the cervical cord is shown in Figure 3.4.2.

The most widely adopted approach to MT-weighted acquisition is the so-called pulsed MT, in which a spoiled gradient echo (2D or 3D) or a spin echo acquisition is modified to accommodate high power, off-resonance, saturation pulses, which are played out just before each excitation. Similar acquisitions are available on most commercial scanners, and MT weighting is often offered as an option with several sequences. More details on MT imaging acquisition are given in Section 3.4.4; examples of acquisition protocols suitable for the spinal cord are also shown in Table 3.4.1.

One of the limitations of the MTR, however, is that it is the result of the combination of several more fundamental quantities, and it is highly dependent on the acquisition parameters.[12] The characteristics of the MT-saturating pulse, including the shape, the amplitude, the duration, and the offset frequency, for example, have a major effect on the measured MTR.[13] Similarly, imaging parameters such as the repetition time (TR) and the excitation flip angle can affect the result.[14]

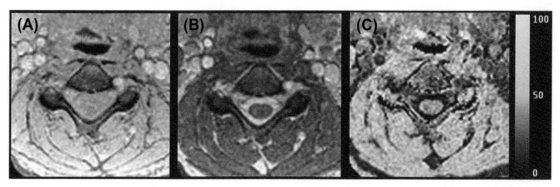

FIGURE 3.4.2   Magnetization transfer ratio (MTR) of the cervical cord in a healthy subject. Two scans, without (A) and with (B) saturation are combined to compute the percentage difference, or MTR (C).

3.4.3 MEASURING MT IN THE SPINAL CORD

The human spinal cord contains segregated sensory and motor pathways that have been difficult to quantify using conventional MRI techniques. Spinal cord lesions are typically more symptomatic than brain lesions and correlate better with the degree of physical disability. MT-MRI provides quantitative values about the degree of damage, while conventional MRI gives a simple volumetric measure of disease burden. Using MT-MRI, a study showed that it is possible to assess demyelination of specific spinal pathways and that signal abnormalities in the dorsal and lateral columns of the spinal cord are correlated with vibration sensation (dorsal) and strength (lateral).[15] Another study also demonstrated that measures of MTR in the dorsal and ventrolateral spinal cord predicted the sensory and the motor disability, respectively.[8]

3.4.3.1 Clinical Relevance of MT-MRI in the Spinal Cord

The structural changes occurring within and outside T_2-visible lesions have been quantified using MT-MRI.[16] As one major advantage of MT is its specificity to demyelination and degeneration, as assessed by histopathology,[17,18] it is especially helpful in identifying microscopic disease activity in normal-appearing brain tissue on conventional MRI scans.[19] MT-MRI of the spinal cord has shown great potential for clinical assessment of patients suffering from demyelinating diseases, such as MS, adrenomyeloneuropathy (AMN), and neuromyelitis optica (NMO).

3.4.3.1.1 Multiple Sclerosis

MS is an inflammatory demyelinating disease of the CNS[20,21] as extensively described in Chapter 1 of this book. MS selectively affects the myelin sheath of the

TABLE 3.4.1   MT Sequence Selection

Sequence	TR (ms)	TE (ms)	MT Prepulse (Offset Frequency)	Scan Time (Matrix)	B_0	References
Three-dimensional spoiled gradient echo	110	13	5-lobed sinc (1.5 kHz)	8 min (368 × 326)	3.0 T	Smith et al.[7]
Three-dimensional gradient echo	28	3.2	Gaussian (1.2 kHz)	5 min (256 × 256)	3.0 T	Cohen-Adad et al.[8]
Three-dimensional gradient echo	50	12	5-lobed sinc (1–63 kHz)	32 min (256 × 228)	1.5 T	Smith et al.[9] Fatemi et al.[10]
Two-dimensional gradient echo	600	25	Gaussian (1.5 kHz)	(128 × 128)	1.5 T	Agosta et al.[118]
Fast spin echo	1600	17	3-lobed sinc (1 kHz)	17.7 min (256 × 192)	1.5 T	Silver et al.[6,11]
Two-dimensional gradient echo	616	22	Gaussian (1.5 kHz)	5.3 min (128 × 256)	1.0 T	Lycklama a Nijeholt et al.[119]
Gradient echo	750	23	Sinc (0.7 kHz)	4.8 min (256 × 180)	0.3 T	Yoshioka et al.[120]

CNS and oligodendrocytes, which causes multifocal demyelinated plaques in the brain, the spinal cord, and the optic tract. MS is characterized by both focal and spatially diffuse lesions of the brain and spinal cord with heterogeneous pathologies. Especially, the spinal cord is a common site of involvement in MS as cord pathology is a major cause of the disability suffered by MS patients.[22] MTR is most commonly used to quantify tissue changes in MS[23] and has been measured in the spinal cord of MS patients.[24–28] Previous studies showed that significant changes in MTR can be detected between controls and MS patients in the spinal cord WM.[11,17,24–26] In MS patient groups, cord MTR decreased in both normal-appearing tissue and lesions, and furthermore correlated with the degree of demyelination and axonal density in the spinal cord,[17,29] similarly found in the brain. A correlation between MTR values and disability has also been observed in the spinal cord of MS patients.[15,27,28] MT-MRI studies in the upper cervical cord showed that diffuse abnormalities measured by MTR are an important contributor to disability,[27,30] implying that the assessment of regional cord damage can contribute to the understanding of the factors associated with the development of disability. Such results show that MTR has greater pathological specificity for changes in myelin content than conventional MRI does. Furthermore, several groups reported that the MTR values in the cord are independent or only partially correlated with focal abnormalities in the brain, suggesting that changes seen in the cord are not merely the result of Wallerian degeneration of the motor tract and do not simply reflect brain pathology.[26,28] This indicates that measuring pathology of the spinal cord using MT-MRI may be a "rewarding exercise in terms of understanding MS pathophysiology".[16]

3.4.3.1.2 Adrenomyeloneuropathy

AMN is a noninflammatory neurodegenerative disease with millimeter-size lesions in the dorsal and lateral columns of the cervical cord.[31] In contrast to MS, conventional MRI has shown no significant changes in patients with AMN other than cord atrophy late in the disease as AMN does not have an overt inflammatory component. Previous studies showed that MTR values are sensitive to cord pathology in the cervical-dorsal columns of AMN patients[9,10] and correlates well with EDSS and quantitative sensory-motor tests.[10] A subsequent study performed by the same group demonstrated for the first time that qMT-derived metrics can be a potential quantitative biomarker to assess and characterize human spinal cord tissues in disease.[7]

3.4.3.1.3 Neuromyelitis Optica

Neuromyelitis optica (NMO), also known as Devic's disease, is an inflammatory demyelinating disease that

selectively affects the optic nerve and the spinal cord.[32] There has long been debate as to whether NMO is a variant of MS. However, clinical, immunological, and pathological characteristics of NMO are increasingly being used to distinguish it from MS.[33–35] In patients with NMO, no brain abnormalities are generally found on the T_2-weighted scans, as one of the supportive criteria for NMO diagnosis is a negative conventional MRI scan of the brain at disease onset.[33] Filippi et al.[36] investigated the occult damage of the normal-appearing brain tissue (NABT) in patients with relapsing NMO using MT-MRI and found no difference between patients and control subjects, whereas MS patients had a significantly lower histogram average MTR and peak height. Rocca et al.[37] reported the abnormal changes in the normal-appearing WM and GM (NAWM/NAGM) in patients with NMO, and found reduced MTR of the NAGM in patients with NMO, which suggested the presence of GM damage in these patients. Despite potential advantages of investigating pathophysiology of NMO, MT-MRI has not been widely used to study the spinal cord in vivo. Recently, a study based on a novel approach to MT-MRI, namely MTCSF,[9] MT-weighted scan normalized to the CSF signal (described further in Section 3.4.3.2), demonstrated that MTCSF values of NMO patients were significantly higher than those of control subjects,[38] suggesting that the assessment of NMO cervical cord damage is feasible using the quantitative capability of MT-MRI.

3.4.3.2 Challenges

MT-MRI of the cervical cord presents technical difficulties, mainly because of the size of its structure and tendency to move during imaging. First of all, around 1 cm in diameter of region of interest requires at least submillimeter spatial resolution to distinguish the small GM and WM structures in the spinal cord. However, acquisition of high-resolution images at 1.5 T or 3 T results in reduced signal-to-noise ratio (SNR) and increased motion sensitivity through longer scan times. Another technical challenge is that the cord is subject to many types of motion such as cardiac pulsation and respiration. Despite availability of various motion correction algorithms, certain types of motion such as out-of-plane motions along the slice direction are more difficult to accurately correct, especially when imaging the cross section of the spinal cord where variations along the cord are slower than in plane. To this end, spinal cord MT-MRI has been mainly limited to assess total disease burden,[27,39] which allows detection of large inflammatory lesions. To overcome such limitations, the MTCSF approach has been developed[9] and utilized in studies with various clinical applications.[10,15] In MTCSF, MT effects are quantified in the spine using cerebrospinal fluid as an internal intensity standard, allowing interindividual comparison of MT-weighted data without the need for a reference scan:

$$\text{MTCSF} = \frac{M_S}{M_{\text{mean}}^{\text{CSF}}(\text{ROI})} \qquad (3.4.2)$$

$M_{\text{mean}}^{\text{CSF}}(\text{ROI})$ is obtained from an automatically selected region of interest (ROI), within the CSF, where no MT is expected to occur, CSF being substantially free water. A study showed tract-specific signal abnormalities in the dorsal and lateral columns of the spinal cord in MS patients using MTCSF.[15] One limitation of MTCSF is its dependency on T_1 and T_2 contrast, which might be altered in the presence of inflammation. For this reason this method is unlikely to be able to distinguish between demyelination and inflammation, and might be limited to clinical applications in which inflammation is known not to occur. Figure 3.4.3 shows a comparison between standard MTR and MTCSF of the cord. As MTCSF is an MT-weighted image scaled by a single value, the image quality appears to be greater than MTR, which instead is a voxel-by-voxel measure where noise contributes to both the nominator and denominator of the fraction.

It should be noted that MTR is a semiquantitative measure that not only depends on the size of the macromolecular pool but also on the exchange rate between the bound and mobile proton pools.[40] To overcome the multiparametric dependence of MTR, qMT may provide a more direct surrogate of myelin content.[41,42] However, estimation of qMT requires assumptions on the number of proton pools in the sample and necessitates multiple MT measurements as well as an independent measurement of T_1.[43] Alternatively, MT-MRI can be combined with diffusion-weighted MRI (DW-MRI). Studies showed that combining those two biomarkers can provide information more specific to WM pathology in MS,[44] spinal cord injury,[8] and amyotrophic lateral sclerosis.[45] Another study demonstrated the high

reproducibility of MT and DW-MRI at 3 T suggesting robust assessment of WM integrity in the human cervical cord.[46]

3.4.4 MT ACQUISITION PROTOCOLS

3.4.4.1 Continuous Wave Irradiation

Off-resonance continuous wave (CW) irradiation was first used to demonstrate MT effects in tissue.[1] In a CW experiment, RF pulses of several seconds with constant amplitude are used to saturate the macromolecular pool. Typically, irradiation is applied with 0.5–10 kHz off resonance. Direct saturation is minimized by the narrow bandwidth of CW irradiation. On the other hand, these experiments are not feasible on clinical systems, since the RF transmitters are not designed for CW operation. The first workers on imaging the MT effect in spinal cord recognized that CW irradiation would not be practical and investigated ways of producing an MT effect with pulsed saturation.

3.4.4.2 Pulsed Irradiation

Pulsed irradiation of shorter duration can be applied either on-resonance or off-resonance. On-resonant saturation is achieved by "transparent" pulses.[47–51] These consist of binomial pulses, such as $1\bar{1}$, or $1\bar{2}1$, whose net effect is zero for long T_2 spins such as those in free water. Here the number refers to the relative tip angle, and the bar means that the angle is reversed, thus $1\bar{1}$ could be 45° immediately followed by −45°. These pulses have no net effect on the mobile protons, while the short T_2 spins such as those in the bound pool are saturated.[47,48] This is because the transverse magnetization decays as soon as it is produced and the z-magnetization is not recovered by the second pulse. Despite their easy implementation and strong signal attenuation, the use of binomial pulses was not established due to their intrinsic direct saturation[52] and lack of flexibility,

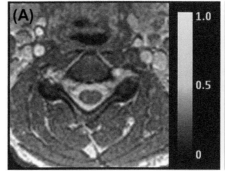
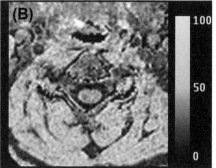

FIGURE 3.4.3 A comparison between MTCSF (A) and MTR (B) in the cervical cord. In MTCSF the signal intensity is normalized by the average signal intensity measured in a region of interest containing CSF. Notice that MTCSF is a normalized MT-weighted image while MTR is a semiquantitative measure.

compared with off-resonance pulses. Currently, off-resonance pulses are exclusively used as more control over the saturation is possible. Off-resonance pulses are typically shaped in Gaussian, or sinc with up to five lobes, with a bandwidth of a few 100 Hz, at frequency offsets of 50 Hz–50 kHz from the free proton-resonance frequency.

Table 3.4.1 summarizes representative protocols, which have been used in the spinal cord MT-MRI studies. However, it should be noted that MT-MRI using pulsed MT is still not a widely established method in the daily clinical routine, especially due to its long acquisition times. In addition, MTR suffers from its difficulty to be reproduced across different studies as it is very sensitive to pulse sequence details and relaxation properties.[53,54] Furthermore, clinical limitations on specific absorption rate (SAR) obstruct a complete saturation of the restricted pool protons, hereby making data interpretation and standardization difficult.[55] Several technical issues including field strength, MT saturation and sequence properties, B1-inhomogeneity, and subject positioning complicate the comparability of MTR values. Recently, a new MT-sensitized method using balanced steady state free precession (bSSFP) was proposed and shown to provide high-resolution images with significantly reduced acquisition times in brain imaging.[56,57] However, it has not yet been performed in the spinal cord.

3.4.5 QUANTITATIVE MODELS OF MT

3.4.5.1 Two-Pool Model

Attempts to provide indices of myelination more reproducible than the MTR led to the introduction of an analytical description of the two-pool model. A simple description can be given by the model proposed by Henkelman et al.,[58] reproduced in Figure 3.4.4. This model was originally developed for a CW irradiation experiment in agar gels, in which RF pulses of several seconds with constant amplitude are used to saturate the macromolecular pool.

In Figure 3.4.4, "A" labels the liquid pool, and "B" labels the macromolecular pool. The density of spins in the two pools is M_0^A and M_0^B, respectively. As the M_0^A is constant and $M_0^A >> M_0^B$, it is often set equal to 1 to normalize the experiment.[58] The shaded portion of the boxes represents the spins in each pool that are saturated, while the white area represent the spins that are in the longitudinal plane, for a given instant of time. The proportion of saturated spins depends on the irradiation history. After the RF irradiation has been turned off, longitudinal relaxation tends to bring the magnetization back to the longitudinal plane, with relaxation rates R_A $(=1/T_1^A)$ and R_B $(=1/T_1^B)$, respectively. The exchange rate constant between the two pools is R, assumed to be symmetrical. As $M_0^A >> M_0^B$, this is a pseudo-first order exchange process with exchange constant from A to B equal to RM_0^B. The rate from B to A is therefore RM_0^A to preserve compartment sizes. The effect of off-resonance irradiation is summarized by the rates of loss of longitudinal magnetization due to RF absorption (R_{RFA} and R_{RFB}), described in more detail in the following paragraphs.

Assuming that the MT effect can be modeled using this two-pool description, the magnetization of either pool can be described by its longitudinal component (M_z^A, M_z^B) and its transverse components (M_x^A, M_y^A, M_x^B, M_y^B). The exchange between pools associated with the transverse components of magnetization can be

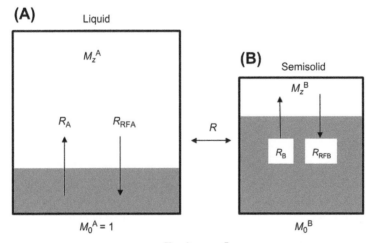

FIGURE 3.4.4 Two-pool model proposed by Henkelman et al.[58] M_0^A and M_0^B represent the fully relaxed values of magnetization associated with the two pools. The shaded areas correspond to the saturated spins at a given time. Each pool is characterized by its own longitudinal relaxation rate (R_A and R_B) and by its rate of loss of longitudinal magnetization due to the RF irradiation (R_{RFA} and R_{RFB}). The exchange rate between the two pools, R, is assumed to be symmetrical. *Source: Adapted with permission from Henkelman RM et al., in Magn Reson Med, Copyright 1993, John Wiley Inc.*

considered negligible due to the extremely short T_2 associated with the macromolecular pool. The coupled Bloch equations for the system can thus be written as follows[58]:

$$\frac{dM_z^A}{dt} = R_A(M_0^A - M_Z^A) - RM_0^B M_Z^A \\ + RM_0^A M_Z^B + \omega_1(t)M_y^A \tag{3.4.3}$$

$$\frac{dM_z^B}{dt} = R_B(M_0^B - M_Z^B) - RM_0^A M_Z^B + RM_0^B M_Z^A \\ - (R_{RFB}(\Delta f, \omega_1(t)))M_Z^B \tag{3.4.4}$$

$$\frac{dM_x^A}{dt} = -\frac{M_x^A}{T_2^A} - 2\pi\Delta f M_y^A \tag{3.4.5}$$

$$\frac{dM_y^A}{dt} = -\frac{M_y^A}{T_2^A} + 2\pi\Delta f M_x^A - \omega_1(t)M_z^A. \tag{3.4.6}$$

where T_2^A represents the transverse relaxation time of the liquid pool, Δf represents the frequency offset of the pulse, while $\omega_1(t)$ is the time-dependent amplitude of the pulse expressed in rads^{-1} (i.e., the angular frequency of precession induced by the pulse).

In the CW case considered by Henkelman et al., $\omega_1(t) = \omega_1$, and the system admits solution in the steady state, i.e., when all the derivatives are equal to zero:

$$M_z^A = \frac{M_0(R_B RM_0^B + R_{RFB}R_A + R_B R_A + R_A RM_0^A)}{(R_{RFA} + R_A + RM_0^B)(R_{RFB} + R_B + RM_0^A) - RRM_0^B}, \tag{3.4.7}$$

where

$$R_{RFA} = \frac{\omega_1^2 T_2^A}{1 + (2\pi\Delta T_2^A)} \tag{3.4.8}$$

$$R_{RFB} = \frac{\omega_1^2 T_2^B}{1 + (2\pi\Delta T_2^B)} \tag{3.4.9}$$

are derived analytically from the steady state solution, and are proportional to the Lorentzian absorption line shape of each pool.

Despite a Lorentzian line shape as the only possible solution for a single T_2, this line shape does not adequately describe the macromolecular component. Henkelman et al. used a Gaussian line shape for agar gel,[58] while Li et al.[59] show that, in CNS tissue, the spectra associated with macromolecular pool are better modeled by a super-Lorentzian, of the form:

$$R_{RFB}(\Delta f, \omega_1) = \omega_1^2\sqrt{2\pi}\Bigg[T_2^B \int_0^1 \frac{1}{|3u^2 - 1|} \\ \exp\left(-2\left(\frac{2\pi\Delta f T_2^B}{3u^2 - 1}\right)^2\right)du\Bigg]. \tag{3.4.10}$$

As typically $2\pi\Delta T_2^A >> 1$, Eqn (3.4.7) can be rewritten, after dividing by R_A, as:

$$M_z^A = \frac{M_0^A\left(R_B\left[\frac{RM_0^B}{R_A}\right] + R_{RFB} + R_B + RM_0^A\right)}{\frac{RM_0^B}{R_A}(R_B + R_{RFB}) + \left(1 + \left[\frac{\omega_1}{2\pi\Delta f}\right]^2\left[\frac{1}{R_A T_2^A}\right]\right)(R_{RFB} + R_B + RM_0^A)}. \tag{3.4.11}$$

Equation (3.4.11) is written in terms of seven parameters: M_0^A (assumed equal to 1), R_A, R_B, RM_0^B, RM_0^A, T_2^A, and T_2^B, but these cannot be uniquely determined.[58] Constraints are imposed typically by keeping R_B fixed at 1 s^{-1},[54,55,58] and by measuring the observed longitudinal relaxation rate of the sample, R_{Aobs} ($=1/T_{1obs}$) independently, linked to R_A by[58]

$$R_A = R_{Aobs} - \frac{RM_0^B(R_B - R_{Aobs})}{R_B - R_{Aobs} + RM_0^A}. \tag{3.4.12}$$

Equation (3.4.11) can thus be fitted, using a nonlinear least squares technique, to a minimum of four measurements, obtained with variable settings of ω_1 and Δf, in a CW experiment.

qMT PARAMETERS

- Liquid pool spin density: M_0^A
- Macromolecular pool spin density: M_0^B
- Bound pool fraction: $f = \frac{M_0^B}{M_0^A + M_0^B}$
- Relative size of the macromolecular pool: $F = \frac{M_0^B}{M_0^A}$
- Exchange rate constant: R
- Forward exchange rate: RM_0^B
- Reverse exchange rate: RM_0^A
- Longitudinal relaxation rate of the liquid pool: R_A

- Longitudinal relaxation rate of the macromolecular pool: R_B
- Transverse relation time of the liquid pool: T_2^A
- Transverse relation time of the macromolecular pool: T_2^B
- By definition, the following relationships between parameters hold:

$$f = \frac{F}{F+1}$$

$$F = \frac{RM_0^B}{RM_0^A}$$

3.4.5.2 Extension to Pulsed MT

As mentioned in Section 3.4.4, CW irradiation is impractical and generally not available for in vivo imaging experiments. In vivo MT-weighted MRI is generally obtained using the so-called pulsed MT acquisition, in which the long period of saturation is replaced by a much shorter irradiation pulse (typically applied just before each excitation pulse) along with intervals without irradiation (during which data is collected). For data from this type of acquisition, Henkelman's equation must be modified to allow for the short duration of the saturation pulses relative to T_1. Under these circumstances Eqns (3.4.3)–(3.4.6) only

where P_{SAT} is the mean square saturating field and γ is the gyromagnetic ratio.

P_{SAT} is equivalent to

$$P_{SAT} = p_2 B_{max}^2 \frac{\tau_{SAT}}{TR'}, \tag{3.4.14}$$

where p_2 is the ratio of the mean square amplitude of the saturation pulse to that of a rectangular pulse of equivalent amplitude, B_{max} is the maximum amplitude of the pulse, τ_{SAT} is its duration, and TR' is the interval between successive pulses.

B_{max} can be computed with knowledge of the equivalent on-resonance flip angle (ϑ) of the pulse, being:

$$\vartheta[°] = \left[\frac{180}{\pi}\right] \gamma p_1 B_{max} \tau_{SAT} \tag{3.4.15}$$

(where p_1 is the ratio of the mean amplitude of the saturation pulse to that of a rectangular pulse of the same amplitude).

By means of the CWPE approximation, Henkelman's steady state model can be straightforwardly applied to the in vivo MRI case, neglecting the imaging elements of the pulse sequence.

Introducing the symbol $F = \frac{M_0^B}{M_0^A}$, known as the relative size of the macromolecular pool, and substituting $RM_0^A = \frac{RM_0^B}{F}$, the equation

$$SI(\omega_1, \Delta f) = \frac{M_0 \left(R_B \left[\frac{RM_0^B}{R_A} \right] + R_{RFB}(\omega_{1\,CWPE}, \Delta f) + R_B + \frac{RM_0^B}{F} \right)}{\left[\frac{RM_0^B}{R_A} \right] (R_B + R_{RFB}(\omega_{1\,CWPE}, \Delta f)) + \left(1 + \left[\frac{\omega_{1\,CWPE}}{2\pi\Delta f} \right]^2 \left[\frac{1}{R_A T_2^A} \right] \right) \left(R_{RFB}(\omega_{1\,CWPE}, \Delta f) + R_B + \frac{RM_0^B}{F} \right)} \tag{3.4.16}$$

admit a numerical solution.[60] In order to provide a computationally efficient approach, a number of approximated signal equations for pulsed MT, all based on the original two-pool model, have been developed.[54,55,61]

For simplicity, here we have rewritten all equations keeping the conventions introduced by Henkelman et al.,[58] wherever possible. However, some authors label the A and B pools as F and R, respectively,[55] or f and m[61] and use the symbol W instead of R_{RFB}.[55,61] The pseudo–first order exchange rates, RM_0^B and RM_0^A, are often referred to as k_f (or simply k) and k_r.

Ramani et al. used a CW power equivalent approximation (CWPE)[54] where the pulse is simply replaced by a CW irradiation with the mean square amplitude that would give the same power over the interval between MT pulses:

$$\omega_{1\,CWPE} = \gamma \sqrt{P_{SAT}}, \tag{3.4.13}$$

can be used to fit directly to data collected using the pulsed MT method. We note that, in order to ease the comparison between the signal equations, we have broken with the terminology of the original paper by Ramani et al.,[54] where the macromolecular fraction f (with $f = F/(F+1)$) was used instead of the relative size of the macromolecular pool F. As $F \ll 1$, the two parameters tend to be similar, and have both been associated with myelin content.

In the attempt to validate it as a myelin marker, $F(f)$ has been measured in animal models of demyelination and axonal loss,[62] suggesting that myelin alone could explain the difference in F measured in gray and WM. These data also support the hypothesis that axonal loss in the absence of demyelination does not affect F.[63] In a postmortem study, f was shown to be strongly associated with a histological measure of myelination obtained by assessing light transmittance on stained MS brain slices.[42] The same paper also demonstrated the ability of that parameter to differentiate between demyelinated and remyelinated lesions, as well as between remyelinated lesions and the normal-appearing white matter.

As Ramani's equation does not explicitly model the effects of the excitation pulses and TR, its description of the MT-weighted signal is valid only when the degree of T_1 weighting in the acquisition sequence is minimal.[64]

Sled and Pike[55,65] proposed a solution derived by approximating the pulse sequence as a series of periods of free precession, CW irradiation, and instantaneous saturation of the free pool.

During each of these periods, Eqns (3.4.3)–(3.4.6) have either an exact or an approximate solution, and these solutions can then be concatenated by imposing the appropriate initial conditions, leading to an expression for the measured signal which is less expensive to compute than numerically integrating the full set of differential equations.

The effect of an MT pulse on the macromolecular pool is modeled as a rectangular pulse whose width is equal to the full width at half maximum (τ_{RP}) of the curve obtained by squaring the instantaneous amplitude of the MT pulse throughout its duration, and whose amplitude is such that the pulses have equivalent average power (rectangular pulse, or RP, approximation). The effect of the pulse on the liquid pool is modeled as an instantaneous fractional saturation of the longitudinal magnetization. Such fractional saturation (S_{1A}) is estimated by solving (numerically) the system of Eqns (3.4.3), (3.4.5) and (3.4.6) when R and R_A are set to 0.

In matrix form,[55] let us consider the longitudinal components of magnetization only:

$$\mathbf{M}_z(t) = \begin{bmatrix} M_z^A(t) \\ M_z^B(t) \end{bmatrix}. \qquad (3.4.17)$$

Instantaneous saturation of the free pool, caused by both MT and excitation pulses, is described by multiplying $\mathbf{M}_z$ by the matrix $\mathbf{S}$ (where θ is the excitation flip angle):

$$\mathbf{S} = \begin{bmatrix} S_{1A} \cos\theta & 0 \\ 0 & 1 \end{bmatrix}. \qquad (3.4.18)$$

The state of the magnetization after a period t_1 (assuming starting time $= t_0$) is given by the solution to the system of Eqns (3.4.3) and (3.4.4) for either free precession (FP) or CW:

$$M_z(t_0 + t_1) = \exp\{A_{CW}t_1\}M_z(t_0) + [I - \exp\{A_{CW}t_1\} \\ \times]A_{CW}^{-1}BM_0 \qquad (3.4.19)$$

$$M_z(t_0 + t_1) = \exp\{A_{FP}t_1\}M_z(t_0) + [I - \exp\{A_{FP}t_1\}] \\ \times A_{FP}^{-1}BM_0, \qquad (3.4.20)$$

with

$$A_{CW} = \begin{bmatrix} -R_A - RM_0^B & RM_0^A \\ RM_0^B & -R_B - RM_0^A - R_{RFB} \end{bmatrix}$$

$$A_{FP} = \begin{bmatrix} -R_A - RM_0^B & RM_0^A \\ RM_0^B & -R_B - RM_0^A \end{bmatrix}$$

$$B = \begin{bmatrix} -R_A & 0 \\ 0 & -R_B \end{bmatrix}.$$

According to Sled and Pike's RP approximation, over the time interval TR$'$ between application of MT pulses (typically the time required to excite and collect data for a single k-space line of a single image slice), $\mathbf{M}_z$ undergoes instantaneous saturation, CW irradiation for a period $\tau_{RP}/2$, FP for a period (TR$' - \tau_{RP}$), and CW for another $\tau_{RP}/2$. After including all three steps, we can impose the equality

$$M_z(TR') = M_z(0), \qquad (3.4.21)$$

and solve for $\mathbf{M}_z$. Recalling that the signal observed at readout is

$$SI(\omega_1, \Delta f) = cM_z^A(TR)S_{1A}\sin\theta, \qquad (3.4.22)$$

(where c is a constant scaling factor) it is thus possible to obtain an analytical expression to model the MT-weighted signal.

Yarnykh[61] proposed a technique that neglects any direct saturation of the liquid pool (by assuming the offset frequency is large enough) and approximates shaped RF pulses by an effective rectangular pulse, with the same duration as the real pulse (τ_{SAT}), and constant amplitude ω_{1eff}:

$$\omega_{1\,eff} = \frac{1}{\tau_{SAT}} \int_0^{\tau_{SAT}} \omega_1^2(t)dt. \qquad (3.4.23)$$

Following an approach similar to that of Sled and Pike,[55] Yarnykh decomposes the sequence into a period of saturation, a delay for spoiling gradients, a readout period, and a relaxation period.

The solutions (in matrix form) obtained for each period are then concatenated to yield an expression for $\mathbf{M}_s$, the magnetization vector immediately before a readout pulse.

The expression is then simplified using a first-order approximation assuming short time intervals and low excitation flip angles. The resulting analytical solution for M_{zs}^F, the z component of the liquid pool magnetization just before the readout pulse, is given by:

$$M_{zs}^A = \frac{1/F + 1(A + R_A s R_{RFB})}{A + (R_A + RM_0^B) s R_{RFB} - \left(R_B + \frac{RM_0^B}{F} + s R_{RFB}\right) \frac{\ln(\cos \alpha)}{TR}}, \quad (3.4.24)$$

where s is the duty cycle and

$$A = R_A R_B + R_A \frac{RM_0^B}{F} + R_B RM_0^B. \quad (3.4.25)$$

Yarnykh expresses the signal intensity relative to the unsaturated case as the MTR:

$$MTR(R_{RFB}) = 1 - \frac{M_{zs}^A(R_{RFB})}{M_{zs}^A(R_{RFB} = 0)} \approx \frac{s R_{RFB}}{P + Qs R_{RFB}}, \quad (3.4.26)$$

with

$$P = \frac{A\left(A - \left(R_B + \frac{RM_0^B}{F}\right) \frac{\ln \cos \alpha}{TR}\right)}{RM_0^B \left(A - \frac{R_B \ln \cos \alpha}{TR}\right)} \quad (3.4.27)$$

$$Q = \frac{A\left(A - (R_A + RM_0^B) \frac{\ln \cos \alpha}{TR}\right)}{RM_0^B \left(A - \frac{R_B \ln \cos \alpha}{TR}\right)}. \quad (3.4.28)$$

The parameters P, Q, and T_2^B can thus be obtained by fitting the model to a series of MTR measurements at different settings of the saturating pulse. $F(f)$ and RM_0^B (k) can be derived with knowledge of R_{Aobs} from

$$P \approx \frac{\left(R_A^{obs} \cdot \frac{F+1}{F} - \frac{(\ln \cos \alpha)}{F}\right)}{TR} \quad (3.4.29)$$

$$Q \approx \left(R_A^{obs} - \frac{(\ln \cos \alpha)}{TR}\right) (RM_0^B)^{-1} + 1. \quad (3.4.30)$$

It has been shown[64,66] that these three approximations yield consistent results, providing that the experimental conditions comply with the basic assumptions.

3.4.5.3 Quantitative MT of the Spinal Cord

Quantitative MT of the spinal cord has been implemented[7] using pulsed MT and the formalism introduced by Sled and Pike, with the modifications introduced by Portnoy et al.[66] Data were obtained using a 3D gradient echo sequence, sinc-shaped MT pulses with fixed amplitude, and 10 offset frequencies, logarithmically sampled between 1 and 64 kHz. Data were obtained from healthy subjects and patients with AMN. The average signal from four regions of interest (lateral columns, dorsal column, and dorsolateral horn GM) was extracted and used to fit the model. F was the only parameter showing significant differences between patients and controls. All the qMT parameters estimated in the WM and GM of cord in healthy controls were consistent with those typically reported for the brain (for the GM the values in the cord were close to those typically found in subcortical structures of the brain).

3.4.5.4 Parameter Interpretation and Validation

Quantitative MT provides a number of parameters, which reflect indirectly some properties of the macromolecular pool and may potentially measure differing pathological substrates. Most research has focused on demonstrating that F reflects myelin content. As reported in the previous session, animal[62,63] and postmortem[42] studies have reached encouraging results, which support the interpretation of F (or f) as a marker of myelination. Despite these observations, F and measures of myelination derived from short T_2 mapping (see Chapter 3.5) appear largely uncorrelated,[67] prompting the debate about which technique better estimates myelin in vivo.

Among the other MT parameters, T_2^B has received little attention, mainly because it appears relatively stable across conditions (healthy subjects vs. patients, WM vs. GM, etc.). Recent observations, however, suggest that this parameter might be sensitive to WM fiber orientation.[68]

Finally, the interpretation of RM_0^B, the pseudo-first order forward exchange rate, is uncertain, as the exact mechanisms of MT are still unknown. Based on results obtained in the cortex of patients with Alzheimer's disease, it has been suggested that it might reflect metabolic changes.[69]

3.4.5.5 Sources of Bias

Since quantitative MT relies on fitting a nonlinear model to a series of MT-weighted images collected using MT pulses of variable amplitude and offset frequency, any imperfection in the time-varying magnetic field (B_1) will result in a deviation from the nominal on-resonance equivalent flip angle (and ω_1), while any imperfection in the static field (B_0) will result in a deviation from the nominal value of Δf. Both effects can introduce a spatially variable bias in the estimated parameters. B_0 inhomogeneity is particularly relevant for spinal cord imaging, due to the vicinity of bone tissue, causing an abrupt change in susceptibility (see Chapter 2.2). B_0 inhomogeneity can be diminished by using the body-coil transmit,[70] although this solution is unlikely to be sufficient to mitigate the problem at field strengths higher than 1.5 T. Ideally the B_1 and B_0 fields should be measured at the same time as the MT acquisition, and used to retrospectively correct the data. Simulations suggest that $F(f)$ is relatively robust to small deviations from the nominal B_0 field, while it is highly sensitive to B_1 inhomogeneities.[71]

3.4.5.6 Beyond the Two-Pool Model

The two-pool model is a simplistic description of WM characteristics, which neglects the existence of multiple water compartments. On the other hand, multicompartmental T_2 mapping[72] yields an estimate of the myelin water fraction (MWF) based on the hypothesis of two or more isolated water compartments (see Chapter 3.5). Attempts to provide a unified view led to the development of four-pool models.[43,73] This approach assumes four communicating proton pools (myelin solids, myelin water, intra/extracellular water, and non-myelin solids), including most of the basic features of the multicompartment T_2 water model and the two-pool MT model. The number of parameters to be fitted makes this type of model impractical for in vivo applications. However, it can be used to predict the behavior of T_2 spectra and MT as a function of myelin content, thus helping the interpretation of changes observed with these quantitative MRI methods based on simplified models of white matter.

3.4.5.7 Reduced Models

The clinical applications of quantitative models of MT described in the previous sessions have been limited so far due to the long acquisition times. The scan time is predominantly affected by the number of data points and/or the signal-to-noise ratio (SNR) of the underlying acquisition required to achieve a sufficient SNR in the calculated maps.

A constraint on the minimum number of images is imposed by the total number of model parameters to be estimated. The number of data points required can thus be decreased by reducing the number of model parameters to a subset of those required to fully fit the model by imposing physically meaningful constraints on the others. Yarnykh and Yuan[74] constrained both, T_2^A and T_2^B, based on the following observations. First, although T_2^A and R_A taken separately may significantly vary, the product $T_2^A R_A$ is fairly constant in CNS tissues, even in the presence of pathology, such as MS lesions.[65,75] Secondly, the reported T_2^B's for the brain, both in vivo an in vitro[65,75] fall into the range of 9.2–12.3 µs with little difference between white and gray matter. By fixing the ratio $T_2^A R_A$ to 0.055 (at 1.5 T) and T_2^B to 11 µs, they were able to reduce the number of MT sampling point to 4 (plus a T_1-mapping scan). Used in combination with a 3D high-resolution acquisition, this strategy was shown to produce high-quality maps of f and RM_0^B (k) in the human brain.

Using further constraints, recently the same group presented a method for mapping f based on two measurements (an MT-weighted and a reference scan), together with the appropriate T_1 and field mapping scans.[76]

Ropele et al.[77] have estimated k_f (RM_0^B) based on the assumption of complete saturation of the macromolecular pool. Under these circumstances, the Eqns (3.4.3)–(3.4.6) reduce to a single differential equation:

$$\frac{dM_z^A}{dt} = R_A\left(M_0^A - M_z^A\right) - k_f M_z^A, \quad (3.4.31)$$

which admits a mono-exponential solution with time constant T_{1sat}, such that

$$\frac{1}{T_{1\,sat}} = R_A + k_f. \quad (3.4.32)$$

In the steady state, the forward exchange rate can be expressed as a function of T_{1sat} and of the MTR:

$$k_f = \frac{MTR}{T_{1\,sat}}. \quad (3.4.33)$$

Although k_f measured using this methods might be sensitive to biological changes, the basic assumption of complete saturation is impossible to ensure, and therefore caution is recommended when interpreting results of in vivo applications.[78]

One of the limitations of the MTR is its dependency on T_1, as well as on the density of macromolecular protons. In some circumstances (e.g., demyelinating lesions) the increase in T_1 can partially mask the decrease in macromolecular density, resulting in an apparent stability of the MTR. Helms et al.[79] proposed a method based on three acquisitions (just one more than a simple MTR computation) to separate the two contributions.

The method is a modification of the T_1-quantification approach based on two 3D acquisitions with differing flip angles.[80] The third, additional, acquisition is an MT-weighted 3D gradient echo sequence.

Helms introduces a series of approximation, which lead the following expression for the signal of the MT-weighted acquisition:

$$S_{MT} \cong A\alpha \frac{R_1 TR}{\alpha^2/2 + \delta + R_1 TR}, \qquad (3.4.34)$$

where α is the excitation flip angle, $R_1 = 1/T_1$, and A is the amplitude of the spoiled gradient echo at the echo time, TE, under fully relaxed conditions ($R_1 TR \gg 1$).

The parameter of interest is δ, the "MT saturation", which describes the signal attenuation imposed by the application of an MT pulse.

The phenomenological term δ is independent of relaxation and can be calculated once A and R_1 are known, and appears to be a sensitive to the presence of demyelination.

A preliminary study applying this method to the cervical cord[81] produced encouraging results, demonstrating feasibility and relatively good intra- and intersubject reproducibility (around 10%).

For cord applications, the substantial decrease in scan time achievable for these reduced models make them attractive alternatives to the full modeling.

3.4.6 MT DATA ANALYSIS METHODS

Most studies based on the use of MT imaging of the cord set out to compare the MTR, or other MT-derived parameters, between patients and healthy subjects. The most popular strategies for extracting the relevant values in a format suitable for statistical analysis are region of interest (ROI) and histogram analysis.

In the context of cord imaging, ROIs are typically defined in the transverse plane. In the first published studies, ROIs tended to be circular and to coincide with a large part of cord transverse area, without any attempt to separate WM and GM,[6] while, more recently, measurements with a more accurate anatomical definition have been presented using high resolution T_1- or proton density-weighted images as anatomical reference.[8,82] Smith et al.[46] combined MTCSF imaging with diffusion tensor imaging (DTI) of the cord. DTI tractography was used to reconstruct the dorsal and the lateral columns, and column-specific MTCSF values were obtained from a group of healthy subjects.

Histogram analysis is an attractive alternative to ROI placement, as it may be more robust to the misregistration between saturated and unsaturated scans.[30] It involves the creation of a frequency distribution showing the proportion of voxels in an image with a given range of signal intensities. The full range is divided into a number of "bins". The histogram counts the number of observations falling in each bin. Usually some numerical features (such as the peak height or the peak location) are selected to characterize the shape of the histogram, and a statistical comparison between patients' and controls' average metrics is performed. This approach is indicated in the presence of diffuse pathology.

3.4.7 CHEMICAL EXCHANGE SATURATION TRANSFER

3.4.7.1 Principle of CEST and Its Applications

CEST has recently emerged as an alternative contrast mechanism for MRI.[83–89] In CEST-MRI, small molecules in solution are saturated by selective RF irradiation. The saturation is transferred to the water pool via labile protons of the solute, such as amide (NH) and hydroxyl (OH),[90–93] as first demonstrated by Wolff and Balaban.[1] Saturated solute protons are repeatedly replaced by nonsaturated water protons, leading to an accumulation of saturated protons in the water pool. After a few seconds of RF irradiation, this gives rise to an observable signal reduction in the water pool. Highest sensitivity to proton transfer is achieved if the exchange rate from solute to water k_{sw} is large and the solute has a high concentration. Z-spectrum[94] or CEST spectrum[95] displays RF saturation effects on water as a function of saturation frequency offset relative to water, which is assigned to be at 0 ppm. The magnitude of the CEST effect is quantified as an MT asymmetry ratio MTR_{asym}

$$MTR_{asym}(\Delta\omega) = \frac{S(-\Delta\omega) - S(\Delta\omega)}{S_0}, \qquad (3.4.35)$$

where $\Delta\omega$ is the shift difference between the irradiation frequency and the water frequency. S and S_0 are the saturated and nonsaturated intensities. An example of Z-spectrum and MTR_{asym} is shown in Figure 3.4.5.

CEST observation of solutes and particles in the millimolar to nanomolar range has been demonstrated both in vitro[84,87,96–100] and in vivo.[90,93,101–103] Zhou et al.[90,104] demonstrated a CEST effect that is based on the magnetization exchange between bulk water and labile endogenous amide protons, detecting endogenous mobile proteins and peptides in biological tissue via chemical exchange, an approach that is known as amide proton transfer (APT) imaging. Especially, given the hydrogen exchange is exponentially proportional to

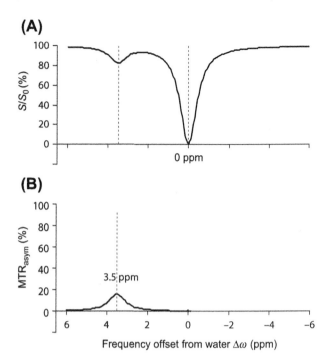

FIGURE 3.4.5 (A) Measurement of normalized water saturation (S/S_0) as a function of irradiation frequency, generating a Z-spectrum (or CEST spectrum). (B) Result of magnetization transfer ratio asymmetry (MTR_{asym}) analysis of the Z-spectrum with respect to the water frequency (0 ppm).

physiological pH, the pH contrast can be generated by measuring the exchange rates. pH-sensitive APT imaging has served as a new metabolic biomarker to clinical imaging for brain tissue.[90,105] Recently, a preliminary study demonstrated that APT imaging is feasible at 7 T and showed contrast between WM and GM in healthy brain tissues as well as abnormal signal in NABT in a small cohort of patients with MS[106] (see also Chapter 2.4).

A drawback to CEST imaging remains the high concentrations required (>10 mM) and the need for strong MR irradiation pulses for presaturation, which are limited by power deposition limitations, or SAR. As another technical challenge, B_0 field inhomogeneity often complicates MTR_{asym} analysis in CEST imaging, which requires accurate identification of water proton peak.[107] In order to resolve this problem, various methods have been suggested[108–111] and successfully used in different clinical applications.[103,106,112] One approach is to acquire images over a range of saturation frequency offsets (Z-spectrum, typically with high saturation power), followed by polynomial or cubic-spline fitting and centering of the Z-spectrum in each voxel.[90,104,113] This may work in vitro or even in vivo if the CEST and water saturation curves are sufficiently separated, as in the case for NH groups in proteins

and peptides. However, such an approach may be less accurate if studies are done in vivo, where the conventional MT effect has been shown to be asymmetric.[114,115] As another approach, Sun et al.[109] reported that B_0 field maps can be used in combination with other information, such as T_1, T_2, and B_1 field maps. This method is suitable for studies with small ranges of B_0 shifts rather than large frequency shifts that are commonplace for in vivo human data. Recently, a separate acquisition with low saturation power, which detects the direct saturation of water, has been used to establish the frequency shift caused by field inhomogeneities for in vivo human data and is termed water saturation shift referencing (WASSR).[108] The minimum in the WASSR Z-spectrum corresponds to the true bulk water resonance and is used to correct shifts caused by B_0 inhomogeneities in the subsequently obtained CEST acquisitions on a voxel-by-voxel basis. In order to reduce total scan time for both CEST and WASSR data acquisition, implementation of the keyhole technique has been suggested.[110]

3.4.7.2 CEST vs. MT

CEST-MRI experiments are performed in a similar manner to MT-MRI, but with important differences. While MT contrast is based on magnetization exchange between cellular solid or semisolid protons and water protons, CEST contrast originates from chemical exchange between labile protons and water protons. In MT-MRI, the broad spectral line shape of the semisolid components can be saturated by a variety of short pulses and saturation over a large frequency range of about ±100 kHz is detected. In contrast, CEST-MRI requires much narrower bandwidth of the RF irradiation in order to be more specific to the resonances of interest such as NH and OH groups. In general, CEST is observed in a small chemical shift range of less than 5 ppm from water, but may also be registered at several 100 ppm depending on the type of CEST agent.

3.4.7.3 CEST in the Spinal Cord

Application of CEST in the spinal cord is still in its infancy despite its promising potential. Recently, Ng et al.[116] showed that the z-spectrum in GM/WM is asymmetrical about the water resonance frequency when using both spin echo (SE)-echo planar imaging (EPI) and gradient echo (GE)-EPI, attributed mainly to the conventional MT and CEST effects. High amplitude of MTR_{asym} was also identified in the frequency range of the amide proton, suggesting feasibility of CEST-MRI in the human spinal cord. In another study by Dula et al.,[117] CEST-MRI was used to calculate the amide proton transfer asymmetry (APT_{asym}) to detect subtle characteristics of MS lesions in the human spinal cord. Similarly to Ng et al., APT_{asym} measures from the healthy controls showed a significant difference between GM and WM. In addition, a WM lesion in MS patients demonstrated a relative decrease in APT_{asym}.

3.4.8 CONCLUSION

The potential specificity of MT imaging makes it attractive for spinal cord imaging in conditions such as MS and AMN. While MTR has been widely applied to the cervical cord, quantitative MT is limited by technical challenges and long scan times. Optimized acquisitions, as well as approaches based on reduced models, allow the scan time to be reduced and/or the precision to be increased. The use of quantitative MT in the spinal cord is therefore expected to grow in the next few years, despite the difficulties related to the geometry and the physiology of the cord.

CEST is another area that is growing fast. Previous studies have shown great promise in assessing various metabolites. The advantages of high saturation efficiency and specificity of CEST will be particularly useful for understanding pathophysiology of neuro-related diseases in spinal cord.

References

1. Wolff SD, Balaban RS. Magnetization transfer contrast (MTC) and tissue water proton relaxation in vivo. *Magn Reson Med.* 1989;10(1):135–144.
2. Mengotti P, D'Agostini S, Terlevic R, et al. Altered white matter integrity and development in children with autism: a combined voxel-based morphometry and diffusion imaging study. *Brain Res Bull.* 2011;84(2):189–195.
3. Pike GB, Hu BS, Glover GH, Enzmann DR. Magnetization transfer time-of-flight magnetic resonance angiography. *Magn Reson Med.* 1992;25(2):372–379.
4. Finelli DA, Hurst GC, Karaman BA, Simon JE, Duerk JL, Bellon EM. Use of magnetization transfer for improved contrast on gradient-echo MR images of the cervical spine. *Radiology.* 1994;193(1):165–171.
5. Filippi M, Rocca MA, Martino G, Horsfield MA, Comi G. Magnetization transfer changes in the normal appearing white matter precede the appearance of enhancing lesions in patients with multiple sclerosis. *Ann Neurol.* 1998;43(6):809–814.
6. Silver NC, Barker GJ, Losseff NA, et al. Magnetisation transfer ratio measurement in the cervical spinal cord: a preliminary study in multiple sclerosis. *Neuroradiology.* 1997;39(6):441–445.
7. Smith SA, Golay X, Fatemi A, et al. Quantitative magnetization transfer characteristics of the human cervical spinal cord in vivo: application to adrenomyeloneuropathy. *Magn Reson Med.* 2009;61(1):22–27.
8. Cohen-Adad J, El Mendili MM, Lehericy S, et al. Demyelination and degeneration in the injured human spinal cord detected with diffusion and magnetization transfer MRI. *NeuroImage.* 2011;55(3):1024–1033.
9. Smith SA, Golay X, Fatemi A, et al. Magnetization transfer weighted imaging in the upper cervical spinal cord using cerebrospinal fluid as intersubject normalization reference (MTCSF imaging). *Magn Reson Med.* 2005;54(1):201–206.
10. Fatemi A, Smith SA, Dubey P, et al. Magnetization transfer MRI demonstrates spinal cord abnormalities in adrenomyeloneuropathy. *Neurology.* 2005;64(10):1739–1745.
11. Silver NC, Good CD, Barker GJ, et al. Sensitivity of contrast enhanced MRI in multiple sclerosis. effects of gadolinium dose, magnetization transfer contrast and delayed imaging. *Brain.* 1997;120(Pt 7):1149–1161.
12. Berry I, Barker GJ, Barkhof F, et al. A multicenter measurement of magnetization transfer ratio in normal white matter. *J Magn Reson Imaging.* 1999;9(3):441–446.
13. Cercignani M, Symms MR, Ron M, Barker GJ. 3D MTR measurement: from 1.5 T to 3.0 T. *NeuroImage.* 2006;31(1):181–186.
14. Finelli DA, Reed DR. Flip angle dependence of experimentally determined T1sat and apparent magnetization transfer rate constants. *J Magn Reson Imaging.* 1998;8(3):548–553.
15. Zackowski KM, Smith SA, Reich DS, et al. Sensorimotor dysfunction in multiple sclerosis and column-specific magnetization transfer-imaging abnormalities in the spinal cord. *Brain.* 2009;132(5):1200–1209.
16. Filippi M, Rocca MA. Magnetization transfer magnetic resonance imaging of the brain, spinal cord, and optic nerve. *Neurotherapeutics.* 2007;4(3):401–413.
17. Mottershead JP, Schmierer K, Clemence M, et al. High field MRI correlates of myelin content and axonal density in multiple sclerosis—a post-mortem study of the spinal cord. *J Neurol.* 2003;250(11):1293–1301.
18. Schmierer K, Scaravilli F, Altmann DR, Barker GJ, Miller DH. Magnetization transfer ratio and myelin in postmortem multiple sclerosis brain. *Ann Neurol.* 2004;56(3):407–415.
19. Dalton CM, Brex PA, Miszkiel KA, et al. Spinal cord MRI in clinically isolated optic neuritis. *J Neurol Neurosurg Psychiatry.* 2003;74(11):1577–1580.
20. Compston A, Coles A. Multiple sclerosis. *Lancet.* 2002;359(9313):1221–1231.
21. Noseworthy JH, Lucchinetti C, Rodriguez M, Weinshenker BG. Multiple sclerosis. *N Engl J Med.* 2000;343(13):938–952.
22. Tench CR, Morgan PS, Jaspan T, Auer DP, Constantinescu CS. Spinal cord imaging in multiple sclerosis. *J Neuroimaging.* 2005;15(suppl 4):94S–102S.
23. Horsfield MA. Magnetization transfer imaging in multiple sclerosis. *J Neuroimaging.* 2005;15(suppl 4):58S–67S.
24. Hickman SJ, Hadjiprocopis A, Coulon O, Miller DH, Barker GJ. Cervical spinal cord MTR histogram analysis in multiple sclerosis using a 3D acquisition and a B-spline active surface segmentation technique. *Magn Reson Imaging.* 2004;22(6):891–895.
25. Rovaris M, Bozzali M, Santuccio G, et al. In vivo assessment of the brain and cervical cord pathology of patients with primary progressive multiple sclerosis. *Brain.* 2001;124(Pt 12):2540–2549.
26. Rovaris M, Bozzali M, Santuccio G, et al. Relative contributions of brain and cervical cord pathology to multiple sclerosis disability: a study with magnetisation transfer ratio histogram analysis. *J Neurol Neurosurg Psychiatry.* 2000;69(6):723–727.
27. Lycklama a Nijeholt GJ, Castelijns JA, Lazeron RH, et al. Magnetization transfer ratio of the spinal cord in multiple sclerosis: relationship to atrophy and neurologic disability. *J Neuroimaging.* 2000;10(2):67–72.
28. Filippi M, Bozzali M, Horsfield MA, et al. A conventional and magnetization transfer MRI study of the cervical cord in patients with MS. *Neurology.* 2000;54(1):207–213.
29. Bot JC, Blezer EL, Kamphorst W, et al. The spinal cord in multiple sclerosis: relationship of high-spatial-resolution quantitative MR

imaging findings to histopathologic results. *Radiology.* 2004; 233(2):531–540.

30. Bozzali M, Rocca MA, Iannucci G, Pereira C, Comi G, Filippi M. Magnetization-transfer histogram analysis of the cervical cord in patients with multiple sclerosis. *AJNR Am J Neuroradiol.* 1999; 20(10):1803–1808.

31. Powers JM, DeCiero DP, Ito M, Moser AB, Moser HW. Adrenomyeloneuropathy: a neuropathologic review featuring its noninflammatory myelopathy. *J Neuropathol Exp Neurol.* 2000; 59(2):89–102.

32. Wingerchuk DM, Lennon VA, Lucchinetti CF, Pittock SJ, Weinshenker BG. The spectrum of neuromyelitis optica. *Lancet Neurol.* 2007;6(9):805–815.

33. Wingerchuk DM, Hogancamp WF, O'Brien PC, Weinshenker BG. The clinical course of neuromyelitis optica (Devic's syndrome). *Neurology.* 1999;53(5):1107–1114.

34. Chan KH, Ramsden DB, Yu YL, et al. Neuromyelitis optica-IgG in idiopathic inflammatory demyelinating disorders amongst Hong Kong Chinese. *Eur J Neurol.* 2009;16(3):310–316.

35. Wingerchuk DM. Neuromyelitis optica: effect of gender. *J Neurol Sci.* 2009;286(1–2):18–23.

36. Filippi M, Rocca MA, Moiola L, et al. MRI and magnetization transfer imaging changes in the brain and cervical cord of patients with Devic's neuromyelitis optica. *Neurology.* 1999;53(8): 1705–1710.

37. Rocca MA, Agosta F, Mezzapesa DM, et al. Magnetization transfer and diffusion tensor MRI show gray matter damage in neuromyelitis optica. *Neurology.* 2004;62(3):476–478.

38. Kim M, Chan A, Mak H, Chan Q, Chan K. *Magnetization Transfer MRI Measurements of Cervical Spinal Cord Abnormalities in Patients with Neuromyelitis Optica.* 2010. Proc ISMRM: 4230, Stockholm, Sweden.

39. McGowan JC, Yang JH, Plotkin RC, et al. Magnetization transfer imaging in the detection of injury associated with mild head trauma. *AJNR Am J Neuroradiol.* 2000;21(5):875–880.

40. McCreary CR, Bjarnason TA, Skihar V, Mitchell JR, Yong VW, Dunn JF. Multiexponential T2 and magnetization transfer MRI of demyelination and remyelination in murine spinal cord. *NeuroImage.* 2009;45(4):1173–1182.

41. Davies GR, Ramani A, Dalton CM, et al. Preliminary magnetic resonance study of the macromolecular proton fraction in white matter: a potential marker of myelin? *Mult Scler.* 2003;9(3):246–249.

42. Schmierer K, Tozer DJ, Scaravilli F, et al. Quantitative magnetization transfer imaging in postmortem multiple sclerosis brain. *J Magn Reson Imaging.* 2007;26(1):41–51.

43. Levesque IR, Pike GB. Characterizing healthy and diseased white matter using quantitative magnetization transfer and multicomponent T(2) relaxometry: a unified view via a four-pool model. *Magn Reson Med.* 2009;62(6):1487–1496.

44. Reich DS, Smith SA, Zackowski KM, et al. Multiparametric magnetic resonance imaging analysis of the corticospinal tract in multiple sclerosis. *NeuroImage.* 2007;38(2):271–279.

45. Cohen-Adad J, El Mendili MM, Morizot-Koutlidis R, et al. Involvement of spinal sensory pathway in ALS and specificity of cord atrophy to lower motor neuron degeneration. *Amyotroph Lateral Scler.* 2013;14(1):30–38.

46. Smith SA, Jones CK, Gifford A, et al. Reproducibility of tract-specific magnetization transfer and diffusion tensor imaging in the cervical spinal cord at 3 tesla. *NMR Biomed.* 2010;23(2):207–217.

47. Hu BS, Conolly SM, Wright GA, Nishimura DG, Macovski A. Pulsed saturation transfer contrast. *Magn Reson Med.* 1992;26(2): 231–240.

48. Schneider E, Prost RW, Glover GH. Pulsed magnetization transfer versus continuous wave irradiation for tissue contrast enhancement. *J Magn Reson Imaging.* 1993;3(2):417–423.

49. Pike GB, Glover GH, Hu BS, Enzmann DR. Pulsed magnetization transfer spin-echo MR imaging. *J Magn Reson Imaging.* 1993;3(3): 531–539.

50. Yeung HN, Aisen AM. Magnetization transfer contrast with periodic pulsed saturation. *Radiology.* 1992;183(1):209–214.

51. Chai JW, Chen C, Chen JH, Lee SK, Yeung HN. Estimation of in vivo proton intrinsic and cross-relaxation rate in human brain. *Magn Reson Med.* 1996;36(1):147–152.

52. Hua J, Hurst GC. Analysis of on- and off-resonance magnetization transfer techniques. *J Magn Reson Imaging.* 1995;5(1):113–120.

53. Cercignani M, Symms MR, Schmierer K, et al. Three-dimensional quantitative magnetisation transfer imaging of the human brain. *NeuroImage.* 2005;27(2):436–441.

54. Ramani A, Dalton C, Miller DH, Tofts PS, Barker GJ. Precise estimate of fundamental in-vivo MT parameters in human brain in clinically feasible times. *Magn Reson Imaging.* 2002;20(10):721–731.

55. Sled JG, Pike GB. Quantitative interpretation of magnetization transfer in spoiled gradient echo MRI sequences. *J Magn Reson.* 2000;145(1):24–36.

56. Bieri O, Scheffler K. Optimized balanced steady-state free precession magnetization transfer imaging. *Magn Reson Med.* 2007; 58(3):511–518.

57. Bieri O, Scheffler K. On the origin of apparent low tissue signals in balanced SSFP. *Magn Reson Med.* 2006;56(5):1067–1074.

58. Henkelman RM, Huang X, Xiang QS, Stanisz GJ, Swanson SD, Bronskill MJ. Quantitative interpretation of magnetization transfer. *Magn Reson Med.* 1993;29(6):759–766.

59. Li JG, Graham SJ, Henkelman RM. A flexible magnetization transfer line shape derived from tissue experimental data. *Magn Reson Med.* 1997;37(6):866–871.

60. Graham SJ, Henkelman RM. Understanding pulsed magnetization transfer. *J Magn Reson Imaging.* 1997;7(5):903–912.

61. Yarnykh VL. Pulsed Z-spectroscopic imaging of cross-relaxation parameters in tissues for human MRI: theory and clinical applications. *Magn Reson Med.* 2002;47(5):929–939.

62. Ou X, Sun SW, Liang HF, Song SK, Gochberg DF. The MT pool size ratio and the DTI radial diffusivity may reflect the myelination in shiverer and control mice. *NMR Biomed.* 2009;22(5):480–487.

63. Ou X, Sun SW, Liang HF, Song SK, Gochberg DF. Quantitative magnetization transfer measured pool-size ratio reflects optic nerve myelin content in ex vivo mice. *Magn Reson Med.* 2009;61(2):364–371.

64. Cercignani M, Barker GJ. A comparison between equations describing in vivo MT: the effects of noise and sequence parameters. *J Magn Reson.* 2008;191(2):171–183.

65. Sled JG, Pike GB. Quantitative imaging of magnetization transfer exchange and relaxation properties in vivo using MRI. *Magn Reson Med.* 2001;46(5):923–931.

66. Portnoy S, Stanisz GJ. Modeling pulsed magnetization transfer. *Magn Reson Med.* 2007;58(1):144–155.

67. Sled JG, Levesque I, Santos AC, et al. Regional variations in normal brain shown by quantitative magnetization transfer imaging. *Magn Reson Med.* 2004;51(2):299–303.

68. Muller DK, Pampel A, Moller HE. *Orientation Dependence of Magnetization Transfer in Human White Matter.* 2010. Proc ISMRM: 2996, Stockholm, Sweden.

69. Giulietti G, Bozzali M, Figura V, et al. Quantitative magnetization transfer provides information complementary to grey matter atrophy in Alzheimer's disease brains. *NeuroImage.* 2012;59(2): 1114–1122.

70. Tofts PS, Steens SC, Cercignani M, et al. Sources of variation in multi-centre brain MTR histogram studies: body-coil transmission eliminates inter-centre differences. *MAGMA.* 2006;19(4):209–222.

71. Cercignani. M, Symms M.R, Boulby P.A, Barker G.J, Quantification of B0 and B1 Effects on the Estimation of MT Parameters at 3.0 T. Proc ISMRM: 3500, Seattle, WA, USA

72. Whittall KP, MacKay AL, Graeb DA, Nugent RA, Li DK, Paty DW. In vivo measurement of T2 distributions and water contents in normal human brain. *Magn Reson Med.* 1997;37(1): 34–43.

73. Stanisz GJ, Kecojevic A, Bronskill MJ, Henkelman RM. Characterizing white matter with magnetization transfer and T(2). *Magn Reson Med.* 1999;42(6):1128–1136.

74. Yarnykh VL, Yuan C. Cross-relaxation imaging reveals detailed anatomy of white matter fiber tracts in the human brain. *NeuroImage.* 2004;23(1):409–424.

75. Morrison C, Henkelman RM. A model for magnetization transfer in tissues. *Magn Reson Med.* 1995;33(4):475–482.

76. Yarnykh VL. Fast macromolecular proton fraction mapping from a single off-resonance magnetization transfer measurement. *Magn Reson Med.* 2012;68(11):166–178.

77. Ropele S, Stollberger R, Hartung HP, Fazekas F. Estimation of magnetization transfer rates from PACE experiments with pulsed RF saturation. *J Magn Reson Imaging.* 2000;12(5):749–756.

78. Henkelman RM, Stanisz GJ, Graham SJ. Magnetization transfer in MRI: a review. *NMR Biomed.* 2001;14(2):57–64.

79. Helms G, Dathe H, Kallenberg K, Dechent P. High-resolution maps of magnetization transfer with inherent correction for RF inhomogeneity and T1 relaxation obtained from 3D FLASH MRI. *Magn Reson Med.* 2008;60(6):1396–1407.

80. Venkatesan R, Lin W, Haacke EM. Accurate determination of spin-density and T1 in the presence of RF-field inhomogeneities and flip-angle miscalibration. *Magn Reson Med.* 1998;40(4): 592–602.

81. Samson RS, Ciccarelli O, Kachramanoglou C, et al. Multi-parameter mapping of the human cervical cord at 3.0 T in less than 20 minutes. *Proc Intl Soc Mag Reson Med.* Montreal, Canada; 2011: 2754.

82. Yiannakas MC, Kearney H, Samson RS, et al. Feasibility of grey matter and white matter segmentation of the upper cervical cord in vivo: a pilot study with application to magnetisation transfer measurements. *NeuroImage.* 2012;63(3):1054–1059.

83. Ward KM, Aletras AH, Balaban RS. A new class of contrast agents for MRI based on proton chemical exchange dependent saturation transfer (CEST). *J Magn Reson.* 2000;143(1):79–87.

84. Goffeney N, Bulte JW, Duyn J, Bryant Jr LH, van Zijl PC. Sensitive NMR detection of cationic-polymer-based gene delivery systems using saturation transfer via proton exchange. *J Am Chem Soc.* 2001;123(35):8628–8629.

85. Zhou J, van Zijl PC. Chemical exchange saturation transfer imaging and spectroscopy. *Progr NMR Spectr.* 2006;48(2–3):109–136.

86. Zhang S, Merritt M, Woessner DE, Lenkinski RE, Sherry AD. PARACEST agents: modulating MRI contrast via water proton exchange. *Acc Chem Res.* 2003;36(10):783–790.

87. Aime S, Barge A, Delli Castelli D, et al. Paramagnetic lanthanide(III) complexes as pH-sensitive chemical exchange saturation transfer (CEST) contrast agents for MRI applications. *Magn Reson Med.* 2002;47(4):639–648.

88. Yoo B, Pagel MD. A PARACEST MRI contrast agent to detect enzyme activity. *J Am Chem Soc.* 2006;128(43):14032–14033.

89. Liu G, Li Y, Pagel MD. Design and characterization of a new irreversible responsive PARACEST MRI contrast agent that detects nitric oxide. *Magn Reson Med.* 2007;58(6):1249–1256.

90. Zhou J, Payen JF, Wilson DA, Traystman RJ, van Zijl PC. Using the amide proton signals of intracellular proteins and peptides to detect pH effects in MRI. *Nat Med.* 2003;9(8):1085–1090.

91. van Zijl PC, Zhou J, Mori N, Payen JF, Wilson D, Mori S. Mechanism of magnetization transfer during on-resonance water saturation. A new approach to detect mobile proteins, peptides, and lipids. *Magn Reson Med.* 2003;49(3):440–449.

92. Zhou J, Lal B, Wilson DA, Laterra J, van Zijl PC. Amide proton transfer (APT) contrast for imaging of brain tumors. *Magn Reson Med.* 2003;50(6):1120–1126.

93. Ling W, Regatte RR, Navon G, Jerschow A. Assessment of glycosaminoglycan concentration in vivo by chemical exchange-dependent saturation transfer (gagCEST). *Proc Natl Acad Sci USA.* 2008;105(7):2266–2270.

94. Bryant RG. The dynamics of water-protein interactions. *Annu Rev Biophys Biomol Struct.* 1996;25:29–53.

95. Ward KM, Balaban RS. Determination of pH using water protons and chemical exchange dependent saturation transfer (CEST). *Magn Reson Med.* 2000;44(5):799–802.

96. Snoussi K, Bulte JW, Gueron M, van Zijl PC. Sensitive CEST agents based on nucleic acid imino proton exchange: detection of poly(rU) and of a dendrimer-poly(rU) model for nucleic acid delivery and pharmacology. *Magn Reson Med.* 2003;49(6): 998–1005.

97. Aime S, Delli Castelli D, Lawson D, Terreno E. Gd-loaded liposomes as T1, susceptibility, and CEST agents, all in one. *J Am Chem Soc.* 2007;129(9):2430–2431.

98. Zhang S, Winter P, Wu K, Sherry AD. A novel europium(III)-based MRI contrast agent. *J Am Chem Soc.* 2001; 123(7):1517–1518.

99. Woods M, Woessner DE, Zhao P, et al. Europium(III) macrocyclic complexes with alcohol pendant groups as chemical exchange saturation transfer agents. *J Am Chem Soc.* 2006;128(31): 10155–10162.

100. Saar G, Zhang B, Ling W, Regatte RR, Navon G, Jerschow A. Assessment of glycosaminoglycan concentration changes in the intervertebral disc via chemical exchange saturation transfer. *NMR Biomed.* 2012;25(2):255–261.

101. Gilad AA, McMahon MT, Walczak P, et al. Artificial reporter gene providing MRI contrast based on proton exchange. *Nat Biotechnol.* 2007;25(2):217–219.

102. van Zijl PC, Jones CK, Ren J, Malloy CR, Sherry AD. MRI detection of glycogen in vivo by using chemical exchange saturation transfer imaging (glycoCEST). *Proc Natl Acad Sci USA.* 2007;104(11):4359–4364.

103. Kim M, Chan Q, Anthony MP, Cheung KM, Samartzis D, Khong PL. Assessment of glycosaminoglycan distribution in human lumbar intervertebral discs using chemical exchange saturation transfer at 3 T: feasibility and initial experience. *NMR Biomed.* 2011;24(9):1137–1144.

104. Zhou J, Tryggestad E, Wen Z, et al. Differentiation between glioma and radiation necrosis using molecular magnetic resonance imaging of endogenous proteins and peptides. *Nat Med.* 2011; 17(1):130–134.

105. Sun PZ, Zhou J, Sun W, Huang J, van Zijl PC. Detection of the ischemic penumbra using pH-weighted MRI. *J Cereb Blood Flow Metab.* 2007;27(6):1129–1136.

106. Dula AN, Asche EM, Landman BA, et al. Development of chemical exchange saturation transfer at 7 T. *Magn Reson Med.* 2011;66(3):831–838.

107. van Zijl PC, Yadav NN. Chemical exchange saturation transfer (CEST): what is in a name and what isn't? *Magn Reson Med.* 2011; 65(4):927–948.

108. Kim M, Gillen J, Landman BA, Zhou J, van Zijl PC. Water saturation shift referencing (WASSR) for chemical exchange saturation transfer (CEST) experiments. *Magn Reson Med.* 2009;61(6): 1441–1450.

109. Sun PZ, Farrar CT, Sorensen AG. Correction for artifacts induced by B(0) and B(1) field inhomogeneities in pH-sensitive chemical exchange saturation transfer (CEST) imaging. *Magn Reson Med.* 2007;58(6):1207–1215.

110. Varma G, Lenkinski RE, Vinogradov E. Keyhole chemical exchange saturation transfer. *Magn Reson Med*. 2012;68(4): 1228–1233.

111. Zhou J, Blakeley JO, Hua J, et al. Practical data acquisition method for human brain tumor amide proton transfer (APT) imaging. *Magn Reson Med*. 2008;60(4):842–849.

112. Zhu H, Gillen J.S, Barker P.B, van Zijl P.C, Zhou J. 3D Amide Proton Transfer (APT) Imaging of the Whole Brain at 3 T 2009. Proc ISMRM: 4475, Honolulu, Hawaii, USA.

113. Stancanello J, Terreno E, Castelli DD, Cabella C, Uggeri F, Aime S. Development and validation of a smoothing-splines-based correction method for improving the analysis of CEST-MR images. *Contrast Media Mol Imaging*. 2008;3(4):136–149.

114. Pekar J, Jezzard P, Roberts DA, Leigh Jr JS, Frank JA, McLaughlin AC. Perfusion imaging with compensation for asymmetric magnetization transfer effects. *Magn Reson Med*. 1996; 35(1):70–79.

115. Swanson SD. Protein mediated magnetic coupling between lactate and water protons. *J Magn Reson*. 1998;135(1):248–255.

116. Ng MC, Hua J, Hu Y, Luk KD, Lam EY. Magnetization transfer (MT) asymmetry around the water resonance in human cervical spinal cord. *J Magn Reson Imaging*. 2009;29(3):523–528.

117. Dula AN, Dortch RD, Landman BA, Gore JC, Smith SA. *Application of Chemical Exchange Saturation Transfer (CEST) Imaging to Examine Amide Proton Transfer (APT) in the Spinal Cord at 3 T*. 2011. Proc ISMRM: 407, Montreal Canada.

118. Agosta, et al. Associations between cervical cord gray matter damage and disability in patients with multiple sclerosis. *Archives of Neurology*. 2007;64(9):1302–1305.

119. Lycklama à Nijeholt GJ, Barkhof F, Castelijns JA, van Waesberghe JH, Valk J, Jongen PJ, Hommes OR. Comparison of two MR sequences for the detection of multiple sclerosis lesions in the spinal cord. *AJNR Am J Neuroradiol*. 1996 Sep;17(8): 1533–1538.

120. Yoshioka H, Nishimura H, Masuda T, Nakajima K, Onaya H, Itai Y. Magnetization transfer contrast imaging of the cervical spine at 0.3 T. *J Comput Assist Tomogr*. 1994 Nov-Dec;18(6): 947–953.

T_2 Relaxation

Cornelia Laule[1,2], *Alex MacKay*[1,3]

[1]Radiology Department [2]Pathology and Laboratory Medicine Department
[3]Physics & Astronomy Department, University of British Columbia, Vancouver, Canada

3.5.1 OVERVIEW

T_2-weighted imaging plays a key role in clinical MR imaging of spinal cord. While T_2 weighting is highly sensitive, it is notoriously unspecific as very different pathological conditions can lead to similar increases in water content that result in similar T_2 increases. Therefore, T_2-weighted imaging should be considered a qualitative clinical tool; however, if the full T_2 decay curve from spinal cord is acquired, there is an opportunity to extract quantitative pathological information about the spinal cord.

This chapter provides an overview of T_2 relaxation and its application to both normal and pathological spinal cord. The aim is to introduce the concept of T_2 relaxation and describe how T_2 can be measured as well as interpreted. We present a summary of significant results obtained from T_2 measurements in the spinal cord and conclude with practical recommendations for the implementation of quantitative T_2 relaxation measurements.

3.5.2 T_2 RELAXATION IN CNS TISSUE

T_2, the spin–spin relaxation time (or transverse relaxation time), describes the irreversible decay of the MR signal in the transverse plane. Immediately following an excitation pulse (e.g., 90°), the MR signal is maximum because all of the protons are aligned with each other. However, the signal strength decays to zero at a rate $(1/T_2^*)$ determined by the magnetic field distribution or the chemical shift distribution of the spins. By following the excitation pulse with a 180° pulse, signal dephasing caused by an inhomogenous magnetic field and/or a chemical shift dispersion can be refocused to produce an echo. The height of this spin echo is determined by irreversible processes; it decreases exponentially with time from the excitation pulse with time constant T_2.

In this chapter we describe T_2 relaxation in two ways, first presenting an intuitive picture of the T_2 process in tissue and then providing a mechanistic description of T_2 relaxation.

3.5.2.1 Intuitive Description of T_2 Relaxation

The complete MR signal from spinal cord tissue contains contributions from protons in water and from protons in nonaqueous tissue. It has been demonstrated[1,2] that the signal from water in central nervous system tissue has T_2 relaxation times greater than 10 ms and that the signal from nonaqueous tissue decays to zero in one ms or less. MRI scanners can readily assess signals with T_2 times longer than 10 ms; therefore, it is possible to accurately characterize T_2 relaxation of the water in the spinal cord by measuring the T_2 decay curve.

T_2 relaxation in the spinal cord is complicated by the fact that within a typical imaging voxel volume of a few cubic millimeter, structure at a cellular level is inhomogenous. For example, glial cells have single plasma membranes while myelinated neurons contain many membranes in close proximity. This microscopic heterogeneity results in different relaxation behaviors for water protons in different environments within a single voxel. From perusal of high resolution cross-sectional electron micrographs of CNS tissue (Figure 3.5.1), one can visualize three distinct water reservoirs: intracellular water, extracellular water, and water trapped between the bilayers of the myelin sheaths. Because water interactions with nonaqueous tissue are most pronounced in myelin due to the tightly confined space between myelin bilayers, myelin water in spinal cord has a relatively short T_2 time of 10–20 ms. Intra- and extracellular water, which is not in as close association with nonaqueous tissue as myelin water, have a longer T_2. Although intra- and extracellular spaces are physically different, they have

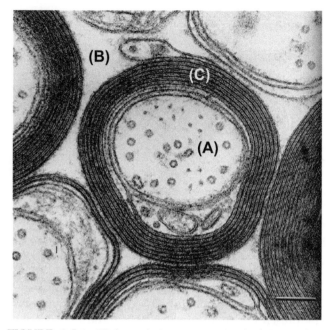

FIGURE 3.5.1 High resolution cross-sectional electron micrographs of CNS tissue. Three distinct water reservoirs are visible: (A) intracellular water, (B) extracellular water, and (C) water trapped between the bilayers of the myelin sheaths. *Source: Reprinted with kind permission from Springer Science+Business Media B.V. Raine CS. Morphology of Myelin and Myelination. In Morell P, ed. Myelin, 2nd ed. New York: Plenum Press, 1984: 12.*

similar T_2s of around 70–90 ms at 1.5 T and cannot be measured separately.[3,4] Therefore, T_2 relaxation measurements in spinal cord yield two T_2 components, one at 10–15 ms and one at approximately 80 ms. The fraction of MR signal in the myelin water component is known as the myelin water fraction (MWF). This fraction, as expected, is substantially larger in white matter than gray matter.[5] In previous studies on fixed brain samples, MWF was found to correlate strongly with histological stains for myelin lipids.[6,7] The MWF in white matter of the spinal cord is approximately twice as large as MWF values in brain,[3,4] which may reflect physiological variations.[8] The term *myelin water imaging* has been used to describe quantitative T_2 relaxation studies focused on the myelin water component.

In addition to the presence of multiple water environments, an even further complication in the spinal cord is that boundaries between water environments are blurred due to translational diffusion. Water molecules in pure water or dilute solutions undergo random motion, moving an average distance of $R = (6D\tau)^{1/2}$ in time τ,[9] where D is the water diffusion coefficient. For a typical MR image obtained with an echo time (TE) = 60 ms, free water in a solution moves over 30 microns. The barriers present in the spinal cord reduce water diffusion coefficients on average to about 1/4 that in free water, and water molecules move on average about 20 microns in 60 ms. Due to diffusion,

parameters derived by MR techniques are averaged over their values during the timescale of the measurement. See Chapter 3.1 for more detailed information of diffusion and diffusion anisotropy in the cord.

3.5.2.2 Mechanistic Description of T_2 Relaxation

For a simple spin system consisting of a molecule with a single proton site, T_2 is understood quantitatively[10,11] in terms of fluctuating magnetic fields produced by adjacent protons undergoing molecular motions. When protons are located on molecules that reorient rapidly due to molecular tumbling and translational diffusion, they produce oscillating magnetic fields. Molecular motions, which are driven by the inherent kinetic energy of the molecules, are characterized by a correlation time, τ_c, which is the time required for the molecule to undergo a substantial reorientation. The fluctuating magnetic fields caused by these molecular motions cause T_2 relaxation. The dependence of T_2 on the correlation time of molecular motions and the Larmor frequency is quantitatively expressed in Eqn (3.5.1). The constant, K, is related to the strength of the interactions between adjacent protons.

$$\frac{1}{T_2} = K\left(\frac{3}{2}\tau_c + \frac{\frac{5}{2}\tau_c}{1 + (\omega_o\tau_c)^2} + \frac{\tau_c}{1 + (2\omega_o\tau_c)^2}\right) \quad (3.5.1)$$

Equation (3.5.1) shows that T_2 is sensitive to rapid molecular motions at the Larmor frequency, ω_o, and twice the Larmor frequency. T_2 is also influenced by low frequency motions that cause the term $3/2 \tau_c$ to become large, thereby explaining why T_2 is particularly sensitive to slow motions. It turns out that for very fast motions, like free water tumbling, the $3/2 \tau_c$ term is negligible and $T_2 = T_1$, which holds for relaxation in cerebrospinal fluid (CSF)[12] (where T_1 is defined as $1/T_1 = K(\tau_c/(1 + \omega_o^2\tau_c^2) + 4\tau_c/(1 + 4\omega_o^2\tau_c^2)))$. In the presence of slow fluctuations below the Larmor frequency (64 MHz at 1.5 T), T_2 is shorter than T_1.

The model for relaxation described herein holds for simple spin systems such as water solutions but is unable to quantitatively characterize relaxation in the spinal cord, which contains multiple proton environments. Relaxation times for water in CNS tissue are strongly influenced by interactions between water and nonaqueous protons attached to lipids, proteins, and nucleic acids. In the spinal cord, water protons interact with other protons attached to molecules moving at a wide range of different frequencies (e.g., low frequencies arising from very slow macromolecular reorientations to high

MECHANISMS OF T_2 RELAXATION IN THE SPINAL CORD

In the healthy spinal cord, two components are distinguishable by T_2 relaxation:

1. a short T_2 component assigned to water between the bilayers of the myelin sheath.
2. a longer T_2 component assigned to water in the intra- and extracellular spaces.

Because myelin water undergoes much more interaction with nonaqueous tissue, it has a shorter T_2 time than that of the intra- and extracellular water components. The myelin water fraction (MWF) is the proportion of spinal cord water with short T_2. The signals from intra- and extracellular water cannot be separated on the basis of T_2 time.

frequencies arising from fast small molecule tumbling). As a consequence, T_2 times are shorter than T_1 times.

3.5.2.3 Measurement of T_2 Relaxation

The first step in a quantitative T_2 study is the acquisition of high-fidelity T_2 decay curves. The T_2 decay curve is a plot of MR signal versus TE (time to echo). The Carr–Purcell–Meiboom–Gill sequence,[13,14] which consists of a 90° excitation pulse followed by a series of equally spaced 180° refocusing pulses, is the most common technique for measuring T_2 times in vivo, typically with 32 echoes from TE of 10 ms to TE of 320 ms. Estimated T_2 times may depend upon the echo spacing of the multi-echo sequence. The echo spacing dependence of T_2 arises due to events that occur during the interval between the 180° refocusing pulses, for example, diffusion of water between regions of different magnetic susceptibility.[15,16] Producing accurate T_2 decay curves in vivo is challenging because it requires accurate refocusing pulses in the presence of magnetic field and radio-frequency field inhomogeneities. An effective solution for single slice approaches (discussed following) is to apply composite rectangular radio-frequency refocusing pulses flanked by large gradient pulses that alternate in sign and decrease in height with echo time.[17] The composite radio-frequency pulses provide robust 180° flip angles and the gradient pulses are required to eliminate contribution to the signal from spins located outside the selected slice. An example of a T_2 decay curve from spinal cord is shown in Figure 3.5.2.

Initial in vivo implementations of T_2 measurements in both brain[18] and spinal cord[3] made use of the

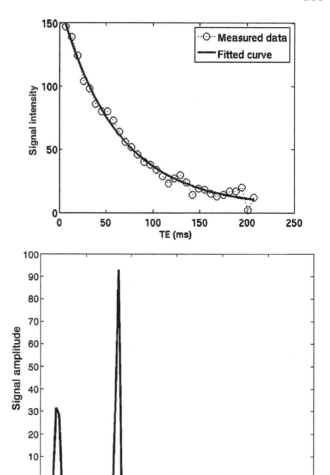

FIGURE 3.5.2 Example of T_2 distribution from spinal cord by Wu et al.[3] *Source: Reprinted from Wolters Kluwer Lippincott Williams & Wilkins.*

previously described rectangular refocusing pulses combined with large-gradient crusher lobes. This approach was sufficient for proof of concept and for addressing focused research questions; however, because it required over 20 min to produce a single slice, it had limited clinical applicability. This 2D multi-echo single slice pulse sequence cannot simply be extended to a multislice acquisition because the various microscopic environments in CNS tissue are affected differently by magnetization transfer resulting from the off-resonance slice selective refocusing pulses from neighboring slices.[19] Several different approaches have since been employed to make myelin water imaging available in a clinically relevant imaging time. These include: a 3D-multiple spin echo sequence,[20] a 3D gradient echo sequence,[21,22] and a TE-prepared spiral sequence.[23–25]

An additional technique that has been proposed to assess myelin water uses steady state sequences.[26] The steady state approach for extracting T_2

information from spinal cord is conceptually very different from the multiple spin echo approach. Multicomponent-driven equilibrium single pulse observation of T_1 and T_2 (mcDESPOT)[26] makes use of three sequences: spoiled gradient echo, inversion-prepared spoiled gradient echo, and balanced steady state free precession. The strength of the mcDESPOT approach is the relatively faster and higher resolution data acquisition; each sequence is run at several different flip angles, and the entire protocol takes about 26 min for cervical cord coverage with $1 \times 1 \times 1.5$ mm^3 isotropic voxels. However, a disadvantage of the mcDESPOT approach is the complex and somewhat constrained analysis, discussed in the following section.

Most myelin water imaging to date has been carried out in brain, and application to the spinal cord presents significant challenges. For example, the well-documented magnetic field inhomogeneities in spinal cord (see Chapter 2.1) are expected to make it very difficult, if not impossible, to use T_2^*-based approaches. To date, only multiple spin echo and steady state sequences have been reported for measuring myelin water in spinal cord.

3.5.2.4 Analysis of T_2 Relaxation

For single-component T_2 relaxation, the T_2 decay curve follows:

$$S(\text{TE}) = S(\text{TE} = 0)e^{\frac{-\text{TE}}{T_2}} \qquad (3.5.2)$$

However, as mentioned before, the water environment in the spinal cord is inhomogenous. The T_2 decay curve contains contributions from myelin water and also intra- and extracellular water; therefore, the T_2 analysis must deal with multiple T_2 components. Equation (3.5.2) then becomes:

$$S(\text{TE}) = \sum S_i e^{\frac{-\text{TE}}{T_{2i}}}. \qquad (3.5.3)$$

Inversion of Eqn (3.5.3) for estimation of component amplitudes and relaxation times, S_i and T_{2i}, is an ill-posed problem, which means that there is not a unique solution.[27] Quite different combinations of S_is and T_{2i}s can fit the data equally well; this is a consequence of the fact that exponential functions, unlike sine waves, do not form an orthogonal basis set. The most conservative approach (and the most common approach in the literature) for solving Eqn (3.5.3) is to minimize the number of a priori assumptions about the solution. The non-negative least squares (NNLS) approach assumes only that (1) the S_is are positive and (2) Eqn

(3.5.3) fits the data.[27] It makes no assumptions about the number of exponential components; this is a fundamental requirement for robust decay curve fitting, since the number of contributing components in the spinal cord is unknown a priori, especially in the presence of pathology. The NNLS algorithm uses χ^2 minimization to fit the relaxation decay curve to a large number of T_2 components. NNLS produces a T_2 distribution consisting of a few discrete spikes; however, most investigators prefer a smooth distribution. A continuous distribution can be achieved by minimizing χ^2 as well as a regularizer. A common regularizer is the sum of the squares of the solution amplitudes—the so-called "small model".[27] An example of a T_2 distribution from spinal cord tissue can be seen in Figure 3.5.2.

The myelin water fraction is defined as the area under the myelin water peak of the T_2 distribution divided by the total area under the T_2 distribution. At 1.5 T, MR signal, $S(T_2)$, with T_2 between 10 and 40 ms, is assigned to myelin water. At 3 T, this region has been contracted to 10–35 ms to minimize contributions from intra- and extracellular water. The geometric mean T_2 (GMT$_2$) time for each peak is estimated by evaluating the following equation:

$$\text{GMT}_2 = e^{\frac{\int S(T_2)\log(T_2)\, dT_2}{\int S(T_2)\, dT_2}} \qquad (3.5.4)$$

where $S(T_2)$ is the T_2 distribution and the integral limits are chosen to cover the T_2 peak of interest. For the intra/extracellular water peak, the integral is usually acquired from 40 to 200 ms. The GMT$_2$ is the mean T_2 on a logarithmic scale. An interesting property of the GMT$_2$ is that it is the reciprocal of the GM$(1/T_2)$.[28]

An alternative approach to dealing with multicomponent relaxation curves is to use nonlinear curve-fitting techniques.[21,29–32] In many applications, researchers have simultaneously fit T_1 and T_2 relaxation times.[30–32] The nonlinear fitting approach requires more a priori information; however, if the a priori information is accurate, this approach may result in more robust solutions.

At magnetic fields larger than 1.5 T, it is well known that, due to dielectric effects,[33] the B_1 field in tissue is not homogenous. As a result, the refocusing pulses in the multi-echo train are not necessarily 180°, and the decay curve no longer follows Eqn (3.5.3). In particular, the early echoes have amplitudes that exhibit an odd/even oscillation.[34] Fortunately, it is possible to understand these oscillations quantitatively in terms of stimulated echoes, which occur after magnetization is temporarily placed along the z axis by suboptimal 180° pulses.[35–37] In fact, it is possible to extract not only the T_2 distribution but also the B_1 distribution by making use of the extended phase graph algorithm.[35–37]

The analysis of mcDESPOT data, instead, involves fitting the data with a constrained model with, typically, two water components. The fitting process is complex, involving at least six parameters, i.e., T_1, T_2, relative amplitudes, and residence times for each component. This fitting process, which may employ a genetic algorithm or stochastic regional contraction, does converge, yielding myelin water maps as well as relaxation time maps and B_0 and B_1 maps. For reasons that are not yet understood, in brain mcDESPOT results differ substantially from multiple spin echo values, but in the spinal cord the two approaches yield similar findings.[38] However, the mcDESPOT analysis method and results derived from it must be interpreted with caution, as discussed in a very recent paper by Lankford and Does.[39] The authors produced theoretical calculations of the Cramer-Rao lower bounds of the variance of fitted model using a variety of model system parameters, meant to mimic those expected in human white matter. The results indicated that mcDESPOT signals acquired at feasibly attainable signal-to-noise ratios cannot provide parameter estimates with useful levels of precision. While precision can be greatly improved by constraining solutions with a priori information, this could lead to biased parameter estimates. The authors concluded that mcDESPOT-derived estimates of two-pool model parameters cannot yet be unambiguously related to specific tissue characteristics.

The use of T_2 relaxation to learn about the spinal cord is an emerging field; to our knowledge only 12 papers have reported quantitative measurements of T_2 in the spinal cord. The following sections summarize preclinical and human T_2 relaxation studies to date.

3.5.3 PRECLINICAL T_2 RELAXATION STUDIES IN THE SPINE

3.5.3.1 Initial Observation of Myelin Water Signal in the Spinal Cord

The first spinal cord T_2 relaxation study that observed a myelin water signal was conducted in the early 1990s by Stewart et al.[1] (Table 3.5.1). At the time of this work, the usefulness of T_2 relaxation to characterize pathology was under debate, but the authors postulated that with not only careful and systematic measurement, but also appropriate analysis, MR relaxation times could indeed yield important information about tissue and tissue pathology. In particular, the goal of their work was to demonstrate that quantitative MR can be used to distinguish the different types of pathology seen in multiple sclerosis (MS). They used a 4320 echo CPMG pulse sequence to measure proton T_2 values in the spinal cord from Hartley guinea pigs inoculated to produce experimental allergic encephalomyelitis (EAE), the animal model of MS. In order to collect a very large number of points for the relaxation decay curve and negate the possible effects of localization techniques, experiments were conducted ex vivo on a modified Bruker SXP 4-100 NMR spectrometer operating at 2.1 T (90 MHz for protons). Up until that point, the majority of previous studies had restricted the tissue proton relaxation decay curves to be composed of one, two, or three discrete exponential components. However, as recent studies analyzed relaxation decay curves in terms of continuous distributions of relaxation times,[27,40,41] the authors suggested that since this approach makes fewer a priori assumptions, it may be more appropriate when trying to characterize the complex nature of tissues.

Stewart et al. analyzed their data using both a nonlinear functional minimization program (Minuit)[42]

T_2 RELAXATION MEASUREMENT AND ANALYSIS

Spin echo techniques: To date, most T_2 measurements in vivo have made use of multiple echo spin echo sequences followed by fitting of the decay curves with multiple exponential components to produce a T_2 distribution. The T_2 distributions from white matter contain at least two peaks that are assigned to myelin water and intra/extracellular water. Histological validation studies provide evidence that myelin water is quantitatively related to myelin content. The advantages of this approach are limited a priori assumptions, however, the technique involves a lengthy data acquisition and is signal-to-noise limited.

Steady state techniques: mcDESPOT has the advantage of more rapid data acquisition and analysis with an explicit model that includes T_1, T_2, as well as exchange parameters. However, results obtained from the steady state approach may be biased due to the constraints required in order to enable the solutions to converge, and caution should be taken when interpreting results. No histological validation studies have been conducted.

TABLE 3.5.1   Summary of Preclinical T_2 Relaxation Studies in the Spinal Cord

Study	Study Population	Sequence	Coil	TR (ms)	TE (ms)	Field Strength (T)	Acquired Voxel Size (In-plane; Thickness)	Acquisition Time (min)
Stewart[1]	Guinea pig ($n = 12$)	4320 echo CPMG	1-cm i.d. four-turn and 6-cm-long solenoid coil	10,000	0.4	2.1	n/a (NMR)	70
Kozlowski[44]	Rat (ex vivo: $n = 10$, in vivo: $n = 1$)	32 echo CPMG	2-cm i.d. four-turn solenoid coil (ex vivo) 3-cm i.d. circular surface coil (in vivo)	1500	6.673	7	100, 78, and 61 µm; 1 mm 117 µm; 1.5 mm	38
Kozlowski[45]	Rat ($n = 15$)	32 echo CPMG	Four-turn, 13-mm i.d. and 20-mm-long solenoid coil	1500	6.673	7	78 µm; 1 mm	38
McCreary[54]	Mouse ($n = 10$)	64 echo spin echo	35-mm-diameter birdcage coil	3000	5	9.4	150 µm; 0.75 mm	6.4
Minty[4]	Cow ($n = 18$)	32 echo CPMG 4320 echo CPMG	TR head coil 1 cm i.d. four-turn and 6-cm-long solenoid coil	3000 10,000	10 0.4	1.5 2.1	0.94 mm; 3 mm n/a (NMR)	25.6 70
Dula[64]	Rat ($n = 6$)	48 echo spin echo	10-mm-diameter loop gap coil	6000	9.2 ms for first 32 echoes, then 50 ms for the last 16 echoes	7	0.78 mm; 2 mm	77
Harkins[66]	Rat ($n = 5$)	32 echo IR-prepped spin echo	38 mm Litz quadrature coil	6000	9 ms for first 24 echoes, then 50 ms for the last 8 echoes	9.4	0.2 mm; 1.5 mm	102.4

i.d. = inner diameter; *All studies used NNLS for analysis. All imaging studies were collected in the axial plane.

where decay curves were fitted by the sum of a *specified* number of exponential components, the optimum number of which was chosen to be the minimum number that adequately described the data, and using a non-negative least squares algorithm (NNLS)[27] whereby no a priori assumptions were introduced about the number of contributing components. Using Minuit, three exponentials provided the best fit to spinal cord data (10 ms (13%), 76 ms (57%), 215 ms (30%)). However, not only did discrete NNLS analyses give lower χ^2 (goodness of fit) values than the nonlinear Minuit discrete treatment, but two spikes were often observed on either side of the T_2 obtained using Minuit, suggesting a distribution of T_2 amplitudes rather than a discrete value. Smooth NNLS solutions consisted of two broad peaks, a small peak with a T_2 near 10 ms and a larger peak near 100 ms. The smooth solutions were examined for features that could possibly distinguish between the normal and abnormal tissue states. The average relaxation time was calculated in a variety of ways including the median, mode, and weighted arithmetic, geometric, and harmonic means. Of these, the weighted geometric mean seemed to be the best indicator of pathology. Stewart et al. determined the marker with the best diagnostic potential was the "integral ratio" of the larger secondary peak size to the smaller fast-relaxing component.

Stewart et al. concluded that the smooth NNLS results support a model with two distinct reservoirs of water in CNS tissue: one with a T_2 near 10–20 ms with approximately 17% of the total water, and the other a broad peak with T_2 from about 50 to 300 ms, which included all the other water. The assignment of the T_2 peak near 10 ms to myelin water was the first of its kind for spinal cord tissue. At the time, findings were in agreement with two other ex vivo studies that examined human and cat brain.[2,41] Furthermore, the amplitude of the myelin water signal decreased with the extent of demyelination, as evidenced by histology, and the absence of change in the short T_2 component after tissue homogenization was consistent with evidence from the literature that homogenization leaves the myelin layers intact.[43] The usefulness of quantitative T_2 assessment was however not deemed to be limited to the study of the myelin water signal, as Stewart et al. stated that the width of the longer T_2 peak associated with the bulk of the water in CNS tissue is a qualitative measure of inhomogeneity in cell size, cytoplasmic content, and extracellular space in the tissue.

3.5.3.2 High-Resolution Myelin Water Maps Reveal Anatomical Distribution of White and Gray Matter in Formalin-Fixed Injured Spinal Cord

Several decades after the myelin water signal was initially observed in spinal cord tissue by Stewart et al., Kozlowski and colleagues used quantitative T_2 measurement to study models of spinal cord injury in rats.[44,45] This group was the first to create spinal cord *myelin water maps*, which highlighted the anatomical distribution of myelin water within the white and gray matter of the spinal cord. Given that white matter damage is largely responsible for the functional loss observed following spinal cord injury and that significant effort has been directed at developing therapies to rebuild myelin at the injury site, Kozlowski et al. were motivated by the potential value of myelin water imaging as a noninvasive myelin marker to assess spinal cord injury treatment.

Their initial pilot study demonstrated the feasibility of high spatial resolution myelin water measurements in both control and dorsal column transection–injured rat formalin-fixed spinal cords ex vivo, and a single control animal in vivo.[44] Myelin water measurements were carried out at 7 T using a 32-echo single-slice, multi-echo CPMG sequence. For ex vivo measurements, a 2-cm inner diameter (i.d.) four-turn solenoid coil was used for pulse transmission and signal reception, while for the in vivo experiment a 3-cm i.d. circular surface coil was employed. Total acquisition time for six averages was 38 min, and very high in-plane spatial resolution was achieved with 100, 78, and 61 μm ex vivo and 117 μm in vivo. Voxel-wise T_2 distributions were calculated from the multi-echo data using NNLS, and myelin water maps were generated by integrating the T_2 distribution regime assigned to myelin water (7.75–20 ms) and dividing the result by the total integral of the T_2 distribution in each pixel. Both in vivo and ex vivo myelin water maps clearly demonstrated the characteristic gray matter "butterfly" shape with the center gray matter portion of the spinal cord showing markedly reduced myelin, while the surrounding peripheral white matter exhibited high signal corresponding to higher myelin content. The average MWF values from in vivo GM and WM were 5% and 24%, respectively, which corresponded well with previously reported values and expected amounts of myelin in rat spinal cord. However, signal-to-noise ratio (SNR) within the in vivo cord was less than optimal, and the authors suggested SNR could be significantly improved by using a small surface RF coil surgically implanted against the spinal cord.[46] Although in vivo reproducibility was not assessed, excellent reproducibility of the myelin water measurements in excised control spinal cords was demonstrated by small standard deviations for MWF and average T_2. Quantitative correlation analysis between MWF and Luxol fast blue staining for myelin revealed a strong relationship between MWF and LFB optical density ($R^2 = 0.95$ for all data, $R^2 = 0.89$ for dorsal white matter only, $R^2 = 0.48$ for lateral white matter only), providing evidence of MWF specificity for myelin.

Myelin water maps from injured cord that underwent dorsal column transection demonstrated injury morphology very well—reduced myelin at the injury site was apparent from the lack of myelin water in the dorsal part of the spinal cord, while lateral and ventral white matter tracts appeared intact on the myelin water images. Examination of images revealed that 5 mm cranially to the injury site large amounts of myelin debris were formed that displayed as increased signal on the myelin basic protein stained images, as well as a high intensity area on the myelin water map. The debris, and corresponding increased myelin staining and myelin water fraction, was still present 18 days post injury, importantly suggesting that myelin water imaging is not specific for only intact myelin, but rather total myelin content, an observation also reported by Webb et al. in peripheral nerve.[47]

3.5.3.3 Temporal Evolution of Myelin Water in Injured Spinal Cord In Vivo

In a follow-up study, Kozlowski et al. demonstrated for the first time that quantitative T_2 can be used to characterize the temporal evolution of white matter damage following dorsal column transection injury in rat spinal cords. In particular, MWF maps were generated with sufficiently high spatial resolution to highlight myelin damage in specific major dorsal column tracts. The authors used a cervical dorsal column transection injury model as it allows for a clean distinction of damaged (degenerating) tracts in the injured spinal cord. In particular, the descending CST degenerated *caudal* to the lesion, while the ascending sensory axons in the gracile fascicle degenerated *cranial* to injury. Formalin-fixed spinal cords from 15 rats were examined in three groups: injury group studied 3 weeks post injury ($n = 5$), injury group studied 8 weeks post injury ($n = 4$), and control group ($n = 6$). Myelin water measurements on excised cord were carried out at 7 T using a four-turn, 13-mm i.d. and 20-mm-long solenoid coil with a 32-echo single-slice, multi-echo CPMG sequence. As in Kozlowski's preliminary study,[44] total acquisition time for six averages with in-plane spatial resolution of $78 \times 78\ \mu m$ was 38 min. Average values of myelin water fraction were calculated in the fasciculus gracilis, fasciculus cuneatus, and the dorsal CST 5 mm cranial, as well as 5 and 10 mm caudal to injury and correlated with histology.

The high resolution myelin water maps showed contrast between the CST and other WM tracks in the dorsal column in control animals (Figure 3.5.3). Corresponding MBP stained sections clearly showed there was less myelin in CST than in the other WM tracks in the dorsal column (particularly in the fasciculus cuneatus, but also the fasciculus gracilis to some degree, as well). Kozlowski et al. found the fasciculus gracilis at 5 mm cranial to injury exhibited a marked reduction in MWF at both 3 and 8 weeks post injury. MWF was also reduced at 3 weeks at 5 and 10 mm caudal to the injury site. At 8 weeks post injury, this

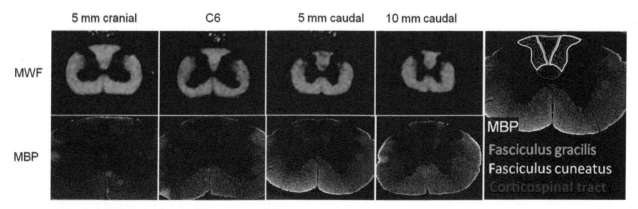

FIGURE 3.5.3 The ex vivo rat spinal cord myelin water maps clearly demonstrate the characteristic gray matter "butterfly" effect with the center gray matter portion of the spinal cord showing markedly reduced myelin, while the surrounding peripheral white matter exhibited high signal. Contrast between the corticospinal tract and other white matter tracts in the dorsal column is also observed, both in the myelin water maps and in the corresponding staining for myelin basic protein. *Source: Images kindly provided by Dr. Piotr Kozlowski, Department of Radiology, University of British Columbia.*

trend was reversed as MWF returned to normal at 5 mm caudal, and increased significantly above the normal level at 10 mm caudal to injury. Despite significant axonal involvement as demonstrated by histological staining, the CST exhibited only small changes in MWF at 3 and 8 weeks, likely due to the presence of myelin debris. The authors noted that at 8 weeks post injury both the CST and the fasciculus gracilis showed *increased* MWF proximal to injury, i.e., cranial in the CST and caudal in the gracilis. They hypothesized that this may have been due to loosening of the myelin sheaths, which, if confirmed by EM, would suggest that MWF, unlike LFB or MBP histological staining, is not only sensitive to the amount of myelin but also to myelin structure. Changes in the fasciculus cuneatus were much less dramatic than in the other two tracts; however, MWF and LFB showed significant reductions, as compared to control, both cranially and caudally to injury at 3 weeks post injury, which were largely reversed at 8 weeks post injury. The authors concluded that MWF was a more sensitive measure of myelin in traumatic spinal cord injury than the diffusion tensor imaging derived measure transverse (radial) diffusivity (see Chapter 3.1), which was also assessed in their study.

3.5.3.4 Monitoring Acute Changes in Myelin Integrity Using a Murine Model of Demyelination with Spontaneous Remyelination

The comparison between MWF and other MR measures is an interesting and ongoing area of research. Another MR parameter, which has often been touted in the literature as a marker for myelin, is the magnetization transfer ratio (MTR). Magnetization transfer imaging (MTI) involves detecting the exchange of magnetization between nonaqueous tissue and water and is typically described by the semiquantitative value MTR[48] (see Chapter 3.4). The large literature on MTI makes it clear that MTR is a very sensitive measure of tissue damage, however, its specificity for myelin has been controversial.[49] While MTR has been associated with myelin,[50] it has also been associated with axonal integrity,[51,52] inflammation,[53] and changes in water content.[49] Given the clear need for an in vivo marker of remyelination to evaluate potential therapies targeting demyelination, further studies and histological validations of MR techniques influenced by myelin are required.

In an attempt to clarify the specificity of MWF and MTR for monitoring acute changes in myelin, McCreary et al. examined a murine model of demyelination and remyelination.[54] The authors modeled focal demyelination with spontaneous remyelination by injecting lysolecithin directly into white matter tracks. Lysolecithin has been shown to solubilize myelin with little axonal damage in mouse spinal cord,[55] and white matter regions demyelinated by lysolecithin injection remyelinate relatively quickly in the mouse.[56] McCreary et al. chose this model as the location of the lesion is known and can be easily located on MRI. Furthermore, the model involves changes in myelin with little edema, and remyelination occurs within weeks, which makes tracking changes using MRI feasible.

For their study, animals were injected with lysolecithin at the dorsal funiculi of the C5 spinal cord. MR imaging was performed 7, 14, 21, and 28 days post injection on a 9.4 T Bruker system using a 35 mm diameter birdcase coil. Seven animals were imaged serially at all four time points, and three additional mice were imaged at each of the four time points, after which they were sacrificed for histological study. MR experiments at the injury site included a 64-echo spin echo with slice thickness of 0.75 mm and in-plane resolution of 150×150 μm and a spin echo with and without a 2 kHz off-resonance pulse for the MT study, with slice thickness of 0.75 mm and in-plane resolution of 78×156 μm. AnalyzeNNLS[57] was used for T_2 analysis, and MTR was calculated as the difference between average signal intensity with and without saturation pulses, normalized to the signal intensity without saturation pulses. The typical myelin water and intra/extracellular water T_2 peaks were observed in the mouse spinal cord, and MWF values of 0.35 for the dorsal column were similar to findings by Kozlowski.[44] The authors also make note of an additional longer T_2 peak, which appeared most frequently at 14 and 21 days post injury. The underlying cause of this additional peak was unknown. The MWF and GMT_2 of the intra/extracellular water significantly decreased at 14 days post injury and then returned to control levels by 28 days, which corresponded to the clearance of myelin debris and remyelination, which was shown by eriochrome cyanine and Oil Red O staining. MTR was also significantly decreased 14 days after lysolecithin injection, however, in contrast to T_2 measures, it remained low over the time course studied. The authors also note that evidence of demyelination shown by both MWF and MTR lagged behind histological confirmation of myelin loss by approximately 1 week, suggesting that MR measures are limited in their ability to detect acute myelin-related changes. In particular, McCreary et al. suggest that the delay in MWF changes in response to demyelination observed in their study was most likely due to the presence of degraded myelin remaining in the lesion, which is supported by the large amount of Oil Red O staining for lipids at 7 days post injury. This hypothesis is supported by a freeze fracture study on macrophages from lysolecithin-induced lesions in rat spinal cord, which showed that phagocytosed myelin initially retained its lamellar structure within vacuoles before eventual lysosomal digestion formed lipid-filled vacuoles.[58] Furthermore, work by Webb et al. found that MWF did not distinguish intact myelin from degraded myelin in rat sciatic nerve.[47] The authors note that partial volume effects may also contribute to the temporal contradiction between MWF and histology as small changes in myelin are difficult to detect over the relatively large volumes required for imaging.

The rather interesting observation of a *decreased* GMT_2 of the intra/extracellular water is opposite to what is typically observed in pathology where T_2 *increases* are often found in areas of injury. The authors note that the pattern of change in T_2 distribution observed in this study was contrary to those predicted by a model of demyelination, inflammation, and axonal loss in peripheral nerve by Odrobina et al.[59] Possible explanations include increased magnetization exchange between myelin and intra/extracellular water due to loss of myelin structure as lysolecithin solubilizes the sheath into discrete lipoprotein units, or the presence of infiltrating macrophages within the lesion, which could increase the amount of non-myelin macromolecules and decrease T_2 values.

McCreary's work was the first to examine the mouse spinal cord using quantitative T_2 relaxation, and was also the first to examine MWF at 9.4 T. The authors showed it is possible to follow a time course of demyelination and repair in a lysolecithin model of spinal cord injury and concluded that MWF more closely reflected the time course of histological evaluation of myelin content than MTR. They suggest differences between MWF and MTR may identify early remyelination.

3.5.3.5 Histogram Analysis and Partial Volume Effects on Myelin Water in Bovine Spinal Cord

Shortly after the work by Kozlowski and McCreary, Minty et al. reported on a combined MRI and NMR study of bovine spinal cord.[4] The authors were the first to present histogram analysis of MWF in spinal cord and demonstrated the influence of partial volume effects on MWF for pixels near tissue boundaries. The study examined 18 fresh bovine spinal cord samples, cut into multiple sections. MRI experiments were conducted using a transmit/receive head coil on a 1.5 T scanner with a single 5-mm-thick slice 32-echo CPMG sequence. Spinal cord samples were arranged such that multiple axial cross sections could be examined simultaneously. Three samples underwent further study on a modified Bruker SXP 4-100 NMR spectrometer operating at 2.1 T (90 MHz) using a 4320-echo CPMG sequence. NNLS was used for decay curve analysis. Myelin water maps from MRI demonstrated that the central gray matter butterfly was clearly resolved as having a lower MWF, with an average value of 8.2%. White matter showed a consistently high myelin water signal, with an average MWF of 30%. Intermediate MWF of <20% was resolved at tissue boundaries and was interpreted by the authors as likely arising from partial volume effects. T_2 distributions from ex vivo bovine spinal cord revealed peak T_2 times and component amplitudes similar to those observed in humans in vivo, which were also examined in Minty's study. NMR measurements found an average MWF of 34% and offered a quantitative validation of findings observed with MRI, as similar component amplitudes and T_2 times were resolved for the same sample.

Measured MWFs in bovine spinal cord white and gray matter were consistent with those found by Kozlowski et al. in rat spinal cord.[44,45] However, the authors noted that spinal cord white matter MWF was considerably higher than values observed in brain tissue.[18,60] An informative discussion was presented that describes potential reasons for the increased spinal cord MWF including: (1) the possibility of additional short T_2 reservoirs; (2) true anatomical variation in myelin content; and (3) the influence of magnetization exchange. NMR analysis did indeed reveal that the short T_2 peak tended to split into two peaks at approximately 8 and 20 ms. It is conceivable that one of the short peaks represents a distinct microanatomical reservoir, such as multilamellar mitochondria. The possibility of true regional differences is supported by ex vivo evidence of an approximate 2.5 times higher myelin content yield from rat spinal cord compared to cerebrum.[8] The potential role of magnetization exchange in MWF estimation raises an important area of research. Minty et al. highlights a simple calculation regarding compartmental mixing times presented by Koenig,[61] which indeed suggests, based on the estimated mixing time of 64 ms for a 10 lamellae fiber, that small nerve fibers would undergo increased myelin water exchange relative to larger fibers, and, as a result, would have artifactually lower

MWF. The authors however go on to state that experimental measurements of myelin water exchange do not support the above conclusion, as two studies have observed significantly longer myelin mixing times of 560 ms in bovine optic nerve at room temperature[62] and 1024 ms in bovine white matter at 37 °C.[63] Furthermore, modeling by Bjarnason et al. demonstrated that although inter-reservoir exchange increases do lead to an underestimation of true myelin content, the estimated reductions in measured MWF were around 10–20%.[63] Minty et al. concluded that, while on the basis of a fiber size argument alone one might expect MWFs measured in structures containing smaller fibers to be somewhat lower, this cannot explain the observed threefold difference between spinal cord and brain MWF. This debate is therefore still open, and further investigations are needed to explain the different behavior of MWFs in the spinal cord compared to the brain.

3.5.3.6 The Effect of Exchange on the T_2 Distribution in Formalin-Fixed Rat Spinal Cord

The role of exchange in determining MWF is currently an exciting and active area of spinal cord research. The interpretation that MWF is measuring water trapped within the myelin lamellae is based on the assumption that exchange between myelin-associated water and water in other compartments, such as inside and outside of the axon, is slow. Several experiments support this theory as slow exchange times have been reported in the literature for bovine optic nerve and bovine white matter.[62,63] However, given that axon diameter, myelin thickness, and fiber packing are known to vary within the central nervous system, the slow exchange assumption may not hold in all white matter regions. Therefore, the assumptions underlying the slow exchange model are worthy of further scrutiny.

Dula et al. recently examined six samples of excised fixed rat spinal cord with quantitative T_2 relaxation and histology.[64] T_2 measurements were performed on a 7 T 16-cm-bore Varian scanner using a 10-mm-diameter loop gap coil. A single 2-mm-thick slice transverse to the long axis of the spinal cord was examined using 48 spin echoes with scan duration of 77 min and nominal in-plane resolution of 40 μm after zero filling. T_2 distributions were estimated using NNLS[27] and regularized with a minimum curvature constraint, which used the generalized cross-validation approach for adjustments.[65] Unlike previous studies that used a definitive boundary for the myelin water range (e.g., 7.75–20 ms at 7 T[44]), Dula et al. used the region of lowest amplitude between

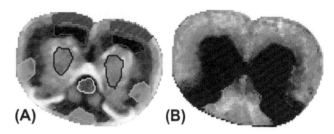

FIGURE 3.5.4 (A) Typical T_2-weighted image showing manually drawn ROIs in gray matter and each of the six white matter tracts: vestibulospinal (pink), funiculus cuneatus (red), rubrospinal (aqua), reticulospinal (blue), funiculus gracilis (green), and dorsal corticospinal (yellow); and (B) myelin water fraction map. *Source: Reprinted with permission from Ref. 61 (Figure 4).*

the two dominant T_2 distribution components (i.e., the nadir between the myelin water and intra/extracellular water T_2 peaks) of each ROI's average distribution as the boundary between the myelin water and other water. Six white matter tracts were selected for analysis, each with unique microscopic characteristics for myelin thickness and axon diameter, but relatively constant myelin volume fraction (Figure 3.5.4). For each sample, histological analysis determined myelin fraction, myelin thickness, and axon diameter from one area within each tract.

MWF values observed by Dula et al. were in agreement with studies by Kozlowski et al. at 7 T.[44,45] Five of six tracts demonstrated relatively similar MWF values ranging from mean (standard deviation) of 0.36 (0.06) to 0.29 (0.05), consistent with the fairly constant myelin volume fraction ranging from 0.61 (0.02) to 0.56 (0.03). The dorsal CST, an area of relatively small axons with thin myelin sheaths, however, showed a much lower MWF of 0.19 (0.02), as well as a reduced myelin volume fraction of 0.51 (0.006). No correlation between MWF and myelin volume was observed ($R^2 = 0.49$, $p = 0.12$ calculated from data presented within the manuscript[64]), however the six white matter tracts were specifically chosen to represent regions with similar myelin content, and therefore inclusion of other white matter areas to increase the dynamic range may lead to a significant correlation. MWF was more closely related to both myelin thickness and axon diameter ($R^2 = 0.75$, $p = 0.03$ and $R^2 = 0.62$, $p = 0.06$, respectively, calculated from data presented within the manuscript[64]). The mean T_2 time of non-myelin "other" water was strongly correlated with myelin thickness and axon diameter ($R^2 = 0.93$, $p = 0.002$ and $R^2 = 0.89$, $p = 0.005$, respectively, calculated from data presented within the manuscript[64]). A magnetization transfer metric, the pool size ratio, was found to be independent of myelin thickness and axon diameter and was therefore considered to be largely independent to magnetization exchange.

Based on the observed relationship between the T_2 parameters with myelin thickness and axon diameter, the authors presented a two-pool model to demonstrate the effect of exchange on the T_2 distribution. The authors' work is based on the fact that water in smaller compartments (such as small, thinly myelinated axons) will have shorter average lifetimes within these compartments, leading to faster intercompartmental exchange rates. In their model, as myelin water lifetime decreased from 500 to 40 ms, the MWF decreased from 0.36 to 0.13 and the mean T_2 of "other" water shifted to shorter times. Consequently, the T_2 distribution from WM with small, densely packed axons with thin myelin may underestimate the myelin content and report short T_2 times for both myelin and other water. The authors also provide an estimate that an axon diameter of ~5 µm is necessary to satisfy a slow-exchange model. Dula et al. conclude that observations from their ex vivo study are consistent with exchange-mediated variation in the T_2 distribution across different white matter tracts. However, the authors go on to state that the possible confounding factors of temperature and chemical fixation cannot be ignored.

3.5.3.7 The Effect of Exchange on the T_2 Distribution in Rat Spinal Cord In Vivo

To address the possible influences of temperature and chemical fixation, a very recent follow-up study by the same group reported findings from in vivo multiexponential T_2 measurements in rat spinal cord.[66] In this study, Harkins et al. provided an interpretation of in vivo T_2 data from four white matter spinal cord tracts using a histology-based finite difference model of water proton exchange and transverse relaxation.

Five rats underwent an inversion-recovery prepped 32-echo multiple spin echo imaging sequence on a 9.4 T 31-cm-bore Varian system with a 38-mm Litz quadrature coil. The application of the inversion pulse served to null signal from cerebrospinal fluid to avoid flow artifacts. A single 1.5-mm-thick slice transverse to the long axis of the spinal cord was examined; scan duration was ~100 min and images had a nominal in-plane resolution of 100 µm after zero filling. Regions of interest from white matter tracts were analyzed using NNLS, however, unlike the voxel-wise approach employed by Dula et al., mean echo magnitudes were estimated from each ROI and then fitted to the sum of decaying exponential functions to minimize bias due to Rician noise. Water components were then distinguished by the local minimum between the two dominant T_2 spectral components (Figure 3.5.5). For histological analysis,

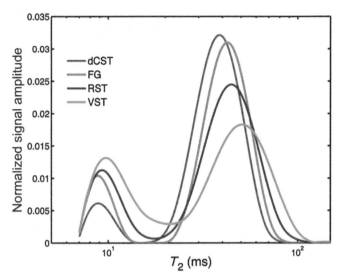

FIGURE 3.5.5   Population-averaged T_2 spectra for four spinal cord tracts (vestibulospinal, funiculus gracilis, rubrospinal, dorsal corticospinal). *Source: Reprinted with permission from Ref. 63 (Figure 3).*

four spinal cord white matter tracts were identified in histology sections originally presented by Dula et al.[64] High resolution images were segmented into regions of myelin, intra-axonal space, and extra-axonal space to determine average myelin thickness and axon radius. Experimental results showed that in contrast to the roughly constant myelin volume across the four regions observed on histology, the MWF varied from 10% to 35%. Furthermore, the MWF, myelin water T_2, and "other" water T_2 all tended to decrease for smaller axons and thinner myelin, an observation that suggests a greater effect of intercompartmental water exchange on transverse relaxation and is consistent with the ex vivo findings of Dula et al.[64]

As the dorsal CST MWF was lower in the Harkins study than that observed by Dula, the authors suggest this may indicate the lower temperature of the ex vivo work reduced water exchange to a greater extent than it was increased by fixation. However, given the relatively smaller number of rats in both studies ($n = 6$, Dula et al.[64]; $n = 5$ Harkins et al.[66]), findings should be interpreted with some caution. Consistency of slice location between the in vivo and ex vivo studies is unknown, and natural variation of myelin content may occur between animals, especially since Dula et al. examined male rats, while Harkins et al. examined females. Furthermore, given the small size of the dorsal CST, its close proximity to gray matter and relatively small number of voxels able to define it (~9, based on figure within Harkins et al.[66]), the possibility of partial volume effects should be considered. Finally, although the samples used for histological analysis were identical for Harkins and Dula studies, the reported measures for myelin thickness from the tracts were not consistent (36% difference for the dorsal CST, 27% difference for the funiculus gracilis), nor was axonal radius (63% difference for the vestibulospinal tract, 71% difference for the rubrospinal tract). Although a higher resolution microscopy was used by Harkins, this difference may also reflect the variation in fiber size and composition within a single tract.

To model T_2 relaxation, echo magnitudes were fit with a finite difference model, as described in detail within the Harkins publication,[66] using input geometry defined by the segmented histology images of each white matter tract. T_2 relaxation was also modeled by fitting the Bloch–McConnell equations to the echo magnitudes for a three-compartment system.[67] The authors argue that in contrast to previous models of multi-echo T_2[62,68,69] using the Bloch–McConnell equations,[67] which (1) assume that each compartment is instantaneously well mixed and (2) neglect tissue heterogeneity, finite difference models do not require the assumption of well-mixed compartments and are naturally well suited to account for variation in the shape and dimension of tissue components, such as myelin thickness and axon diameter. The finite difference simulation was run for all tracts in one of three conditions: (1) no intercompartmental water exchange, (2) diffusion-limited exchange, and (3) permeability-limited exchange (large enough to allow rapid mixing of the myelin water for all tracts).

The finite difference models, which incorporate either a finite diffusion coefficient in the myelin compartment or define a finite permeability at each compartment boundary, were fitted significantly better than the Bloch–McConnell model, which incorporated water exchange but not intracompartment diffusion or intratract variation in axon/myelin dimensions. The finite difference model was, however, unable to determine whether water exchange in spinal white matter is mediated by the rate of water diffusion within the myelin or at the boundary of myelin. The authors also noted that the modeled myelin water lifetime ranged from 43 ms for the dorsal CST to 150 ms for the vestibulospinal tract.

Harkins et al. conclude both exchange and anatomical heterogeneity was necessary to account for the variation of the observed MWF between white matter tracts in the rat spinal cord. However, the authors do state that exchange properties of myelin water may be different between brain and spinal cord. Consequently, more work is needed to determine the impact of water exchange throughout central nervous system white matter, and this continues to be an active and exciting area of research.

WHAT CAN WE LEARN FROM PRECLINICAL MODELS ABOUT T_2 IN THE SPINAL CORD?

- Healthy mammalian spinal cord contains up to three water compartments: myelin water, intra/extracellular water, and CSF (partial volume from the spinal canal)
- Myelin water fraction more closely follows histologically derived myelin content than MTR
- Myelin water fraction is unable to distinguish between intact myelin and myelin debris
- Water movement between compartments (exchange) can result in lower measured myelin water fractions and shorter T_2 times; nerve tracts with thinner myelin sheaths and smaller axon diameters show more evidence of exchange
- Magnetization transfer measurements in the cord (Chapter 3.4) are less affected by myelin water exchange

---

3.5.4 HUMAN T_2 RELAXATION STUDIES IN THE SPINAL CORD

3.5.4.1 Initial In Vivo Observation of Myelin Water Signal

The first human in vivo T_2 relaxation study on spinal cord was published by Wu et al.[3] (Table 3.5.2). While the technique had previously been applied in vivo to the brain,[18,70] technical challenges had limited the implementation of multi-echo T_2 relaxation to study the spinal cord. Given that spinal cord myelin damage occurs in many diseases and conditions, including multiple sclerosis and spinal cord injury, the successful development and application of a possible in vivo marker to assess pathology and treatment response was highly significant. The aim of their pilot study was to optimize an inversion recovery multiple spin echo sequence for estimating spinal cord MWF. Wu et al.'s technical note reports the scan–rescan reproducibility of the short T_2 myelin water signal in healthy controls, as well as preliminary measurements in diseased cord.

MR experiments were conducted on six healthy controls and four people with demyelinating disease on a 1.5 T GE MR system using a single-element posterior neck surface coil with high sensitivity in the cervical spinal cord. The body coil was used to transmit radiofrequency pulses for excitation. A 32-echo CPMG

TABLE 3.5.2 Summary of Human T_2 Relaxation Studies in the Spinal Cord

Study	Study Population	Sequence	Coil	TR (ms)	TE (ms)	Field (T)	Acquired Voxel Size (In-plane; Thickness)	Acquisition Time (min)
Wu[3]	Healthy controls (n = 6), demyelinating disease (n = 4)	32 echo IR-prepped CPMG	Single-element posterior neck surface coil	3000	7.2	1.5	1.4–1.6 mm; 5 mm	13
Smith[71]	Healthy controls (n = 6)	16 echo spin echo	Body coil excitation and a 16-channel neurovascular coil (eight head elements, two bilateral c-spine elements, six anterior-posterior lower c-spine/upper thoracic elements) for reception	Minimum TR = 2500 ms, cardiac gated	10	3	1 mm; 5 mm	4.5–5
Minty[4]	Healthy controls (n = 17)	32 echo IR-prepped CPMG	Body coil for radio frequency (RF) pulse transmission and a phased array spine coil for signal detection	3000	10	1.5	1.88 × 0.94 to 2.18 × 1.09; 5 mm	25.6
Laule[76]	Healthy controls (n = 24), primary progressive multiple sclerosis (n = 24)	32 echo IR-prepped CPMG	Transmit/receive head coil	3000	10	1.5	1.72 × 0.86 mm; 5 mm	13.3
MacMillan[5]	Healthy controls (n = 30)	3D 32 echo multi-echo	Phased array spine coil, using only the first four elements for best localization of the cervical SC	1300	10	3	0.7 mm; 5 mm	20
Kolind[38]	Healthy controls (n = 7)	mcDESPOT	Eight-channel torso-array radio frequency coil	SPGR 5.0, bSSFP 3.5, IR-SSFP 4.6	SPGR 2.2, bSSFP 1.7, IR-SSFP 1.7	1.5	1 mm; 1.5 mm	26

*All studies used NNLS for analysis except for Smith (mono-exponential fit) and Kolind. All imaging studies were collected in the axial plane except for Minty and Kolind (sagittal).

sequence was developed and included the application of a 1250 ms inversion pulse before the 90° excitation pulse to null the signal from cerebrospinal fluid. Two averages of a single 5-mm-thick axial slice were collected at the level of the third cervical vertebra for controls and at a level of lesion for the people with demyelinating disease. Healthy controls were imaged multiple times on different days to assess scan–rescan reproducibility. As the spatial resolution in the images did not permit demarcation between white and gray matter, regions of interest encircled the entire spinal cord. Partial volume effects were then minimized by the application of intensity thresholding to remove peripheral voxels. NNLS was used for voxel-wise decay curve analysis. Mean healthy control MWF was 26.8% and was reproduced reasonably well with the scan–rescan coefficient of variation ranging from 3% to 10% across the six subjects. Subjects with demyelinating disease had a mean MWF of 20%.

The initial publication by Wu et al. demonstrated the feasibility of human in vivo spinal cord myelin water imaging. Given the relatively low field strength of 1.5 T, large voxel size of 1.5×1.5 mm^2 in-plane resolution, and given the challenges present during in vivo scanning of the spinal cord such as CSF flow, cardiac and respiratory motion, the reproducibility of <10% was promising. The authors recommended that further technical improvements and clinical studies were needed, and they concluded that if the necessary spatial resolution could be achieved with reasonable scan times, MWF measurements should play a key role in guiding trials of myelin repair and/or protection in lesions of the spinal cord.

3.5.4.2 Optimization of Image Contrast by Relaxation Assessment

Several years after the study by Wu, Smith et al. measured T_2 relaxation in the cervical cord at 3 T.[71] Rather than focusing on myelin water, this study sought to quantitatively determine the relaxation time constants. Their motivation was twofold: accurate assessment of relaxation time may be useful for (1) investigating pathology and (2) derivation of experimental parameters to optimize image contrast. During the time of this publication the use of higher field MR systems was becoming more common. The authors point out that as relaxation rates are field dependent, experimental parameters must be re-optimized to take full advantage of the benefits of higher field strength. Furthermore, the assumption that spinal cord white and gray matter relaxation rates are identical to those found in brain tissue may not be valid given differences in tissue composition and structure. Therefore, their aim was to determine relaxation time for white and gray matter in the spinal cord, as well as optimize sequence

parameters for maximal image contrast between white and gray matter, and between CSF and white matter.

Six healthy controls were examined using a Philips 3 T system with body coil excitation and a 16-channel neurovascular coil (eight head elements, two bilateral c-spine elements, six anterior-posterior lower c-spine/upper thoracic elements) for reception. T_2 relaxation data was measured using a 16-echo spin-echo sequence (TE = 10–160 ms) with a single 5-mm-thick slice centered at C3 at an in-plane resolution of 1.0×1.0 mm^2, reconstructed to 0.5×0.5 mm^2. To eliminate CSF in-flow effects associated with cardiac pulsation in the longer echo T_2 acquisitions, the sequence was cardiac gated with a minimum TR of 2.5 s leading to a scan time of 4.5–5 min. Unlike Wu et al., and previous T_2 work in animal models, which used multiple exponentials to characterize T_2 decay in spinal cord, Smith et al. employed a mono-exponential fit to only the eight even echoes to decrease possible stimulated echo contributions. Qualitatively, mean T_2 maps showed little visual contrast between white and gray matter. Likewise, no quantitative T_2 difference was found between white and gray matter (73 vs. 76 ms) nor between left and right lateral column white matter (73 vs. 72 ms). The authors note that their calculated spinal cord T_2 times were similar to those observed by Lu et al. at 3 T who employed an 8-echo CPMG experiment with likely a mono-exponential fit,[72] in particular for frontal white matter. This observation is perhaps surprising given the structural differences (fiber size and packing) between spinal cord tissue and frontal white matter, however, experimental data needs to be interpreted with caution as T_2 decay curves were treated as mono-exponential when in reality their behavior is more complex.

Smith et al. also conducted simulations to demonstrate optimal imaging parameters for conventional spinal cord imaging in the clinic. They used the steady state signal equations for spin echo and inversion recovery from Haacke et al.[73] to simulate the effect of TE and TR on white/gray contrast and also white/CSF contrast. Simulations found that spin echo showed the greatest gray/white matter contrast at very short TE and TR greater than 3000 ms, while optimal white/CSF contrast was at longer TE (>100 ms) and long TR. The authors concluded that relaxation values measured in their study should be useful in parameter optimization for clinical spinal cord imaging at 3 T, as well as in quantitative methods such as MR spectroscopy metabolite concentration measurement.

3.5.4.3 Sagittal Acquisition Demonstrates Myelin Water Sensitivity to White Matter Distribution along the Entire Cord Length

To achieve greater volumetric coverage than the single slice axial myelin water imaging approach used by

Wu et al., Minty et al. employed a sagittal multi-echo T_2 relaxation acquisition for in vivo human study.[4] This was the first, and is to date the only, study to acquire MWF data along the entire length of cervical, thoracic, and lumbar cord. Given the varying contributions of white and gray matter along the length of the spinal cord (Figure 3.5.6), superior-inferior variation in MWF would be expected.

Seventeen healthy controls underwent MR imaging on a 1.5 T GE MR system using a sagittal 5-mm-thick single-slice 32-echo CPMG sequence with four averages. As CSF is a major complicating factor in spinal cord imaging[74] and its presence can affect transverse relaxation measurements, an inversion pulse was included prior to the 90° excitation pulse. The authors explain that for a sequence involving inversion recovery (IR) at a finite pulse repetition time (TR), the calculation of inversion time (TI) requires consideration of the saturation effects that occur due to repeated pulse structure. They assumed a CSF T_1 of 4500 ms based on Haacke et al.,[73] and by accounting for saturation effects, determined a theoretical TI of 1153 ms; a TI of 1200 ms was chosen for their study. Voxel size ranged from 0.94×1.9 mm^2 to 1.1×2.2 mm^2.

ROIs were drawn on the spinal cord adjacent to landmarked vertebrae (C2–T12) where the vertical dimension of the ROI was the height of the adjacent vertebral body, while the width was that of the spinal cord less one to two voxels on the anterior and posterior margins to minimize partial voluming at the spinal cord periphery. T_2 decay curves were analyzed using NNLS. MWF was compared to white matter area fractions derived from segmentation of photomicrographs from a neuroanatomy textbook.[75] Photomicrographs were segmented in two ways: (1) white matter area over the total cord area in the axial plane of corresponding spinal cord locations and (2) with the lateral margins of the spinal cord truncated to approximate the volume that would be measured using MRI assuming a 5-mm-midline sagittal slice.

MWF varied along the length of the spinal cord (Figure 3.5.7). Minty et al. report a global consistency between MWF and "white matter area fraction" resolving similar local minima at C6–C7 (the cervical enlargement), and trending toward a global minimum distally in T11 (consistent with the beginning of the lumbar enlargement). The highest MWF values were observed in the thoracic cord (28.7%) consistent with the expectation of a small contribution of gray matter to total signal in a midline sagittal slice through the thoracic area. Cervical MWF (21.8%) was slightly smaller than other studies (25.3%,[76] 26.4%[3]), which the authors suggest may be due to their study's increased relative GM content due to the use of a 5-mm-sagittal slice through the approximately 10-mm-diameter cervical SC. Assuming the slice was midline, the imaged volume excluded WM on the lateral margins of the cervical cord, thereby increasing the relative GM content of the slice. MWF

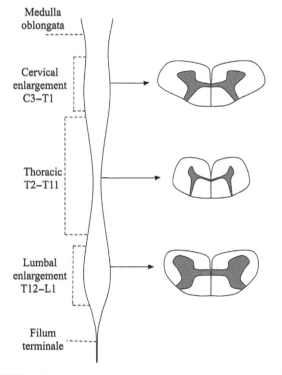

FIGURE 3.5.6 A cartoon depicting regional variation of spinal cord size (not to scale) and changes in white matter to gray matter ratios at different spinal cord levels. The left side of the image depicts the whole spinal cord and the right side contains representative axial sections through the indicated regions of the spinal cord. When a 5-mm-midline sagittal slice is used in a spinal cord MRI, more WM is proportionally excluded than GM. *Source: Reprinted with permission from Ref. 4.*

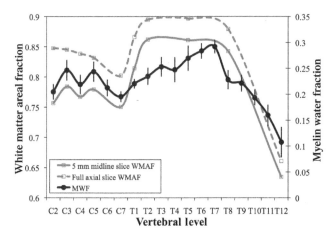

FIGURE 3.5.7 Average MWFs for various cord segments compared with WM areal fractions (WMAFs) determined from image segmentation of axial photomicrographs. When the WMAFs were determined using segmentation corresponding to a 5-mm-midline slice used in the MRIs, similar shapes were observed in the curves for C2–C7 when compared with MWFs. Standard error shown. *Source: Reprinted with permission from Ref. 4.*

distal to T11 (i.e., at T12 and L1) continued to show good agreement with expectation; however, there was increased error in these measurements, reflecting both a natural increase in the variation of white matter content in this area and the difficulty in keeping the spinal cord within the imaged volume due to the shrinking diameter of the cona medullaris, where the spinal cord terminates.

While sagittal acquisition clearly has the advantage of permitting a much greater volumetric coverage, Minty et al. present a nice discussion on the limitations of the sagittal scanning plane, in particular the cost of partial voluming a 5-mm voxel across the WM/GM interface at best, and across the SC/CSF interface at worst. Partial voluming is a limitation of all MRI techniques, which can have negative consequences for the multi-echo T_2 experiment and MWF accuracy. However, as the authors point out, achieving the anatomic coverage (full length of the spinal cord) in an axial scan plane using a single-slice technique under in vivo conditions is not feasible in terms of data acquisition.

The authors also discussed technical challenges associated with the inversion recovery-prepped sequence and SNR. Some of the challenges exacerbated in the quantitative multi-echo technique used by Minty et al. include: an imaging protocol that required prolonged patient immobility, a physiological area that was challenging to image (CSF flow, truncation artifact due to sharp spinal cord borders), and the use of a phased array spine coil (which caused decreased signal homogeneity). The authors highlight that the pulsatile flow of CSF was a particular concern because nulling signal from CSF required the delivery of an effective inversion pulse, which, even when delivered adequately, imparted a further cost in SNR relative to conventional in vivo relaxation experiments. Given that SNR is an important factor in accurate T_2 determination, Minty et al. also presented a simulation whereby the effects of low SNR on T_2 analysis were investigated. Synthetic 32 echo data was created and Rician noise was added to the data at SNR levels of 1000, 400, 200, 100, and 50. MWFs were computed using NNLS and compared to a known input value. They found that a loss of T_2 distribution resolution and an increase in MWF variance was observed as SNR decreased, particularly when SNR fell below 100. However, the authors still suggest that two distinct peaks need not be resolved for robust MWF determination as long as one can assume a model for spinal cord white matter that assigns a range of T_2 values in the T_2 distribution consistent with data collected at higher SNR, and providing any pathology affecting T_2 times substantially is absent. Finally, a nice discussion (already summarized in the preclinical section) is presented that suggests potential

reasons for the increase MWF in spinal cord relative to brain, whereby the authors conclude that higher MWF in spinal cord were primarily due to higher myelin content.

This study marked the successful implementation of an inversion recovery multi-echo sequence on a phased array spine coil for the purposes of sagittal T_2 relaxation measurements in human spinal cord in vivo. MWF measured in this study exhibited sensitivity to the WM distribution expected in the spinal cord. The authors state the potential applications of T_2 measurement in the spinal cord, both in characterizing disease processes like multiple sclerosis and in monitoring proposed neuroregenerative therapies over time, should encourage future research in this area.

3.5.4.4 Longitudinal Assessment of Myelin Water in Primary Progressive Multiple Sclerosis Demonstrates Myelin Loss over 2 Years

The first, and thus far only, longitudinal assessment of T_2 relaxation in human spinal cord was conducted by Laule et al.[76] who serially examined individuals with primary progressive multiple sclerosis (PPMS) over 2 years. Involvement of the spinal cord in PPMS is common and likely an important element in disability.[77] Given Wu et al.'s preliminary work that found reduced MWF in MS cervical cord, in conjunction with other studies that have indicated abnormalities in cervical cord area[78,79] that progress over a relatively short period of time,[78] the goal of Laule et al.'s work was to investigate longitudinal MWF changes in PPMS. Their aim was to assess T_2 relaxation in response to a proposed disease-modifying therapy that may enable better understanding of the relationship between disability and spinal cord metrics in PPMS.

MR images were acquired using a 1.5 T GE system using a standard transmit-receive head coil. For T_2 relaxation measurement a single 5-mm-slice 32-echo relaxation sequence with a preparatory inversion recovery pulse (TI = 1200 ms) to null signal from CSF was collected. The single slice was obliquely chosen perpendicular to the spinal cord at the C2–C3 level with voxel size of 1.72×0.86 mm. Twenty-four PPMS subjects and 24 age- and sex-matched controls were examined at baseline, year 1 and year 2. Seven controls underwent two scans at one visit with subject repositioning between scans to determine measurement reproducibility. Voxelwise T_2 decay curves were analyzed using NNLS.[27] ROIs, drawn by two separate observers (blinded to subject type and scan time) around the outer boundary of the spinal cord on the first echo of the T_2 relaxation data, were mapped onto MWF maps, whereby the mean MWFs were determined from the contributing voxels within that ROI.

Inter- and intraobserver coefficients of variation (COV) were very good for MWF (<5%, <2.5%, respectively) and scan–rescan COV was also good at 8%. MWF maps revealed reduced MWF in the gray matter relative to white matter, and the characteristic butterfly pattern was visible in the center of the spinal cord (Figure 3.5.8). Areas of reduced MWF were visually evident in PPMS, despite no lesions being present at or adjacent to the slice of interest. Baseline MWF was 11% lower in PPMS relative to controls (0.225 vs. 0.253, $p = 0.12$). The authors state that given the relatively small number of subjects scanned, the detection of differences was limited; at least double the sample size would be needed to detect any significant difference with a power of 0.9 using their data. The MWF values for control subjects obtained by Laule et al. were similar to those observed by Wu and colleagues[3] (0.268), are in agreement with those reported by MacMillan et al. using a higher field strength of 3 T (0.25 for C4 level),[5] and are slightly higher than those observed by Minty et al. (0.22 (0.02) for cervical cord).[4] The observed trend of an 11% lower MWF in PPMS at baseline compared to controls is smaller than the findings of Wu et al. who observed a 25% reduction in cervical cord MWF in a group of only four subjects with MS, but are in agreement with findings from a postmortem study that reports an average 13% lower white matter volume for upper cervical cord in MS.[80] PPMS spinal cord MWF decreased by 10.5% over 2 years, while control spinal cord MWF showed no change. Changes in MWF observed for the PPMS group were not correlated with changes in cervical cord volume, which the authors also examined. There was also no effect of treatment on change in MWF in PPMS subjects.

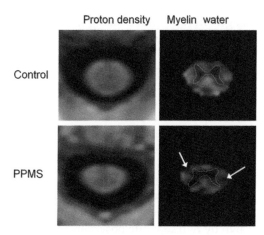

FIGURE 3.5.8 Conventional magnetic resonance and corresponding myelin water image of cervical cord for a primary progressive multiple sclerosis subject and matched control with more obvious suggestion of the butterfly appearance of the gray matter on the myelin water image (lines). Areas of reduced myelin water are noted in the primary progressive multiple sclerosis subject (arrows).

The authors conclude that myelin-associated water can be reliably assessed over a relatively short period of time and that quantitative assessment of T_2 relaxation may help quantify changes in the spinal cord due to evolving MS. Although cord atrophy was not correlated with decreased MWF, decreases in cervical cord area may be caused by a combination of axonal loss and demyelination. The authors note that the lack of correlation of MWF changes with EDSS progression and with treatment may reflect the relatively small sample size, the slower-than-expected clinical progression in the clinical trial overall, and the variability of the MWF measurement. Nevertheless, their findings suggest that progressive demyelination may contribute to cervical cord abnormalities in PPMS, and larger longitudinal studies with increased volumetric coverage are warranted. Since cervical cord MWF decreases by about 5% per year in PPMS, T_2 relaxation would be a promising candidate for assessment of putative PPMS therapies.

3.5.4.5 Multislice T_2 Relaxation Assessment at 3 T Reveals In Vivo Myelin Water Distinction of Gray and White Matter, and Age Dependence

Clinical applicability of MWF would require significant reductions in scan time and greater volumetric coverage, and would benefit from increased signal to noise at higher field strength. The first multislice report, and the first in vivo 3 T implementation, examining myelin water was conducted by MacMillan et al.[5] In their normative study the authors sought to apply a new 3D multi-echo T_2 relaxation sequence in the cervical spinal cord with sufficient axial resolution to distinguish gray and white matter. The authors performed a scan–rescan reliability assessment of MWF and GMT$_2$, and investigated age-related differences in T_2 measures in healthy subjects.

MR experiments were conducted on 12 young adults (aged 21–30 years) and 18 older adults (aged 51–75 years) with a phased array spine coil, using only the most superior four elements for best localization of the cervical SC, on a Philips 3.0T system. The 3D-T_2 volume was centered at the C5 vertebral body to collect eight 5-mm-thick axial slices, with an in-plane resolution of 0.7×0.7 mm^2 for a scan duration of 20 min. Unlike the study by Smith et al., a triggered or navigated acquisition sequence was not used as the scan time would need to reach more than 30 min to maintain the appropriate minimum TR. Scan–rescan repeatability was also examined by acquiring a second MRI scan within one week in a subset of the older subjects. Voxel-wise decay curve analysis was conducted with NNLS.

Axial MWF maps of young adults exhibited excellent contrast between gray and white matter in the characteristic butterfly pattern, while demarcation was less notable on the intra/extracellular GMT_2 maps and not clearly visible on the global GMT_2 maps. The authors also noted that MWF maps of the younger healthy adults tended to exhibit the expected pattern of gray and white matter more often than the older adults, prompting the need to use a T_2-weighted image for more accurate ROI placement in the older cohort. Quantitative results (Figure 3.5.9) revealed a much higher average white matter MWF of 0.30 in comparison to gray matter with 0.05, in agreement with work by Kozlowski et al.[44] and Minty et al.[4] Global GMT_2, reflecting the mean T_2 of all water, was shorter in white matter than gray matter due to the contribution of the short-T_2 myelin water reservoir in white matter. Intra/extracellular GMT_2, reflecting the mean T_2 of the intra/extracellular water pool, was longer in white matter than gray matter.

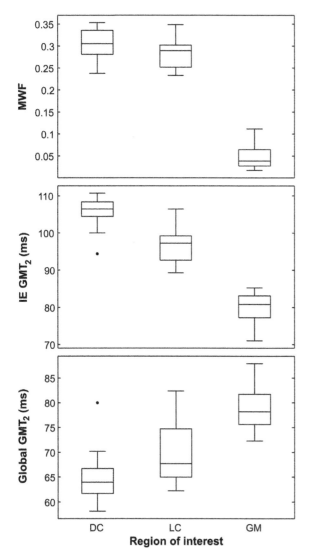

FIGURE 3.5.9 Myelin water fraction (MWF), intra- and extracellular and global geometric mean T_2 in the spinal cord white matter regions (dorsal column (DC), lateral columns (LC)) and gray matter (GM). *Source: Reprinted with permission from Ref. 5.*

MacMillan's observations of gray/white matter differences for GMT_2 measures is in contrast to previous work by Smith et al.[71] who observed no quantitative T_2 difference between white and gray matter. However, several key methodological differences must be kept in mind when comparing findings between the Smith and MacMillan studies. Smith et al. employed a mono-exponential fit to 8 of 16 collected echoes, while MacMillan used an analysis approach that made no a priori assumptions about the number of exponential components to fit 32 echo data. Mono-exponential behavior does not sufficiently characterize the T_2 decay in white matter, and collection of data at longer echo times (320 vs. 160 ms) will provide additional data points to more accurately characterize the T_2 of intermediate components. Therefore, the work by MacMillan et al. is a more accurate representation of T_2 times for spinal cord.

Comparison of dorsal and lateral white matter revealed no significant difference in MWF or global GMT_2, however, intra/extracellular GMT_2 was significantly longer in white matter from the dorsal column. Good reproducibility was observed for all measures, with no significant differences between the data from the two scans and the mean difference between the two scans not significantly different from zero as demonstrated by a Bland–Altman plot. Average reliability coefficients were 0.74 for MWF, 0.66 for intra/extracellular GMT_2, and 0.74 for global GMT_2, within the range reported for a similar study of MWF in brain.[81] Several age-related differences were noted; in particular, older subjects showed a 12% reduction in MWF and 5% shorter intra/extracellular GMT_2 (Figure 3.5.10). The finding of reduced MWF with age is consistent with a postmortem histology study that observed small myelinated fiber density strongly decreased in the cervical spinal cord with age from 19 to 90 years.[82] The authors suggest a more in-depth study of sensory or motor conduction and myelin water imaging would help to elucidate the relationship between myelin degradation and loss of nerve function due to age or disease.

The work by MacMillan and colleagues marked the first time that MWF was measured in the gray matter and white matter separately in the human cervical spinal cord in vivo. This was also the first in vivo human spinal cord MWF measurement at 3 T and the first multislice MWF acquisition in the spinal cord. The authors noted that there was a greater difference in T_2 times between gray and white matter when measuring the intra/extracellular water alone as compared to the entire water distribution, which is an important property that can be exploited in the development of new imaging sequences to improve gray/white matter contrast. Furthermore, the age-related changes in MWF and intra/extracellular GMT_2 times, but not in global

GMT$_2$ times, indicate that multi-echo T_2 relaxation measures are sensitive to changes in myelin integrity and cell morphology that may not be apparent on conventional T_2-weighted images.

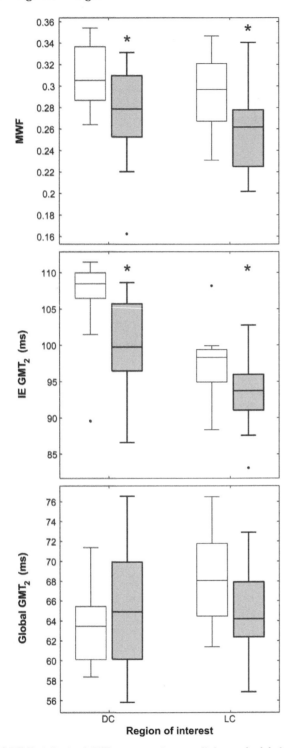

FIGURE 3.5.10 MWF, intra- and extracellular and global geometric mean T_2 in the dorsal and lateral column white matter in younger and older healthy adults. Stars indicate where older adult data (shaded gray) is significantly different from younger adult data. *Source: Reprinted with permission from Ref. 5.*

3.5.4.6 Steady State Technique Provides Increased Volumetric Coverage and Higher Resolution for T_2 Relaxation Measurement

The recent work by Kolind and Deoni[38] using the mcDESPOT technique is a very different approach to the measurement of T_2 relaxation in spinal cord. mcDESPOT provides much larger spinal cord coverage at higher resolution in about the same imaging time as the more conventional multiple spin echo approaches for measuring T_2 relaxation. In addition to extracting a myelin water fraction, mcDESPOT provides values of T_1 and T_2 for two predefined components: (1) myelin water and (2) the free water (both intra and extracellular) components as well as a measure of exchange between these two water reservoirs. As discussed in the introduction, the mcDESPOT technique collects spoiled gradient echo and steady state free precession acquisitions at a wide range of flip angles. The analysis includes extraction of B_0 and B_1 maps that are used to correct the results for artifacts due to B_0 and B_1 inhomogeneities.

The Kolind study focused on the cervical spinal cord using a 3D sagittally acquired acquisition that produced 120 1.5 mm axial slices with 1×1 mm in-plane resolution covering from C1 to C7 in seven healthy volunteers. The data acquisition involved collection of 21 different image contrasts in approximately 26 min. The characteristic butterfly shape of the gray matter in the cervical cord was clearly visible in the myelin water maps. The average MWF measured across the entire cervical spinal cord was 20.5% in agreement with values obtained in previous spin echo studies by Minty[4] and MacMillan[5] but slightly lower than that obtained in the Wu and Laule studies.[3,76] The coefficient of variation of the spinal MWF across the seven volunteers was 2.6%. Cervical spinal cord gray matter MWF averaged 10.9 (1.1)% while white matter MWF averaged 25.1 (1.3)%. The white matter MWF found with mcDESPOT agreed well with previous work in both animals and humans, while the gray matter was slightly higher than found by other studies 3–8%.[4,44,45,64] Unlike the preclinical study by Dula et al.,[64] this study did not find significant differences in MWF between dorsal, lateral, and ventral columns. Finally, the Kolind study investigated the variation of MWF along the spinal cord and found that the MWF for C2–C5 was significantly larger than that for C6–C7, which is consistent with the known reduction in white matter area in the cervical cord enlargement. The MWF reduction at C6–C7 was accompanied by a significant increase in the global T_1, which may also reflect the increased relative amount of gray matter at the enlargement.

While the results from the two techniques for measuring T_2 relaxation in the spinal cord are quite similar, the mcDESPOT approach is fundamentally different from the multiple spin echo approach.

Advantages of the mcDESPOT approach are extended coverage in the same acquisition time, the extraction of many more parameters, and the existence of an explicit accommodation for the effect of water exchange. A disadvantage of the mcDESPOT approach is the complex and somewhat constrained analysis.[39] More research is required before we shall fully understand the differences between these two approaches for measuring MWF.

WHAT CAN WE LEARN FROM HUMAN T_2 RELAXATION STUDIES IN THE SPINAL CORD?

- MWF varies along the length of the spinal cord and agrees with the white matter area fraction as determined by histology
- It is easier to do T_2 measurements in the cervical cord than on the thoracic or lumbar regions
- Quantitative assessment of T_2 is sensitive to changes in cervical cord myelin water fraction in primary progressive multiple sclerosis over 2 years
- T_2 relaxation measurement at 3 T reveals in vivo myelin water distinction of gray and white matter
- Compared to younger individuals, older healthy adults have reduced myelin water in the cervical cord

---

3.5.5 HOW TO COLLECT AND ANALYZE T_2 DATA FROM THE SPINAL CORD

Because the majority of the literature on T_2 in the spinal cord has employed spin echo techniques, the following section refers to multiple spin echo approaches only. Readers who wish to work with steady state approaches (e.g., mcDESPOT) are referred to Kolind and Deoni.[38] Most of the following relates to in vivo imaging of human spinal cord.

3.5.5.1 Acquisition

Coils: The conventional approach for T_2 relaxation measurement is to use the body coil for transmission and phased array surface coils for receiving. However, since high signal to noise is important for accurate T_2 measurement, coils that provide higher signal from the spinal cord will result in improved T_2 measurements, and therefore more research should be dedicated to the development of coils optimized for high resolution, high SNR, and cord imaging (see Chapter 2.1).

Sequence: Due to the presence of magnetic field inhomogeneity in the spinal canal, a multiple spin echo sequence is recommended for cord T_2 measurement. It is unlikely that T_2^* approaches could provide accurate MWF in the cord. Using a series of single TE acquisitions would be prohibitively time consuming and would also expose the T_2 decay curve to diffusion and exchange effects and is therefore not recommended. Some investigators[3,4] have used a preinversion pulse with a TI time of about 1.2 s at 1.5 T to null the CSF signal and thereby minimize artifacts arising from CSF flow. If this approach were to be applied at 3.0 T, a slightly longer TI would be required to account for the increase in CSF T_1 at the higher field strength (appropriate optimization would be recommended). For most MR scanners, pulse programming is required to generate sequences that yield accurate T_2 decay curves.

Generally, 3D sequences are superior to 2D approaches, both for SNR considerations and also to minimize potential artifacts due to magnetization transfer from off-resonance slice selections. To minimize aliasing in 3D sequences with few slices, slice oversampling, i.e., acquisition of up to 1.8 times the number of required slices, is strongly recommended. Figure 3.5.11 shows a pulse sequence diagram for a 3D multiple spin echo sequence.

Minimum TE time: The echo train must contain a "sufficient" number of echoes at short TEs to accurately characterize myelin water, which has a T_2 around 10–20 ms at 1.5 and 3 T. Minimum TE should be 10 ms or less. If the refocusing pulses are not perfect $180°$ pulses, then the echo spacing must be equal otherwise complex stimulated echo patterns may

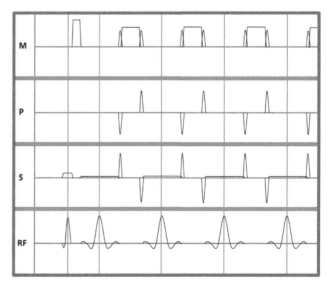

FIGURE 3.5.11 MR pulse sequence for the first few echoes of a 3D multi-spin echo sequence for acquisition of the T_2 decay curve. M, P, and S stand for measurement, phase, and slice, respectively.

occur that are, practically speaking, uncorrectable. It should also be noted that the measured T_2 time may depend upon echo spacing.[83]

Length of echo train: The length of the echo train should be long enough to accurately define the longest T_2 components. Two or four echo T_2 measurement sequences are not recommended for the spinal cord[84] because they contain insufficient information to characterize the relaxation and also the results vary substantially for different choices of echo times. For optimal results, the echo train should extend to three times the longest T_2 time and until the acquired signal has amplitude smaller than the noise. Practically speaking, a minimum configuration for the spinal cord is 32 echoes at echo spacing of 10 ms. If one wishes to accurately characterize long T_2 components due to edema or inflammation, more echoes should be acquired. To extend the echo train length without incurring a specific absorption ratio that is prohibitively high, the echo spacing can be increased for the later echoes.[85] However, if the imaging volume has inhomogenous B_1, then changing the echo spacing could make it effectively impossible to correct for stimulated echo artifacts.[37]

When the echo train length is so long that the signal mean has decreased to less than the noise, then problems may arise due to the existence of Rician noise in magnitude images. Rician, or Rayleigh, noise cannot be easily distinguished from a long T_2 signal. One approach to overcome the problem with Rician noise is to collect real and imaginary data and phase correct the images. Another approach is to discard data points where the signal has decayed to less than one standard deviation of the noise.

TR: For spin echo sequences, the effective TR begins at the last 180° pulse. When the effective TR is less than 1 s the measured MWF may differ from that measured at longer TR times (unpublished observations in brain). To be more specific, for a 32-echo spin echo sequence with spacing 10 ms and TR 1000 ms, the effective TR is $1000 - 310 \text{ ms} = 690 \text{ ms}$. Reasonable results have been obtained from the spinal cord at 3.0 T with effective TR time of ~ 700 ms.[5]

Scan plane: Spinal cord images are best displayed in the axial (or transverse) plane. Axial plane voxel size should be 1×1 mm or less for determination of gray/white matter boundaries and delineation of different white matter tracts. Accurate T_2 measurement is easier to accomplish in the cervical spinal cord because sequences for the thoracic or lumbar spinal cord require both small voxel size in the spinal cord and large FOV to avoid image fold-over artifacts. This in turn has the unwanted effect of lengthening the scan time.

Sequence options: It is not appropriate to make use of saturation bands when collecting T_2 measurements from the spinal cord because the saturation bands act as magnetization transfer pulses that preferentially affect the myelin water signal.[19] The use of cardiac or peripheral triggering to collect echo decay trains at the same point in the cardiac cycle would potentially result in improved data. However, for realistic TR times over 1000 ms, gating generally will require waiting two R-to-R intervals, which may result in prohibitively long imaging times.

Sequence optimization for improved signal to noise: For quantitative analysis, T_2 decay curves must have high signal-to-noise ratios with the minimum acceptable noise standard deviation being approximately 1% of the signal strength at the shortest echo time.[86,87] There are a number of ways to increase SNR in the spinal cord including: increasing the number of averages and increasing the voxel size by changing the slice thickness. More advanced strategies include collecting real and imaginary signals and phase unwrapping the images to gain up to 40% in signal to noise by using only the real image for T_2 fitting. Also, SNR gain can come from the optimization of the RF coil design (see Chapter 2.1).

Sequence optimization for speed: If the images have sufficient signal to noise, parallel imaging is recommended to shorten the imaging time (see Chapter 2.1).

3.5.5.2 Analysis

Decay curve fitting: Because there are at least two distinguishable water reservoirs in the spinal cord, the analysis of T_2 decay curve data must be capable of resolving multiple T_2 components. Single component treatments are incapable of accurately fitting decay curves from cord. Because it is generally not known a priori how many T_2 components exist in a cord voxel, the analysis technique should not be biased toward a fixed number of components. While normal cord is expected to exhibit two T_2 components, in pathology, for example, cord lesions, there may be more than two T_2 components.

To date, 91% of spin-echo T_2 studies of the spinal cord have employed the non-negative-least-squares (NNLS) algorithm with regularization. If, during data collection, the refocusing pulse was more than a few degrees off 180°, stimulated echo artifacts will be evident in the T_2 decay as an odd–even oscillation in the earlier echoes of the decay curve. Stimulated echo artifacts may be corrected by using the extended phase graph algorithm.[35–37] If not corrected, the extracted myelin water fractions may be artificially low.[37]

Recently, Bjarnason and Mitchell developed AnalyzeNNLS,[57] a software designed specifically for multiexponential decay image analysis that has a user-friendly graphical user interface and can analyze data from many MR manufacturers. AnalyzeNNLS is a simple, platform independent analysis tool that was created using the extensive mathematical and visualization libraries in Matlab and released as open source code allowing scientists to evaluate, scrutinize, improve, and expand. AnalyzeNNLS does not deal with stimulated echo artifacts, and therefore caution should be used when applying AnalyzeNNLS at 3 T or higher.

Regularization: When applying regularized NNLS, a decision is made with regard to the amount of smoothing to be applied to the T_2 distribution by changing the relative proportions of the regularizer to the least square quantity being minimized. This topic has not been well researched to date. A rule of thumb in the field has been to add sufficient smoothing to obtain a T_2 distribution with separate myelin water and intra/extracellular water peaks. While the resulting MWF values are only slightly dependent upon the amount of smoothing, it is recommended that the amount of smoothing be held fixed for all spinal cord data acquired from a given pulse sequence and MR scanner.

Input T_2 times and MWF boundaries: Another topic not well researched in the literature is the optimal choice of the optimal number of T_2 times to insert into the NNLS analysis of the T_2 decay curve, as well as what limits to use for myelin water fraction determination. For typical data from human spinal cord, a lower MWF limit of 1–1.5 times the minimum TE time has been used most often. The extracted MWF will depend upon this limit, especially for noisy data. In animal studies with very high signal to noise in the decay curve, much lower T_2 limits may be used. The upper T_2 limit should be 2 s or longer to ensure that CSF components make minimal contribution to the intra/extracellular peak. The number of T_2 points used in the analysis determines the computer time required for analysis. Values for the number of T_2 points used in NNLS studies of white matter vary from 40 to 120. For MWF measurements in spinal cord, it may be best to use a larger number of T_2 points since due to the small size of the spinal cord, few voxels have to be analyzed and computational time is brief. The window chosen for determination of MWF generally extends from the shortest T_2 point up to 35 ms (3.0 T) or 40 ms (1.5 T) for in vivo measurements. Ex vivo measurements in formalin-fixed tissue require a shorter upper T_2 limit. Changes in this window will change the values of MWF. When regularization is used, the myelin water peak is often pushed against the lowest T_2 time. At 3.0 T, the intra/extracellular peak can have signal below 40 ms.

Filters: Several investigators working with MWF in brain and spinal cord have applied filters to either the initial T_2-weighted images[64,88] or to the extracted myelin maps.[76] Optimal choices for filters have not yet been established in the literature; most investigators do not use filters.

3.5.5.3 Spinal Cord T_2 Relaxation "Cookbook" for T_2 Decay Curve Measurement in Humans In Vivo

ACQUISITION	
Coil	• More research is required for development of optimal coils • High SNR is desirable
Sequence	• Axial/transverse plane • 3D Spin echo (T_2) recommended • Gradient echo (T_2^*) not recommended
TR/TE	• Minimum TR effective >700 ms • Minimum TE ≤10 ms • Constant echo spacing
# of echoes	• T_2 decay curve should ideally extend until signal reaches noise level
Resolution	• Voxel sizes $\leq 1 \times 1 \times 5$ mm^3
Options	• Parallel imaging recommended • No saturation bands

ANALYSIS	
Decay curve fit	• Analysis must enable multiple components • Analysis should not require a priori assumptions about the number of T_2 components • Analysis should deal with Rician noise • NNLS recommended
NNLS	• T_2 input times should start at 1–1.5* minimum TE and extend to over 2 s • Optimal # of input T_2 times depends on length of decay curve, size of dataset, and available computer time • Regularization recommended—adjust smoothing to get separate peaks for myelin water and intra/extracellular • Boundaries for myelin water nominally 10–30 (or 40) ms and for intra/extracellular water 30 (or 40)–200 ms

3.5.6 CONCLUDING REMARKS

As noted previously, to date there have been few T_2 relaxation studies in the spinal cord. This is largely because T_2 relaxation acquisition and analysis sequences are not yet available on clinical MR scanners. A distinct advantage of doing T_2 relaxation in the spinal cord is that it provides information relating to the myelination state of the spinal cord that has important medical applications. Furthermore, compared to EPI based techniques such as DTI and fMRI, T_2 relaxation in the spinal cord is much less affected by the B_0 inhomogeneity present in the spinal canal. For these reasons, we predict that the future of T_2 relaxation in the spinal cord will be bright.

References

1. Stewart WA, MacKay AL, Whittall KP, Moore GR, Paty DW. Spin–spin relaxation in experimental allergic encephalomyelitis. Analysis of CPMG data using a non-linear least squares method and linear inverse theory. *Magn Reson Med.* 1993;29(6):767–775.

2. Fischer HW, Rinck PA, Van Haverbeke Y, Muller RN. Nuclear relaxation of human brain gray and white matter: analysis of field dependence and implications for MRI. *Magn Reson Med.* 1990; 16(2):317–334.

3. Wu Y, Alexander AL, Fleming JO, Duncan ID, Field AS. Myelin water fraction in human cervical spinal cord in vivo. *J Comput Assist Tomogr.* 2006;30(2):304–306.

4. Minty EP, Bjarnason TA, Laule C, Mackay AL. Myelin water measurement in the spinal cord. *Magn Reson Med.* 2009;61(4): 883–892.

5. MacMillan EL, Madler B, Fichtner N, et al. Myelin water and T_2 relaxation measurements in the healthy cervical spinal cord at 3.0 T: repeatability and changes with age. *Neuroimage.* 2011;54(2): 1083–1090.

6. Laule C, Leung E, Li DK, et al. Myelin water imaging in multiple sclerosis: quantitative correlations with histopathology. *Mult Scler.* 2006;12(6):747–753.

7. Laule C, Kozlowski P, Leung E, Li DK, Mackay AL, Moore GR. Myelin water imaging of multiple sclerosis at 7 T: correlations with histopathology. *Neuroimage.* 2008;40(1):1575–1580.

8. Smith ME, Sedgewick LM. Studies of the mechanism of demyelination. Regional differences in myelin stability in vitro. *J Neurochem.* 1975;24(4):763–770.

9. Einstein A. Motion of suspended particles in stationary liquids required from the molecular kinetic theory of heat. *Ann Phys.* 1905; 17:549–560.

10. Callaghan PT. *Principles of Nuclear Magnetic Resonance Microscopy.* Oxford: Oxford University Press; 1991.

11. Bloembergen N, Purcell EM, Pound RV. Relaxation effects in nuclear magnetic resonance absorption. *Phys Rev.* 1948;73(7):679.

12. Bottomley PA, Foster TH, Argersinger RE, Pfeifer LM. A review of normal tissue hydrogen NMR relaxation times and relaxation mechanisms from 1–100 MHz: dependence on tissue type, NMR frequency, temperature, species, excision, and age. *Med Phys.* 1984; 11(4):425–448.

13. Carr HY, Purcell EM. Effects of diffusion on free precession in nuclear magnetic resonance experiments. *Phys Rev.* 1954;94(3):630–639.

14. Meiboom G, Gill D. Modified spin echo method for measuring relaxation times. *Rev Sci Instrum.* 1958;29(8):688–691.

15. Ye FQ, Martin WR, Allen PS. Estimation of brain iron in vivo by means of the interecho time dependence of image contrast. *Mag Reson Med.* 1996;36(1):153–158.

16. Stefanovic B, Pike GB. Human whole-blood relaxometry at 1.5 T: assessment of diffusion and exchange models. *Magn Reson Med.* 2004;52(4):716–723.

17. Poon CS, Henkelman RM. Practical T_2 quantitation for clinical applications. *J Magn Reson Imaging.* 1992;2(5):541–553.

18. MacKay A, Whittall K, Adler J, Li D, Paty D, Graeb D. In vivo visualization of myelin water in brain by magnetic resonance. *Magn Reson Med.* 1994;31(6):673–677.

19. Vavasour IM, Whittall KP, Li DK, MacKay AL. Different magnetization transfer effects exhibited by the short and long T_2 components in human brain. *Magn Reson Med.* 2000;44(6):860–866.

20. Meyers SM, Laule C, Vavasour IM, et al. Reproducibility of myelin water fraction analysis: a comparison of region of interest and voxel-based analysis methods. *Magn Reson Imaging.* 2009;27(8): 1096–1103.

21. Du YP, Chu R, Hwang D, et al. Fast multislice mapping of the myelin water fraction using multicompartment analysis of T_2^* decay at 3 T: a preliminary postmortem study. *Magn Reson Med.* 2007;58(5):865–870.

22. Lenz C, Klarhofer M, Scheffler K. Feasibility of in vivo myelin water imaging using 3D multigradient-echo pulse sequences. *Magn Reson Med.* 2011;68(2):523–528.

23. Oh J, Han ET, Lee MC, Nelson SJ, Pelletier D. Multislice brain myelin water fractions at 3 T in multiple sclerosis. *J Neuroimaging.* 2007;17(2):156–163.

24. Oh J, Han ET, Pelletier D, Nelson SJ. Measurement of in vivo multi-component T_2 relaxation times for brain tissue using multi-slice T_2 prep at 1.5 and 3 T. *Magn Reson Imaging.* 2006;24(1): 33–43. Epub 2005 Dec 2019.

25. Nguyen TD, Wisnieff C, Cooper MA, et al. T_2 prep three-dimensional spiral imaging with efficient whole brain coverage for myelin water quantification at 1.5 tesla. *Magn Reson Med.* 2012;67(3):614–621.

26. Deoni SC, Rutt BK, Arun T, Pierpaoli C, Jones DK. Gleaning multicomponent T_1 and T_2 information from steady-state imaging data. *Magn Reson Med.* 2008;60(6):1372–1387.

27. Whittall KP, MacKay AL. Quantitative interpretation of NMR relaxation data. *J Magn Reson.* 1989;84(1):134–152.

28. Bjarnason TA. Proof that gmT2 is the reciprocal of gmR2. *Concepts Magn Reson.* 2011;38A(3):128–131.

29. Armspach JP, Gounot D, Rumbach L, Chambron J. In vivo determination of multiexponential T_2 relaxation in the brain of patients with multiple sclerosis. *Magn Reson Imaging.* 1991;9(1):107–113.

30. Lancaster JL, Andrews T, Hardies LJ, Dodd S, Fox PT. Three-pool model of white matter. *J Magn Reson Imaging.* 2003;17(1):1–10.

31. Vermathen P, Robert-Tissot L, Pietz J, Lutz T, Boesch C, Kreis R. Characterization of white matter alterations in phenylketonuria by magnetic resonance relaxometry and diffusion tensor imaging. *Magn Reson Med.* 2007;58(6):1145–1156.

32. Deoni SC, Rutt BK, Arun T, Pierpaoli C, Jones DK. Gleaning multi-component T_1 and T_2 information from steady-state imaging data. In: *ISMRM; 2008;* Toronto, Canada. 2008:240.

33. Schick F. Whole-body MRI at high field: technical limits and clinical potential. *Eur Radiol.* 2005;15(5):946–959.

34. Vold RL, Vold RR, Simon HE. Errors in measurements of transverse relaxation rates. *J Magn Reson.* 1973;11(3):283–298.

35. Hennig J. Multiecho imaging sequences with low refocusing flip angles. *J Magn Reson.* 1988;78(3):397–407.

36. Lebel RM, Wilman AH. Transverse relaxometry with stimulated echo compensation. *Magn Reson Med.* 2010;64(4):1005–1014.

37. Prasloski T, Madler B, Xiang QS, Mackay A, Jones C. Applications of stimulated echo correction to multicomponent T_2 analysis. *Magn Reson Med.* 2011;67(6):1803–1814.

38. Kolind SH, Deoni SC. Rapid three-dimensional multicomponent relaxation imaging of the cervical spinal cord. *Magn Reson Med.* 2011;65(2):551–556.

39. Lankford CL, Does MD. On the inherent precision of mcDESPOT. *Magn Reson Med.* 2013;69(1):127–136.

40. Kroeker RM, Henkelman RM. Analysis of biological NMR relaxation data with continuous distributions of relaxation times. *J Magn Reson.* 1986;69(2):218–235.

41. Menon RS, Allen PS. Application of continuous relaxation time distributions to the fitting of data from model systems and excised tissue. *Magn Reson Med.* 1991;20(2):214–227.

42. James F, Roos M. Minuit – a system for function minimization and analysis of the parameter errors and correlations. *Comput Phys Commun.* 1975;10(6):343–367.

43. Norton W, Cammer W. Isolation and characterization of myelin. In: Morell P, ed. *Myelin.* 2nd ed. New York: Plenum Press; 1984: 147–195.

44. Kozlowski P, Liu J, Yung AC, Tetzlaff W. High-resolution myelin water measurements in rat spinal cord. *Magn Reson Med.* 2008; 59(4):796–802.

45. Kozlowski P, Raj D, Liu J, Lam C, Yung AC, Tetzlaff W. Characterizing white matter damage in rat spinal cord with quantitative MRI and histology. *J Neurotrauma.* 2008;25(6):653–676.

46. Yung AC, Kozlowski P. Signal-to-noise ratio comparison of phased-array vs. implantable coil for rat spinal cord MRI. *Magn Reson Imaging.* 2007;25(8):1215–1221.

47. Webb S, Munro CA, Midha R, Stanisz GJ. Is multicomponent T_2 a good measure of myelin content in peripheral nerve? *Magn Reson Med.* 2003;49(4):638–645.

48. Wolff SD, Balaban RS. Magnetization transfer contrast (MTC) and tissue water proton relaxation in vivo. *Magn Reson Med.* 1989;10(1): 135–144.

49. Vavasour IM, Laule C, Li DK, Traboulsee AL, MacKay AL. Is the magnetization transfer ratio a marker for myelin in multiple sclerosis? *J Magn Reson Imaging.* 2011;33(3):713–718.

50. Schmierer K, Scaravilli F, Altmann DR, Barker GJ, Miller DH. Magnetization transfer ratio and myelin in postmortem multiple sclerosis brain. *Ann Neurol.* 2004;56(3):407–415.

51. van Waesberghe JH, Kamphorst W, De Groot CJ, et al. Axonal loss in multiple sclerosis lesions: magnetic resonance imaging insights into substrates of disability. *Ann Neurol.* 1999;46(5):747–754.

52. Fisher E, Chang A, Fox RJ, et al. Imaging correlates of axonal swelling in chronic multiple sclerosis brains. *Ann Neurol.* 2007; 62(3):219–228.

53. Gareau PJ, Rutt BK, Karlik SJ, Mitchell JR. Magnetization transfer and multicomponent T_2 relaxation measurements with histopathologic correlation in an experimental model of MS. *J Magn Reson Imaging.* 2000;11(6):586–595.

54. McCreary CR, Bjarnason TA, Skihar V, Mitchell JR, Yong VW, Dunn JF. Multiexponential T_2 and magnetization transfer MRI of demyelination and remyelination in murine spinal cord. *Neuroimage.* 2009;45(4):1173–1182.

55. Hall SM. The effect of injections of lysophosphatidyl choline into white matter of the adult mouse spinal cord. *J Cell Sci.* 1972;10(2): 535–546.

56. Jeffery ND, Blakemore WF. Remyelination of mouse spinal cord axons demyelinated by local injection of lysolecithin. *J Neurocytol.* 1995;24(10):775–781.

57. Bjarnason TA, Mitchell JR. AnalyzeNNLS: magnetic resonance multiexponential decay image analysis. *J Magn Reson.* 2010;206(2): 200–204.

58. Tipperman R, Kasckow J, Herndon RM. The fine structure of macrophages in lysolecithin-induced demyelination: a freeze-fracture study. *J Neuropathol Exp Neurol.* 1984;43(5):522–530.

59. Odrobina EE, Lam TY, Pun T, Midha R, Stanisz GJ. MR properties of excised neural tissue following experimentally induced demyelination. *NMR Biomed.* 2005;18(5):277–284.

60. Gareau PJ, Rutt BK, Bowen CV, Karlik SJ, Mitchell JR. In vivo measurements of multi-component T_2 relaxation behaviour in guinea pig brain. *Magn Reson Imaging.* 1999;17(9):1319–1325.

61. Koenig SH, Brown 3rd RD, Spiller M, Lundbom N. Relaxometry of brain: why white matter appears bright in MRI. *Magn Reson Med.* 1990;14(3):482–495.

62. Stanisz GJ, Kecojevic A, Bronskill MJ, Henkelman RM. Characterizing white matter with magnetization transfer and T_2. *Magn Reson Med.* 1999;42(6):1128–1136.

63. Bjarnason T, Vavasour I, Chia C, MacKay A. Characterization of the NMR behaviour of white matter in bovine brain. *Magn Reson Med.* 2005;54(5):1072–1081.

64. Dula AN, Gochberg DF, Valentine HL, Valentine WM, Does MD. Multiexponential T_2, magnetization transfer, and quantitative histology in white matter tracts of rat spinal cord. *Magn Reson Med.* 2010;63:902–909.

65. Golub G, Heath M, Wahba G. Generalized cross-validation as a method for choosing a good ridge parameter. *Technometrics.* 1970; 21(2):215–223.

66. Harkins KD, Dula AN, Does MD. Effect of intercompartmental water exchange on the apparent myelin water fraction in multiexponential T_2 measurements of rat spinal cord. *Magn Reson Med.* 2012;67(3):793–800.

67. McConnell HM. Reaction rates by nuclear magnetic resonance. *J Chem Phys.* 1958;28(3):430–431.

68. Levesque IR, Pike GB. Characterizing healthy and diseased white matter using quantitative magnetization transfer and multicomponent T_2 relaxometry: a unified view via a four-pool model. *Magn Reson Med.* 2009;62(6):1487–1496.

69. Zimmerman JR, Brittin WE. Nuclear magnetic resonance studies in multiple phase systems: lifetime of a water molecule in an adsorbing phase of silica gel. *J Chem Phys.* 1957;61(10):1328–1333.

70. Laule C, Vavasour IM, Moore GRW, et al. Water content and myelin water fraction in multiple sclerosis: a T_2 relaxation study. *J Neurol.* 2004;251(6):284–293.

71. Smith SA, Edden RA, Farrell JA, Barker PB, Van Zijl PC. Measurement of T_1 and T_2 in the cervical spinal cord at 3 tesla. *Magn Reson Med.* 2008;60(1):213–219.

72. Lu H, Nagae-Poetscher LM, Golay X, Lin D, Pomper M, van Zijl PC. Routine clinical brain MRI sequences for use at 3.0 Tesla. *J Magn Reson Imaging.* 2005;22(1):13–22.

73. Haacke E, Brown R, Thompson M. *Magnetic Resonance Imaging: Physical Principles and Sequence Design.* John Wiley & Sons Canada Ltd; 1999.

74. McGowan JC. Technical issues for MRI examination of the spinal cord. *J Neurol Sci.* 2000;172(Suppl 1):S27–S31.

75. Riley H. *Atlas of the Basal Ganglia, Brain Stem and Spinal Cord Based on Myelin-Stained Material.* Williams & Wilkins; 1943.

76. Laule C, Vavasour IM, Zhao Y, et al. Two-year study of cervical cord volume and myelin water in primary progressive multiple sclerosis. *Mult Scler.* 2010;16(6):670–677.

77. Lycklama-a-Nijeholt GJ, van Walderveen MA, Castelijns JA, et al. Brain and spinal cord abnormalities in multiple sclerosis. Correlation between MRI parameters, clinical subtypes and symptoms. *Brain.* 1998;121(Pt 4):687–697.

78. Stevenson VL, Leary SM, Losseff NA, et al. Spinal cord atrophy and disability in MS: a longitudinal study. *Neurology.* 1998;51(1): 234–238.

79. Bieniek M, Altmann DR, Davies GR, et al. Cord atrophy separates early primary progressive and relapsing remitting multiple sclerosis. *J Neurol Neurosurg Psychiatry.* 2006;77(9):1036–1039.

80. Gilmore CP, DeLuca GC, Bo L, et al. Spinal cord atrophy in multiple sclerosis caused by white matter volume loss. *Arch Neurol.* 2005;62(12):1859–1862.

81. Vavasour IM, Clark CM, Li DK, Mackay AL. Reproducibility and reliability of MR measurements in white matter: clinical implications. *Neuroimage.* 2006;32(2):637–642.

82. Terao S, Sobue G, Hashizume Y, Shimada N, Mitsuma T. Age-related changes of the myelinated fibers in the human corticospinal tract: a quantitative analysis. *Acta Neuropathol.* 1994;88(2): 137–142.

83. Stefanovic B, Sled JG, Pike GB. Quantitative T_2 in the occipital lobe: the role of the CPMG refocusing rate. *J Magn Reson Imaging*. 2003;18(3):302–309.

84. Whittall KP, MacKay AL, Li DK. Are mono-exponential fits to a few echoes sufficient to determine T_2 relaxation for in vivo human brain? *Magn Reson Med*. 1999;41(6):1255–1257.

85. Skinner MG, Kolind SH, Mackay AL. The effect of varying echo spacing within a multiecho acquisition: better characterization of long T_2 components. *Magn Reson Imaging*. 2007;25(6): 834–839.

86. Fenrich FR, Beaulieu C, Allen PS. Relaxation times and microstructures. *NMR Biomed*. 2001;14(2):133–139.

87. Graham SJ, Stanchev PL, Bronskill MJ. Criteria for analysis of multicomponent tissue T_2 relaxation data. *Magn Reson Med*. 1996; 35(3):370–378.

88. Jones CK, Whittall KP, MacKay AL. Robust myelin water quantification: averaging vs. spatial filtering. *Magn Reson Med*. 2003; 50(1):206–209.

Atrophy

Mark A. Horsfield[1], Massimo Filippi[2]

[1]Department of Cardiovascular Sciences, University of Leicester, Leicester, UK [2]Institute of Experimental Neurology, Division of Neuroscience, San Raffaele Scientific Institute, Vita-Salute San Raffaele University, Milan, Italy

3.6.1 HISTORICAL PERSPECTIVE

Since the early days of X-ray computerized tomography (CT) in the late 1970s, it has been possible to visualize the spinal cord in cross-section in vivo, and to make quantitative measurements of the cord diameter. Early studies required the introduction of an iodinated contrast agent into the cerebrospinal fluid (CSF) by means of a lumbar puncture, in a procedure known as computed myelography.[1,2] Cord atrophy was clearly visible, and the normal range of cord size in the cervical region as measured on CT was established early on (Figure 3.6.1).

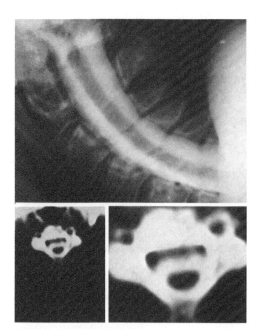

FIGURE 3.6.1 Pioneering work in assessing cord atrophy from X-ray computerized tomography (CT) scans. Atrophy at the C4 level. *Source: From Ref. 1, reprinted with permission.*

Early quantitative measurements made from magnetic resonance imaging (MRI) scans also established the normal range of cord diameters in the cervical and thoracic regions. MRI has considerable advantages over CT scanning: there is no ionizing radiation involved, and the natural contrast between the cord and the CSF-filled space is much greater so that contrast agent in the arachnoid space is not needed. Whether from CT scans or from MRI, linear size measurements in the anterior-posterior (A-P) and left-right (L-R) directions were made manually by either using a rule held against a radiographic film or using a computer image analysis system. Computerized systems were also used to draw around the cord in order to assess its cross-sectional area.

While the measurement of cross-sectional areas was shown to be feasible, manual delineation of the cord raises the issue of whether such measurements are reliable. It was recognized early on that human perception of the location of the boundary between the cord parenchyma and the CSF is heavily influenced by the brightness and contrast settings of the radiographic film or digital display, and that standardization was needed if assessment consistency was to be achieved.[3] The development of standardized methods for quantitative analysis, and preferably at least some automation, aims to reduce the variability of repeated measures by a single assessor (intraobserver reproducibility) or between different assessors (interobserver reproducibility). If a method can be developed that is completely automated, then the only influence on the measurements is the repeatability of the scanning technique (the so-called scan-rescan variability). An evaluation of all of these types of error is needed for a spinal cord atrophy measurement technique to become established and accepted as reliable.

This also brings up the question of how reliable such measures need to be in practice, which is of course

207

dependent on the context of the measurement. Changes in spinal cord cross-sectional area may occur at a very slow rate, of the order of a few percent per year, which makes challenging the detection of change in relatively short longitudinal studies, or in cross-sectional studies at the early stages of disease. In order to keep patient sample sizes manageably small, it is imperative to employ the most reliable and robust techniques that are currently available, and to continue to improve on existing methods.

3.6.2 MRI SCANNING CONSIDERATIONS

Successful segmentation of the spinal cord relies on there being a good demarcation of the boundary between the cord parenchyma and the surrounding CSF. In T_1-weighted imaging, the CSF will be darker than the cord due its long T_1, while in T_2-weighted imaging, the CSF will be brighter due to its long T_2. Either type of scan can therefore, in principle, be employed in atrophy measurements. In order to recommend one particular type of scan, other considerations must therefore be brought into play.

First is the spatial resolution that can be achieved. The highest spatial resolution is normally achieved by using a three-dimensional (3D) acquisition, with two spatial dimensions being phase encoded and one dimension being frequency encoded. This allows the MR signal to be acquired from the whole imaging volume throughout the imaging sequence, maximizing signal-to-noise ratio (SNR) and leading to the best possible spatial resolution. This type of acquisition requires a very short repetition time (TR) that is really only compatible with gradient-echo pulse sequences and T_1-weighted imaging. While it is possible to perform 3D acquisition of T_2-weighted images, 3D T_2 pulse sequences are still normally less SNR efficient than T_1-weighted sequences, and they rely on multiple-echo rapid acquisition with relaxation enhancement (RARE) with very long echo trains, which are prone to blurring fine detail, and artifacts at feature boundaries.[4]

However, T_2-weighted imaging may be desired for other reasons, for example to look for focal hyperintensities in the cord that are indicative of pathology. One potential problem is that pathology causing hyperintensity near the edge of the cord could confound segmentation algorithms, leading to an underestimation of cord area in that region. Because of the shape of the spinal cord, with only slow changes in the cross-section along its length, it is feasible to assess atrophy on T_2-weighted multislice cord images acquired axially and with relatively poor resolution in the slice (head-foot) direction. Nevertheless, care must be taken in regions where the cord does not pass perpendicularly through the image plane, because where the cord passes at an angle through

the slice, the boundary will appear blurred because the boundary position varies through the image slice.

3D T_1-weighted acquisition is normally performed with the frequency-encoded direction being head-foot, and the stored image planes are therefore either sagittal or coronal. Since the cord cross-section is viewed in the axial plane, the scans must therefore be reformatted into axial, and at this point it is prudent to use a multiplanar reconstruction (MPR), with free selection of the resampled plane orientation, to make sure that the cord axis is truly perpendicular to the reconstructed planes at the most important anatomical location, such as the cervical region. Loss of image quality on reformatting of 3D acquired images can be completely avoided if sinc interpolation is used.

MR images are prone to motion artifacts, and the cervical region of the cord can suffer particularly badly. Because of the way that MR image data are collected, gross motion of the patient often appears as replications of the image features, or "ghosts", that are superimposed on top of the image at intervals over the field of view. The main causes are breathing, swallowing, or movement caused by discomfort of the patient during long scans. In particular, in the thoracic region, cardiac motion and pulsation of the major vessels are issues. The artifacts caused by breathing, swallowing, and cardiac motion can be greatly reduced by using "saturation bands" that cover the anterior portion of the chest and abdomen away from the cord. In saturation bands, radiofrequency (RF) pulses are repeatedly applied in conjunction with a magnetic field gradient to select and dephase the signal from the moving tissue so that it cannot corrupt the region of interest. CSF pulsation can cause bright signal that is misplaced and can appear

---

ACQUISITION FOR ATROPHY MEASUREMENTS

- 3D scans → isotropic resolution (1 mm or less) and high SNR
- Use saturation bands on the chest and abdomen to suppress image artifacts from breathing and swallowing
- Make use of parallel imaging for fast acquisition (see Chapter 2.1)
- T_1 weighted → CSF dark and spinal cord bright
  - MP-RAGE (Siemens), 3DFFE (Philips), SPGR (GE)
- T_2 weighted → CSF bright and spinal cord dark
  - SPACE (Siemens), VISTA (Philips), and CUBE (GE)
  - Hyperintensities due to white matter pathology could confound cord segmentation

superimposed on the cord. Flow-compensated sequences greatly alleviate the problem, and these work by "gradient moment nulling" so that spins moving with a fairly constant velocity do not experience a phase shift relative to stationary spins, and therefore do not appear spatially misplaced.[5]

3.6.3 SEMIAUTOMATED ATROPHY MEASUREMENT

All methods for estimating spinal cord atrophy from MRI scans have, at their heart, a way of determining the location of the boundary between the cord parenchyma and the surrounding material. For much of the length of the cord, it is bordered by CSF, although there are many anatomical levels where the cord surface touches the surface of the spinal canal. This leads to a loss of the distinctive boundary as the surrounding tissues may have a very similar intensity to the cord. Furthermore, although the cord is roughly ovoid in cross-section, the shape changes from a more circular shape in the upper cervical region to a flattened elliptical shape in the mid-lower cervical region, becoming more circular again in the thoracic region before tapering out to the conus in the upper lumbar region (Figure 3.6.2). With the high spatial resolution that is now available from modern MRI scanners, the dorsal and ventral nerve roots that come from the cord at regular intervals, passing through the intervertebral foramina, are increasingly visible on thin-slice images and can further confound segmentation software. Nevertheless, the cord is a long, thin, curved cylinder of irregular cross-section, with a convex or only slightly concave boundary and with a cross-sectional shape that changes only slowly along its length. These properties can be used to good effect when segmenting the cord, and can help to overcome the problems associated with marginal spatial resolution and poor and inconsistent contrast.

Cord segmentation methods can be divided roughly into those that use cord shape information and those that do not. The methods that do not use shape information have tended to concentrate on measuring the cord at a specific anatomical level, particularly in the midcervical region. This is because, with normal neck flexion, at this level the spinal cord is usually surrounded completely by CSF, or there is only a small region where the cord abuts the border of the spinal canal. There is good cord–CSF contrast, and the division between them involves the selection of an intensity threshold.

3.6.3.1 Intensity Threshold Selection

With the spatial resolution of the order of 0.8–1.0 mm that is achievable on modern MRI scanners, the shape of the cord is easily judged by the human eye. Nevertheless, at the boundary between the cord and the CSF, there is a so-called partial-volume effect that blurs the boundary because an image voxel contains a mixture of parenchyma and CSF, with the proportion of each being determined by the position of the boundary within the voxel (Figure 3.6.3).

When an image pixel contains a 50% mixture of cord and CSF, the intensity should be midway between the intensity of pixels that contain pure cord and that for pure CSF. Thus, the threshold to separate the two is logically set halfway between these intensities.[3] This forms the basis of the cord area measurement method developed by Losseff et al.,[6] which involves selection of the intensity threshold by defining two regions of interest (ROIs), one surrounding just the cord and the other surrounding the whole of the intravertebral space. With the intensity threshold set, it should be a simple matter to outline the cord by following a contour of isointensity at the cord surface. Contour following may be problematic when the cord touches the surface of the spinal canal, with the contour "spilling out" into adjacent structures; hence, the Losseff method is specifically used at the C2–C3 level, where the cord is usually centered within the canal.

3.6.3.2 Edge Detection

The location of the edge of the cord may also be determined in another way. The intensity difference between the cord and CSF, together with the inherent blurring and finite pixel size in MR images, means that there is a gradient in intensity at the boundary. The true edge position is therefore most likely to be the point of maximum intensity gradient magnitude. This definition of the edge has the advantage that it is relatively insensitive to small variations in image intensity over the image field of view, such as occur due to the nonuniform reception properties of the RF coils. The spinal cord can be segmented over an extended region at the C2 level using edge detection, as was demonstrated by Tench et al.[7] (Figure 3.6.4).

3.6.3.3 Incorporating Shape Information

Because the cord has a cylindrical shape with a closed boundary, this topological information can be used to make the segmentation of the cord more robust. Furthermore, the shape varies smoothly both around the circumference of the cylinder and in the head-foot direction, with no abrupt changes in cross-section. Both of these properties can help segmentation algorithms to

FIGURE 3.6.2 Changing cross-sectional shape of
the spinal cord illustrated on four axial views and one
sagittal view of a T2-weighted image. It changes from
a fairly circular shape in the upper cervical region (the
most cranial margin of C0), to a flattened elliptical
shape in the mid-lower cervical region (C2—C6), and becomes more circular again in the thoracic region (T9
—T10) before tapering out in the upper lumbar region.
The cord has been segmented and outlined using the
method in Ref. 11.

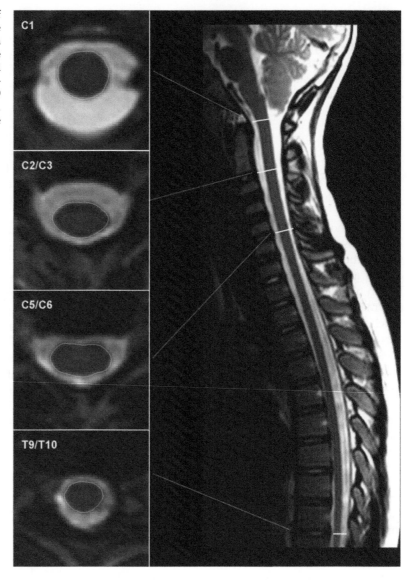

overcome problems such as image artifacts that can
overlie the cord, poor contrast due to CSF pulsation,
and the cord touching the surface of the spinal canal
and abutting structures that are of very similar brightness to the cord.

In order to produce smooth outline shapes, a common
approach is to use an active contour method, such as a
"snake",[8] which is a way to define a smooth curve that
is attracted to image features such as edges, but in which
sharp bends are penalized. Individual axial slices from
the cord image may be analyzed independently, as
was done by Deng et al.[9] A total energy term is
composed of a weighted sum of both "external" and
"internal" components. The external energy encapsu-
lates the attraction of the contour to the edges of image
features; it is computed from the intensity gradient
and is at a minimum when the contour lies on a steep

intensity gradient. The internal energy is a property of
the shape of the contour and is minimized when the contour is a smooth uniform curve. Minimizing the total
energy is a balance between maintaining a smooth shape
whilst conforming to the edges of features present in the
image; this smoothness helps to prevent the contour
from spreading into adjacent structures, or wandering
when the contrast at the edge of the cord is poor. The
method was reliable enough to detect atrophy of a few
percent.

The extension of the active contour into three dimensions is the active surface. Treating the cord as a single
3D structure whose surface is to be found, rather than
as individual two-dimensional (2D) slices, has the
potential to further improve reliability. Coulon et al.[10]
developed a method that could segment the cord over
the whole of the cervical region. Although the reliability

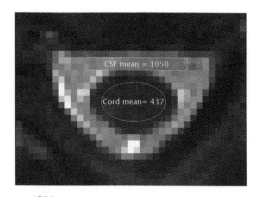

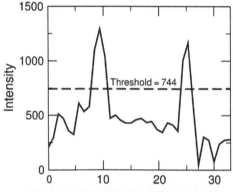

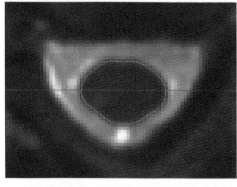

FIGURE 3.6.3 T_2-weighted axial section through the spinal cord at the C2–C3 level. Spatial resolution is 0.93 mm × 0.93 mm in plane, with a slice thickness of 3.0 mm. Top: The placement of regions of interest (ROIs) within the cerebrospinal fluid (CSF) and parenchyma, carefully positioned to avoid partial volume. The mean intensity within each region is used to calculate the intensity threshold that is midway between them. Middle: A trace through the cord at the position shown in the lower picture illustrates that the threshold separates the parenchyma in the central portion of the plot from the peaks in intensity in the arachnoid space. Lower: The same cord image but interpolated to emphasize the partial volume effect, with a contour of iso-intensity plotted around the cord, the contour level being set from the calculated threshold.

was not as great as when cord area was measured just at the C2–C3 level using Losseff's method, this paper nevertheless showed the potential of active surface models.

An active surface model has been pursued in our own work,[11] but it incorporates a number of modifications to improve both the speed of processing and the reliability.

First, the cord surface is defined, as in the work by Deng et al.[9] (in 2D), by a B-spline radius generator, which is a much more compact way of representing the surface. The cord centerline is also defined by a spline interpolator. Smoothness around the circumference is ensured by applying filtering to the Fourier representation of the cord shape, removing any high-spatial-frequency Fourier coefficients. Finally, smooth transitions in shape along the cord are enforced by fitting to spatial variation of the Fourier coefficients along the cord using a polynomial least-squares fitting procedure, and re-estimating the coefficients by interpolation of the fitted polynomial curve. The order of the polynomials and the number of Fourier coefficients together determine the number of degrees of freedom, which is set to be a compromise between the fidelity of the surface shape and the robustness and speed of the surface extraction. Even with a high number of degrees of freedom, the whole process of cord segmentation is quite fast (typically less than 5 min), while a "believable" representation of the cord shape can be achieved with surprisingly few degrees of freedom (Figure 3.6.5).

In 3D active surface methods, the image intensity gradient is again used to generate a "force" to drive the active surface to the true cord surface. The use of 3D Sobel operators[13] is a convenient way to generate image intensity gradient information. The operators result in three images showing intensity gradients in the x, y, and z directions, although these images need to be intensity scaled in order to take account of any differences in pixel spacing in the three directions. The gradient images can be separately interpolated to estimate the gradient vector at any subpixel spatial location. When the active surface is aligned with the cord surface, the local image intensity gradient vector should be normal to the active surface.

Using the types of method that take into account the cord topology to apply an appropriate degree of smoothing, the spinal cord can be extracted and its cross-sectional area quantified with reproducibility comparable to, if not better than, the traditional Losseff method. Several studies have shown the value of such measures in demonstrating differences between clinical phenotypes in MS, and in measuring small changes in longitudinal studies in relatively small patient cohorts.

3.6.4 TOWARD THE FULLY AUTOMATED

All the methods for cord segmentation described in this chapter require some degree of user interaction: it is common for the user to indicate the approximate position of the cord by placing a set of point landmarks at the center of the cord, on a range of slices that covers the volume of interest. Fully automated analysis would

FIGURE 3.6.4 (A) Axial image of the cord surrounded by cerebrospinal fluid (CSF) at the C2 level. (B) Edges automatically detected; pixels are highlighted where the intensity gradient is locally maximal. (C) The boundary between the cord and CSF has been identified by the operator to form a region of interest around the cord. *Source: From Ref. 7, reprinted with permission.*

remove any subjectivity, making the atrophy measures operator independent and patient repositioning and scanner operation the only sources of measurement error. If identification of the cord could be accomplished automatically and reliably, many segmentation schemes could become fully automatic.

The method presented by Gray et al.[14] is a fully automated two-stage process using the Fuzzy C-Means clustering algorithm. The first stage identifies the spinal canal by selecting the largest fuzzy-connected component near the center of the image field of view. From this, the centerline of the canal is extracted as the centroid of this feature. The second step segments the CSF from the spinal cord. While this was a preliminary study, it illustrates that it is, in principle, possible to estimate cord atrophy in a fully automated procedure.

afforded by imaging at high field strength now make this feasible, and a gray matter fraction of around 25% has been reported in healthy controls when using a 7.0 T scanner to image the cervical cord, using manual segmentation.[15] A slightly smaller gray matter fraction of about 17% has been reported using a semiautomated segmentation technique applied to images acquired at 3.0 T, using an optimized 3D gradient-echo pulse sequence.[16] Separate assessment of gray matter and white matter atrophy may become an important research area, as it has in the brain, because it might contribute to a better understanding of the pathological mechanisms leading to cord atrophy in different neurological conditions, for example by determining whether cord volume loss is due to white matter (i.e., demyelination and axonal loss) rather than gray matter (i.e., neuronal loss) injury.

3.6.5 GRAY AND WHITE MATTER VOLUMENTRY

Separate measurement of the gray and white matter cross-sectional areas or volumes requires segmentation of these two tissues in the cord images. The excellent gray and white matter contrast and spatial resolution

3.6.6 WHAT SHOULD WE MEASURE?

Most atrophy assessments have measured the cord cross-sectional area, normally at a particular spinal level, such as the C2–C3 disk.[6] For measures over an extended cord segment, the cord volume has also been suggested

FIGURE 3.6.5 Spinal cord contours obtained using an active surface method (Horsfield et al.[11]) at three levels on a T_1-weighted image. Top row: top of C2; middle row: C3–C4; and bottom row; C7–C8. The column labels indicate the numbers of Fourier shape coefficients used to describe the outline shape. A convincing outline of the cord can be seen at all levels with 13 coefficients, while increasing to them to 31 can lead to an uneven outline, as seen at the C2 level. Choosing the optimum is a compromise between robustness and shape fidelity.

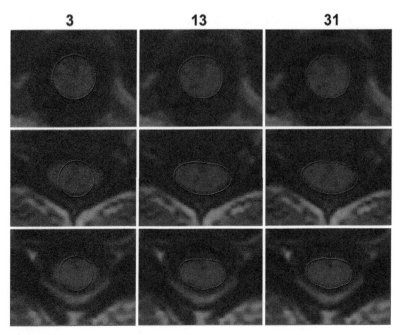

as a possible outcome. However, this has the potential to introduce an unnecessary source of variability, since the volume will be more or less proportional to the length of cord segment defined. Any variability in the definition of the superior or inferior extent of the cord segment will give commensurate errors in volume. Instead, the average cross-sectional area over the segment should be reported, which will be largely insensitive to the variation in cord extent landmarks.

If image planes are acquired perpendicular to the cord centerline, or if a multiplanar reconstruction is performed to resample them to this orientation, then the area of an ROI surrounding the cord is the cord area. However, over an extended length, the cord curves and therefore does not remain perpendicular to the scan planes along its whole length. It is therefore an advantage if a cord segmentation method intrinsically generates the path of the cord centerline, since then the true perpendicular area can be generated easily along the whole cord.[10]

Of course, the spinal cord varies in both length and cross-sectional area in the normal population, which should be taken into account when assessing differences between individuals or in group analysis. Normalization can use head size as a factor that is not affected by disease to scale the cord areas. This can be as a total intracranial volume (TICV)[17] or as a typical cranial cross-sectional area measured from MRI scans.[11] However, it may also be possible to use the anatomy of the cord, such as the cross-sectional area of the spinal thecal sac, or the cord length as the normalization factor.[18]

METHODS FOR MEASURING SPINAL CORD AREA

- Intensity thresholding: optimal threshold chosen based on mean cord parenchyma and CSF intensities (e.g., Losseff)[6]
- Edge detection: cord surface defined by maximum intensity gradient (e.g., Tench)[7]
- Active contour and surface: shape information used to constrain segmentation (e.g., Coulon,[10] Deng,[9] and Horsfield[11])

3.6.7 THE CLINICAL NEED FOR ATROPHY MEASUREMENT

The spinal cord is a clinically eloquent site in the central nervous system, which is often affected by inflammatory and neurodegenerative processes leading to irreversible tissue loss. Several neurological conditions, such as multiple sclerosis (MS),[19,20] demyelinating

inflammatory myelopathies,[21] amyotrophic lateral sclerosis (ALS),[22] and spinal cord injury (SCI),[23] lead to severe cord atrophy. Since the spinal cord is the main pathway for information connecting the brain with the peripheral nervous system, spinal cord atrophy has a major impact on patients' clinical status.

In MS, focal and diffuse damage occurs in the brain and spinal cord, and MRI is the most sensitive tool to detect changes in tissue integrity over time.[20,24] Spinal cord damage has the potential to affect dramatically the functional outcome of patients with MS. The spinal cord is frequently involved in this disease, with conventional MRI scans showing focal cord lesions in up to 90% of patients with an established form of the disease.[25] Cord pathology plays an important role in the development of irreversible clinical disability in MS, and the quantification of cord atrophy[26–28] might provide useful surrogate markers to monitor disease progression, either natural or modified by treatment. The following are the main results derived from the quantification of cord atrophy in patients with MS.

3.6.7.1 Cord Atrophy and Clinical Phenotypes

Cord tissue loss is present in all MS disease clinical phenotypes, but it is more pronounced in the progressive[12,29–34] than in the relapsing-remitting (RR)[12,35,36] forms of the disease (RRMS), with no differences between patients with primary progressive MS (PPMS) and those with secondary progressive MS (SPMS).[37] Studies of patients at presentation with clinically isolated syndromes (CIS) suggestive of MS have provided conflicting results, since some of them did not find atrophy in the cervical portion of the cord,[12,38] while others did.[39] Differences in the methods applied to quantify atrophy and in the clinical and MRI characteristics of the subjects enrolled in these studies might explain, at least in part, these discrepancies. This notion is also supported by the results of the study of Brex et al.,[39] who found that the spinal cord area was significantly smaller in the subgroup of CIS patients with an abnormal brain MRI compared to healthy controls, whereas no cord atrophy was detected in CIS patients with a normal brain MRI.

Recently, Rocca et al.[12] applied the active surface method that has been described here in a multicenter study, including a large sample of MS patients spanning the major disease clinical phenotypes, and found that cervical cord atrophy was more pronounced in patients with the progressive forms of the disease and in those with long-lasting disease in comparison to those in the early phase. Furthermore, cervical cord atrophy was less pronounced in patients with benign MS (BMS) compared to those with SPMS with relatively shorter disease duration, thus helping to explain the more

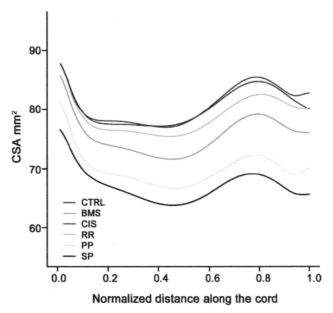

FIGURE 3.6.6   Spinal cord cross-sectional area plotted along the cord between the superior margin of C2 and the inferior border of C5 for different clinical MS subtypes and healthy controls. BMS: benign multiple sclerosis; CIS: clinically isolated syndrome; CTRL: control; PP: primary progressive MS; RR: relapsing-remitting MS; SP: secondary progressive MS. Distance along the cervical cord was normalized by dividing it by the subject's cervical cord between the two landmarks. *Source: From Ref. 12, reprinted with permission.*

favorable disease course of BMS. In the same study, plots of spinal cord area from C2 to C5 for the different disease clinical phenotypes were also derived to determine whether a specific level of the cord rather than the entire length is particularly sensitive to MS-related atrophy. This analysis showed that the curves for BMS, PPMS, and SPMS patients were well separated from each other and from those of the remaining study groups, while this was not the case of the curve for RRMS patients, which tended to overlap with those of CIS and healthy controls in some portions of the cervical cord (Figure 3.6.6). These variations according to location for RRMS patients might help to explain the discrepancies between the results of previous studies when they assessed this particular clinical phenotype, since some studies found cord atrophy in RRMS, while others did not.[6,17,35]

Only one clinical study measured the volume of the gray matter of the cervical cord in patients with RRMS and found no atrophy of this compartment in this clinical phenotype.[40]

3.6.7.2 Topography of Cord Atrophy

Pathologic and lesion-based studies have consistently demonstrated that atrophy more frequently affects the cervical rather than the lower segments of the cord.[27,41]

Only a few studies have explored the distribution of atrophy across the whole cord to determine the regional susceptibility to irreversible tissue loss. Klein et al.[34] have evaluated the whole spinal cord volume from C1 to T12 using a 3.0 T scanner and found a trend toward decreased spinal cord volume at the level of the upper cervical cord in PPMS and SPMS compared to healthy controls. The opposite trend, toward increased spinal cord volume, was found throughout the cervical and thoracic cord in RRMS and CIS patients compared to healthy controls, suggesting in these groups the possible influence of inflammation or edema on cord volume. Recently, by segmenting the entire cervical cord from 3D T_1-weighted images, a method has been developed that allows a voxel-based assessment of cord atrophy to be performed.[42] The method has shown that compared to controls, RRMS patients' atrophy was localized to a few clusters in the posterior cord. Conversely, SPMS patients showed a widespread pattern of cord atrophy, predominantly in the posterior and lateral cord columns.[42]

3.6.7.3 Longitudinal Evaluation of Cord Atrophy

Several longitudinal studies have assessed the evolution of cervical cord atrophy. A decrease of cord cross-sectional area has been described in patients with RRMS[43] and progressive MS,[31,33,44–47] whereas no changes were detected in CIS patients during one year of follow-up.[39] In RRMS patients, the mean annual rate of cervical cord area loss was estimated as 0.812 mm^2 in a 3-year follow-up.[43] SPMS patients had an atrophy rate of 1.63% per year over a 2-year period,[47] whereas in PPMS patients, an 11% reduction of cervical cord area was detected during a 5-year follow-up.[31] In a 2.4-year study including patients with RRMS, SPMS, and PPMS, cord area decreased at follow-up at a similar rate in all three patient groups.

Only two studies have assessed cord atrophy modifications following treatment in patients with MS. In a 4-year follow-up study, Lin et al.[45] showed that patients who started treatment with interferon beta 1a early (baseline) developed less cord atrophy than those who started treatment after 24 or 36 months from study initiation. Another study demonstrated that in PPMS patients, the rate of cervical cord atrophy progression diminishes after treatment with riluzole.[48]

3.6.7.4 Clinical Correlations

Several cross-sectional[6,12,30,33,34,44,49] and longitudinal[31,45,46,50] studies have found relatively strong correlations between disability (usually measured using the Expanded Disability Status Scale [EDSS] score) and cervical cord atrophy. Recently, Rocca et al.[12] showed that the normalized cross-sectional area correlated with EDSS ($r = -0.49$), with a differential effect among disease clinical phenotypes: no association in either CIS or BMS, but an association in RRMS ($r = -0.30$), SPMS ($r = -0.34$), and PPMS ($r = -0.27$).

Other studies, which have investigated the independent roles of measures of brain and cervical cord damage in predicting disability, have shown that cervical cord atrophy is a significant independent predictor of disability,[51] particularly in the progressive phenotypes of the disease.[32]

In line with the results of a study of pathology,[41] cervical cord atrophy has also been associated with disease duration,[12,33,49] supporting the notion of a cumulative effect over time of the neurodegenerative pathological processes leading to tissue loss.

3.6.7.5 Correlations with Brain T_2 Lesion Volume and Other MRI Measures

Only moderate correlations have been found between cervical cord atrophy and conventional and advanced MRI measures of brain damage,[45,46,51] suggesting that degenerative and inflammatory processes typical of MS affect the cord and the brain with dynamics that are partially independent.

Pathological studies, which assessed predominantly SPMS and PPMS patients, have demonstrated convincingly that individual lesions play a minor role in local atrophy.[41,52] In line with this, a recent study[12] showed that cord atrophy was not influenced by the presence of lesions. These results suggest that Wallerian degeneration of long fiber tracts, rather than local damage to the tracts, is one of the main factors leading to tissue loss in the cord of patients with MS.

3.6.7.6 Atrophy in Diseases Other than MS

In one study involving 19 patients with spinal cord injury, spinal cord atrophy was shown to correlate with motor and sensory deficits.[23] Notably, Lundell et al. showed that anterio-posterior width (APW) and left-right width (LRW) of the cord can be used to assess sensory and motor function independently. In another study, atrophy was shown to correlate with American Spinal Injury Association (ASIA) score in a chronic spinal cord injury population, independently from DTI and magnetization transfer measurements.[53] Spinal cord atrophy has also been demonstrated in patients with amyotrophic lateral sclerosis.[54] Notably, Cohen-Adad et al. showed an association between muscle deficits and local spinal cord atrophy, suggesting that atrophy is a sensitive biomarker for lower motor neuron degeneration. The authors tested the specificity of atrophy at a given vertebral level (between C4 and C7) in relation to muscle deficits and motor-evoked potentials using a stepwise linear regression model. They demonstrated that deficit of the deltoid muscle (at the C5 spinal level, equivalent to the C4 vertebral level) was associated with atrophy at the C4 vertebral level, and that deficit of the abductor pollicis brevis or adductor digiti minimi (at the C8 spinal level, equivalent to the C7 vertebral level) was associated with atrophy at the C7 vertebral level.

3.6.8 SUMMARY

Measures of spinal cord atrophy are of clinical significance in a number of neurological disorders, including MS, ALS, and spinal cord injury. Spinal cord atrophy is one of the long-term sequelae of MS, particularly in the more disabling forms of the disease, with the cervical cord being most affected. The main cause is thought to be Wallerian degeneration as a result of changes that occur in the brain, rather than tissue loss due to primary cord pathology. In spinal cord injury and ALS, functional deficits of spinal origin have been shown to correlate with the degree of atrophy at corresponding vertebral levels.

Several groups have developed methods for semiautomated measurement of atrophy, with segmentation based on the intensity contrast between the cord parenchyma and the surrounding CSF.[3,6,7,9–11,13,17] Some of these methods are implemented in a commercially available software package.[55] With modern high-field MRI scanners, acquiring high-resolution images of the spinal cord is relatively straightforward, particularly in the cervical region. Semiautomated analysis of the axially reformatted images, either at a specific level such as the C2–C3 disk[6] or along an extended segment of the cord,[11,45] should be reliable enough to detect atrophy rates of a few percent per year in relatively short-term studies with reasonably sized cohorts of subjects. Improvements in accuracy will undoubtedly come with the better spatial resolution achievable using scanners with 3.0 T field strength[16] or higher.[15] Fully automated analysis of the spinal cord cross-sectional area, and even separate quantification of gray and white matter volumes, should be achievable in the near future.

References

1. Thijssen H, Keyser M, Horstink M, Meijer E. Morphology of the cervical spinal cord on computed myelography. *Neuroradiology.* 1979;18(2):57–62.
2. Yu Y, Duboulay G, Stevens J, Kendall B. Morphology and measurements of the cervical spinal cord in computer-assisted myelography. *Neuroradiology.* 1985;27(5):399–402.

3. Seibert C, Barnes J, Dreisbach J, Swanson W, Heck RJ. Accurate CT measurement of the spinal cord using metrizamide—physical factors. *AJR*. 1981;136(1):777–789.

4. Constable R, Gore J. The loss of small objects in variable TE imaging—implications for FAS, RARE and EPI. *Magn Reson Med*. 1992;28(1):9–24.

5. Ehman R, Felmlee J. Flow artifact reduction in MRI—a review of the roles of gradient moment nulling and spatial presaturation. *Magn Reson Med*. 1990;14(2):293–307.

6. Losseff N, Webb S, ORiordan J, et al. Spinal cord atrophy and disability in multiple sclerosis—a new reproducible and sensitive MRI method with potential to monitor disease progression. *Brain*. 1996;119(3):701–708.

7. Tench C, Morgan P, Constantinescu C. Measurement of cervical spinal cord cross-sectional area by MRI using edge detection and partial volume correction. *JMRI*. 2005;21(3):197–203.

8. Kass M, Witkin A, Terzopoulos D. Snakes—active contour models. *Int J Comput Vision*. 1987;1(4):321–331.

9. Deng X, Ramu J, Narayana P. Spinal cord atrophy in injured rodents: high-resolution MRI. *Magn Reson Med*. 2007;57(3):620–624.

10. Coulon O, Hickman S, Parker G, et al. Quantification of spinal cord atrophy from magnetic resonance images via a B-spline active surface model. *Magn Reson Med*. 2002;47(6):1176–1185.

11. Horsfield MA, Sala S, Neema M, et al. Rapid semi-automatic segmentation of the spinal cord from magnetic resonance images: application in multiple sclerosis. *NeuroImage*. 2010;50(2):446–455.

12. Rocca M, Horsfield M, Sala S, et al. A multicenter assessment of cervical cord atrophy among MS clinical phenotypes. *Neurology*. 2011;76(24):2096–2102.

13. Duda R, Hart P. *Pattern Classification and Scene Analysis*. New York: John Wiley & Sons; 1973.

14. Gray W, Cuzzocreo J, Smith S, et al. Automated segmentation of high resolution spinal cord MRI. In: *16th Annual Meeting of the Organization for Human Brain Mapping (HBM)*. Barcelona, Spain; 2010: 1361.

15. Sigmund EE, Suero GA, Hu C, et al. High-resolution human cervical spinal cord imaging at 7 T. *NMR Biomed*. 2012;25(7):891–899.

16. Yiannakas MC, Kearney H, Samson RS, et al. Feasibility of grey matter and white matter segmentation of the upper cervical cord in vivo: a pilot study with application to magnetisation transfer measurements. *NeuroImage*. 2012;63(3):1054–1059.

17. Mann R, Constantinescu C, Tench C. Upper cervical spinal cord cross-sectional area in relapsing remitting multiple sclerosis: application of a new technique for measuring cross-sectional area on magnetic resonance images. *J Magn Reson Imaging*. 2007;26(1):61–65.

18. Healy BC, Arora A, Hayden DL, et al. Approaches to normalization of spinal cord volume: application to multiple sclerosis. *J Neuroimaging*. 2012;22(3):E12–E19.

19. Agosta F, Filippi M. MRI of spinal cord in multiple sclerosis. *J Neuroimaging*. 2007;17(S1):46S–49S.

20. Bakshi R, Thompson AJ, Rocca MA, et al. MRI in multiple sclerosis: current status and future prospects. *Lancet Neurol*. 2008;7(7):615–625.

21. Wingerchuk DM. Neuromyelitis optica. *Int MS J*. 2006;13(2):42–50.

22. Turner MR, Grosskreutz J, Kassubek J, et al. Towards a neuroimaging biomarker for amyotrophic lateral sclerosis. *Lancet Neurol*. 2011;10(5):400–403.

23. Lundell H, Barthelemy D, Skimminge A, Dyrby TB, Biering-Sorensen F, Nielsen JB. Independent spinal cord atrophy measures correlate to motor and sensory deficits in individuals with spinal cord injury. *Spinal Cord*. 2011;49(1):70–75.

24. Filippi M, Rocca M, Arnold D, et al. EFNS guidelines on the use of neuroimaging in the management of multiple sclerosis. *Eur J Neurol*. 2006;13(4):313–325.

25. Nijeholt G, van Walderveen M, Castelijns J, et al. Brain and spinal cord abnormalities in multiple sclerosis—correlation between MRI parameters, clinical subtypes and symptoms. *Brain*. 1998;131(4):687–697.

26. Bjartmar C, Kidd G, Mork S, Rudick R, Trapp B. Neurological disability correlates with spinal cord axonal loss and reduced N-acetyl aspartate in chronic multiple sclerosis patients. *Ann Neurol*. 2000;48(6):893–901.

27. Gilmore C, DeLuca G, Bo L, et al. Spinal cord atrophy in multiple sclerosis caused by white matter volume loss. *Arch Neurol*. 2005; 62(12):1859–1862.

28. Gilmore C, Bo L, Owens T, et al. Spinal cord gray matter demyelination in multiple sclerosis—a novel pattern of residual plaque morphology. *Brain Pathol*. 2006;16(3):202–208.

29. Kidd D, Thorpe J, Thompson A, et al. Spinal cord MRI using multiarray coils and fast spin-echo 2: findings in multiple sclerosis. *Neurology*. 1993;43(12):2632–2637.

30. Filippi M, Campi A, Colombo B, et al. A spinal cord MRI study of benign and secondary progressive multiple sclerosis. *J Neurol*. 1996;243(7):502–505.

31. Ingle G, Stevenson V, Miller D, Thompson A. Primary progressive multiple sclerosis: a 5-year clinical and MR study. *Brain*. 2003; 126(11):2528–2536.

32. Furby J, Hayton T, Anderson V, et al. Magnetic resonance imaging measures of brain and spinal cord atrophy correlate with clinical impairment in secondary progressive multiple sclerosis. *Mult Scler J*. 2008;14(8):1068–1075.

33. Laule C, Vavasour I, Zhao Y, et al. Two-year study of cervical cord volume and myelin water in primary progressive multiple sclerosis. *Mult Scler J*. 2010;16(6):670–677.

34. Klein J, Arora A, Neema M, et al. A 3T MR imaging investigation of the topography of whole spinal cord atrophy in multiple sclerosis. *Am J Neuroradiol*. 2011;32(6):1138–1142.

35. Rashid W, Davies G, Chard D, et al. Upper cervical cord area in early relapsing-remitting multiple sclerosis: cross-sectional study of factors influencing cord size. *J Magn Reson Imaging*. 2006;23(4): 473–476.

36. Bieniek M, Altmann D, Davies G, et al. Cord atrophy separates early primary progressive and relapsing remitting multiple sclerosis. *J Neurol Neurosurg Psychiatry*. 2006;77(9):1036–1039.

37. Rovaris M, Bozzali M, Santuccio G, et al. In vivo assessment of the brain and cervical cord pathology of patients with primary progressive multiple sclerosis. *Brain*. 2001;124(12):2540–2549.

38. Zivadinov R, Banas A, Yella V, et al. Comparison of three different methods for measurement of cervical cord atrophy in multiple sclerosis. *Am J Neuroradiol*. 2008;29(2):319–325.

39. Brex P, Leary S, O'Riordan J, et al. Measurement of spinal cord area in clinically isolated syndromes suggestive of multiple sclerosis. *J Neurol Neuropsychiatry Neurosurg*. 2001;70(4):544–547.

40. Agosta F, Pagani E, Caputo D, Filippi M. Associations between cervical cord gray matter damage and disability in patients with multiple sclerosis. *Arch Neurol*. 2007;64(9):1302–1305.

41. Evangelou N, DeLuca G, Owens T, Esiri M. Pathological study of spinal cord atrophy in multiple sclerosis suggests limited role of local lesions. *Brain*. 2005;128(1):29–34.

42. Valsasina P, Horsfield MA, Rocca MA, et al. Spatial normalization and regional assessment of cord ctrophy: voxel-based analysis of cervical cord 3D T1-weighted images. *Am J Neuroradiol*. 2012; 33(11):2195–2200, 1012.

43. Rashid W, Davies G, Chard D, et al. Increasing cord atrophy in early relapsing-remitting multiple sclerosis: a 3 year study. *J Neurol Neurosurg Psychiatry*. 2006;77(1):51–55.

44. Stevenson V, Leary S, Losseff N, et al. Spinal cord atrophy and disability in MS—a longitudinal study. *Neurology*. 1998;51(1): 234–238.

45. Lin X, Tench C, Turner B, Blumhardt L, Constantinescu C. Spinal cord atrophy and disability in multiple sclerosis over four years: application of a reproducible automated technique in monitoring disease progression in a cohort of the interferon beta-1a (Rebif) treatment trial. *J Neurol Neurosurg Psychiatry.* 2003;74(8): 1090–1094.

46. Agosta F, Absinta M, Sormani MP, et al. In vivo assessment of cervical cord damage in MS patients: a longitudinal diffusion tensor MRI study. *Brain.* 2007;130(8):2211–2219.

47. Furby J, Hayton T, Altmann D, et al. A longitudinal study of MRI-detected atrophy in secondary progressive multiple sclerosis. *J Neurol.* 2010;257(9):1508–1516.

48. Kalkers NF, Barkhof F, Bergers E, van Schijndel R, Polman C. The effect of the neuroprotective agent riluzole on MRI parameters in primary progressive multiple sclerosis: a pilot study. *Mult Scler J.* 2002;8(6):532–533.

49. Edwards S, Gong Q, Liu C, et al. Infratentorial atrophy on magnetic resonance imaging and disability in multiple sclerosis. *Brain.* 1999;122(2):291–301.

50. Sastre-Garriga J, Ingle G, Rovaris M, et al. Long-term clinical outcome of primary progressive MS: predictive value of clinical and MRI data. *Neurology.* 2005;65(4):633–635.

51. Cohen A, Neema M, Arora A, et al. The relationships among MRI-defined spinal cord involvement, brain involvement, and disability in multiple sclerosis. *J Neuroimaging.* 2012;22(2):122–128.

52. Bergers E, Bot J, De Groot C, et al. Axonal damage in the spinal cord of MS patients occurs largely independent of T2 MRI lesions. *Neurology.* 2002;59(11):1766–1771.

53. Cohen-Adad J, El Mendili MM, Lehérici S, Pradat PF, Blancho S, Rossignol S, Benali H. Demyelination and degeneration in the injured human spinal cord detected with diffusion and magnetization transfer MRI. *NeuroImage.* 2011;55(3):1024–1033.

54. Cohen-Adad J, El Mendili MM, Morizot-Koutlidis R, et al. Involvement of spinal sensory pathway in ALS and specificity of cord atrophy to lower motor neuron degeneration. *Amyotroph Lateral Scler.* 2013;14(1):30–38.

55. Image analysis software package Jim. Xinapse Systems Ltd. http://www.xinapse.com/Manual; 2013 Accessed 11.13.

PART IV

IMAGING SPINAL CORD FUNCTION

4.1

Spinal Cord fMRI

Paul E. Summers[1], Jonathan C.W. Brooks[2], Julien Cohen-Adad[3]

[1]Department of Biomedical, Metabolic and Neural Sciences, University of Modena and Reggio Emilia, Modena, Italy; and Department of Radiology, European Institute of Radiology, Milan, Italy

[2]Clinical Research Imaging Centre (CRiCBristol), University of Bristol, Bristol, UK

[3]Institute of Biomedical Engineering, Polytechnique Montreal; Functional Neuroimaging Unit, CRIUGM, Université de Montréal, Montreal, QC, Canada

4.1.1 BLOOD OXYGENATION LEVEL DEPENDENT

4.1.1.1 Basic Principles

Functional magnetic resonance imaging (fMRI) allows noninvasive detection of neuronal activity. fMRI based on the blood oxygenation level dependent (BOLD) contrast mechanism was first introduced in 1990.[1,2] The basic principle behind the BOLD effect is that following neuronal activation, metabolic demand for oxygen induces a local increase in blood flow and blood volume. However, this blood supply far exceeds actual oxygen requirements, yielding a transient increase of oxyhemoglobin in the venous compartment and thus a relative decrease in the concentration of deoxyhemoglobin (HbR). Given that deoxyhemoglobin has paramagnetic properties, its presence induces local variations of the magnetic field imposed by the MR scanner, yielding a faster transverse relaxation mechanism (here we focus on the so-called T_2^* decay, but T_2 decay is also implicated, see, e.g., Bandettini et al.[3]). Since deoxyhemoglobin concentration is reduced following neuronal activation, there is less distortion of the local magnetic field, so local protons will experience slower transverse dephasing, resulting in a higher T_2^*-weighted MR signal.

Signal changes arising in BOLD fMRI are relatively small, typically less than 5% of the resting MR signal level in the brain, but may be detected by repeating stimulation (so-called "blocks" or "events") and rest periods several times, followed by statistical analysis (or inference) to distinguish task-correlated responses from noise.

The BOLD effect is widely used in the neuroimaging community, with more than 20,000 papers having been published to date using this technique (MEDLINE search, April 2013). Several reviews of the BOLD effect and its application in brain fMRI are available.[4–8] FMRI was applied for the first time in the spinal cord at 1.5 T using a motor task,[9] and has since been shown to be technically feasible in both humans[9–23] and animals.[23–28] However, results from the spinal cord remain controversial due to their low reproducibility.[16,29]

4.1.1.2 Neurovascular Coupling

Given that fMRI relies on hemodynamic changes to infer neuronal activity, it is worth understanding some basic properties of blood regulation (see also Chapter 4.3). BOLD signal exists because oxygenated blood supply far exceeds the actual demand of activated neurons. Two theories explain this phenomenon. The first suggests that the enzymes responsible for metabolizing the oxygen to produce adenosine triphosphate (ATP) saturate, leaving residual oxygen (i.e., nonmetabolized) to be washed out in the venous compartment where BOLD signal is recorded.[30] The second theory suggests that the low rate of oxygen diffusion through the blood brain barrier necessitates a disproportionate increase of blood flow compared to the amount of consumed oxygen.[31] An implication of the first theory is that one should observe a saturation of metabolic rate of oxygen (MRO_2) when blood flow is increased. According to the second theory, one should observe a proportional relationship between the two parameters. Hoge et al. have demonstrated the existence of a linear relationship between cerebral blood flow and MRO_2 using hypercapnia, thereby supporting the hypothesis of restricted oxygen diffusion.[32]

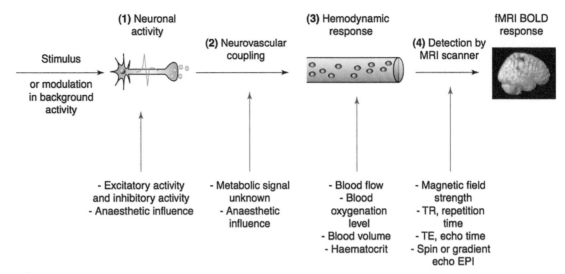

FIGURE 4.1.1 Illustration of the neurovascular coupling yielding the BOLD effect. Potential factors that can influence the detected BOLD response are listed. *Source: Reproduced with permission from Arthurs and Boniface.* [107]

> Given the strong dependence of the BOLD signal on vascular parameters (blood flow, blood volume), fMRI *does not* provide an absolute measure of metabolic changes associated with neuronal activity. Percentage BOLD signal changes should be interpreted with care, as they do not directly relate to neuronal activity (Figure 4.1.1).

4.1.1.2.1 Neurovascular Coupling in the Spinal Cord

As in the brain, spinal neurons require energy supplied by ATP and so are dependent on the delivery of oxygen via blood flow. To study this relationship, Marcus et al. induced a metabolic response in the lumbosacral spinal cord following stimulation of the femoral and sciatic nerves in dog, lamb, and sheep.[33] They concurrently measured blood flow using microelectrodes, detecting a 50% local blood flow increase in the ipsilateral gray matter but no significant blood flow increases in the ipsilateral white matter nor in the whole contralateral region. The authors therefore concluded that the hemodynamic response following a metabolic stimulus is extremely localized in terms of vascular reaction close to the activated neurons. This observation has since been confirmed by intrinsic optical imaging studies in the cervical[34] and lumbar[35] spinal cord of rats.

Complementary insight into blood flow control comes from a study by Nix et al., who compared vascular reactivity between the spinal cord and the brain in the rat.[36] They used microelectrodes to measure arterial partial pressure of O_2 (P_{O_2}) changes to a CO_2 challenge ("hypercapnia"). A brisker vascular response was observed in the cord compared to the brain, leading the authors to conclude that "spinal cord blood flow regulation is somewhat more sensitive to CO_2 than is that in the brain cortex". We could hypothesize that vascular coupling is tighter in the spinal cord than that in the brain, yielding less washout of deoxyhemoglobin and therefore lower BOLD effect.

4.1.1.2.2 Hemodynamic Response Function

The timing of the BOLD response depends on the coupling between oxygen demand from neurons and the vascular response.[37] The temporal profile of this response is characterized by a hemodynamic response function (HRF), whose height, shape, and phase (relative to the onset of oxygen demand) are a fundamental component in the modeling process commonly used in fMRI analysis. A canonical HRF, available in most fMRI processing packages (e.g., SPM, FSL, AFNI) is typically used for analyzing brain fMRI data. Despite this common usage, the HRF is known to vary across brain regions,[38] and one human study has demonstrated a slower HRF in the spinal cord compared to the brain canonical HRF.[18] Given the contradictory results from human in vivo studies using fMRI and more direct experimental animal studies using e.g., laser Doppler blood flow,[36] characterizing the HRF in the spinal cord in response to various stimuli warrants further investigation.

4.1.1.3 Different Tasks—Different Neuronal Systems in the Spinal Cord

Both motor and sensory neuronal systems are of interest as targets for fMRI studies of the spinal cord. As yet, the majority of motor studies have focused on hand movement or finger tapping, while painful

TABLE 4.1.1 Different Motor and Sensory Tasks Used for Spinal Cord BOLD fMRI, with Sequence Type

Type	Task/Stimulus	Pulse Sequence	TE	Orientation	References
Motor	Fist clenching	FLASH (GE)	40 ms	Axial	Yoshizawa et al.[9]
Motor	Fist clenching (squeezing ball)	FLASH (GE)	30 ms	Sagittal, axial	Stroman, Nance & Ryner[108]
Motor	Forearm, wrist, and finger flexion	GE-EPI	50 ms	Sagittal, axial	Madi et al.[21]
Motor (voluntary + stimulated)	Fist clenching, finger flexing	Multishot GE-EPI	50 ms	Sagittal, axial	Backes, Mess & Wilmink[19]
Motor, sensory	Tongue flexion, Smiling, Puckering lips (motor), touch (sensory)	GE-EPI	60 ms	Coronal, sagittal	Komisaruk et al.[109]
Motor	Finger flexing	GE-EPI	50 ms	Axial	Govers et al. (2007)[10]
Motor	Finger tapping	GE-EPI	15 ms	Axial	Ng et al. (2008)[42]
Motor	Finger tapping	GE-EPI	32 ms	Sagittal	Maieron et al.[11]
Motor	Finger flexing	TSE GE-EPI	35 ms 20 ms	Sagittal	Bouwman et al.[16]
Motor	Fist clenching (squeezing rubber ball)	GE-EPI	40 ms	Transverse	Giulietti et al.[18]
Motor, monitoring of physiological processes	Fist clenching, effect of cardiac cycle	GE-EPI	40 ms	Sagittal	Piché et al.[39]
Sensory	Application of pressure on fingertip	GE-EPI	50 ms	Sagittal	Stracke et al.[12]
Sensory, monitoring of physiological processes	Noxious thermal, effect of cardiac and respiratory cycle	GE-EPI	45 ms 24 ms	Axial	Brooks et al.[14]
Sensory	Noxious thermal	GE-EPI	40 ms	Axial	Eippert et al.[21]
Sensory	Noxious thermal, brushing (nonpainful)	GE-EPI	23 ms	Axial	Summers et al.[17]
Sensory	Touch (contact with object)	1-shot GE-EPI 4-shot GE-EPI	27.6 ms 23 ms	Axial	Giuletti et al.[110]
Sensory	Noxious thermal, punctate (nonpainful)	GE-EPI	39 ms	Axial	Brooks et al.[40]
Sensory, monitoring of physiological processes	Noxious thermal, punctate (nonpainful)	GE-EPI	39 ms	Axial	Kong et al.[111]
Manipulation of physiological parameters	Hypercapnia	GE-EPI	30 ms	Axial	Cohen-Adad et al.[15]

and nonpainful thermal, brushing, and electrical stimuli have been used in sensory studies (see Table 4.1.1). There remains considerable scope to develop appropriate paradigms for the full range of movements and variety of sensory receptors that involve the spinal cord.

4.1.1.3.1 Motor Tasks

The hand has been the preferred target for motor tasks as it can be used with relatively little co-motion of more proximal muscles that might result in bulk movement of the spinal cord. Fist clenching may be expected to yield a functional response over a large extent of the spinal cord due to its involvement of the muscles of the forearm and all the digits of the hand and their coordinated motion. Unsurprisingly, it was used in the first spinal fMRI study[9] and has been the basis for characterizing the temporal features of the spinal BOLD response.[18,41] It should be noted that motor tasks will inevitably involve both a motor and a proprioceptive/sensory component. Through finger tapping experiments, researchers have investigated spinal cord responses specific to the complexity[42] and speed[11] of performing finger movements. Both greater complexity and higher rate were associated with greater BOLD responses.

Leg movements are of particular interest for spinal cord injury studies and locomotor rehabilitation but are difficult to achieve without inducing task-related movement that may induce false positive results.

4.1.1.3.2 Sensory Stimulation

Different classes of afferent nerve fibers convey sensory information from the body surface, muscles, and viscera to the spinal cord. These fibers are specialized, in that some respond preferentially to light touch, vibration, stretch, moving stimuli, or temperature and others to potentially tissue-damaging stimuli (so called nociceptors).

The role of the spinal cord in the processing of painful stimuli has been an active area of investigation with electrical, laser, and thermal stimuli being applied in imaging experiments. Studies comparing noxious and non-noxious electrical stimuli in rats[26,27] have shown notably higher reproducibility and sensitivity of BOLD responses to noxious stimuli. A similar distinction has been observed in humans between noxious laser heating and innocuous brush strokes to the dorsum of the hand.[17] These findings correspond well with prior reports in animal models using autoradiography and invasive measurements.[43,44] In agreement with known neuroanatomical pathways, increased BOLD signal has been observed primarily ipsilateral to the side of nociceptive stimulation.[40] A first investigation of the influence of placebo modulation of spinal responses to painful sensory stimuli has been reported by Eippert et al.[21] Rather limited effort has gone into BOLD studies of non-nociceptive stimuli in their own right. Tactile stimulation (vibration at the finger tips at 3 Hz) has been shown to produce activation of the cervical cord in humans.[12]

4.1.2 CHALLENGES IN fMRI OF THE SPINAL CORD

FMRI of the spinal cord is much more challenging than that in the brain.[10,29,45,46] While investigations reporting successful results have been published, the reproducibility of these data is questionable.[11,14,18,26,27] In this light, it seems worth understanding why detecting the BOLD effect is so challenging in the spinal cord, given that neuroscientists have used this technique in the brain for more than 20 years.

4.1.2.1 Spatial Localization of the BOLD Signal

For a given paradigm (motor, sensory), where should you expect BOLD signal to occur? This question is important, as it helps to validate fMRI results by assessing the sensitivity and spatial specificity of statistical maps. To address this question we need to consider several aspects of the anatomy and physiology.

4.1.2.1.1 Cross-Sectional Distribution of Gray Matter Specialization

The primary synaptic connections in the motor and sensory systems of the spinal cord are distributed as illustrated in the Annex (Figures 7–14). In general the cell bodies and synapses of motor neurons are located in the ventral horn. In contrast, sensory neurons have their cell bodies located in the dorsal root ganglion outside the spinal cord and rely on interneurons, with which they form synaptic connections in the dorsal horn, to relay sensory information to supraspinal regions. From the spinal cord, the motor system gives rise to the ventral nerve roots, while sensory information is carried via the dorsal nerve roots.

4.1.2.1.2 Vertebral/Spinal Nerve Equivalence

Motor stimulation paradigms involving a particular muscle or muscle group (collectively known as a myotome) or sensory stimulation of a particular region of the skin (served by a single spinal nerve, and referred to as a dermatome) will be associated with cord activity corresponding to the representative nerve root (ventral—motor, dorsal—sensory). It is thus established neurophysiological practice to describe the position of such spinal cord responses in terms of the corresponding spinal nerve root ("spinal" or "segmental" level). Unfortunately, an important discrepancy has emerged in that spinal cord fMRI results are typically analyzed and interpreted relative to the vertebral level. This can be problematic as the spinal and vertebral levels are not anatomically matched. Although there is a gross model for finding spinal nerve entries relative to vertebral levels (see Annex), this correspondence is not entirely accurate as there is intersubject variability. In short, the human spinal column (vertebral bones, ligaments, and intervertebral discs) grows at a more rapid pace and in response to different forces than the human spinal cord. As a result the spinal cord is considerably shorter than the spinal column in adults (less so in infants), and the nerve roots tend to exit the spinal canal considerably lower than the position of their entry/exit from the spinal cord. Concerning the cervical cord, it is worth noting that the nerve roots for the 2nd to 7th spinal nerves exit at or above the level of their corresponding vertebral bodies, but the 8th cervical nerve root is not associated with a vertebral body and exits immediately below the 7th cervical and above the 1st thoracic vertebral body. Thereafter the spinal nerves exit below, and sometimes some distance from, the level of their associated vertebral body.

Recent studies have investigated this issue by performing structural imaging of nerve rootlets and by finding the correspondence between spinal and vertebral levels.[47] Moreover, the spinal nerves are not comprised of a single unit but rather as a series of rootlets fanning out over some rostral-caudal extent. A consequence of this structural formation is that a given nerve root can be expected to form synapses across a relatively extended segment of the spinal cord (Figure 4.1.2). For any given subject, the exact distribution of spinal rootlets is rarely known and is likely to vary across subjects, leading to variability in response location along the spinal cord within the territory of a given nerve root.

4.1.2.1.3 Distribution of Neuronal Activity in Response to Sensory/Motor Stimulus

The spatial distribution of neuronal activity in the axial and rostro-caudal dimensions is likely to further vary across individuals as the location of dermatome boundaries and polysynaptic pathways differ slightly between individuals.[48–50] The contribution from descending modulation was also shown to vary, hence motor tasks can elicit variable distribution of activity across subjects.[51]

Moreover, most motor tasks are not "purely motor" as they also involves sensory inputs. For example, a ball-squeezing task also involves sensory inputs from the palm and fingers as well as proprioceptive inputs.

4.1.2.1.4 Ipsi/Contralaterality

Although consistent ipsilateral activation has been reported,[11,14,40,41] its poor reproducibility has also been noted.[9,10,19,29] Ipsilateral neurons of the spinal cord are expected to activate predominantly when performing motor or sensory tasks. However, contralateral motorneurons and interneurons are also involved through various crossed spinal pathways.[49] Thus, lateralization of activity is not a clear-cut issue.

Further complicating the differentiation of ipsi- and contralateral activity are partial volume effects (voxels can include both right and left sides). To minimize the effect of partial volume effect, axial acquisition with high in-plane resolution is recommended.

Previous studies in the brain have also raised possibility of a "blood stealing" effect in which "negative BOLD" signal is recorded in an inactive area near the site of increased metabolic demand. This effect is caused by the reduction in blood supply (hence decrease of T_2^*-weighted signal), due to an increase of blood flow in a neighboring vasculature area where neuronal activation occurs.[52] As the anterior arterial supply to the spinal cord is carried by a midline vessel, the scope exists for steal even in the contralateral cord, as well as distal to the cord along the longitudinally running posterior arteries. However, intrinsic optical imaging techniques applied in the rat spinal cord, which directly measure the relative proportions of deoxygenated and oxygenated blood through light reflectance, revealed a predominantly ipsilateral response to right and left forepaw electrical nerve stimulation.[34] Furthermore, Sasaki et al. did not find any evidence for vascular stealing, suggesting that in the anesthetized rat normal neurovascular coupling leads to ipsilateral increased blood flow following stimulation, without apparent compensatory changes in the contralateral cord.

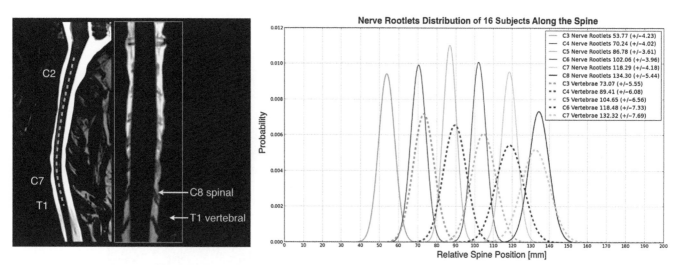

FIGURE 4.1.2 Correspondence between vertebral and spinal levels. Left panel shows a coronal section of the spinal cord with nerve rootlets emerging from the spinal cord (minimum intensity projection reconstruction following the curvature of the cervical spinal cord). The yellow arrow points to the upper limit of the C8 nerve rootlets attachment with the spinal cord; the white arrow points to the same rootlets as they enter the foramina between the C7 and T1 vertebrae. The right panel shows a spatial distribution of spinal versus vertebral levels in 16 subjects. *Source: Courtesy of David Cadotte and Michael Fehlings.*[47]

4.1.2.1.5 *Venous Drainage*

At first sight, studies reporting BOLD responses "outside" the spinal cord[10,15,19,27,53] may be a concern. Curiously, however, the venous organization of the spinal cord, coupled with the use of gradient echo EPI, may in fact favor such results, at least as far as those responses adjacent to the cord surface.

A number of brain fMRI studies have shown that BOLD signal changes are greatest in large venules and superficial draining veins.[54–56] This effect is illustrated in Figure 4.1.3, which compares BOLD activation map and susceptibility-weighted imaging in the same subject: larger BOLD responses are detected at the location of big veins. Because the spinal cord gray matter is surrounded by white matter, large activation signals could therefore be detected several millimeters from the gray matter activation site.[57–59]

It has been argued that the BOLD response in superficial veins should be attenuated because of their orientation parallel to the static magnetic (B_0) field,[29] while radicular veins running perpendicular to B_0 should exhibit a maximal response. This argument neglects the role of crossing elements in the venous plexus linking the draining veins and collecting blood from the emergence of the radicular veins at the cord surface. Whether anastomotic connections are the sole cause of these task-correlated signals at the periphery of the spinal cord remains to be established. If indeed these anastomotic connections do have a significant role, differences in their distribution may further exacerbate intersubject variability in fMRI response localization.[10] This could also explain why the spatial location of cardiac-related signal was shown to be invariant within subjects but highly variable across subjects.[39]

Although these large-vessel BOLD responses are not false positives per se, the interest in them is limited in standard fMRI studies, where we aim to map neuronal activity with high spatial specificity. Although some have advocated excluding such large vein activations,[57–59] doing so is not routine practice in brain fMRI. The combination of voxel sizes (typically 27 mm^3) and smoothing kernels (FWHM ~5–8 mm) used in brain studies, coupled with the presence of cortical gray matter immediately below the brain surface, means that responses in draining veins tend to be included and give an apparent co-localization of the activation epicenter and BOLD signal. In spinal cord fMRI, the in-plane resolution of voxels is commonly 1 mm, the gray matter is generally separated from the surface, and little or no smoothing is typically applied. Thus, BOLD signal changes in large pial draining veins will tend to be more clearly separated from the source gray matter than in brain studies.

One pragmatic approach to minimizing the influence of draining veins would be to exclude tissues outside the cord, however, it is likely that the imaging point spread function and any applied spatial smoothing could introduce superficial activity in draining veins back into the cord. Perhaps of more practical use would be the combination of both cord segmentation and group analysis techniques (see following as well as Chapter 4.2), both of which would tend to reduce the influence of surface draining veins.

Methods to achieve better spatial specificity include the use of other contrast mechanisms such as blood flow and MION-based volume measurements in animals,[60–62] the use of higher magnetic field[56,63] and spin echo sequences, as they are more specific to the

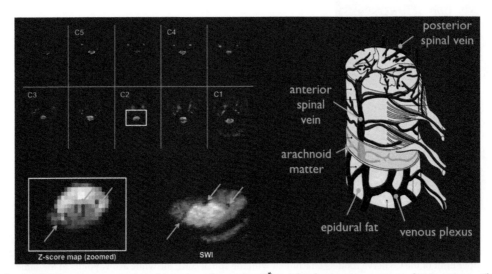

FIGURE 4.1.3 Large BOLD responses occur in big veins when using T_2^*-weighted contrast, as assessed using susceptibility-weighted imaging (SWI), where veins appear darker. BOLD responses were induced using hypercapnic challenge.[15]

microvascular compartment and hence reveal responses closer to the activation epicenter.[64–66] However, spin echo sequences are also less BOLD sensitive than gradient echo sequence, which is problematic for spinal cord fMRI[16,67,68] where high image noise makes detection of small signal changes more difficult.

4.1.2.2 Signal Change and Sensitivity

The process used to identify sites of activation relies on statistically distinguishing a task-related signal change from the inherent noise in the signal as repeated images are made over time. The smaller the signal change relative to the noise, the lower sensitivity to BOLD responses. A number of factors have been implicated in reducing the BOLD sensitivity of fMRI in the spinal cord relative to the brain: (1) neurovascular coupling; (2) signal and noise properties of the images; and (3) confounding factors such as task-related motion.

4.1.2.2.1 Neurovascular Coupling

The basic process of an increase in local oxygen metabolism in response to an increase in neuronal activity, with consequent increase in blood flow and blood volume, have been shown to mirror in the spinal cord the events that give rise to a BOLD response in the brain. That is not to say, however, that the degree of blood flow and blood volume changes, or the extent of BOLD signal changes are the same as in the brain. It may be, in fact, that BOLD signal changes are lower in the spinal cord.

As noted earlier, a brisker vascular response was observed in the cord compared to the brain,[36] which could imply that there is a tighter coupling between oxygen demand and perfusion increase in the spinal cord, and therefore lower relative decrease of HbR (and therefore less BOLD signal increase).

Other factors not specific to the spinal cord but that could also affect BOLD responses are:

- Baseline perfusion and vascular reactivity strongly determine the dynamic range of the BOLD signal.[69,70] They may notably be influenced by age,[71] general vascular health,[72] and caffeine intake.[73]
- Level of arousal and task performance, e.g., subject doesn't properly perform the requested task.
- Habituation effects, which implies less neuronal firing after repeating the same task during an experimental paradigm.[74]

4.1.2.3 Signal and Noise Properties of the Images

A basic fMRI experiment involves creating a temporal series of images in which some images are acquired during rest and others during the task. The analysis then treats each voxel in the images individually so we can consider the statistical analysis as one of distinguishing the signal change (the contrast) from the noise fluctuations over time in the signal of a voxel. What is important in fMRI is, therefore, the so-called "contrast-to-noise ratio" (CNR) between the mean signal from the set of time points obtained during rest (S_{rest}) and those obtained during activity (S_{active}) relative to the noise in the time series. The BOLD signal change ($\Delta S = S_{active} - S_{rest}$) in response to the task is typically expressed as a percentage of the resting signal intensity ($\%\Delta S$), which can be divided by 100 to give the fractional signal change:

$$\%\Delta S = 100 \times \Delta S / S_{rest}$$

The CNR can be expressed as follows:

$$CNR = \Delta S / \sigma_{tNoise}$$

where σ_{tNoise} is the standard deviation of the noise in the resting time series. Expressed in this form, it is clear that low noise, high signal, and large percentage signal changes will all favor a high value of the t-statistic (and hence the detection of a significant difference). As noted in the previous section, percentage signal changes in spinal BOLD studies may well be smaller than those recorded in the brain. Further increasing the difficulty of fMRI measurements in the spinal cord, the underlying signal available tends to be lower, and the noise higher, than in the brain. Both these considerations count toward lower sensitivity to task-related BOLD responses.

From the above, it is clear that the signal and noise characteristics of an fMRI image have an important impact on the sensitivity to detect BOLD activations.[75–78] In rapid imaging techniques such as EPI, the image signal-to-noise ratio (SNR_0), also called static SNR, is primarily associated with system and thermal noise intrinsic to the MR signal. It represents the SNR of individual images reflecting the condition of the system at the time the image is acquired.

In a study comparing BOLD responses in the spinal cord versus in the brain,[15] SNR_0 was 67 ± 8 in the brain and 39 ± 4 in the spinal cord (mean $\pm$ SD across subjects), using an EPI acquisition with voxel size equal to $1.5 \times 1.5 \times 4 mm^3$. The significantly lower SNR_0 in the spinal cord may contribute to the lower BOLD sensitivity encountered at the spinal level (see also Chapter 2.1).

Chief amongst the factors contributing to the lower SNR_0 in the spinal cord is the lower sensitivity of receiver coils in this region (see Chapter 2.1). Further notable contributions to low SNR_0 are susceptibility artifacts due to the differing tissues (airways/lungs, bone, muscle, and CSF) that lie in close proximity to the spinal cord. Magnetic susceptibility differences between these structures produce inhomogeneities in the static magnetic field in and around the spinal cord that may induce distortions and signal dropout in gradient echo images. Strategies to increase SNR_0 therefore include better coils, and maximizing the shim quality prior to scanning. The choice of imaging parameters can also play an important role (e.g., voxel size, slice thickness, choice of imaging bandwidth).

4.1.2.3.1 Temporal SNR and Physiological Noise

Temporal SNR (tSNR) is defined as the ratio of a voxel's average signal over a period of time divided by its standard deviation[79]: $tSNR = S_{rest}/\sigma_{tNois}$ (see Figure 4.1.4). In addition to the factors that contribute to SNR_0, the tSNR encompasses noise due to factors that change over time. Some of these relate to instrumental factors and physiological variations (see Chapter 4.2) over the period of the fMRI time series. Low tSNR in the spinal cord results both from low image SNR_0 and large signal variability due to physiological noise (arising from CSF, spinal cord and blood pulsation, swallowing, cardiac and respiration-induced susceptibility effects, etc. see chapter 4.2). Given that the goal of fMRI is to detect subtle signal variations across time, the level of tSNR is a good indicator of the sensitivity to detect BOLD signal change in an fMRI experiment. We therefore recommend calculating tSNR at the earliest possible opportunity (i.e., in preliminary data) and reporting it along with BOLD fMRI results. This allows a prospective power analysis to be performed for study design, and allows other researchers to assess the level of significance of the results.

How to Calculate Temporal SNR (tSNR)?

- Motion correct (using spline interpolation, otherwise smoothing introduced by trilinear interpolation will overestimate the tSNR)
- Detrend (high pass filtering)
- Compute the mean and standard deviation (std) over time for each voxel and generate a spatial map of tSNR (mean/std)
- Draw an ROI in the cord (either the whole cord or the gray matter if distinguishable), and then calculate the mean tSNR within the mask (spatial average)

At 3 T using standard coils, tSNR was found to be 35 ± 8 in the brain and 14 ± 2 in the spinal cord,[15] roughly half the values for SNR_0 in the same study. This further reduces the sensitivity of fMRI in the spinal

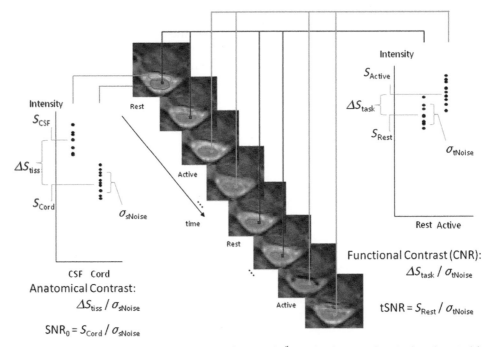

FIGURE 4.1.4 Calculation of temporal SNR. The above pictures show axial T_2^*-weighted views of a spinal cord, typical for fMRI experiments. For a single voxel followed through a time series of images, the difference in intensities between active and rest periods gives rise to the Functional Contrast that is evaluated statistically in fMRI studies (right side). The ratio of the mean signal value from the time points in one condition (typically rest) to their standard deviation defines the temporal signal-to-noise ratio (tSNR). These concepts are analogous to those used in distinguishing between two anatomical regions (tissues) in a single image (left side), where Anatomical Contrast depends on the difference in signal values between the tissues relative to their noise, and the (static) SNR of each tissue is given by the ratio of the mean signal value to the standard deviation of signal values from that tissue.

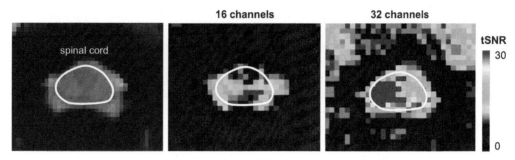

16 channels   **32 channels**

FIGURE 4.1.5 Effect of RF coil on the tSNR. In the cervical spinal cord (white ROI), tSNR was 13.9 when using the 16-channel coil (12-channel head + 4-channel neck) and 24.7 using the 32-channel coil. *Source: Modified from Ref. 15.*

cord compared to the brain. The use of highly sensitive coils can make a substantial improvement in image SNR, thereby improving the sensitivity to detect BOLD responses (see Figure 4.1.5).

4.1.2.3.2 Task-Related Motion

It is important to appreciate that even a submillimeter motion that happens in synchrony with the task paradigm can produce apparent task-related BOLD activity, which can either obscure the true pattern of activity or produce false positive activations. Even a simple hand motor task, performed inappropriately, can induce movement of the upper arm, which could then be transferred to the shoulders and the rest of the upper body. Motor paradigms are more prone to task-related motion, but aversive responses to noxious stimuli and changes of muscle tone in sensory tasks could also produce such effects. For tasks that might involve back muscles, the risk of movement of the upper part of the body, including the spinal cord, is clear. Bulk limb movements, such as lower limb locomotion tasks, because of the need for compensatory postural changes, are particularly likely to produce gross subject motion during fMRI acquisition that make data interpretation more difficult.[80]

Changes in muscle tone or body habitus over the course of an fMRI study that are not task correlated will, on the other hand, tend to increase the variance over the time series with the effect of reducing sensitivity. A common cause is that the head supports of most scanners leave the head balanced near the occiput (back of the head) and thus prone to a nodding motion as the muscles of the neck relax, as well as side-to-side rotations. A recent study showed that using cervical collars or vacuum bags that conform to the head/neck of the subject substantially minimize motion in the spinal cord.[81] A cushion that conforms to the length of the neck, as well as side cushions, can also serve to this purpose.

It cannot be stressed enough that experimenters must look closely at their data and be vigilant for potential task-related motion. Typical signatures of task-related

motions are: (1) high t-scores at high intensity boundaries (e.g., between the spinal cord and CSF), and (2) symmetric positive/negative signal change (see Figure 4.1.6).

4.1.3 DATA ACQUISITION

4.1.3.1 Field Strength

Image SNR scales approximately linearly with magnetic field strength, hence, using a higher field magnet should, in principle, provide higher sensitivity to detect BOLD responses (see Chapter 2.4). As well, at higher field strengths, susceptibility effects are also increased. Given that the BOLD effect is based on a susceptibility change, due to variation of paramagnetic deoxyhemoglobin concentration, higher field strength also improves the sensitivity in detecting BOLD signal changes in T_2^*-weighted contrast.[56,63]

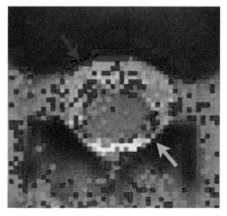

FIGURE 4.1.6 Typical signature of false positives caused by task-related motion. Red pixels are correlated with the task and blue pixels are anticorrelated with the task ($P < 0.05$). When a structure moves with the task, one edge of the picture will show "positive" activation while the opposite edge will show "negative" activation (see arrows). This effect is emphasized at high contrast boundaries, e.g., bone and spinal cord (dark) versus CSF (bright). On this example task-related motion is observed at two interfaces: CSF/bone (arrows) and CSF/spinal cord. *Source: Modified with permission from Moffitt et al.[68]*

Unfortunately, the effects of differences in susceptibility between static tissues (e.g., bone and CSF) or between tissues and air are similarly increased at higher magnetic fields. These effects are typically seen as artifacts, such as signal dropout (due to intravoxel dephasing in T_2^*-weighted imaging) and image distortions (see Chapter 2.3). Moreover, at higher field strengths, the contribution of physiological noise—as opposed to thermal noise in the image—is also higher.[82] Both these phenomena act to reduce temporal and image SNR with consequent reduction in BOLD sensitivity. Reducing the impact of static susceptibility differences can be sought through shim optimization and the use of small voxels.

4.1.3.2 Shimming

Shimming of the magnetic field is crucial for reducing B_0 inhomogeneities, which give rise to geometric distortions and signal drop out in EPI. Shimming problems are exacerbated due to presence of vertebral bodies and spinous processes adjacent to the cord, which are separated from one another by intervertebral discs.[83] Furthermore, if the goal is to cover both the brain and spinal cord in a single scan, this poses an even more significant challenge, as the shim algorithm will tend to be weighted toward the region with a large single tissue type (i.e., the brain), leaving largely suboptimal shim coefficients in the spinal region. Chapter 2.2 covers shimming methods for spinal cord MRI; Chapters 3.1 (diffusion imaging) and 5.1 (MR spectroscopy) also discuss the importance of shimming well, therefore here we will only mention a useful practice to adopt where possible, which is to limit the shim volume to encompassing mainly the spinal cord (see Figure 12 of chapter 3.1).

4.1.3.3 Gradient Echo versus Spin Echo

Using spin echo sequences (T_2-weighted) improves spatial specificity over gradient echo sequences (T_2^*-weighted) due to the refocusing pulse that nulls signals from the extravascular compartment.[56,63] Spin echo sequences are, however, substantially less sensitive for detecting responses to neuronal activity.[3,56,65] Quantitative measurements have shown a factor of three reduction in functional CNR for spin echo studies versus those using gradient echoes.[65] The use of spin echoes for spinal cord fMRI is controversial. While some studies have led to recommending its use,[46] others did not detect reliable BOLD signals in the spinal cord.[16,67,68]

4.1.3.4 CSF Suppression

The CSF surrounding the spinal cord complicates fMRI studies: firstly, for the artifacts that arise from its motion,[84] and secondly, for the high contrast between CSF and cord tissue that occurs at the echo times used for BOLD studies. The latter can give rise to pronounced partial volume effects and in some cases Gibbs ringing artifacts. Flow rephasing in the slice direction can be applied to reduce signal variation due to CSF.[85,86] To further reduce in-flow effect from the CSF, spatially selective saturation pulse superior and inferior to the target volume can be employed.[21]

Use of the FLAIR strategy to reduce CSF contamination was examined,[68] but the low SNR and poor temporal efficiency of the scans appeared to negate any benefits obtained. A recently demonstrated alternative for CSF suppression is the use of a DANTE (Delays Alternating with Nutation for Tailored Excitation) pulse train in conjunction with a standard gradient echo readout, which reduces signal from flowing spins (e.g., blood, CSF) and can produce modest increases in spinal cord tSNR; in preliminary experiments it has also been shown to increase BOLD sensitivity.[87]

4.1.3.5 Spatial Resolution and Spatial Coverage

To determine the distribution of activity along the longitudinal axis of the spinal cord, a sagittal[12,45,88] or coronal acquisition may be preferable as it allows the longest extent to be covered with the fewest slices, allowing more time points to be acquired in a given period. Axial scans on the other hand allow greater flexibility in balancing of high in-plane resolution with greater slice thickness.[9–11,18,19,26–28,41,42,68,80] Some further comments are warranted in consideration of how the choice of orientation interrelates with the choice of voxel sizes—in particular, slice thickness as one seeks to optimize sensitivity while providing the requisite spatial coverage and resolution.

4.1.3.5.1 Sagittal Orientation

Sagittal orientation offers the benefits of extensive spinal coverage using only a few slices.[12,45,86,88] Sagittal orientation favors isotropic resolution (e.g., $2 \times 2 \times 2$ mm^3), which imposes less bias for the spatial mapping of BOLD responses. Due to the limited SNR, however, one disadvantage of having isotropic voxels is the difficulty to reach high spatial resolution in the spinal cord cross section.

4.1.3.5.2 Axial Orientation

Most studies have used an axial orientation with relatively large slice thickness and high in-plane resolution.[9–11,18,19,26–28,41,42,68,80] A typical voxel size is $1 \times 1 \times 5$ mm^3. The main advantage of high in-plane resolution is to be able to discriminate the gray and white matter in the cross-sectional plane (i.e., axial plane), as well as the laterality (right versus left) and the

Resolution

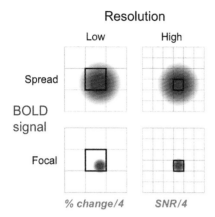

FIGURE 4.1.7 Voxel size should be optimized depending on the spatial PSF of the BOLD response. If the BOLD response is spread, then low resolution is better, because it provides higher SNR. If the BOLD response is focal, then high resolution is better, otherwise the voxel will include "non-activated" tissue and the effect size will be reduced.

anteroposterior location (e.g., ventral versus dorsal horn). These considerations are of great importance for spinal cord fMRI, where the ultimate goal is to investigate specific neuronal responses to a given stimulus (sensory, motor, noxious, etc.).

The optimal in-plane resolution is driven by the point spread function (PSF) of the BOLD response (as illustrated in Figure 4.1.7). For a PSF that is small, having big voxels would decrease the effect size of the detected response due to an averaging effect. In that case, having small voxels would be optimal. Contrariwise, for a large PSF, big voxels would be more advantageous as SNR increases with voxel size. Uncertainty about both the spatial extents and scales of neuronal responses to given stimuli in the spinal cord suggests further investigation on the BOLD PSF in the spinal cord, as has been explored in the brain.[89]

4.1.3.5.3 Slice Thickness

Thicker slices provide higher SNR (slice thickness is directly proportional to image SNR). A typical slice thickness used in spinal cord fMRI is 5 mm. A disadvantage of thicker slices is the occurrence of signal dropout in gradient echo EPI due to intravoxel dephasing. One workaround is to acquire thinner slices (thereby reducing intravoxel dephasing and signal dropout in the individual slices) and then average these slices together during preprocessing of the data.[90] Figure 4.1.8 shows that this strategy substantially decreases the amount of signal dropout. This approach comes at the cost of longer TR, because more slices are required to cover the same region. Alternatively, some researchers have used relatively thick slices but sought simply to avoid the regions of inhomogeneity associated with the spinal processes and discs.[15,18] This is achieved by aligning the slices with the centers of the vertebrae and allowing large gaps between the slices. This of course imposes variable slice gaps across individuals and foregoes continuous coverage of the spinal cord extent.

4.1.3.6 Echo Time

The amount of T_2^*-weighting is driven by the echo time (TE), which is set by the user. Maximum BOLD CNR is achieved when $TE \sim T_2^*$.[91] Hence, optimal TE can be chosen by measuring the T_2^* prior to spinal fMRI experiment using a multiple echo sequence.[16,18] Note that the T_2^* measures will depend on the voxel size, therefore slice position and resolution parameters should be kept the same as for the fMRI experiment. It should be noted that due to the large B_0 field inhomogeneity in the spinal cord, it is difficult to choose an appropriate single TE value. In this case one should favor short TE in order to minimize signal dropout. Also to

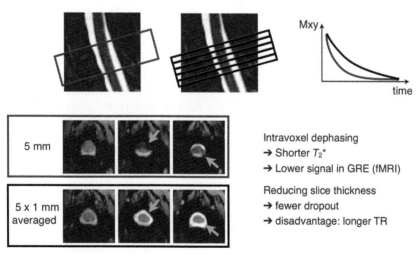

Intravoxel dephasing
→ Shorter T_2^*
→ Lower signal in GRE (fMRI)

Reducing slice thickness
→ fewer dropout
→ disadvantage: longer TR

FIGURE 4.1.8　Illustration of the combination of thinner slices to reduce signal dropout while maintaining SNR in gradient echo EPI.

be recognized, complex relationships arise when identifying the vascular and parenchymal compartments. For example, at 3 T, maximum signal change was found at TE = 21.5 in the vascular compartment and at TE = 41.5 ms in the parenchymal compartment.[92] Alternatively, multiple echo sequences can be employed[93] as they seem to be appropriate in areas prone to B_0 inhomogeneities as shown in the brain.[94]

4.1.3.6.1 Flip Angle and Repetition Time

When using long repetition times (>3 times the average tissue T_1) the signal intensities in gradient-echo images are dominated by the echo time, which being relatively long for BOLD images tends to favor the tissue contrast between tissues and CSF (T_2^*-weighting). Shorter TRs however will increase T_1-weighting contrast. An optimization of the signal received can be achieved by suitable choice of the flip angle based on the tissue T_1 and TR (defined by the Ernst angle relationship). Because the T_1 of CSF is longer than that of spinal cord, optimizing the Ernst angle for the spinal cord will create partial saturation in the CSF. This will reduce the CSF-tissue contrast and so reduce Gibb's and pulsation artifacts. Variation of CSF intensities due to different inflow velocities on the other hand might be reduced by using very small flip angles, at the cost however of diminishing the tissue signal of interest.

In practice there is very little disadvantage for going to shorter TR, as the increased number of signal averages outweighs the reduction in longitudinal magnetization, though at extremely short TR (<300 ms) the choice of flip angle becomes more important.

4.1.3.7 Saturation Bands

If the SAR limit allows it, spatially selective saturation bands can be used to minimize pulsatile blood flow[21] and respiration artifacts. For axial slices, the bands are best placed posterior and anterior to the target region, i.e., in the phase-encoding direction.[21] Saturations bands can also be used as "outer volume suppression" in combination with the reduced field of view technique to decrease susceptibility distortions (see Chapter 2.3). It should be noted, however, that saturation bands "cost" time (i.e., take up time during the TR) so would reduce the total number of slices that can be acquired for a given TR.

4.1.3.8 Cardiac/Respiratory Gating

Cardiac and respiratory gating or breath-holding have been used to a limited extent.[19] However, these approaches are not without their drawbacks: the scan time is prolonged; cardiac or respiratory period variations can introduce differential T_1 effects between time points in the functional time series; and heart and breathing rates can be affected by tasks and so correlate with the experimental paradigm, especially for painful stimuli.

4.1.3.9 Number of Time Points

Given a tSNR measurement (based on pilot data), and a target effect size (eff, expressed in percent change, based on pilot data) it is possible to predict the minimum number of samples (N) needed to reach a significant detection of the BOLD signal change.[79] We can write:

$$N = \frac{2}{R(1-R)} \left(\frac{erfc^{-1}(P)}{TSNR \cdot eff} \right)^2$$

where $erfc^{-1}$ is the inverse of the complementary error function (available in most mathematical software), P is the statistical threshold controlling the false positive rate (also called P-value), and R is the ratio of time points in the "ON" period to the total number of time points (typically 0.5 for balanced designs).

We encourage researchers to perform such power analysis in order to appropriately choose the number of time points for their fMRI experiments.

4.1.4 DATA PROCESSING

4.1.4.1 Motion Correction

Motion correction aims at co-registering all volumes in an fMRI time series to compensate for subject motion. Typically for the brain, each volume is registered to a target image (e.g., the first volume or the mean volume). Registration is generally performed by estimating a rigid-body transformation matrix, i.e., three translations and three rotations, yielding 6 degrees of freedom (dof). Such rigid-body transformation is not appropriate for spinal cord time series as the motion may not be rigid. Not only is this due to the articulated anatomy of the spine, which can bend within an fMRI acquisition if, e.g., subjects swallow or tilt their head, it is also a consequence of susceptibility changes in the lungs inducing B_0 field distortions in nearby tissue. These latter fluctuations tend to shift the image along the phase-encoding direction (typically anteroposterior for axial slices). The image shift is greater closer to the lungs, therefore the resulting displacement is not rigid, e.g., more distortion occurs at C7 versus C2 level.

For axial acquisitions, we therefore advise performing a slice-by-slice motion correction. That is, instead of estimating a rigid-body transformation for the whole volume, a transformation is estimated for each slice independently. Typically, a transformation with 2 dof is estimated (translation along X and Y). This approach assumes no translation along Z, which is a fair assumption given that subjects in supine position rarely move in the rostro-caudal direction, i.e., along the bore. Optionally, rotation about Z can be added to the transformation (yielding 3 dof). However, adding the Z rotation might reduce the robustness of the algorithm, due to the cylindrical symmetry of the spinal cord in the axial plane; therefore, having a FOV sufficiently large to include some asymmetric structures (bones, muscles) could improve the robustness. In counterpoint, motion between the cord and surrounding structures is possible, which is an argument for estimating the 2-dof transformations with a cropped FOV that only includes the cord. Practically, the motion correction process for axial slices can be implemented using standard tools such as FSL (FLIRT), SPM (spm_realign), or AFNI (AIR) within a Matlab or shell wrapper. The following is an example code based on FLIRT (mcflirt):

MOTION CORRECTION ALGORITHM FOR SPINAL CORD

- Crop the image to include only the spinal canal and bony structures():
  ```
  fslroi data data_crop x nx y ny z nz
  ```
- Split the data along Z:
  ```
  fslsplit data_crop data_crop_split −z
  ```
- Perform motion correction for each slice. Here we show an example for slice #4 (the wrapper should loop across all slices). Note that in the following example the transformation is both estimated and applied. As mentioned previously, it is advised to only estimate the transformation, then combine it with other corrections (e.g., distortion correction, template registration) in order to minimize the number of interpolations. Here the spline interpolation is used as it produces the least blurring (compared to trilinear interpolation):
  ```
  mcflirt -in data_crop_split0004 −o
  data_crop_split0004_moco −cost
  normcorr -2d −spline_final
  ```
- Merge data back along Z dimension:
  ```
  fslmerge −z data_moco
  data_crop_split0000_moco
  data_crop_split0001_moco
  data_crop_split0002_moco...
  ```

If acquisition is sagittal, affine transformation with 12 dof (3 translations, 3 rotations, 3 scaling, and 3 shearing) is advisable in order to minimize the effect of a nonrigid motion due to B_0-field fluctuation close to the lungs.

We strongly recommend researchers to test and compare several motion-correction strategies and then choose which one works best based on the following assessments: (1) qualitatively, by streaming each volume of your fMRI data as a video (e.g., using "fslview"); (2) quantitatively, by computing the standard deviation over time of the fMRI time series. An ROI encompassing the spinal cord can be manually drawn in order to calculate the mean standard deviation for each motion correction strategy and guide the choice of the best method.

4.1.4.2 Correcting for Susceptibility Artifacts

Correcting for distortions caused by structural susceptibility variations is optional, but recommended if you wish to overlay your statistical maps on anatomical images. Methods for correcting susceptibility artifacts include phase-based field mapping and reversed gradient methods and are extensively described in Chapter 2.3. Here, a nonlinear transformation matrix is output and should be combined with the motion-correction matrix estimated in the previous step. This doesn't, however, address spin history effects, whereby the susceptibility-induced differences may depend on (1) position in the cardio-respiratory cycle and (2) relative position.

4.1.4.3 Temporal and Spatial Filtering

High pass filtering removes low frequency drifts caused by the MRI system. See Chapter 4.2 for more details on filtering.

Spatial filtering (or smoothing) can improve sensitivity to detect activation. Typically for a $1 \times 1 \times 5$ mm acquisition, a 2 D Gaussian kernel with 2 mm FWHM is often used. Care is warranted, however, as too much smoothing can reduce the sensitivity to detect BOLD signal if the point spread function of the BOLD signal is small compared to the kernel size of the spatial filter (see Figure 4.1.9). This problem is analogous to the choice of voxel size.

4.1.4.4 Statistical Inference

Functional neuroimaging data typically consist of a series of volumes acquired during the course of an experiment. The task of statistical inference is to determine whether a given voxel was "activated" during the experiment. The most widely used approach for estimating activity in fMRI data is the general linear model (GLM), which is implemented in freely available software such as SPM, FSL and AFNI. The principle behind the GLM is a linear regression between the measured signal at each voxel (a time series) and a set of functions

FIGURE 4.1.9 Optimal smoothing depends on the spatial point spread function (PSF) of the BOLD signal. If the BOLD response is spread (big PSF), then smoothing is better, because it will lower the noise (assuming noise is not spatially-correlated). If the BOLD response is focal (small PSF), then smoothing is not advised, because it will average out the signal from surrounding "non-activated" voxels and the effect size will be reduced.

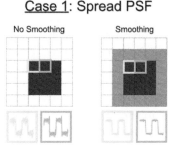

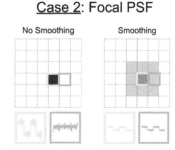

that the experimenter chooses and hopes explain signal variance in the time series. These functions must be carefully chosen for their contributions to the measured time series (Y). As illustrated in Figure 4.1.10, the modeling functions attempt to encompass signal variation caused by the BOLD response (the regressor of interest, X, containing the task paradigm convolved by the HRF), other factors such as physiological fluctuations, system drifts, subject motion (regressors of noninterest, D), and any residual (ε) considered as a random noise term. The weight (or effect size, β) of the regressor of interest may then be expressed as z- or t-score, and the null hypothesis tested to assess whether the regressor of interest can explain MRI signal variation. The signal Y can be modeled as follows:

$$Y = \beta X + \lambda D + \varepsilon$$

In this model, one assumes that ε is independent and identically normally distributed (i.i.d.). If ε was not i.i.d., the variance of the estimator would be underestimated, thus leading to a biased t-score and therefore altering activation detection sensitivity.[95,96] In the case of spinal fMRI, cardiac-cycle-related signal variations significantly contribute to the total variance of time series.[14] Hence, when modeling Y with the GLM one must take cardiac signal into account, otherwise the residuals

ε would include cardiac fluctuations leading to colored residuals, i.e., there would be temporal autocorrelations within residuals leading to a biased t-score. There are various strategies to model or minimize the effect of physiological fluctuations. These strategies are described in depth in Chapter 4.2.

4.1.4.5 Group Analysis

Typically in a brain study all subjects are registered to a template (e.g., the MNI template) in order to produce a spatial statistical map. Whilst spinal fMRI data is amenable to group analysis, this approach is more difficult as (1) there is no standard template of the spinal cord, preventing the use of a normalization procedure as usually done in the brain and (2) the normalization techniques used in the brain are less suited for images of the vertebral column. A few groups have created their own spinal cord template by averaging images from the subjects within the study.[21,97] Going further, a normalization procedure proposed by Stroman et al. consists of straightening the cord using manual delineation of the central canal, followed by a homothetic transformation in the rostro-caudal direction to account for variation in the size and separation of the vertebrae between subjects.[88] A recent study by Fonov et al.[98]

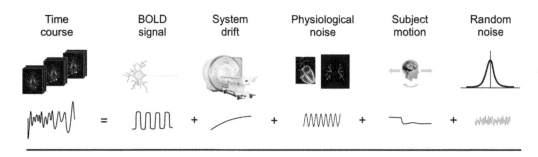

FIGURE 4.1.10 General linear model (GLM) applied to fMRI data.

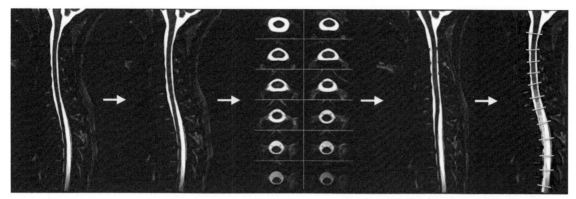

FIGURE 4.1.11   Pipeline for spinal cord template registration. An anatomical data (T_2-weighted turbo spin echo) is denoised and intensity normalized, then the spinal cord and CSF are automatically segmented to allow nonlinear registration to a labeled template generated from 17 subjects: the MNI-Poly-AMU template. For more information see Fonov et al.[98]

used state-of-the-art methods for generating a template of the spinal cord and registering multimodal images to it (see Figure 4.1.11). Despite encouraging progresses, registering spinal cord EPI data to T_2 templates remains a challenging task and is the subject of current investigations.

4.1.4.6 Presenting Results

Whilst fMRI of the brain is well established, spinal cord fMRI is a rapidly evolving field. Hence, researchers have the responsibility to present their results in a comprehensive and unbiased way. In order to allow the reviewer or reader of an article to assess the quality of the data and the likelihood for confounding effects (task-related motion, thresholding issues, etc.), we recommend the following:

- Report tSNR measurements and describe how tSNR was calculated (see above).
- Show all your data. Don't show only slices that have interesting "blobs". If space is an issue, it is possible to show every other slice or to reformat the data to coronal or sagittal orientation. This is important for assessing the occurrence of false positives (specificity). Also, it provides more information to the community, helping other researchers to reproduce the study and compare the quality of their results to published material.
- Show positive *and* negative t-scores, in order to assess the presence of deactivation and task-related motion (see section "challenges of fMRI of the spinal cord").
- The use of extensive masking in many studies prevents assessment of the spatial specificity of the reported activations. In many previous studies, masks were essentially drawn over the spinal cord, making it impossible to assess the number of false positives outside of the spinal cord, i.e., where neuronal activation was unlikely to occur. Although automatic masking procedures are used routinely in brain studies, their use is problematic in the spinal cord where assessment of false positives is needed as a validation tool. Spinal cord fMRI is still at a developmental stage, and researchers need to assess the validity of published results.

- The question often arises: *how should one report the time course of BOLD-related signal change in the spinal cord?* A commonly used method is to threshold the t-statistical maps (e.g., at $p = 0.01$) and to average the time course of voxels passing the threshold. This technique is invalid. Voxels that pass a given threshold are de facto correlated with the experimental paradigm, hence selecting only those voxels when producing an average time course will give a completely biased representation of the data. Instead, we recommend the calculation of the average time course to be driven by the underlying anatomy, not by the statistical results. To do so, the researcher can identify a region that is expected to be activated (hypothesis driven) by creating an ROI based on the mean EPI or based on the coregistered anatomical image, and then average the time course within *every voxel in this region*. Percent signal change should similarly be reported from the ROI. A combination of both the statistical and anatomical approaches is possible, but details of the methodology need to be reported. Note that the ROI should be the smallest consistent with the hypothesized response to avoid diluting the signal change.
- Correction for multiple comparisons: see Chapter 4.2.

4.1.5 CONCLUSIONS

The poor sensitivity and reproducibility of fMRI in the spinal cord highlights the importance of better understanding the low-level physical and physiological processes giving rise to the MR signal of interest, as well as further improving technical and analytical methods. Some of the areas where further investigation is needed in order to strengthen the basis for spinal cord BOLD fMRI include:

- Characterization of oxidative metabolism in spinal neurons[99]
- Characterization of neurovascular coupling at the spinal level, which might differ from that in the brain[36]
- Investigation of the influence of anesthetics on neuronal and vascular response[100,101]
- Linking the recruitment of activated fibers (in case of motor or sensory stimuli) with the number of activated neurons
- Modeling the link between vascular response and MRI signal[102]
- Relating the size of BOLD signal responses to recorded behavior
- Standardizing methods for measuring and reporting statistically significant areas of activity
- Optimizing the use of pulse sequences, e.g., using multi-echo techniques to increase the sensitivity of activation detection[94,103]
- Designing dedicated coils for improved sensitivity[104]
- Optimizing the processing of spinal fMRI data given the relative importance of physiological-related noise in spinal fMRI time series[14,105]

Other imaging modalities (e.g., DW-MRI, transcranial magnetic stimulation, positron emission tomography, etc.) could add useful information for investigating spinal cord fMRI.[106]

In conclusion, we believe that fMRI of the spinal cord is still developing, and despite an increasing number of high impact publications demonstrating its use, it requires further validation via studies of test-retest reproducibility, standardization, and corroboration of results by multiple groups using similar acquisition and analysis techniques.

4.1.6 RECIPE

Parameters	Values	Comments
Slice orientation	Axial	Perpendicular to the cord
FOV	96 × 96 mm	Reducing the FOV in the phase-encoding direction (along with the number of phase lines) can aid in minimizing susceptibility artifacts. Needs suppression technique (e.g., sat band) or 2D selective RF pulse to avoid aliasing

Parameters	Values	Comments
Matrix	64 × 64	Yielding 1.5 mm in-plane resolution
Slice thickness	5 mm	
Acceleration[1]	2	GRAPPA (Siemens), SENSE (Philips), ARC (GE) Not advised if using reduced FOV technique (e.g., <32 phase lines) or if g-factor is high (see chapter 2.1)
N slices	20	Depends on the desired coverage
Slice order	Interleave	To minimize cross-talk
PE direction	A-P	May also benefit from P-A ("blip-down") acquisition
TR	3000 ms	
TE	30 ms	Depends on the calculated T_2^*
Partial Fourier	Off	Can be used to reduce TE
Shimming	Automatic, z-shim and dynamic shimming if possible	Adjust the shim box to the spinal cord (see Figure 13 in Chapter 3.1)
Fat suppression	SPAIR	
BW/pixel	∼2000 Hz	Set to minimize echo spacing and hence susceptibility distortions
Saturation bands	1 or 2	Placed anteriorly and posteriorly to the spine (see recipe in Chapter 3.1)

[1] Be aware that acceleration is only possible if there is adequate coil coverage in the phase-encoding direction. With the typical neck coil (anterior and posterior elements), there is enough coverage for acceleration of 2. However, for thoracic or lumbar imaging, there is usually only a spine array matrix posteriorly, therefore not enough coil element if phase-encoding direction is A-P. In that case, acceleration is not advised.

References

1. Ogawa S, et al. Brain magnetic resonance imaging with contrast dependent on blood oxygenation. *Proc Natl Acad Sci USA*. 1990; 87(24):9868–9872.
2. Kwong KK, et al. Dynamic magnetic resonance imaging of human brain activity during primary sensory stimulation. *Proc Natl Acad Sci USA*. 1992;89(12):5675–5679.
3. Bandettini PA, et al. Spin-echo and gradient-echo EPI of human brain activation using BOLD contrast: a comparative study at 1.5 T. *NMR Biomed*. 1994;7(1–2):12–20.
4. Raichle ME. Cognitive neuroscience. Bold insights. *Nature*. 2001; 412(6843):128–130.
5. Bandettini PA, Ungerleider LG. From neuron to BOLD: new connections. *Nat Neurosci*. 2001;4(9):864–866.
6. Logothetis NK. The neural basis of the blood-oxygen-level-dependent functional magnetic resonance imaging signal. *Philos Trans R Soc Lond B Biol Sci*. 2002;357(1424):1003–1037.
7. Heeger DJ, Ress D. What does fMRI tell us about neuronal activity? *Nat Rev Neurosci*. 2002;3(2):142–151.

8. Nair DG. About being BOLD. *Brain Res Brain Res Rev*. 2005;50(2): 229–243.

9. Yoshizawa T, et al. Functional magnetic resonance imaging of motor activation in the human cervical spinal cord. *NeuroImage*. 1996;4(3 Pt 1):174–182.

10. Govers N, et al. Functional MRI of the cervical spinal cord on 1.5 T with fingertapping: to what extent is it feasible? *Neuroradiology*. 2007;49(1):73–81.

11. Maieron M, et al. Functional responses in the human spinal cord during willed motor actions: evidence for side- and rate-dependent activity. *J Neurosci*. 2007;27(15):4182–4190.

12. Stracke CP, et al. Interneuronal systems of the cervical spinal cord assessed with BOLD imaging at 1.5 T. *Neuroradiology*. 2005;47(2): 127–133.

13. Stroman PW, et al. Noninvasive assessment of the injured human spinal cord by means of functional magnetic resonance imaging. *Spinal Cord*. 2004;42(2):59–66.

14. Brooks JC, et al. Physiological noise modelling for spinal functional magnetic resonance imaging studies. *NeuroImage*. 2008; 39(2):680–692.

15. Cohen-Adad J, et al. BOLD signal responses to controlled hypercapnia in human spinal cord. *NeuroImage*. 2010;50(3): 1074–1084.

16. Bouwman CJ, et al. Spinal cord functional MRI at 3 T: Gradient echo echo-planar imaging versus turbo spin echo. *NeuroImage*. 2008;43(2):288–296.

17. Summers PE, et al. A quantitative comparison of BOLD fMRI responses to noxious and innocuous stimuli in the human spinal cord. *NeuroImage*. 2010;50(4):1408–1415.

18. Giulietti G, et al. Characterization of the functional response in the human spinal cord: impulse-response function and linearity. *NeuroImage*. 2008;42(2):626–634.

19. Backes WH, Mess WH, Wilmink JT. Functional MR imaging of the cervical spinal cord by use of median nerve stimulation and fist clenching. *AJNR Am J Neuroradiol*. 2001;22(10):1854–1859.

20. Madi S, et al. Functional MR imaging of the human cervical spinal cord. *AJNR Am J Neuroradiol*. 2001;22(9):1768–1774.

21. Eippert F, et al. Direct evidence for spinal cord involvement in placebo analgesia. *Science*. 2009;326(5951):404.

22. Valsasina P, et al. Spinal fMRI during proprioceptive and tactile tasks in healthy subjects: activity detected using cross-correlation, general linear model and independent component analysis. *Neuroradiology*. 2008;50(10):895–902.

23. Majcher K, et al. Functional magnetic resonance imaging within the rat spinal cord following peripheral nerve injury. *NeuroImage*. 2007;38(4):669–676.

24. Cohen-Adad J, et al. Investigations on spinal cord fMRI of cats under ketamine. *NeuroImage*. 2009;44(2):328–339.

25. Lawrence J, Stroman PW, Malisza KL. Comparison of functional activity in the rat cervical spinal cord during alpha-chloralose and halothane anesthesia. *NeuroImage*. 2007;34(4):1665–1672.

26. Lilja J, et al. Blood oxygenation level-dependent visualization of synaptic relay stations of sensory pathways along the neuroaxis in response to graded sensory stimulation of a limb. *J Neurosci*. 2006;26(23):6330–6336.

27. Zhao F, et al. BOLD and blood volume-weighted fMRI of rat lumbar spinal cord during non-noxious and noxious electrical hindpaw stimulation. *NeuroImage*. 2008;40(1):133–147.

28. Endo T, et al. Reorganization of sensory processing below the level of spinal cord injury as revealed by fMRI. *Exp Neurol*. 2008; 209(1):155–160.

29. Giove F, et al. Issues about the fMRI of the human spinal cord. *Magn Reson Imaging*. 2004;22(10):1505–1516.

30. Fox PT, et al. Nonoxidative glucose consumption during focal physiologic neural activity. *Science*. 1988;241(4864):462–464.

31. Gjedde A, Kuwabara H, Hakim AM. Reduction of functional capillary density in human brain after stroke. *J Cereb Blood Flow Metab*. 1990;10(3):317–326.

32. Hoge RD, et al. Linear coupling between cerebral blood flow and oxygen consumption in activated human cortex. *Proc Natl Acad Sci USA*. 1999;96(16):9403–9408.

33. Marcus ML, et al. Regulation of total and regional spinal cord blood flow. *Circ Res*. 1977;41(1):128–134.

34. Sasaki S, et al. Optical imaging of intrinsic signals induced by peripheral nerve stimulation in the in vivo rat spinal cord. *NeuroImage*. 2002;17(3):1240–1255.

35. Brieu N, et al. Characterization of the hemodynamic response in vivo rat lumbar spinal cord by intrinsic optical imaging and laser speckle microscopy. *J Neurosci Methods*. 2010;30:191(2):151–157.

36. Nix W, et al. Comparison of vascular reactivity in spinal cord and brain. *Stroke*. 1976;7(6):560–563.

37. Logothetis NK, et al. Neurophysiological investigation of the basis of the fMRI signal. *Nature*. 2001;412(6843):150–157.

38. Aguirre GK, Zarahn E, D'Esposito M. The variability of human, BOLD hemodynamic responses. *NeuroImage*. 1998;8(4):360–369.

39. Piché M, et al. Characterization of cardiac-related noise in fMRI of the cervical spinal cord. *Magn Reson Imaging*. 2009;27(3):300–310.

40. Brooks JC, et al. Stimulus site and modality dependence of functional activity within the human spinal cord. *J Neurosci*. 2012; 32(18):6231–6239.

41. Stroman PW, Ryner LN. Functional MRI of motor and sensory activation in the human spinal cord. *Magn Reson Imaging*. 2001; 19(1):27–32.

42. Ng MC, et al. Cervical spinal cord BOLD fMRI study: modulation of functional activation by dexterity of dominant and non-dominant hands. *NeuroImage*. 2008;39(2):825–831.

43. Porro CA, et al. Functional activity mapping of the rat spinal cord during formalin-induced noxious stimulation. *Neuroscience*. 1991; 41(2–3):655–665.

44. Coghill RC, Mayer DJ, Price DD. The roles of spatial recruitment and discharge frequency in spinal cord coding of pain: a combined electrophysiological and imaging investigation. *Pain*. 1993; 53(3):295–309.

45. Bouwman CJ, et al. Spinal cord functional MRI at 3 T: gradient echo echo-planar imaging versus turbo spin echo. *NeuroImage*. 2008;43(2):288–296.

46. Stroman PW. Magnetic resonance imaging of neuronal function in the spinal cord: spinal FMRI. *Clin Med Res*. 2005;3(3):146–156.

47. Cadotte D, et al. Creating an MRI anatomic atlas of the human cervical spine: implications for spinal fMRI. In: *Proceedings of the Annual Meeting of the Organization for Human Brain Mapping (OHBM)*. Beijing, China; 2012:5345.

48. Baldissera F, et al. Excitability changes in human corticospinal projections to forearm muscles during voluntary movement of ipsilateral foot. *J Physiol*. 2002;539(Pt 3):903–911.

49. Jankowska E. Interneuronal relay in spinal pathways from proprioceptors. *Prog Neurobiol*. 1992;38(4):335–378.

50. Porro CA, Cavazzuti M. Spatial and temporal aspects of spinal cord and brainstem activation in the formalin pain model. *Prog Neurobiol*. 1993;41(5):565–607.

51. Lemon RN. Descending pathways in motor control. *Annu Rev Neurosci*. 2008;31:195–218.

52. Shmuel A, et al. Sustained negative BOLD, blood flow and oxygen consumption response and its coupling to the positive response in the human brain. *Neuron*. 2002;36(6):1195–1210.

53. Cohen-Adad J, et al. Investigations in functional MRI of the spinal cord of cats. *NeuroImage*. 2009;44(2):328–339.

54. Mandeville JB, Marota JJ. Vascular filters of functional MRI: spatial localization using BOLD and CBV contrast. *Magn Reson Med*. 1999;42(3):591–598.

55. Zhao F, Wang P, Kim SG. Cortical depth-dependent gradient-echo and spin-echo BOLD fMRI at 9.4T. *Magn Reson Med*. 2004; 51(3):518–524.

56. Duong TQ, et al. Microvascular BOLD contribution at 4 and 7 T in the human brain: gradient-echo and spin-echo fMRI with suppression of blood effects. *Magn Reson Med*. 2003;49(6): 1019–1027.

57. Ogawa S, et al. On the characteristics of functional magnetic resonance imaging of the brain. *Annu Rev Biophys Biomol Struct*. 1998;27(1):447–474.

58. Malonek D, Grinvald A. Interactions between electrical activity and cortical microcirculation revealed by imaging spectroscopy: implications for functional brain mapping. *Science*. 1996; 272(5261):551–554.

59. Turner R. How much cortex can a vein drain? Downstream dilution of activation-related cerebral blood oxygenation changes. *NeuroImage*. 2002;16(4):1062–1067.

60. Smirnakis SM, et al. Spatial specificity of BOLD versus cerebral blood volume fMRI for mapping cortical organization. *J Cereb Blood Flow Metab*. 2007;27(6):1248–1261.

61. Zhao F, et al. Pain fMRI in rat cervical spinal cord: an echo planar imaging evaluation of sensitivity of BOLD and blood volume-weighted fMRI. *NeuroImage*. 2009;44(2):349–362.

62. Leite FP, et al. Repeated fMRI using iron oxide contrast agent in awake, behaving macaques at 3 Tesla. *NeuroImage*. 2002;16(2): 283–294.

63. Gati JS, et al. Experimental determination of the BOLD field strength dependence in vessels and tissue. *Magn Reson Med*. 1997; 38(2):296–302.

64. Hulvershorn J, et al. Spatial sensitivity and temporal response of spin echo and gradient echo bold contrast at 3 T using peak hemodynamic activation time. *NeuroImage*. 2005;24(1):216–223.

65. Parkes LM, et al. Quantifying the spatial resolution of the gradient echo and spin echo BOLD response at 3 Tesla. *Magn Reson Med*. 2005;54(6):1465–1472.

66. Zhao F, et al. Cortical layer-dependent BOLD and CBV responses measured by spin-echo and gradient-echo fMRI: insights into hemodynamic regulation. *NeuroImage*. 2006;30(4):1149–1160.

67. Jochimsen TH, Norris DG, Moller HE. Is there a change in water proton density associated with functional magnetic resonance imaging? *Magn Reson Med*. 2005;53(2):470–473.

68. Moffitt MA, et al. Functional magnetic resonance imaging of the human lumbar spinal cord. *J Magn Reson Imaging*. 2005;21(5): 527–535.

69. Stefanovic B, et al. The effect of global cerebral vasodilation on focal activation hemodynamics. *NeuroImage*. 2006;30(3):726–734.

70. Vazquez AL, et al. Vascular dynamics and BOLD fMRI: CBF level effects and analysis considerations. *NeuroImage*. 2006;32(4): 1642–1655.

71. Richter W, Richter M. The shape of the fMRI BOLD response in children and adults changes systematically with age. *NeuroImage*. 2003;20(2):1122–1131.

72. D'Esposito M, Deouell LY, Gazzaley A. Alterations in the BOLD fMRI signal with ageing and disease: a challenge for neuro-imaging. *Nat Rev Neurosci*. 2003;4(11):863–872.

73. Chen Y, Parrish TB. Caffeine's effects on cerebrovascular reactivity and coupling between cerebral blood flow and oxygen metabolism. *NeuroImage*. 2009;44(3):647–652.

74. Bandettini PA, et al. Characterization of cerebral blood oxygenation and flow changes during prolonged brain activation. *Hum Brain Mapp*. 1997;5(2):93–109.

75. Bellgowan PS, et al. Improved BOLD detection in the medial temporal region using parallel imaging and voxel volume reduction. *NeuroImage*. 2006;29(4):1244–1251.

76. Bodurka J, et al. Mapping the MRI voxel volume in which thermal noise matches physiological noise–implications for fMRI. *NeuroImage*. 2007;34(2):542–549.

77. Parrish TB, et al. Impact of signal-to-noise on functional MRI. *Magn Reson Med*. 2000;44(6):925–932.

78. Triantafyllou C, et al. Comparison of physiological noise at 1.5 T, 3 T and 7 T and optimization of fMRI acquisition parameters. *NeuroImage*. 2005;26(1):243–250.

79. Murphy K, Bodurka J, Bandettini PA. How long to scan? The relationship between fMRI temporal signal to noise ratio and necessary scan duration. *NeuroImage*. 2007;34(2):565–574.

80. Kornelsen J, Stroman PW. fMRI of the lumbar spinal cord during a lower limb motor task. *Magn Reson Med*. 2004;52(2): 411–414.

81. Yiannakas MC, et al. Feasibility of grey matter and white matter segmentation of the upper cervical cord in vivo: a pilot study with application to magnetisation transfer measurements. *NeuroImage*. 2012;63(3):1054–1059.

82. Triantafyllou C, et al. Physiological noise in gradient echo and spin echo EPI at 3 T and 7 T. In: *Proceedings of the 17th Annual Scientific Meeting of the International Society for Magnetic Resonance in Medicine*. Honolulu, USA; 2009:122.

83. Cooke FJ, et al. Quantitative proton magnetic resonance spectroscopy of the cervical spinal cord. *Magn Reson Med*. 2004;51(6): 1122–1128.

84. Friese S, et al. B-waves in cerebral and spinal cerebrospinal fluid pulsation measurement by magnetic resonance imaging. *J Comput Assist Tomogr*. 2004;28(2):255–262.

85. Eippert F, et al. Activation of the opioidergic descending pain control system underlies placebo analgesia. *Neuron*. 2009;63(4): 533–543.

86. Xie G, et al. Reduction of physiological noise with independent component analysis improves the detection of nociceptive responses with fMRI of the human spinal cord. *NeuroImage*. 2012; 63(1):245–252.

87. Li L, et al. Cerebrospinal fluid (CSF) flow suppressed spinal cord functional MRI using multi-slice DANTE-EPI. In: *Proceedings of the 20th Annual Scientific Meeting of the International Society for Magnetic Resonance in Medicine (ISMRM)*. Melbourne, Australia; 2012:615.

88. Stroman PW, Kornelsen J, Lawrence J. An improved method for spinal functional MRI with large volume coverage of the spinal cord. *J Magn Reson Imaging*. 2005;21(5):520–526.

89. Polimeni JR, et al. Laminar analysis of 7T BOLD using an imposed spatial activation pattern in human V1. *NeuroImage*. 2010;52(4):1334–1346.

90. Glover GH. 3D z-shim method for reduction of susceptibility effects in BOLD fMRI. *Magn Reson Med*. 1999;42(2):290–299.

91. Menon RS, et al. 4 Tesla gradient recalled echo characteristics of photic stimulation-induced signal changes in the human primary visual cortex. *Magn Reson Med*. 1993;30(3):380–386.

92. Triantafyllou C, Wald LL, Hoge RD. Echo-time and field strength dependence of BOLD reactivity in veins and parenchyma using flow-normalized hypercapnic manipulation. *PLoS One*. 2011;6(9): e24519.

93. Posse S, et al. Enhancement of BOLD-contrast sensitivity by single-shot multi-echo functional MR imaging. *Magn Reson Med*. 1999;42(1):87–97.

94. Poser BA, Norris DG. Investigating the benefits of multi-echo EPI for fMRI at 7 T. *NeuroImage*. 2009;45(4):1162–1172.

95. Lund T, et al. Non-white noise in fMRI: Does modelling have an impact? *NeuroImage*. 2006;29(1):54–66.

96. Dagli MS, Ingeholm JE, Haxby JV. Localization of cardiac-induced signal change in fMRI. *NeuroImage*. 1999;9(4):407–415.

97. Stroman PW, Figley CR, Cahill CM. Spatial normalization, bulk motion correction and coregistration for functional magnetic resonance imaging of the human cervical spinal cord and brainstem. *Magn Reson Imaging*. 2008;26(6):809–814.

98. Fonov V, Cohen-Adad J, Collins DL. Spinal cord template and a semi-automatic image processing pipeline. In: *Proceedings of the 21st Annual Scientific Meeting of the International Society for Magnetic Resonance in Medicine (ISMRM)*. Salt Lake City, USA; 2013: 1119.

99. Cannon MS, Gelderd JB. Spinal cord vasculature of the rat: a histochemical study of the metabolism of arteries and arterioles. *Stroke*. 1983;14(4):611–616.

100. Sicard K, et al. Regional cerebral blood flow and BOLD responses in conscious and anesthetized rats under basal and hypercapnic conditions: implications for functional MRI studies. *J Cereb Blood Flow Metab*. 2003;23(4):472–481.

101. Martin C, et al. Investigating neural-hemodynamic coupling and the hemodynamic response function in the awake rat. *NeuroImage*. 2006;32(1):33–48.

102. Buxton RB, et al. Modeling the hemodynamic response to brain activation. *NeuroImage*. 2004;23(suppl 1):S220–S233.

103. Chen NK, et al. Functional MRI with variable echo time acquisition. *NeuroImage*. 2003;20(4):2062–2070.

104. Bodurka J, Ledden P, Bandettini P. SENSE optimized sixteen element receive array for cervical spinal cord imaging at 3T. In: *Proceedings of the 16th Annual Scientific Meeting of the International Society for Magnetic Resonance in Medicine (ISMRM)*. Toronto, Canada; 2008 p. 1078.

105. Stroman PW. Discrimination of errors from neuronal activity in functional MRI of the human spinal cord by means of general linear model analysis. *Magn Reson Med*. 2006;56(2):452–456.

106. Harel NY, Strittmatter SM. Functional MRI and other non-invasive imaging technologies: providing visual biomarkers for spinal cord structure and function after injury. *Exp Neurol*. 2008;211(2):324–328.

107. Arthurs OJ, Boniface S. How well do we understand the neural origins of the fMRI BOLD signal? *Trends Neurosci*. 2002;25(1): 27–31.

108. Stroman PW, Nance PW, Ryner LN. BOLD MRI of the human cervical spinal cord at 3 tesla. *Magn Reson Med*. 1999;42(3): 571–576.

109. Komisaruk BR, Mosier KM, Liu WC, et al. Functional localization of brainstem and cervical spinal cord nuclei in humans with fMRI. *AJNR Am J Neuroradiol*. 2002;23(4):609–617.

110. Giulietti G, Summers PE, Ferraro D, Porro CA, Maraviglia B, Giove F. Semiautomated segmentation of the human spine based on echoplanar images. *Magn Reson Imaging*. 2011;29(10): 1429–1436.

111. Kong Y, Jenkinson M, Andersson J, Tracey I, Brooks JC. Assessment of physiological noise modelling methods for functional imaging of the spinal cord. *Neuroimage*. 2012;60(2): 1538–1549.

Physiological Noise Modeling and Analysis for Spinal Cord fMRI

Jonathan C.W. Brooks

Clinical Research and Imaging Centre (CRICBristol), University of Bristol, Bristol, UK

4.2.1 WHAT IS PHYSIOLOGICAL NOISE?

Physiological noise can be defined as any signal change occurring in an image that is due to the subject and that is of no interest. Equally, movement of the subject (e.g., bulk movement of the cord) and *indirect* movement of structures of interest (e.g., caused by arterial pulsation or cerebrospinal fluid (CSF) flow) could also be included in this heading. For the purpose of this discussion, I will limit my attention to those signal changes arising from cardiac and respiratory processes, and how they influence the recorded signal on blood oxygenation level-dependent (BOLD)-based functional images, and not consider correction for bulk movement.

4.2.1.1 Where Does Physiological Noise Come from?

Krüger et al.[1] proposed that physiological noise derives from processes that depend on cortical metabolism (e.g., cerebral blood flow, changes in PaCO$_2$, cerebral blood volume, and consumption of oxygen) and physiological processes such as cardiac output and respiratory rate, which produce arterial pulsatility,[2,3] drive CSF flow,[4] and induce time-varying changes in the main magnetic field (B_0).[5] These processes are interdependent (e.g., chemoreceptors in the brainstem will record changes in the amount of CO$_2$ in the blood and, via sympathetic outflow, increase breathing rate). Equally, there is link between cardiac and respiratory function. An example of this is the connection between cardiac output (stroke volume) and the respiratory cycle, the so-called "respiratory pump"[6] (increased cardiac output during inspiration). One implication of this coupling is that processes driven by cardiac pulsatility, such as CSF flow,

will have a dependence on both the cardiac and respiratory cycles. This phenomenon has been investigated using magnetic resonance imaging (MRI) techniques in the brainstem[7] and spinal cord,[8] and it must be considered when attempting to account for sources of physiological noise in functional imaging experiments.

4.2.1.2 Why is Physiological Noise Important?

As described in Chapter 4.1, the detection of task-related signals in functional MRI (fMRI) is assessed by statistical inference, and it is typically performed by using the general linear model (GLM), which can be expressed via the following equation:

$$Y = \beta \cdot X + \varepsilon \qquad (4.2.1)$$

where Y is the measured time course of a given voxel, X is the experimental design (e.g., the paradigm convolved with a hemodynamic response function), β are the weights or amplitudes of the fitted components in the design, and ε is the residual (i.e., the amount "left over" after the optimal model fit has been obtained). As pointed out in Chapter 4.1, the structured background signal measured in an fMRI experiment includes physiological noise, which can degrade the t-statistic (by inflating the residual term ε) if not properly taken into account.

Physiological noise may be the dominant source of noise in an fMRI experiment. Whilst raw signal to noise increases linearly with field strength,[9] physiological noise increases with the square of the field strength,[10] and as a consequence there is an asymptotic limit to the temporal signal-to-noise ratio (TSNR)[11] that can be achieved at higher field strength.[1,12,13] TSNR is the ratio of the mean signal intensity recorded from a time series of functional images, divided by the standard deviation of that signal. Hence, the best chance for detecting the small ($\sim$1–2%) signal changes associated with functional activity will be in regions of high TSNR (i.e., where the baseline signal is high compared to its variance). In the theoretical model suggested by Krüger and Glover, two contributions to physiological noise were described: a component that induces changes via BOLD-like mechanisms (characterized by a constant c_1, a relaxation rate R_2^*, and the echo time (TE) of the experiment), and a non-BOLD component that depends only on a constant c_2 and the intrinsic signal intensity S. The relationship between these quantities, their dependence on field strength, and their impact on TSNR was further explored by Triantafyllou et al.,[13] as discussed in this chapter.

$$TSNR = \frac{SNR_0}{\sqrt{1 + \lambda^2 \cdot SNR_0^2}},$$
$$\text{where } \lambda^2 = c_1^2 \cdot \Delta R_2^{*2} \cdot TE^2 + c_2^2 \qquad (4.2.2)$$

where SNR_0 is the image SNR (see Chapters 2.1 and 4.1). Equation (4.2.2) shows (as expected) that at high SNR_0, TSNR will tend toward an asymptotic value given by $1/\lambda$.

It is important to note that the influence of physiological noise depends not only on the intrinsic SNR_0 but also on the voxel size, with smaller voxels being less affected than larger ones (relative to the contribution from thermal noise). Equally, not all cortical or subcortical regions will be similarly affected by physiological noise. Krüger and Glover[1] demonstrated distinct spatial patterns of physiological noise affecting brain images: it is increased in gray relative to white matter. Furthermore, when imaging more inferior (ventral) regions of the brain, around the thalamus, mesial temporal lobes, and brainstem, there is an increased contribution from the extrinsic (cardiac and respiratory) noise sources, due to the presence of large vessels (e.g., the Circle of Willis) and the closer proximity to the lungs.

When attempting to record functional signal from the spinal cord, one is faced with a great many challenges, not the least of which is the relative size of the structure of interest to the surrounding sources of physiological noise. The presence of relatively large spinal arteries and veins close to the surface of the cord (see Chapter 4.3) will contribute noise and potentially hinder the accurate localization of activity (see Chapter 4.1). Another significant source of noise arises from CSF in-flow effects[7] in the subarachnoid space surrounding the cord, which will be prominent on single-shot image acquisitions using typical repetition times (TRs $\leq$3 s) and flip angles close to the Ernst angle ($\sim$80°). Left unaccounted for, the various sources of physiological noise each contribute to the measured signal in the fMRI experiment and will reduce the TSNR, placing strict demands on the

experimental paradigm (i.e., an increased signal averaging and an increased number of stimuli). When combined with intrinsically low raw signal to noise (due to receive coil coverage and the need for relatively small voxel volumes), it is apparent that physiological noise may be the "dominant" signal in spinal FMRI experiments.

4.2.1.3 The Noise Characteristics of fMRI Data

In an early study,[14] the power spectrum of resting fMRI data from the brain was shown to have significant power at low frequencies; this is generally referred to as "$1/f$-like" noise (i.e., increased power at low frequencies). The presence of low-frequency noise has implications for analyzing fMRI data as the statistical models that are typically used assume that each sample of activity (i.e., each volume) is independent of other measurements in the experiment, and that the noise is equally distributed across the frequency range sampled. Clearly in the case of fMRI data, the observation of increased power at low frequencies would invalidate this assumption, as the noise is not equally represented at all frequencies. Another characteristic of fMRI data is that they are temporally autocorrelated,[3] which put simplistically means that preceding data points can predict subsequent data–invalidating the assumption of independence. The low-frequency energy in the spectrum of fMRI time-series data and temporal autocorrelation are thought to be due to the presence of physiological noise[3] and synchronized low-frequency neuronal activity across widespread brain regions.[15] Several techniques for assessing and correcting for temporal autocorrelation exist,[16,17] and their importance for spinal fMRI data will be discussed in this chapter.

Brooks et al.[18] investigated the presence of physiological noise in single-shot echo-planar imaging (EPI) data acquired from the human spinal cord with a short TR (200 ms) and no task (i.e., a resting experiment), by using an explorative technique based on independent component analysis.[19] These data revealed structured signals that were spatially and temporally distinct, and they had characteristic frequencies indicating that they derived from cardiac (around 1 Hz) and respiratory (around 0.3 Hz) processes. A component arising due to the interaction between cardiac and respiratory processes,[8,20] and very low-frequency signals[21] in the CSF surrounding the cord (Figure 4.2.1), were also observed.

4.2.2 TIME DOMAIN FILTERING

Temporal filtering is frequently applied during preprocessing of fMRI data, and it aims to remove signals from the data that are unrelated to the experiment (e.g.,

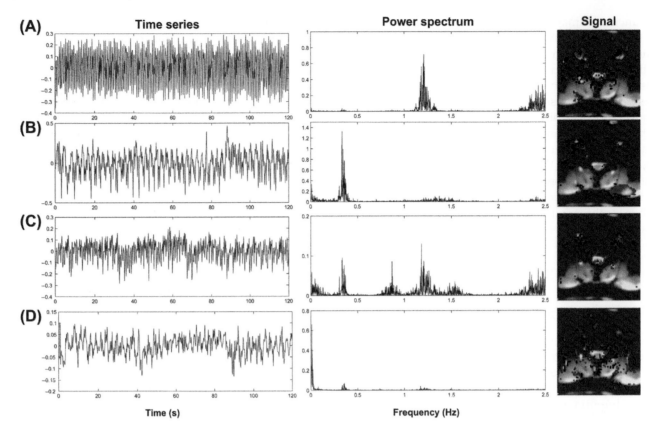

FIGURE 4.2.1   Main ICA-derived signal components (and associated power spectra) detected with critically sampled (TR = 200 ms) spinal cord EPI data: (A) cardiac, (B) respiratory, (C) interaction of cardiac and respiratory, and (D) low (<0.1 Hz) frequency. The time courses and spatial distributions are estimated from resting fMRI data, and reveal clear cardiac-related (~1 Hz) signal around the major vessels (carotid and vertebral arteries) plus cardiac-driven CSF flow effects in the subarachnoid space surrounding the spinal cord. Respiratory effects (0.33 Hz) were found in the muscle of the neck, but they were also found to interact with cardiac effects and were distributed around the spinal cord. Low-frequency components, due to either uncorrected motion or B- or C-waves, were also detected. For clarity, only the first 120 s of each time course are shown. *Source: Reproduced from Ref. 18 with permission.*

low-frequency drift due to scanner hardware considerations, or high-frequency signals arising from physiological processes). Two methods that are typically applied are high-pass filtering (HPF) and low-pass filtering (LPF), or a combination of the two: band-pass filtering (BPF). The first of these, high-pass filtering, can be achieved by applying a filter to the time-series data prior to estimation with the GLM or by including low-frequency cosine waveforms in the GLM—a linear combination of which will account for low-frequency signals in fMRI data (Figure 4.2.2). Almost all fMRI analysis packages will use an HPF as it will generally improve the obtained estimates for the parameters of interest by removing slow drifts from the fMRI time series that would otherwise remain as unmodeled variance in the data (increasing the variance of the residuals).

The second type of filter, the LPF, aims to remove high-frequency signals from the data, leaving the lower frequencies of typical fMRI designs unaffected. While the use of an LPF might seem an intuitive approach to removing physiological signals that are of higher

frequency than the experimental paradigm, there are two significant problems with its application: (1) physiological signals are typically undersampled due to the relatively long TR (e.g., 3–5 s) used in fMRI experiments (i.e., they are not "critically sampled") and thus may be aliased to low frequencies overlapping with the experimental paradigm; and (2) an LPF increases the smoothness of the time-series data, which has the effect of reducing the independence of time points, effectively reducing the number of independent samples in the data set. If the reduction of degrees of freedom is not accounted for in the applied statistical modeling,[22] this will lead to artificially inflated t- and Z-scores, and it is illustrated and described in Figure 4.2.3.

4.2.3 APPROACHES FOR REDUCING THE EFFECTS OF PHYSIOLOGICAL NOISE

Several techniques for minimizing the effect of physiological noise have been described, and they can be divided into three broad groups: (1) those

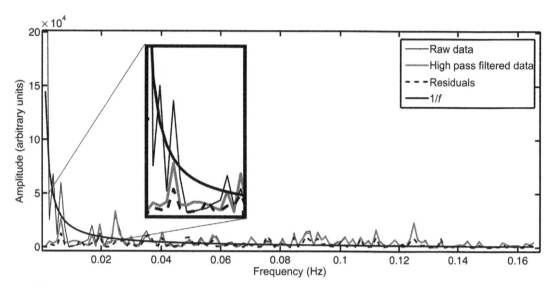

FIGURE 4.2.2 Power spectrum of spinal fMRI data acquired from the whole cervical cord (TE = 39 ms, TR = 3 s, resolution 1.33 × 1.33 × 4 mm, flip angle 80°, field strength 3 T). Increased power at low frequencies can be seen in the sharp rise at the left side of the power spectrum, and the line representing $1/f$ is shown to demonstrate the dependence of the power on frequency. The impact of high-pass filtering is shown, reducing the power below 0.02 Hz, and the power spectrum of the residuals is also shown to illustrate the effect of prewhitening (similar power across the studied frequency range).

that rely on the independent measurement of some physiological parameter (e.g., cardiac waveform or chest wall position), (2) those that require additional image acquisitions to measure the impact of physiological noise and then remove them from the experimental data, and (3) those that alter the data acquisition to attempt to minimize artifacts due to physiological processes.

4.2.3.1 External Physiological Measurements

One approach to taking account of the presence of physiological signals in an FMRI time series is to make a direct measurement of the subject's physiology, and then attempt to remove the corresponding signal from the data. Typically, the biological processes that one is most interested in are the cardiac and respiratory cycles, although other physiological parameters might also be of interest, such as galvanic skin response (GSR), pupil diameter (measured with an eye-tracking apparatus), noninvasive blood pressure, end-tidal CO_2, and arterial blood flow (measured with transcranial Doppler sonography). Considering the simplest case of cardiac and respiratory data, the relevant waveforms can be obtained via photoplethysmography (pulse oximetry) or electrocardiogram (ECG) leads, and pneumatic respiratory bellows, respectively. These data normally would be acquired using a commercial physiological monitoring unit, and the results recorded in real time via an analog-to-digital convertor attached to a personal computer. A typical setup is shown in Figure 4.2.4.

4.2.3.1.1 Data Logging

An important requirement of the independent measurement techniques is that the physiological waveforms should be recorded alongside the timing of the image acquisition, and this is typically achieved by recording "scanner" or "volume" triggers (or transistor–transistor logic (TTL) pulses) on the same computer used to log the physiological traces. The various traces can be seen in Figure 4.2.4, which in this case were sampled at a rate of 100 Hz—which is sufficient to accurately represent these waveforms. In practice, when recording electrophysiological signals such as ECG or electromyogram (EMG), the sampling rate is normally higher to enable artifacts induced by gradient switching to be filtered from the traces. It should be noted that in the case of some waveforms, the absolute magnitude of the recorded signal may be important (e.g., chest wall position measured via respiratory bellows), and this may place limits on the monitoring apparatus to be used. For example, the physiological signals recorded by the scanner's own monitoring equipment may be arbitrarily scaled for display purposes, making them unsuitable for subsequent physiological signal estimation.

4.2.3.1.2 Do I Need to Buy a Dedicated Physiological Recording System?

In most scanners, it is possible to obtain the trace of the physiological signal that is meant to be used for gating (e.g., respiratory trace or pulse oximetry). However, it may not be straightforward to then synchronize these traces to the actual timing of the data, or in some cases the physiological traces are not appropriately sampled.

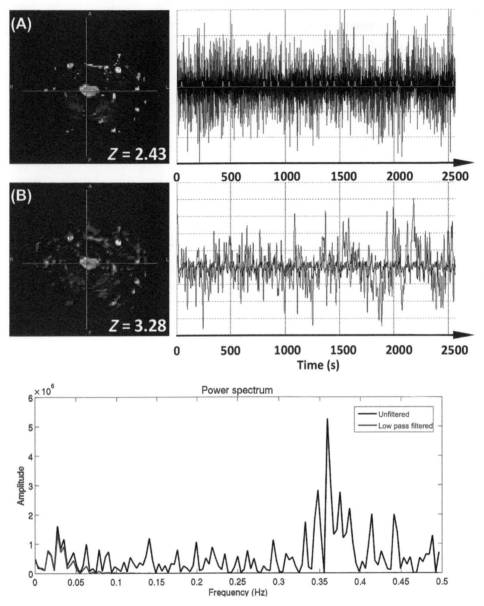

FIGURE 4.2.3   Illustration of the undesired effects of low-pass filtering. Data are from a single subject's spinal fMRI experiment, with the time-series data and resultant statistical maps (threshold $Z > 2.3$). The only difference between (A) and (B) is that the latter had a low-pass filter applied (cutoff 0.1 Hz). It is clear that the time series are temporally smoothed by this procedure—and the effect on the power spectrum is shown below. The action of the LPF is to remove 80% of the noise associated with this experiment, increasing the Z-score of the "activated" voxels in the cord (if not adjusting for loss of degrees of freedom in the model) and, more importantly, dramatically increasing the false-positive detection rate in the nonneuronal tissue of the neck (e.g., in the trachea and vertebral bodies). It should be clear that application of a more modest LPF (cutoff 0.3 Hz) would still lead to artificial inflation of statistics. The reality is that the data (as acquired) are the time series in (A), and thus the confidence of detecting activation is lower than if the "acquired" time-series data were as in (B).

For example, in some scanners, the internal clock used for sampling the signal may not be the same as the one used for timing the image acquisition; as a result, a temporal drift may appear between the two signals (the physiological signal and data acquisition signal), making the physiological traces useless for physiological noise correction. Custom setups can provide a workaround (e.g., output the volume trigger from the scanner given at each TR, and input it into the internal physiological monitoring system of the scanner). In conclusion, it may be easier to buy an external device for monitoring physiological traces, and such a device may also offer other possibilities (e.g., end-tidal CO_2 and skin conductivity measurements).

4.2.3.1.3 Defining the "Phase"

Most of the techniques discussed in this chapter rely on the definition of cardiac or respiratory phase. In this

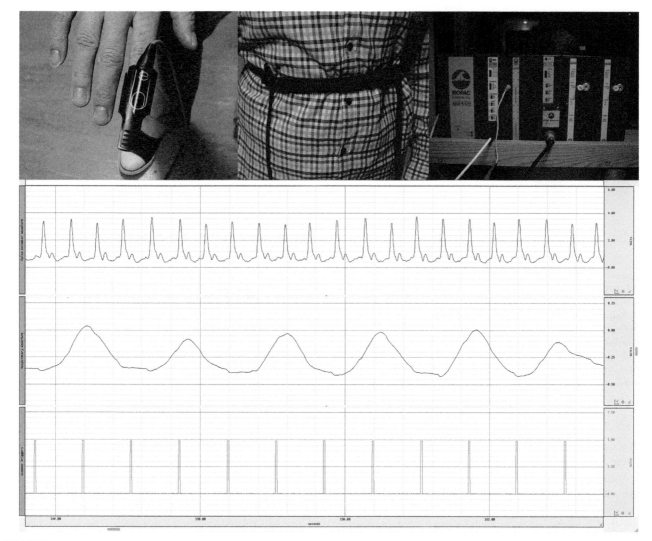

FIGURE 4.2.4 Typical setup for acquiring physiological data during scanning. The pulse oximetry probe and respiratory bellows are connected to a BIOPAC (MP150) analog-to-digital converter, which itself is connected to a personal computer. The recorded waveforms are shown below, with pulse oximetry (red), respiratory waveform (blue), and scanner triggers (green). It is critical to log this information on a single computer, as any drift in the sampling rate will be self-corrected.

context, "phase" refers to some measure of position within the cardiac or respiratory cycle, and it is illustrated here. The cardiac phase is relatively straightforward to measure, as it can be defined as the time of an event (say, acquisition of an imaging slice) relative to the preceding cardiac event (the R-wave or peak in pulse oximetry tracing), divided by the time interval between the surrounding cardiac events. The respiratory phase depends on both the timing of the slice acquisition relative to the respiratory events—from the start of inspiration (inhalation) to the end of expiration (exhalation)—and the depth of breathing. In other words, the effect of lung volume (or chest wall position) on the static magnetic field (B_0) when taking small breaths is not equivalent to that produced when breathing deeply.[5,57] So the respiratory phase cannot be assigned by simply recording the respiratory trace and working out the slice timing relative to the detected peaks. One way to correctly assign respiratory phase is to construct a histogram of all bellows recordings taken during an experiment,[23] then the phase may be calculated by summing up all of the bellows recordings up to the value recorded at the time of interest (e.g., the acquisition time of a given slice), and then dividing by the sum of all histogram values (see Figure 4.2.5). The resulting fraction of the total histogram area defines a phase between 0 and π, and the sign of the phase depends on whether, at the time of the slice acquisition, the subject was inhaling (positive sign) or exhaling (negative sign). Note that, in general, phase is represented as a value between 0 and 2π, or $-\pi$ and $+\pi$, which can then be used to indicate how far along the periodic process you are.

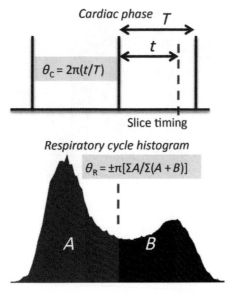

FIGURE 4.2.5 Schematic illustration of a phase definition using physiological waveforms. The cardiac phase is determined by measuring the position on the cardiac cycle, relative to the timing of the surrounding pulse oximetry peaks. The respiratory phase is defined by using a histogram-equalized transfer function,[23] and it requires that the amplitude of the respiratory bellows signal is recorded accurately. *Source: Reproduced from Ref. 24 with permission.*

4.2.3.1.4 k-Space-Based Techniques

In an early report, Hu et al.[25] proposed a method for removing quasiperiodic physiological signals from time-series fMRI data by using a low-order Fourier expansion and the recorded k-space data. As mentioned in earlier chapters, k-space refers to the raw time-domain signal that is recorded by the scanner and subsequently converted into images via the two-dimensional (2D) Fourier transform. For each point in k-space, the timing of the slice acquisition is used to calculate a phase, which is then fed into a Fourier expansion (as discussed in this chapter) to model the effect of the physiological signals ($y_{\text{phys}}(t)$) present in the data:

$$
y_{\text{phys}}(t) = \sum_{n=1}^{N} a_n^{\text{ca}} \sin(n\theta_{\text{ca}}) + b_n^{\text{ca}} \cos(n\theta_{\text{ca}})
$$
$$
+ a_n^{\text{re}} \sin(n\theta_{\text{re}}) + b_n^{\text{re}} \cos(n\theta_{\text{re}}) \qquad (4.2.3)
$$

where $n = 1, \ldots N$ ($N = 4$, typically); the coefficients $a_n^{\text{ca/re}}$ and $b_n^{\text{ca/re}}$ are to be determined; and θ_{ca} and θ_{re} are the cardiac and respiratory phases, respectively.

A series of physiological regressors (or waveforms) are computed, and a nonlinear least-squares fit is obtained to determine the parameter estimate (or amplitude) of each regressor (Figure 4.2.6). The fitted parameters thus define the "weight" of each regressor, which can be used to model out the physiological signal from the data. Subsequently, the corrected k-space data are Fourier transformed to produce the time series of images, with the effect of physiological variation hopefully removed.

4.2.3.1.5 Image-Space Based Techniques

A modification to the Fourier-based modeling of physiological noise was originally proposed by Josephs et al.,[26] which instead of using k-space data performed the correction in image space. Subsequently, Glover et al.[23] published a similar method for image-based physiological noise removal, called RETROICOR (RETROspective Image CORrection). In keeping with the approach of Hu et al., RETROICOR also uses a low-order Fourier expansion to model the quasiperiodic physiological signals present in fMRI time-series images. Whilst theoretically identical to the method of Hu et al., the image-space version is more straightforward to implement, and it does not suffer from the spatial blurring that may be introduced when correcting k-space data. In practice, this technique has been shown to outperform the k-space implementation, because although the correction will perform well near the center of k-space, it will affect signal throughout the reconstructed image (causing blurring); near the edges of k-space, where signal to noise is low, the correction may not be so effective (due to a poor fit to the Fourier basis functions), meaning that fine-grained changes due to physiological noise may not be corrected for.

In a recent study, Brooks et al.[18] extended the RETROICOR model to include higher order Fourier terms, as well as terms that account for interactions between cardiac and respiratory processes and aim to model out signal fluctuations associated with these interactions. These modifications were found to be necessary for fMRI experiments looking at signal in the brainstem[27] and spinal cord.[18] While the cardiac and respiratory phases can explain significant sources of noise in fMRI time series, it is also possible to model second-order changes associated with variation in the cardiac and respiratory cycles. The rate and depth of breathing will alter the concentration of CO_2 present in the blood, which has a measurable effect on MR signal.[28] One approach to account for this signal change is to record the amount of CO_2 in the expired breath, called end-tidal CO_2, and include this as a regressor in your experimental design; an alternative is to include the "minute volume" or "respiratory volume per unit time" (RVT) in the analysis.[29] Variation in heart rate (HR) has also been shown[30,31] to explain "noise" in brain-imaging data (Figure 4.2.7); however, as with all regressors, one should be careful when removing associated signals from fMRI data that may be correlated with your experimental design. In practice, including RVT and HR as nuisance regressors in a physiological noise model (PNM) has been shown to produce modest reductions in the variance of spinal cord fMRI data,[24] and in the

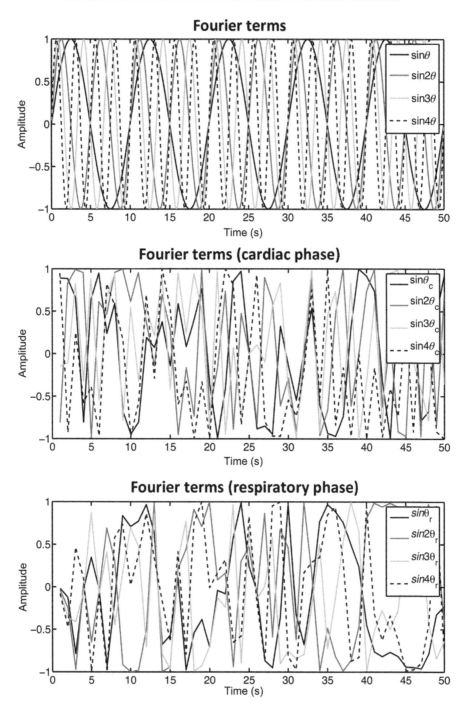

FIGURE 4.2.6 Creation of physiological noise regressors using a low-order Fourier expansion. The effects of physiological noise are approximated by using the cardiac and respiratory phases (determined from the measurements taken from the subject) to create a set of physiological noise regressors from a combination of sine and cosine terms (here, only sine terms are shown). The amplitude, or parameter estimate, for each term is adjusted by the general linear model (GLM) to best fit the data at each voxel. Examples of the nuisance regressors are added to the model to account for cardiac (middle) and respiratory (lower) effects. For comparison, the sinusoidal waveforms obtained with monotonically increasing phases are shown (top).

case of experiments utilizing painful stimuli, nonzero correlation between HR and the experimental design has been shown to have a negative impact on activation statistics.[32]

4.2.3.1.6 FIR Function-Based Methods

The techniques described in this chapter all use a model (e.g., Fourier expansion) to approximate the expected signal changes induced by physiological

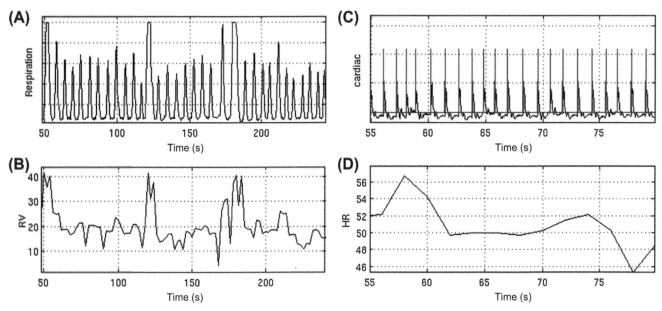

FIGURE 4.2.7 Example of physiological time courses for one subject, showing (A) respiration belt measurements, (B) the calculated respiratory variation (RV), (C) the cardiac cycle with triggers, and (D) the calculated heart rate. Note that (A, B) are displayed on a different time scale from (C, D). *Source: Reproduced from Ref. 31 with permission.*

processes, and thus results will depend on the suitability of the chosen model. The approach, described by Deckers et al.,[33] makes no assumption about the general shape of the physiological signal, only that the signals are periodic. By defining the start and end points of cardiac and respiratory cycles as the detected peaks in the physiological signals, the timing of each data point can be allocated to a separate time interval or "bin" (see Figure 4.2.8).

This approach is analogous to modeling each physiological response with a FIR function, where data acquired at similar time points in the respective physiological cycles are assumed to have a similar signal change. By including separate regressors for each time interval (or bin), whose weight is one (1) for those images falling into the relevant time window, one can build up a complete set of regressors that aims to model the cardiac and respiratory signals. The limitations of this approach are that it does not account for differences in the depth of breathing, and the arbitrarily chosen number of intervals or bins will have a large influence on the obtained results. In other words, to adequately model rapid physiological signal change requires high numbers of bins, but this reduces the number of data points contributing to each regressor, potentially leading to reduced accuracy in estimating the effect while at the same time incurring a large penalty in the number of lost degrees of freedom.

4.2.3.2 Calibration Scan Techniques

Alternatives to using physiological data to identify regions affected by physiological noise have been proposed. One such approach was proposed by de Zwart et al.,[34] and it aims to remove non-task-related correlations within the region of interest and the remaining brain areas. By identifying the region(s) of interest using a standard fMRI analysis, the temporal signal from the same region is extracted from a resting data set and used to identify an extended network of brain regions correlating with the seed. Resting correlation data are thresholded at an arbitrary (but high) correlation coefficient to define a mask that excludes the seed area. The time course of activity within this mask is extracted from the experimental fMRI data, orthogonalized[a] to the design, and incorporated in the final GLM to estimate activity. While this approach increased t-scores by approximately 10% in the seed area by removing correlated fluctuation from the data, it requires additional scan data (lasting 1–2 min) and assumes that none of the large-scale fluctuation seen in either the resting or experimental data is related to the stimulation paradigm. Given the existence of widespread correlation across several brain areas (e.g., visual, motor, and association cortices) associated with resting state networks,[35] such an assumption must be treated with some caution.

---

[a]To remove correlation between two variables. In the context of fMRI data analysis, orthogonalizing one regressor (with regard to one or more other regressors) changes the other regressor(s) so that they are no longer correlated with the original regressor *(Source: Ref. 10).*

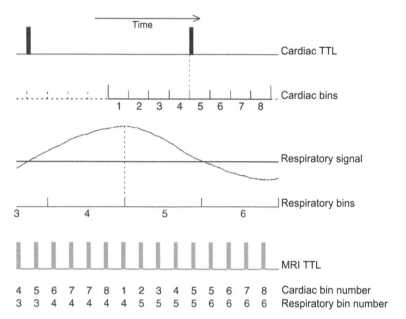

FIGURE 4.2.8 Schematic representation of the filtering method. Both the cardiac cycle (CC) and respiratory cycle (RC) are subdivided into bins. In the example shown here, eight bins are used for both cardiac and respiratory filtering. Information about CC and RC timing is derived from physiological monitoring data, acquired using a pulse oximeter and respiratory bellows, respectively. Filtering for CC and RC is performed independently. MRI data are assigned to a bin based on their acquisition time relative to the nearest event. *Source: Reproduced from Ref. 33 with permission.*

A similar approach to removing noise sources due to variation in the CSF signal from spinal fMRI data was proposed by Brooks et al.[18] In this technique, the average signal from voxels demonstrating the largest (top 20%) variance across the fMRI time series is averaged and fed back as a nuisance regressor into the model used to detect activation. These voxels inevitably lie in the subarachnoid (CSF) space surrounding the cord, and so should not be correlated with stimulus timings, but as a precaution the CSF time course is normally orthogonalized to the design. This relatively simple technique has been shown to produce dramatic reductions in the residuals obtained after fitting the GLM in voxels inside the cord.[24]

A potential solution to the problem of defining signal components related to physiological processes unrelated to neuronal activity is the use of independent component analysis (ICA) to identify noise from critically sampled fMRI data. Piche et al.[36] acquired spinal fMRI data with a short TR (250 ms) while subjects performed a hand-clenching task. By identifying the dominant cardiac frequency from photoplethysmograph data, a band-pass filter was constructed and applied to the critically sampled (for definition, see Section 4.2.2) EPI data. The corresponding pattern of signal variation in the filtered data can be seen in Figure 4.2.9; it is clear that cardiac effects are mostly confined to the CSF space on the ventral and dorsal aspects of the spinal cord, where signal variation is as high as 60% of the mean.

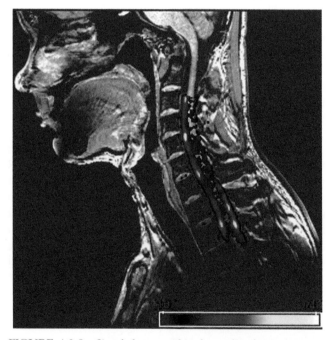

FIGURE 4.2.9 Signal change within the cardiac frequency range overlaid on the T_1 anatomical image in one subject. The color scale indicates the percentage of signal change relative to the mean value of all voxels included in the mask (see methods). The highest peaks are found in the CSF, but note that decreasing the threshold also shows signal changes within the spinal cord. *Source: Reproduced from Ref. 36 with permission.*

Patterns of signal variation identified by filtering the time-series data were then compared to the components detected by a spatial ICA.[37] Coherence analysis identified one or more components that were similar to the cardiac frequency, and these tended to overlap with variance maps from the filtered data. These components tended to be fairly consistent between subjects and across runs within the same subject, suggesting that they could be "filtered out" from the time series of an fMRI experiment. However, it should be noted that the cardiac signal is rarely (if ever) sampled critically in typical fMRI experiments, as the TR tends to be relatively long (TR >1 s). Consequently, signals oscillating at cardiac frequencies will be aliased into the low-frequency range of the experimental design, making unambiguous identification of cardiac components difficult. However, in the study by Brooks et al.,[18] the spatial patterns of cardiac components were found to be similar when comparing critically sampled (TR = 200 ms) and undersampled (TR = 3 s) data, suggesting that techniques such as CORSICA[37] or MELODIC[19] may be useful in identifying signal components that could then be incorporated into the GLM. The CORSICA method was notably applied to detect BOLD responses to painful stimulations in the human cervical spinal cord.[38]

4.2.3.3 Gating-Based Methods

When thinking about the source of physiological noise in fMRI time-series data, it is apparent that cardiac sources are the dominant signal.[2,36] One approach to minimizing cardiac-related signal variation is to gate the acquisition of images to the cardiac cycle.[39,40] An unavoidable consequence of gating is that the time between successive samples is no longer governed by the TR, but instead by the subjects' own heart rate, which can be quite variable and may also depend on the applied stimulus.[41] Variation in the effective TR will give rise to partial saturation effects due to different amounts of longitudinal relaxation occurring between repeated acquisition of the same image slice. A method for correcting partial saturation differences has been reported[39,40] that relies on taking a measurement of the apparent T_1 relaxation time for each voxel, and combining this with the effective TR to correct the measured signal. See Eqn 4.2.4:

$$S_{i,n} = A_{i,n} \cdot \left[1 - \exp\left(- t_n / T_{1,i} \right) \right] \quad (4.2.4)$$

where $S_{i,n}$ is the measured signal for the ith voxel, $A_{i,n}$ is the signal amplitude in the absence of T_1 relaxation, t_n is the interval between successive volumes, and $T_{i,n}$ is the tissue-dependent longitudinal relaxation rate (to be determined).

There are several limitations to this approach: (1) the assumption of a single T_1 value for each voxel may be incorrect in the presence of partial volumes of gray and white matter and CSF in each voxel (typical volumes >27 mm^3), (2) imperfect realignment of fMRI data will increase the problems associated with point (1), and (3) there is the potential confound of stimulation-related changes in the heart rate, which might lead to bias in the applied correction across the time series.

4.2.4 MODELING PHYSIOLOGICAL NOISE

The main concern when attempting to correct for the presence of physiological noise in fMRI data is the impact on the estimation of functional signal, and improvements in the statistics associated with the measurement. All of the techniques described in this chapter constitute some type of filtering process, which will typically have the effect of smoothing in the time domain. When attempting to accurately model signal in an fMRI experiment and estimate the significance of the signal change, one needs to take account of the temporal smoothing introduced by filtering and the loss of degrees of freedom. One simple approach to achieving this is to incorporate physiological regressors in the same model ("X"; see Eqn (4.2.1)) used to estimate activation.[26,42] This has the advantage of allowing the GLM apportion variance to each of the different regressors included in the model, but also intrinsically adjusts the resultant statistics to account for filtering the time-domain signal.[22] One important consideration when using the GLM to determine the strength of activation and model out the physiological (nuisance) regressors is the ability to model each slice independently. The reason why this is important is because the physiological processes induce time-dependent signal fluctuation in the MR signal, so to adequately account for their influence, it is important to associate the appropriate phase measurement with each slice, rather than assign an average phase to each volume. While a method for preprocessing fMRI data is available in Analysis of Functional Neuroimages (AFNI) (i.e., 3dRetroicor), FSL (FMRIB Software Library, Oxford, UK, http://www.fmrib.ox.ac.uk/fsl) incorporates slice-specific correction in the GLM so that it correctly adjusts for loss of degrees of freedom (see Figure 4.2.10).

Equally important for obtaining reasonable estimates of activity when using parametric modeling within the GLM is the requirement for the time points in the fMRI data to be *independent and identically distributed*. As discussed in this chapter, fMRI data will typically demonstrate temporal autocorrelation, invalidating a key assumption behind the applied statistical model. However, these serial correlations can be minimized or

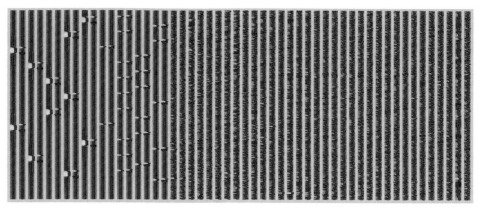

FIGURE 4.2.10   The slice-specific design matrix used to model activity within a single slice of spinal fMRI data with FEAT (part of FSL). In this representation of the model, time runs from top to bottom. The first 18 regressors relate to the applied stimuli. The next 33 are derived from the physiological noise model (PNM), and they comprise eight sine–cosine pairs derived from the cardiac phase, the same number as for the respiratory phase; a further 16 from the interaction terms; and a cerebrospinal fluid regressor, which is orthogonalized to the first 18 regressors (the experimental design).

removed by prewhitening the data[17] either by using autoregressive models or by removing physiological noise.[43] A recent study[24] investigated the improvement in spinal fMRI activation data when including a PNM in conjunction with prewhitening. Activation statistics across 18 subjects were compared for four different applied models: (B) basic experimental design only (there were four different stimuli), (BF) basic design with prewhitening, (BP) basic design with PNM, and (BPF) basic design with PNM and prewhitening.

Prewhitening always reduced the total number of active voxels in both the cord and CSF, but when comparing the ratio of the normalized voxel count in the cord to that in the CSF, we can see that the ratio (goodness, "G") increased when including both a PNM and prewhitening. The reason for this increase could be increased putative "true" positives in the cord, a reduction in the putative "false" positives in the CSF space surrounding the cord, or a combination of the two (Figure 4.2.11).

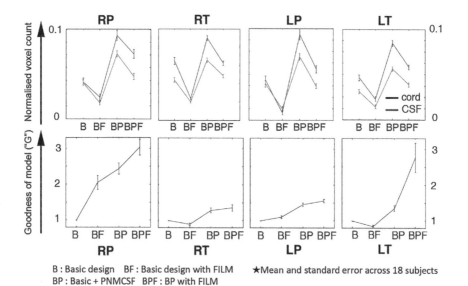

B : Basic design   BF : Basic design with FILM   ★Mean and standard error across 18 subjects
BP : Basic + PNMCSF   BPF : BP with FILM

FIGURE 4.2.11   How prewhitening affects first-level statistics. Upper panel: The graphs demonstrate the effect of using different modeling approaches (B, BF, BP, and BPF) to estimate spinal cord activity in response to four different types of stimulation (RP = punctate stimulation of the right arm, RT = painful thermal stimulation of the right arm, LP = punctate stimulation of the left arm, and LT = painful thermal stimulation of the left arm). Plots show activated voxel numbers (thresholded at $p < 0.01$, uncorrected) in the cord (blue) and cerebrospinal fluid (CSF; red) areas for the four different models for each of the four different stimuli (normalized by the total voxel number in the anatomical region of interest selected for each subject). The graphs show that including a PNM increased voxel counts in both CSF and the cord (on average), but that including a prewhitening step decreases activated voxel counts. Lower panels: to assess the benefit of each modeling approach, a goodness ratio ("G") was defined. G is the ratio of the number of activated voxels in the cord relative to that in the CSF, normalized to the corresponding numbers found with the basic design. Including both a PNM and FILM prewhitening increased G compared to the other three models. *Source: Reproduced from Ref. 24 with permission.*

Another way to assess the improvement obtained when including a PNM when modeling spinal fMRI data is to measure how much variance is removed from the data by including a PNM. The TSNR captures this information by, for each voxel, dividing the mean signal from time-series data by its temporal standard deviation.[11] High TSNR will, therefore, be conducive to detecting small signal changes, as is the case in BOLD fMRI.[44,45] An example data set is shown in Figure 4.2.12, with the raw TSNR from the spinal cord and brainstem shown on the sagittal section, along with a TSNR map obtained after removing stimulus-related activation with a model that included prewhitening and a PNM. The increase in TSNR can be visualized from the percentage change map, which has 10% as its lower cutoff, and reveals increases of up to 100% in the cord (average increase is $32 \pm 22\%$), giving a mean cord TSNR value of 28.3 compared to the original value of 22.5.

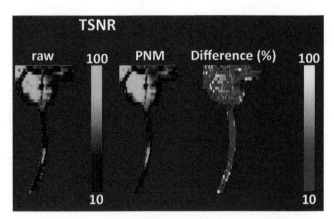

FIGURE 4.2.12 Improvements obtained when correcting for physiological noise. The temporal signal-to-noise ratio (tSNR) from a representative echo-planar imaging data set (sequence parameters are given in the legend for Figure 4.2.2) is shown before and after physiological noise modeling (to remove its effects). The average tSNR in the cord is 22 before correction and 28 afterward, an increase of 32% (in some areas, the increases are closer to 100%). Increased tSNR improves the chance of detecting small signal changes, but it can also reduce the scanning time and number of stimuli required to detect an effect (potentially reducing false negatives).

CORRECTING PHYSIOLOGICAL NOISE

- Acquisition techniques
  - Gating (problematic)
  - Decrease voxel size (but already SNR limited)
- Preprocessing techniques
  - Filtering (low-pass filtering *not* recommended)
  - *k*-space-based (RETROICOR—possible blurring effects; low SNR at edges of *k*-space may cause poor fit)
  - Image based (RETROICOR) → software available (AFNI)
- Modeling techniques
  - Temporal autocorrelation (autoregressive models, prewhitening, and precoloring) → software available (AFNI, SPM, BrainVoyager, and FSL)
  - Image based (PNM) → software available (FSL)

4.2.5 GROUP ANALYSIS

Various strategies for spatial normalization and registration of spinal cord functional imaging data have been published,[46–50,58] but as yet no consensus has been reached on the optimal approach for group analysis. In our laboratory, two different approaches have been explored: (1) slice-by-slice normalization in 2D, and (2) a 3D multistep normalization to T_1-structural images. These are described in this section.

4.2.5.1 2D Slice-by-Slice Registration

In situations where you have limited coverage of the spinal cord, say in the cervical region, it is possible to obtain a reasonable co-registration between subjects by using 2D registration. The approach is limited to acquisitions where slices are positioned to be in equivalent anatomical locations across all subjects; see Figure 4.2.13.

The technique relies on manual identification of the cord outline, although in practice this could be done in a semiautomated fashion,[48] and alignment to the template cord performed using a four-degrees-of-freedom transformation (i.e., translation and scaling). The template cord will typically be the subject demonstrating the lowest amount of spinal curvature, with high cord intensity relative to the CSF. Typical results obtained via this approach are shown in Figure 4.2.14.

4.2.5.2 3D Multistep Registration

The 3D approach is closer to typical normalization strategies employed in group analysis of brain fMRI data, and it will be more suitable for data acquired either contiguously or with a small interslice gap. The whole registration pipeline is illustrated in Figure 4.2.16.

1. Correct for susceptibility-induced distortion between the cord as it is captured on the T_2^*-weighted EPI and the cord on the subject's high-resolution T_1-weighted structural image (see Chapter 2.3). In our laboratory, we find this is a necessary step for all EPI to structural

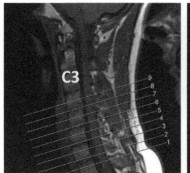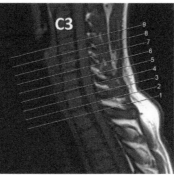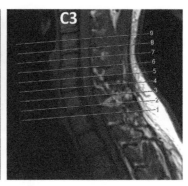

FIGURE 4.2.13   Slice positioning relative to anatomical landmarks. Two-dimensional slice-by-slice registration to a standard template for subsequent group analysis requires that slices be located in the same position for each subject. In this case, the landmark was the intervertebral disc between the C6 and C5 vertebrae, the slice thickness was fixed (4 mm), and the interslice gap was adjusted to provide similar alignment for each subject.

registration and makes use of a slice-by-slice 2D transformation (translations only), which is applied in conjunction with the scanner space transformation (the so-called sqform), which takes the structural images into the space of the functional data. As with the 2D approach described in Section 4.2.5.1, alignment between the two scans (EPI and structural) is achieved by manually segmenting the spinal cord on the two data sets (to define two cord masks), but it could be achieved equally well by semiautomatic segmentation.[50,51] Using the two cord masks, a simple 2D transformation (*X* and *Y* translation only) is used to bring the distorted EPI data into alignment with each subject's structural scan (see Figure 4.2.15). In practice, this first step is applied to functional data before analysis, as it removes susceptibility-related displacement of the cord and improves the results of anisotropic smoothing of fMRI data by aligning adjacent slices to one another.

2. Determine the transformation between an individual subject and the nominated standard, which again is typically chosen on the basis of cord geometry and image quality (clearly, a subjective process). Because of anatomical heterogeneity between each subject's structural data and the standard cord, nonlinear

registration (e.g., FNIRT in FSL, or spatial normalization in SPM) is used to determine the amount of local warping necessary to obtain a good match between the data sets.

3. Combine the linear transformation relating the EPI data to the structural data from the within-subject registration (six-degrees-of-freedom affine transformation, upscaling) to the nonlinear transformation. The final transformation is then applied to the parameter estimate and variance maps are obtained following step 1 to allow inference at the group level (Figure 4.2.16).

4.2.6 DEFINING A STATISTICAL THRESHOLD (*P*-VALUE)

The accurate interpretation of functional activity in any fMRI experiment depends on the reported level of significance. Conventional methods for group analysis of functional imaging data increase statistical power by combining results from several subjects, which are transformed into standard space (as discussed here). Recent reports[46,50,51] have proposed methods for group normalization; however, the problem remains to define a

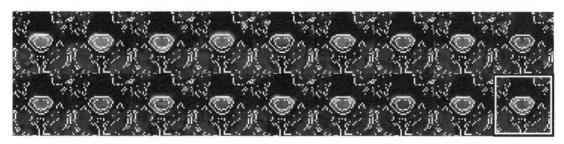

FIGURE 4.2.14   Result of two-dimensional slice-by-slice registration to standard. The nominated standard cord is located in the bottom right corner. In all images, the white outline is determined from the high-intensity boundaries on the standard cord and superimposed on the remaining 17 subjects' images following registration to the standard. Visual inspection of the cord outline (from the standard) and the underlying images provides a means to assess matching for each subject to the standard.

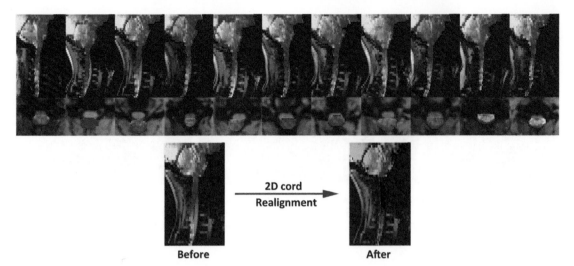

FIGURE 4.2.15 Gross effects of susceptibility differences on spinal EPI data. When overlapping axially acquired EPI data onto high-resolution structural images it is apparent that there is significant displacement of the cord in the phase-encoding (y) direction, leading to an anatomical mismatch (shown here for 11 subjects). By manually drawing the outline of the cord on both EPI and downsampled structural data it is possible to bring the cord back into alignment with the structural (shown for a single subject).

statistical threshold that is corrected for multiple comparisons. Multiple comparisons in neuroimaging relate to statistical inference (i.e., testing for the presence of task-related signal) made at the voxel level. For each individual inference, a p-value is chosen, typically 0.05, meaning that there is less than a 5% chance to find a positive activation when in fact there is none (the sensitivity or false-positive rate). When testing for the presence of activation in multiple voxels, the chance of finding at least one false positive becomes much higher (because of the large number of voxels being tested). Typical voxel numbers in a spinal fMRI experiment range from several hundred to a few thousand, and while these numbers are small when compared to the tens to hundreds of thousands of voxels sampled in a brain fMRI experiment, there is still a significant multiple-comparisons problem.[10]

4.2.6.1 Bonferroni Correction

One approach to correcting for multiple comparisons is to adjust the statistical threshold to account for the family-wise error (FWE) rate. Whilst the relatively small cord volume and consequently low number of statistical comparisons performed in spinal cord fMRI analysis suggest that a Bonferroni correction[10] would be suitable, the low SNR in spinal fMRI leads to intrinsically low t-scores, and no voxels survive this conservative approach. As a direct consequence, almost all reported spinal fMRI results are based on uncorrected statistical thresholds, which limits their interpretation.

4.2.6.2 Regions of Interest Analysis

Alternate approaches include performing a region of interest analysis, where activity is assessed by pooling

voxels in predefined anatomical masks,[46,52] and statistical comparison is made by using a repeated-measures ANOVA. This approach is suitable for group analyses, including studies comparing activity within or between groups[53]; however, the interpretation of the data relies heavily on the suitability of the selected regions of interest, and it may limit the conclusions that can be drawn (e.g., activity within a hemicord cannot be uniquely attributed to motor or sensory processing).

4.2.6.3 Defining False-Positive Detection Rates from Resting Data

One approach to estimating false-positive detection rates is to acquire resting data in addition to experimental data acquired using applied stimuli,[45] and then calculate the number of "activated" voxels from the resting data using the experimental design. By averaging across the group, the expected false-positive rate can be estimated, and the actual number of activated voxels compared to this level to provide a yes-no decision on whether the activated volume exceeds what you might expect by chance. One limitation of this approach is that it does not provide any information about the spatial pattern of activity; however, it may provide a useful first test when examining if a given paradigm produces activation anywhere in the cord.

4.2.6.4 Correcting for the Number of Functional Cord Subunits

One alternative approach is to define a corrected threshold based on the number of independent "units"

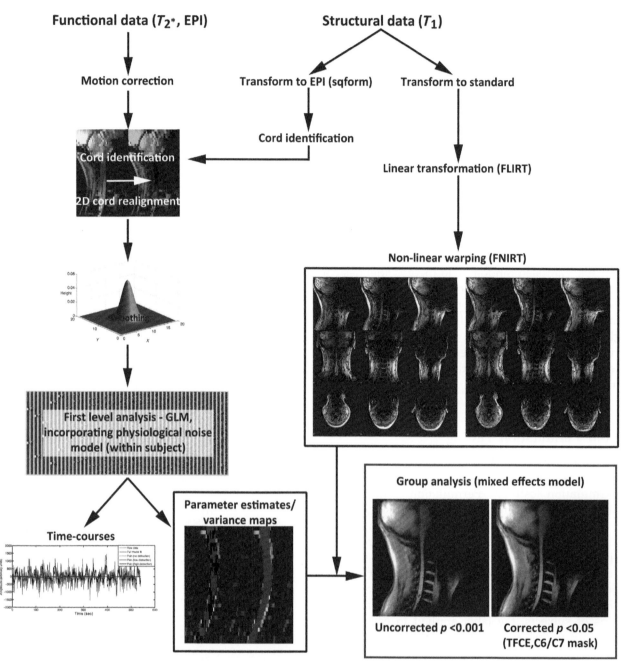

FIGURE 4.2.16 Flowchart for spinal fMRI data processing (single subject) and group analysis. Starting from the functional data (EPI), 2D motion correction is performed to bring all slices into alignment, and the cord is then manually identified on the average image computed from the time series. Similarly, after transforming the structural T_1 image of the subject into the space of the EPI (a "highres2epi" transform), the cord is manually identified. 2D realignment brings the displaced cord (on the EPI) into alignment with the structural data, and functional data are smoothed with an anisotropic filter (FWHM = 2 mm in-plane (x, y), 8 mm through plane (z)). Slice-specific parameter estimates and variance maps for the experimental stimuli are obtained by modeling with a design incorporating a physiological noise model (PNM) in the general linear model (GLM) in FEAT. To facilitate group analysis, subjects' T_1-structural data are registered to the standard cord via an affine transformation (FLIRT) followed by nonlinear warping (FNIRT). The final transformation combines the inverse of the highres2epi transform along with the structural-to-standard transform (linear and nonlinear) to bring the parameter estimates and variance maps into standard space, from which group analysis can be performed. Statistical inference was performed using a repeated-measures ANOVA design with permutation testing using RANDOMISE with a cord mask, and results in the expected location were ipsilateral to the side of stimulation reported using a corrected $p < 0.05$. FEAT, FLIRT, FNIRT, and RANDOMISE are part of the FMRIB Software Library (FSL, http://www.fmrib.ox.ac.uk/fsl).

examined within the cord. In other words, in an experiment comparing activity between the left and right sides of the cords, one approach to defining a corrected threshold would be to divide the normal statistical threshold ($p = 0.05$) by the number of slices multiplied by the number of hemicords.[46] This approach could be extended to cord quadrants if the experimental question related to comparison of dorsal versus ventral activity within hemicords, and it may provide a useful first approximation to determining corrected thresholds.

4.2.6.5 Gaussian Random Field Theory

The most common approach used in brain fMRI experiments, Gaussian random field theory,[54] defines corrected voxel or cluster thresholds based on the smoothness and volume of the data. Unfortunately, such an approach is generally not applicable when studying the small cylindrical volumes associated with spinal fMRI experiments, due to the small number of voxels used to estimate smoothness (particularly in the transverse plane).

4.2.6.6 Permutation Testing

A more robust and potentially more sensitive approach to group analysis of spinal cord fMRI data is permutation testing.[55] Permutation testing can be applied to most group designs (e.g., a single-group average, two-group paired t-test, and repeated-measures ANOVA) and relies on the interchangeability of labels applied to subjects in the model. Here, a label implies group membership for a given subject, and it is used when computing the test statistic. For example, when comparing activity within two groups of subjects, the label applied to each subject implies membership in a particular group (A or B); if the labels are switched (or permuted) for the first subjects in either group (A1ΔB1), a new test statistic can be computed. By permuting the labels repeatedly, the distribution of test statistics is constructed, to which the test statistic obtained with the original labeling (chosen by the experimenter) can be compared and a significance level computed.[55,56] Permutation testing is a nonparametric technique, as it builds the distribution of the test statistic using the data itself by performing many (i.e., thousands of) permutations of the labels in the model. One major advantage of this approach is that it lends itself to accurate statistical inference when examining small, nonspherical volumes, as is the case in spinal cord fMRI analysis, where the recorded parameter estimates may not be normally distributed.

4.2.7 CONCLUSIONS

Spinal cord fMRI has developed from a technique that relies on nonstandard approaches to data acquisition and analysis to a method that can be performed in a research setting with minimal modification to the experimental setup. One critical component to analysis of spinal fMRI data is the correction for physiological noise, which if not accounted for may obscure the measurable signal. Whilst recorded t- and Z-scores are still low at the subject level (and unlikely to survive correction for multiple comparisons), the development of methods for group analysis of spinal cord fMRI is now beginning to show that activity, in this most difficult of areas to image, can be detected and is consistent across a group of subjects.

References

1. Krüger G, Glover GH. Physiological noise in oxygenation-sensitive magnetic resonance imaging. *Magn Reson Med.* 2001;46(4):631–637.
2. Dagli MS, Ingeholm JE, Haxby JV. Localization of cardiac-induced signal change in fMRI. *NeuroImage.* 1999;9(4):407–415.
3. Purdon P, Weisskoff R. Effect of temporal autocorrelation due to physiological noise and stimulus paradigm on voxel-level false-positive rates in fMRI. *Hum Brain Mapp.* 1998;6(4):239–249.
4. Greitz D, Franck A, Nordell B. On the pulsatile nature of intra-cranial and spinal CSF-circulation demonstrated by MR imaging. *Acta Radiol.* 1993;34(4):321–328.
5. Raj D, Anderson AW, Gore JC. Respiratory effects in human functional magnetic resonance imaging due to bulk susceptibility changes. *Phys Med Biol.* 2001;46(12):3331–3340.
6. Lin T. Physiology of the circulation. In: Pinnock C, Lin T, Smith T, eds. *Fundamentals of Anaesthesia.* London: Greenwich Medical Media; 1999:331–360.
7. Klose U, Strik C, Kiefer C, Grodd W. Detection of a relation between respiration and CSF pulsation with an echoplanar technique. *J Magn Reson Imaging.* 2000;11(4):438–444.
8. Friese S, Hamhaber U, Erb M, Kueker W, Klose U. The influence of pulse and respiration on spinal cerebrospinal fluid pulsation. *Invest Radiol.* 2004;39(2):120–130.
9. Buxton RB. *Introduction to Functional Magnetic Resonance Imaging.* 2nd ed. Cambridge University; 2009.
10. Huettel SA, Song AW, McCarthy G. *Functional Magnetic Resonance Imaging.* Sinauer Associates Inc; 2009.
11. Parrish TB, Gitelman DR, LaBar KS, Mesulam MM. Impact of signal-to-noise on functional MRI. *Magn Reson Med.* 2000;44(6):925–932.
12. Hutton C, Josephs O, Stadler J, et al. The impact of physiological noise correction on fMRI at 7 T. *NeuroImage.* 2011;57(1):101–112.
13. Triantafyllou C, Hoge RD, Krueger G, et al. Comparison of physiological noise at 1.5 T, 3 T and 7 T and optimization of fMRI acquisition parameters. *NeuroImage.* 2005;26(1):243–250.
14. Weisskoff R, Baker J, Belliveau J, et al. *Power Spectrum Analysis of Functionally Weighted MR data: What's in the Noise?* New York: Proc Soc Magn Reson Med; 1993.
15. Biswal B, Yetkin FZ, Haughton VM, Hyde JS. Functional connectivity in the motor cortex of resting human brain using echo-planar MRI. *Magn Reson Med.* 1995;34(4):537–541.
16. Bullmore E, Long C, Suckling J, et al. Colored noise and computational inference in neurophysiological (fMRI) time series analysis: resampling methods in time and wavelet domains. *Hum Brain Mapp.* 2001;12(2):61–78.

17. Woolrich MW, Ripley BD, Brady M, Smith SM. Temporal autocorrelation in univariate linear modeling of FMRI data. *NeuroImage*. 2001;14(6):1370–1386.

18. Brooks JCW, Beckmann CF, Miller KL, et al. Physiological noise modelling for spinal functional magnetic resonance imaging studies. *NeuroImage*. 2008;39(2):680–692.

19. Beckmann CF, Smith SM. Probabilistic independent component analysis for functional magnetic resonance imaging. *IEEE Trans Med Imaging*. 2004;23(2):137–152.

20. Frank LR, Buxton RB, Wong EC. Estimation of respiration-induced noise fluctuations from undersampled multislice fMRI data. *Magn Reson Med*. 2001;45(4):635–644.

21. Friese S, Hamhaber U, Erb M, Klose U. B-waves in cerebral and spinal cerebrospinal fluid pulsation measurement by magnetic resonance imaging. *J Comput Assist Tomogr*. 2004;28(2):255–262.

22. Jezzard P, Matthews PM, Smith SM. *Functional MRI*. USA: Oxford University Press; 2003.

23. Glover GH, Li TQ, Ress D. Image-based method for retrospective correction of physiological motion effects in fMRI: RETROICOR. *Magn Reson Med*. 2000;44(1):162–167.

24. Kong Y, Jenkinson M, Andersson J, Tracey I, Brooks JCW. Assessment of physiological noise modelling methods for functional imaging of the spinal cord. *NeuroImage*. 2012;60(2):1538–1549.

25. Hu X, Le TH, Parrish T, Erhard P. Retrospective estimation and correction of physiological fluctuation in functional MRI. *Magn Reson Med*. 1995;34(2):201–212.

26. Josephs O, Howseman A, Friston K. Physiological noise modelling for multi-slice EPI fMRI using SPM. In: *Proceedings of the 5th Annual Meeting of ISMRM*. Vancouver; 1997, 1682.

27. Harvey AK, Pattinson KTS, Brooks JCW, Mayhew SD, Jenkinson M, Wise RG. Brainstem functional magnetic resonance imaging: disentangling signal from physiological noise. *J Magn Reson Imaging*. 2008;28(6):1337–1344.

28. Wise RG, Ide K, Poulin MJ, Tracey I. Resting fluctuations in arterial carbon dioxide induce significant low frequency variations in BOLD signal. *NeuroImage*. 2004;21(4):1652–1664.

29. Birn RM, Smith MA, Jones TB, Bandettini PA. The respiration response function: the temporal dynamics of fMRI signal fluctuations related to changes in respiration. *NeuroImage*. 2008;40(2):644–654.

30. Shmueli K, van Gelderen P, de Zwart JA, et al. Low-frequency fluctuations in the cardiac rate as a source of variance in the resting-state fMRI BOLD signal. *NeuroImage*. 2007;38(2):306–320.

31. Chang C, Cunningham JP, Glover GH. Influence of heart rate on the BOLD signal: the cardiac response function. *NeuroImage*. 2009; 44(3):857–869.

32. Kong J, Kaptchuk TJ, Polich G, et al. Expectancy and treatment interactions: a dissociation between acupuncture analgesia and expectancy evoked placebo analgesia. *NeuroImage*. 2009;45(3):940–949.

33. Deckers RHR, van Gelderen P, Ries M, et al. An adaptive filter for suppression of cardiac and respiratory noise in MRI time series data. *NeuroImage*. 2006;33(4):1072–1081.

34. de Zwart JA, Gelderen PV, Fukunaga M, Duyn JH. Reducing correlated noise in fMRI data. *Magn Reson Med*. 2008;59(4):939–945.

35. Beckmann CF, DeLuca M, Devlin JT, Smith SM. Investigations into resting-state connectivity using independent component analysis. *Philos Trans R Soc Lond B Biol Sci*. 2005;360(1457):1001–1013.

36. Piché M, Cohen-Adad J, Nejad MK, et al. Characterization of cardiac-related noise in fMRI of the cervical spinal cord. *Magn Reson Imaging*. 2009;27(3):300–310.

37. Perlbarg V, Bellec P, Anton J-L, Pélégrini-Issac M, Doyon J, Benali H. CORSICA: correction of structured noise in fMRI by automatic identification of ICA components. *Magn Reson Imaging*. 2007;25(1):35–46.

38. Xie G, Piché M, Khoshnejad M, et al. Reduction of physiological noise with independent component analysis improves the detection of nociceptive responses with fMRI of the human spinal cord. *NeuroImage*. 2012;63(1):245–252.

39. Guimaraes AR, Melcher JR, Talavage TM, et al. Imaging subcortical auditory activity in humans. *Hum Brain Mapp*. 1998;6(1):33–41.

40. Malinen S, Schürmann M, Hlushchuk Y, Forss N, Hari R. Improved differentiation of tactile activations in human secondary somatosensory cortex and thalamus using cardiac-triggered fMRI. *Exp Brain Res*. 2006;174(2):297–303.

41. Tousignant-Laflamme Y, Rainville P, Marchand S. Establishing a link between heart rate and pain in healthy subjects: a gender effect. *J Pain*. 2005;6(6):341–347.

42. Corfield DR, Murphy K, Josephs O, et al. Cortical and subcortical control of tongue movement in humans: a functional neuroimaging study using fMRI. *J Appl Physiol*. 1999;86(5):1468–1477.

43. Lund TE, Madsen KH, Sidaros K, Luo W-L, Nichols TE. Non-white noise in fMRI: does modelling have an impact? *NeuroImage*. 2006;29(1):54–66.

44. Murphy K, Bodurka J, Bandettini PA. How long to scan? The relationship between fMRI temporal signal to noise ratio and necessary scan duration. *NeuroImage*. 2007;34(2):565–574.

45. Summers PE, Ferraro D, Duzzi D, Lui F, Iannetti GD, Porro CA. A quantitative comparison of BOLD fMRI responses to noxious and innocuous stimuli in the human spinal cord. *NeuroImage*. 2010; 50(4):1408–1415.

46. Brooks JCW, Kong Y, Lee MC, et al. Stimulus site and modality dependence of functional activity within the human spinal cord. *J Neurosci*. 2012;32(18):6231–6239.

47. Eippert F, Finsterbusch J, Bingel U, Büchel C. Direct evidence for spinal cord involvement in placebo analgesia. *Science*. 2009; 326(5951):404.

48. Giulietti G, Summers PE, Ferraro D, Porro CA, Maraviglia B, Giove F. Semiautomated segmentation of the human spine based on echoplanar images. *Magn Reson Imaging*. 2011;29(10):1429–1436.

49. Horsfield MA, Sala S, Neema M, et al. Rapid semi-automatic segmentation of the spinal cord from magnetic resonance images: application in multiple sclerosis. *NeuroImage*. 2010;50(2):446–455.

50. Stroman PW, Kornelsen J, Lawrence J. An improved method for spinal functional MRI with large volume coverage of the spinal cord. *J Magn Reson Imaging*. 2005;21(5):520–526.

51. Eippert F, Bingel U, Schoell ED, et al. Activation of the opioidergic descending pain control system underlies placebo analgesia. *Neuron*. 2009;63(4):533–543.

52. Maieron M, Iannetti GD, Bodurka J, Tracey I, Bandettini PA, Porro CA. Functional responses in the human spinal cord during willed motor actions: evidence for side- and rate-dependent activity. *J Neurosci*. 2007;27(15):4182–4190.

53. Agosta F, Valsasina P, Rocca MA, et al. Evidence for enhanced functional activity of cervical cord in relapsing multiple sclerosis. *Magn Reson Med*. 2008;59(5):1035–1042.

54. Worsley KJ, Evans AC, Marrett S, Neelin P. A three-dimensional statistical analysis for CBF activation studies in human brain. *J Cereb Blood Flow Metab*. 1992;12(6):900–918.

55. Nichols TE, Holmes AP. Nonparametric permutation tests for functional neuroimaging: a primer with examples. *Hum Brain Mapp*. 2002;15(1):1–25.

56. Smith SM, Nichols TE. Threshold-free cluster enhancement: addressing problems of smoothing, threshold dependence and localisation in cluster inference. *NeuroImage*. 2009;44(1):83–98.

57. Verma T, Cohen-Adad J. Effect of Respiration on the B0 Field in the Human Spinal Cord at 3T. *Magn Reson Med*. 2014. http://dx.doi.org/10.1002/mrm.25075.

58. Fonov V, Cohen-Adad J, Collins DL. Spinal cord template and a semi-automatic image processing pipeline. In: *Proceedings of the 21st Annual Scientific Meeting of the International Society for Magnetic Resonance in Medicine (ISMRM)*. Salt Lake City, USA; 1996:1119.

Mapping the Vasculature of the Spinal Cord

Walter H. Backes[1], Robbert J. Nijenhuis[2]

[1]Department of Radiology, Maastricht University Medical Center, Maastricht, The Netherlands [2]Department of
Radiology, University Medical Center Utrecht, Utrecht, The Netherlands

4.3.1 RATIONALE

Spinal cord blood vessels are millimeter- to submillimeter-sized blood vessels that are hard to visualize in the human body.[1,2] In vivo imaging of spinal cord arteries and veins was until recently only possible using invasive catheter-based angiography, which involves a radiation burden and needs to be performed by experienced specialists. Noninvasive imaging of spinal cord blood vessels had only recently become available in a robust way using computed tomography[3] (CT) and magnetic resonance (MR) angiography.[4,5] It was mainly from clinical research in aortic aneurysm surgery that the request came to develop noninvasive visualization of spinal cord arteries to avoid the risk of paraplegia induced by damaging the spinal cord blood supply.[6,7] Traditional MR angiography techniques at that time (prior to 2000) were not able to depict normal intradural arteries and were restricted to the visualization of pathologically dilated arteries and veins.[8] Today, techniques have strongly improved vessel-to-background contrast because they use relatively fast contrast-enhanced imaging techniques that are now able to depict and differentiate normal spinal cord arteries from veins.[9]

In this chapter, the relevant vascular anatomy of the spinal cord is first briefly outlined. Then, a technique of fast contrast-enhanced MR angiography is described to image normal spinal arteries and veins. Finally, the possible confounding effect of the variable and unpredictable course of spinal cord veins in relation to the blood oxygen level–dependent (BOLD) effect of spinal cord functional MR imaging (fMRI) will be addressed.

4.3.2 VASCULAR ANATOMY

To understand the thoracolumbar spinal cord vasculature, it is useful to divide the spinal cord vasculature into the supplying arterial part (inlet) and draining venous part (outlet) (see Figure 4.3.1). In this section, a general outline of the spinal cord vasculature will be given as can be imaged with human invasive or noninvasive angiography techniques. In this context, it is important to notice that interindividual anatomic variation is the rule rather than the exception (also see Chapter 4.1 regarding the intersubject variability of BOLD responses).

ANATOMY OF THE SPINAL CORD VASCULATURE

- Anterior cord surface: one spinal artery and one median vein that runs in the anterior median sulcus
- Posterior cord surface: one or two very small posterolateral spinal arteries and one "median" vein. The course of the posterior median vein is more tortuous and is not strictly median as compared to the anterior median vein

---

4.3.2.1 Spinal Cord Arteries

The supplying pathway starts in the aorta and continues with a segmental artery that branches into a number of trunks. Its posterior trunk then forms the radicular artery, which supplies the nerve root. At specific,

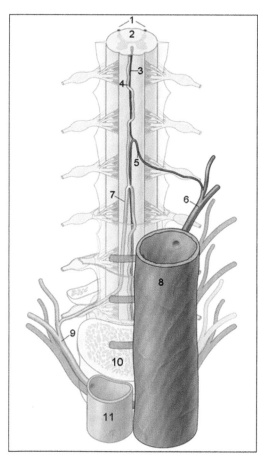

1. Posterior lateral spinal arteries
2. Spinal cord
3. Anterior spinal artery
4. Anterior median vein
5. Great anterior radiculomedullary artery (i.e., Adamkiewicz artery)
6. Segmental artery
7. Great anterior radiculomedullary vein
8. Aorta
9. Segmental vein
10. Vertebra
11. Vena cava

FIGURE 4.3.1   Coronal anatomical drawing of the largest inlet artery and outlet vein of the thoracolumbar spinal cord. The largest supplier of the thoracolumbar spinal cord, which is therefore considered the most important, is the Adamkiewicz artery. This inlet artery, or great anterior radiculomedullary artery, originates from a posterior branch of a segmental artery and connects to the anterior spinal artery with an ascending and descending branch. The descending branch is larger and has a typical hairpin turn. On the posterior cord surface, there are two laterally located spinal arteries. Venous drainage of the anterior cord surface is preformed by a large collecting anterior median vein, which in turn drains the blood to a radiculomedullary vein. The largest of the outlet veins on the anterior cord surface is the great anterior radiculomedullary vein (GARV), which connects to a segmental vein that eventually merges with the vena cava. Note the anatomical similarities in the configuration between the Adamkiewicz artery and the GARV, which both exhibit a hairpin-like configuration. However, the Adamkiewicz artery is normally thinner, has a shorter intradural span, and is located more cranially than the GARV. *Source: With permission reprinted from Ref. 9.*

interindividually different levels, the radicular artery continues its route toward the midline of the anterior cord surface (i.e., the anterior radiculomedullary artery (ARA)) and there connects to the anterior spinal artery (ASA) with an ascending and descending branch. The downward branch has a hairpin-shaped configuration. The largest ARA is known as the Adamkiewicz artery (AKA; diameter 0.5–1.0 mm).[1,2] Due to the opposing blood flow directions, watershed regions may manifest; these are regions between two entering ARAs where there will be very little or even no flow in either direction. The ASA varies strongly in diameter (0.2–0.8 mm)[1,2] along its trajectory (the midthoracic part is thinnest, and the lumbar part is thickest) and distributes blood to the anterior two-thirds of the cord tissue by central and pial branches. On the posterior cord surface, the

spinal arteries are usually paired and located posteriolaterally. They receive their supply also from posterior branches of the segmental arteries (i.e., the posterior radiculomedullary arteries). The diameter of these arteries is less than 0.5 mm[1,2] and can be depicted only occasionally using catheter angiography.

4.3.2.2 Spinal Cord Veins

On the anterior cord surface, there is one collecting vein located medially, the anterior median vein (diameter 0.4–1.5 mm)[1,2] that runs next to the ASA. Posteriorly, there is also one collecting vein (diameter ≤ 2 mm).[1,2] Its course, however, is not strictly medial and is often more tortuous (Figures 4.3.1 and 4.3.5). Both of these veins drain the cord by radiculomedullary

TABLE 4.3.1 Fast Spinal Cord MR Angiography Protocol

Field strength	1.5 or 3.0 T
Coil	Synergy spine phased-array coil
Pulse sequence	3D fast gradient recalled echo, with centric k-space filling
Repetition time, echo time, and flip angle	6.0 ms or less, 1.7 ms or less, and 20–35°
Directions	Frequency-encoding craniocaudal (CC); phase-encoding anterior-posterior (AP); sagittal slices
Field of view	Up to 50 cm CC/40–70% reduction AP
Acquisition time	40–60 s per dynamic phase
Contrast administration	0.2–0.3 mmol Gd-DTPA/kg body weight, injected at 3 ml/s
Voxel size	~1.0 × 1.0 × 1.2 mm
Precontrast	Similar acquisition for subtraction
Dynamic phases	≥ 2
Scan delay	Scan delay time of acquisition is set to filling of abdominal aorta; determined by MR fluoroscopy (Figure 4.3.3) with 2 ml test bolus

veins, which have a spatial configuration comparable to that of the radiculomedullary arteries. Often, the radiculomedullary veins have a longer intradural trajectory than the radiculomedullary arteries.

TECHNIQUES TO MAP THE VASCULATURE OF THE SPINAL CORD

- Intraarterial catheter-based (X-ray) angiography (arteries and veins)
- Contrast-enhanced MR angiography (arteries and veins)
- Susceptibility-weighted imaging (veins)
- CT angiography (arteries and veins)

4.3.3 MR ANGIOGRAPHY

Currently, the best minimally invasive approach to depict the (normal) spinal cord vasculature using MRI is to employ contrast-enhanced MR angiography. Two contrast-enhanced three-dimensional (3D) MR angiography approaches appear successful for the localization of the AKA. The difference between these two approaches is that one technique uses a strong (i.e., temporarily high-concentration) bolus (gadolinium), of which mainly the first passage is captured during a period of 20–60 s. Table 4.3.1 lists the MR angiography protocol advised by Nijenhuis and coworkers.[5,9] For the second approach, a long and slow contrast injection (≤1 ml/s)

FIGURE 4.3.2 Example of transverse susceptibility-weighted images of the spinal cord veins. Shown are phase (A) and minimum-intensity-magnitude (B) images at the T12 level. Depicted spinal cord veins are the anterior median vein (arrowheads), posterior median vein (white arrows), right anterior radiculomedullary vein (small arrows), and posterior radiculomedullary vein (curved arrows). The spinal cord itself is difficult to identify on the phase image; the white (dark) spots in the phase (magnitude) image are the spinal cord veins. *Source: With permission reprinted from Ref. 10.*

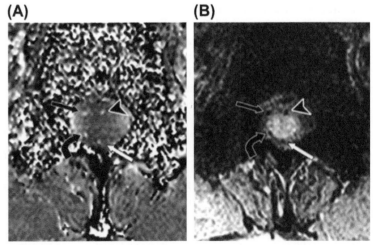

(A)   **(B)**

is used with lengthy acquisition times of 4–6 min (i.e., a decrease in pixel size and slice thickness). The main advantage of the strong-bolus technique is that it may provide separation of intradural arteries and veins, whereas the slow-bolus technique does not allow this temporal differentiation. However, the slow-bolus technique enables the acquisition of images with higher spatial resolution and thereby anatomical differentiation. Both techniques rely on intravenous contrast administration and spoiled gradient echo pulse sequences with ultrashort echo times and repetition times.

An alternative MRI method to detect the spinal cord venous vasculature is susceptibility mapping via an endogenous contrast (deoxyhemoglobin, which is contained in venous blood), which is paramagnetic and therefore induces faster T_2^* decay, which is associated with signal loss.[10] An example is provided in Figure 4.3.2.

Acquisition times for a 3D image data set are usually less than 60 s, which is approximately six times longer than the expected spinal cord arteriovenous transit time (~ 10 s). However, by accurately timing the arrival of the contrast bolus in the aorta (MR fluoroscopy in Figure 4.3.3) and by synchronizing the acquisition of centric k-space sampling, it is possible to optimally exploit the period of approximately 10 s during which the strongest signal difference exists between arteries and veins (Figure 4.3.4). In this way, a first-phase 3D angiogram can be obtained in which arteries should appear brighter than veins. Dynamically acquiring a second-phase image will additionally provide an angiogram in which arteries and veins appear more or less equally enhanced. Second-phase images may also serve to identify the vertebral levels by enhancing the vertebral bodies.

4.3.4 INLET ARTERIES OR OUTLET VEINS?

As inlet arteries and outlet veins of the spinal cord are similarly configured, an ideal MR angiography protocol should be able to discern arteries from veins.

4.3.5 SPINAL CORD VEINS AND THE BOLD EFFECT

One of the weakest points of spinal cord fMRI is its poor axial localization capabilities of signal response (see Chapter 4.1). The exact localization of the spinal

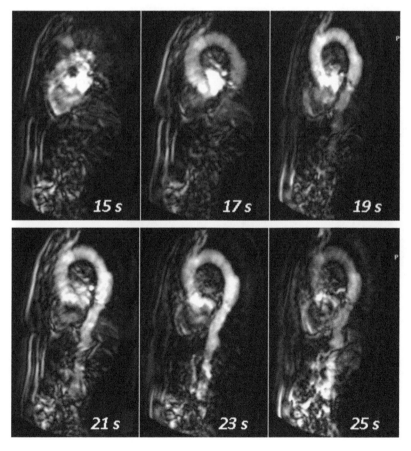

FIGURE 4.3.3 Sagittally oriented thick single slice to determine the delay between injection of 2 ml contrast agent in an antecubital vein and its arrival in the distal abdominal aorta. In this example, 23 s is the optimal delay before starting the MR fluoroscopy sequence. *Source: With permission reprinted from Ref. 9.*

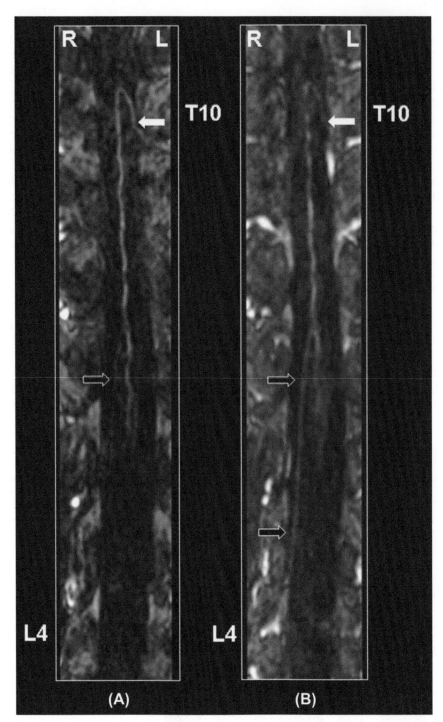

FIGURE 4.3.4 Differentiation of inlet artery and outlet vein using the fast MR angiography protocol. Curved coronal multiplanar reformations of the anterior cord surface in the first (A) and second (B) dynamic phases of MR angiography. The images show the Adamkiewicz artery (white arrow) at vertebral level T10 (left) and the great anterior radiculomedullary vein (black arrows) at vertebral level L4 (right). Note the similar hairpin configuration. Nevertheless, differentiation between artery and vein is possible due to the differences in enhancement; the artery is brightest in the first phase (A) and diminishes in the second phase (B), while the vein increases in the second phase. Furthermore, the vein has a longer intradural trajectory and is located more caudally compared to the artery. Acquisition voxel size: $1.0 \times 1.0 \times 1.2$ mm. *Source: With permission reprinted from Ref. 7.*

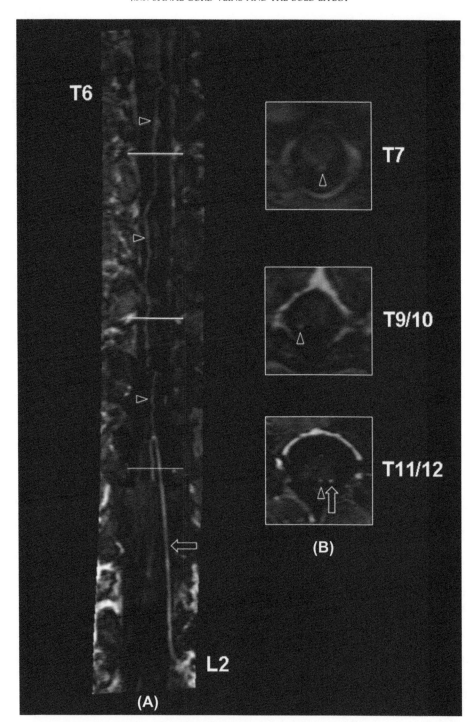

FIGURE 4.3.5 Visualization of a spinal cord vein at the posterior surface using the slow-imaging protocol. Coronal sections of the posterior cord surface (A) and transverse sections through the spinal cord at different vertebral levels (B). The collecting vein (black arrowheads) as well as the draining radiculomedullary vein (black arrow) are depicted. Note that the collecting vein has a tortuous course (A) and its position varies relative to the midline of the cord along its longitudinal trajectory (B). Acquisition voxel size: $0.5 \times 0.5 \times 0.6$ mm.

cord BOLD response is, of course, related to the details of the venous anatomy of the spinal cord. The longitudinal localization of cord responses to somatosensory, motor, or temperature stimuli seems pretty well in agreement with the known functional neuroanatomy of the spinal cord. However, current approaches for reproducibly localizing the cord activation in more detail have not been very successful in lateralizing the cord response to unilateral stimuli, especially in single subjects (as opposed to group studies). From basic neurobiology, we know the existence of interneurons between different parts of the cord and the potential activation of inhibitory neurons at the contralateral side of the cord, although one would expect a dominant (not fully lateralized) ipsilateral BOLD response to unilateral stimuli. For instance, in the study by Maieron et al.,[11] where responses to a motor paradigm were most prominent for the ipsilateral cord, bilateral activation was demonstrated.

The most straightforward explanation for this lack of axial localization is the poor spatial resolution that we use for functional imaging in combination with the irregular venous anatomy. In Figure 4.3.5, you can see the large draining veins from the posterior cord surface as obtained from a slow MR angiography protocol. Note the dorsal tortuous configuration and the variable lateralization of this vein relative to the cord's midline along its trajectory. It could very well be that neuronal activation gives rise to signal changes in small venules inside the cord that are too small to be detected. The larger draining vein is sufficiently large to be detected, but responses are likely to be detected at the opposite side of the cord. One way to circumvent this problem is by using much higher spatial resolutions than are used now for fMRI. Moreover, this emphasizes the need for indepth knowledge of the (venous) vascular anatomy of the spinal cord. In addition, other approaches can provide more spatial specificity to microvasculature as opposed to bigger draining veins (see Chapter 4.1).

CLINICAL APPLICATIONS OF SPINAL CORD MR ANGIOGRAPHY

- Diagnosis of spinal cord vascular abnormalities
- Treatment follow-up
- Localization of spinal cord feeding arteries, for instance in aortic surgery

---

4.3.6 OUTLOOK

The main shortcoming of current MR approaches for spinal cord angiography is its limited spatial resolution, which does allow the depiction of the major inlet arteries or outlet veins but generally fails to locate additional feeders and the smaller vessels inside the cord. In theory, imaging could improve when changing to a 3 T magnet as it offers better signal-to-noise characteristics that can be used to better depict smaller vessels.

The applicability of 3 T MR angiography has already been demonstrated by Bley et al.[12] However, the main advantage of a 1.5 T system still is the ability to use a homogeneous field of view up to 50 cm, which is not yet available for clinical 3 T systems. Achieving such a large field of view is currently challenging for high-field systems. Moreover, the stronger field inhomogeneities near the vertebral bodies at 3 T give rise to susceptibility artifacts that can counteract the gain in the signal-to-noise ratio. At this moment, a major technological challenge is to be taken to improve beyond 1.5 or 3 T MRI systems for spinal cord angiography in humans.

References

1. Lasjaunias P, Berenstein A, TerBrugge KG, eds. *Spinal and Spinal Cord Arteries and Veins*. Berlin: Springer-Verlag; 2001.
2. Thron A. *Vascular Anatomy of the Spine*. Oxford: Oxford University Press; 2002.
3. Takase K, Sawamura Y, Igarashi K, et al. Demonstration of the Adamkiewicz artery at multi-detector row helical CT. *Radiology*. 2002;223(1):39–45.
4. Yamada N, Takamiya M, Kuribayashi S, Okita Y, Minatoya K, Tanaka R. MRA of the Adamkiewicz artery: a preoperative study for thoracic aortic aneurysm. *J Comput Assist Tomogr*. 2000;24(3):362–368.
5. Nijenhuis RJ, Mull M, Wilmink JT, et al. MR angiography of the great anterior radiculomedullary artery (Adamkiewicz artery) validated by digital subtraction angiography. *AJNR Am J Neuroradiol*. 2006;27(7):1565–1572.
6. Kawaharada N, Morishita K, Fukada J, et al. Thoracoabdominal or descending aortic aneurysm repair after preoperative demonstration of the Adamkiewicz artery by magnetic resonance angiography. *Eur J Cardiothorac Surg*. 2002;21(6):970–974.
7. Nijenhuis RJ, Jacobs MJ, Schurink GW, Kessels AG, van Engelshoven JM, Backes WH. Magnetic resonance angiography and neuromonitoring to assess spinal cord blood supply in thoracic and thoracoabdominal aortic aneurysm surgery. *J Vasc Surg*. 2007;45(1):71–77.
8. Pattany PM, Saraf-Lavi E, Bowen BC. MR angiography of the spine and spinal cord. *Top Magn Reson Imaging*. 2003;14(6):444–460.
9. Backes WH, Nijenhuis RJ. Advances in spinal cord MR angiography. *AJNR Am J Neuroradiol*. 2008;29:619–631.
10. Ishizaka K, Kudo K, Fujima N, Zaitsu Y, Yazu R, Tha KK, Terae S, Haacke EM, Sasaki M, Shirato H. Detection of normal spinal veins by using susceptibility-weighted imaging. *J Magn Reson Imaging*. 2010;31(1):32–38.
11. Maieron M, Iannetti GD, Bodurka J, Tracey I, Bandettini PA, Porro CA. Functional response in the human spinal cord during willed motor actions: evidence for side- and rate-dependent activity. *J Neurosci*. 2007;27(15):4182–4190.
12. Bley TA, Duffek CC, François CJ, Schiebler ML, Acher CW, Mell M, Grist TM, Reeder SB. Presurgical localization of the artery of Adamkiewicz with time-resolved 3-Tesla MR angiography. *Radiology*. 2010;255(3):873–881.

PART V

SPECTROSCOPY

Single Voxel MR Spectroscopy in the Spinal Cord: Technical Challenges and Clinical Applications

Bhavana S. Solanky[1], Enrico De Vita[2, 3]

[1]NMR Research Unit, Department of Neuroinflammation, Institute of Neurology, University College, London, UK

[2]Lysholm Department of Neuroradiology, National Hospital for Neurology and Neurosurgery, London, UK

[3]Academic Neuroradiological Unit, Department of Brain Repair and Rehabilitation, Institute of Neurology, University College London, London, UK

5.1.1 MAGNETIC RESONANCE SPECTROSCOPY

5.1.1.1 Introduction

In the large majority of applications MRI focuses on detecting proton signal, in particular the signal from water protons. It therefore provides information about anatomical structure and the biophysical state of tissue water.

Magnetic resonance spectroscopy (MRS) can be seen as an alternative or complementary technique to MRI as it provides chemical and biophysical information that can be extracted from molecules other than water, and from nuclei other than ^{1}H (with ^{13}C and ^{31}P and ^{23}Na being the most common). The main targets of in vivo ^{1}H MRS are metabolites, including neurotransmitters such as glutamate (Glu), aspartate, or gamma-aminobutyric acid (GABA) in the central nervous system (CNS).

In fact whilst the first 2D (MRI) image was produced in 1973,[1,2] the discovery of MRS, originally referred to as nuclear magnetic resonance (NMR), long predates the use of MRI and led to the pioneers, Felix Bloch and Edward Purcell, being awarded the 1952 Nobel Prize in Physics.[3,4]

The aim of MRS is to quantify the concentrations of specific molecules and compounds containing the nucleus of interest in well-defined volumes of interest (VOIs) in the sample or subject. As almost all spinal cord MRS studies have been performed on ^{1}H, the rest of this section will assume that ^{1}H is the detected nucleus.

5.1.1.2 Basic Principles of MRS

A number of textbooks and reviews on the principles of MRS are available.[5,6] Only a very brief overview is presented here.

- *Metabolite.* Indicates any substance produced during metabolism
- *ppm (parts per million).* The unit used to measure chemical shift. The proton chemical shift range is 0–15 ppm. By using these units, the chemical shift for a specific proton does not depend on the B_0 of the scanner. At 3 T, 1 ppm corresponds to ~128 Hz
- *Chemical Shift Imaging.* MR technique aimed at producing images of metabolite concentrations. It works by effectively acquiring an MRS spectrum from each of many physical locations over a 2D grid or over a 3D volume
- *Shielding constant.* Determined by the electronic environment of a nucleus. Indicates the discrepancy between the applied magnetic field

- and the local magnetic field experienced by an individual proton
- *Spectral resolution.* By definition, the resolution in an MR spectrum (frequency step between neighboring points on the horizontal axis) is determined in the first instance by the inverse of the actual data readout duration. By extension this term is used to indicate the ability to resolve neighboring peaks in a spectrum (e.g., it increases/decreases when peaks are narrower/broader)

5.1.1.2.1 Chemical Shift

The physical principle underlying MRS is that a proton will experience a slightly different magnetic field depending on its chemical environment. This is because the electrons spinning around the nucleus create their own tiny magnetic field, shielding the nucleus from the main magnetic field $\mathbf{B_0}$.

The keyword here is *shielding* and refers to the difference between an externally applied magnetic field ($\mathbf{B_0}$) and the actual field B_{0k} experienced by each particular proton (identified by the subscript "k"):

$$B_{0k} = B_0 \cdot (1 - \sigma_k) \tag{5.1.1}$$

where the shielding constant σ_k is independent of B_0.

Given the different shielding constants, the resonance frequencies (Larmor frequencies [$\omega_{Lk} = \gamma B_k$]) of protons belonging to different molecules will vary. The signal collected from a VOI in the sample/subject is Fourier transformed to display the signal on a frequency axis: different chemical environments will appear at different places (frequencies) in the spectrum. The frequency difference from a reference compound is dubbed *chemical shift*, expressed in parts per million (ppm) (i.e., at 3 T 1 ppm is ~128 Hz). By convention, the frequency axis on which metabolite resonances are displayed is inverted such that lowest frequencies are on the right. The 0 ppm point is where the methyl (CH_3) protons of DSS (4,4-dimethyl-4-silapentane-1-sulfonic acid) resonate: these protons are highly shielded by their electron-dense environment, and most other metabolite protons experience less shielding (i.e., greater magnetic fields), have positive chemical shift, and appear to the left of DSS on the spectra.

An example of human brain spectrum from parietal gray matter is shown in Figure 5.1.1. For instance the methyl protons of *N*-acetyl-aspartate (NAA) resonate at 2.01 ppm and free water protons at 4.7 ppm.

5.1.1.2.2 Spin–Spin Coupling

Many biological molecules contain several protons. Because protons possess a small magnetic moment (spin) themselves, they influence each other, thus they affect the magnetic field experienced by nearby protons; this effect is known as *spin–spin coupling*.[a]

In the liquid state this spin–spin interaction is typically canceled through space interaction due to rapid molecular tumbling. In chemical bonds, instead, spin–spin interaction through electrons does not average to zero and is responsible for the "splitting" of resonance lines. This coupling is expressed in units of Hz as it is independent of the externally applied B_0 and only varies with the number (and type) of bonds between the protons.

Each proton will be affected by the spin state of nonmagnetically equivalent protons[b] in the same molecule. Due to the different chemical shifts and coupling constants, each molecule will display one or a number of peaks (or "resonances") on the MRS frequency axis, its MRS "signature".

For instance, any proton that is not coupled to another proton would show a "singlet" resonance, i.e., a single peak in the MRS spectrum. This is not the case for coupled spins, for example in lactate, a group of magnetically equivalent protons (CH_3) is coupled to the CH proton. The proton in CH can be in one of two states, parallel and antiparallel to B_0, each affecting the CH_3 protons slightly differently. The CH_3 singlet therefore experiences a "splitting" and appears in a spectrum as a "doublet" of peaks, each with half of the area it would have had if there had been no coupling. The CH proton resonance is in turn coupled to the three protons of CH_3 and affected by their individual spin states, which means that the CH spectrum will therefore show four lines (quartet) with intensity ratios 1:3:3:1 (corresponding to one configuration for all spins up, three possible configurations for two up one down, three configurations for two down one up, and one configuration for all down). For a CH proton coupled to a CH_2 group, we would see instead a "doublet of doublets" that would form a "triplet" of peaks with ratios (1:2:1).

Spin–spin couplings and the multiplets they produce in relation to the underlying molecular structure are thus extremely useful, together with chemical shift information, to identify and assign resonances.

[a]Heteronuclear coupling also exists, e.g., between ^1H and ^{13}C.

[b]Magnetically equivalent nuclei have the same chemical shifts (chemically equivalent), plus they have same coupling constants with all other coupled nuclei. For instance, CH_3 protons are magnetically equivalent; therefore, if uncoupled they will appear as a singlet. They have a different chemical environment from CH protons, thus they have a different chemical shift.

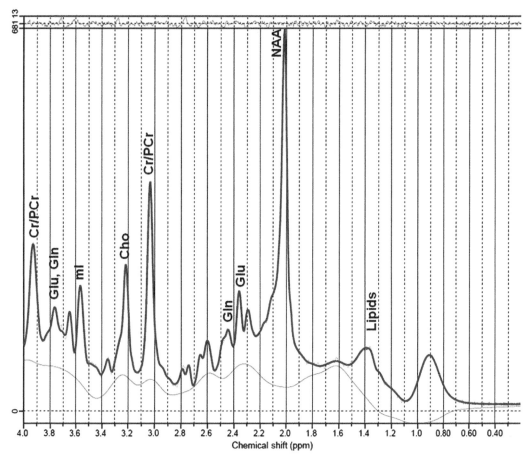

FIGURE 5.1.1   Spectrum acquired at 3 T from a 15.6 ml VOI in the parietal GM of a 32-year-old female. TR = 2 s, TE = 30, NSA = 256. SNR ~ 95, FWHM 4.7 Hz; the peaks from the most prominent brain metabolites are labeled. The spectrum is shown as displayed in the standard output from LCModel with estimated metabolite concentrations on the right-hand side.

High resolution spectra allowing split resonances to be fully resolved can often be obtained on ex vivo tissue extracts or homogenized solutions at high magnetic field (7 T–14 T).

In vivo MRS spectra have limited resolution and in many cases the line splitting cannot be directly observed. In any case, knowledge of the theoretical splitting allows better modeling of the observed signal.

5.1.1.2.3 Aim of MRS Spectral Analysis

Once an MRS spectrum is collected the aim of the MRS spectroscopist is to correctly identify the resonances in the spectrum and assign them to the corresponding molecules. The greater the concentration of a particular molecule in the VOI, the greater the amplitude of its corresponding MRS signature (resonances). By measuring peak amplitudes, after correct assignment it is possible to calculate the absolute or relative concentration of the molecules from which these peaks originate.

This procedure can give direct and detailed information on the biochemistry within the VOI in a wholly

noninvasive fashion. Whilst single-point MRS gives a snapshot view of metabolite concentrations at a specific moment in time, repeated measurements can also be carried out to provide, for instance, dynamic metabolic information.

5.1.1.2.4 Features of MRS Spectra

The main complication in the spectral analysis is that the MRS signatures of many molecules do partially overlap, and this causes an uncertainty associated with each frequency (as explained following), which makes the assignment procedure potentially equivocal.

One of the characteristics of each resonance peak, in fact, is its *linewidth* (often calculated as the full width at half maximum, FWHM) that depends on its T_2^* (apparent transverse relaxation time constant), related to the compounded effect of local and macroscopic magnetic field inhomogeneities. While the effects of inhomogeneities that are stationary in time can be reversed or accounted for with appropriate acquisition techniques, local magnetic field fluctuations are randomly variable in time and are inherent to the system under study.

As in MRI, MRS data quality can also be characterized by a signal-to-noise ratio (SNR) value, expressing the ratio between resonance peaks arising from a chosen compound and random noise occurring equally at all spectral frequencies.

In addition to random noise, the analysis will be complicated by signals arising from molecules and compounds that are not expected or taken into account explicitly (often this is the case for extremely broad resonances from macromolecules resulting in nonflat spectral baselines).

The ability to discriminate resonances will increase as peak linewidths are minimized and SNR maximized. Linewidths can be improved by optimizing the uniformity of the local magnetic field over the VOI (shimming) prior to the acquisition of MRS data (see Section 5.1.2.2). SNR will depend on the acquisition parameters: choice of echo time (TE) and repetition time (TR), acquisition bandwidth (BW), as well as the volume of the VOI (VOI_{volume}) and the number of spectral averages (N_{avg}) collected.

Similarly to MRI, for a singlet resonance peak this can be generally expressed as:

$$\text{SNR} \sim \sqrt{\frac{N_{avg}}{BW}} \cdot VOI_{volume} \cdot e^{\frac{-TE}{T_2}} \cdot \left(1 - e^{\frac{-TR}{T_1}}\right) \qquad (5.1.2)$$

with T_1 and T_2 being the longitudinal and transverse relaxation times, respectively.

In other words, SNR increases linearly with VOI_{volume}, but only with the square root of N_{avg}. Knowledge of T_1 of the substance of interest can allow optimization of SNR per unit time, though in some instances long TRs are preferable to provide insensitivity to pathological T_1 changes. Reduced TE also allows better SNR, however the contribution to the spectra of short-TE macromolecules results in rolling spectral baselines and complicates quantification. Lower readout bandwidths give an SNR advantage, however, the BW cannot be arbitrarily chosen and needs to be large enough to span across the frequencies of resonances from all detectable metabolites.

5.1.1.2.5 Basics of Localized MRS Data Acquisition

The first MRS spectra ever acquired were collected as a rapidly decaying signal or free induction decay (FID). This was measured immediately following a nonspatially selective excitation of a sample in an external (uniform and stationary) B_0 magnetic field. The excitation consisted of a magnetic field (B_1) perpendicular to the B_0 direction and oscillating or rotating at the Larmor frequency corresponding to it. It is therefore common to refer to this magnetic field as a radiofrequency (RF) pulse. In this experiment the FID, contains information from the whole sample experiencing the applied magnetic field B_1.

However, often it is necessary to define the volume from which the signal originates. The simplest way to achieve a spatial localization of the collected signal is by making sure that the excitation pulse is "on resonance" only for a selected VOI as follows.

The B_1 pulse can be designed to excite only a narrow slab of a sample exactly as in MRI by applying at the same time a magnetic field that has the same direction of B_0 but varies in space, i.e., a magnetic field gradient. Employing three subsequent B_1 pulses with gradients along three orthogonal directions defines a 3D VOI where the three slabs overlap. One of the most commonly employed sequences is equivalent to a double-echo spin-echo and employs B_1 pulse with typical flip angles of 90°, 180°, 180° and was originally suggested in 1984 with the acronym of PRESS (point resolved spectroscopy).[7] If the three B_1 pulses are all producing 90° flip angles another extremely common MRS sequence is produced, commonly referred to with the acronym of STEAM (stimulated echo acquisition mode[8]), where it is only the resulting stimulated echo that contains the localized spectral information desired. (Note: See Section 5.1.3.5 for a discussion of the relative merits of these two sequences in relation to spinal cord MRS.)

Signal from multiple VOIs from a slab or volume of tissues can also be collected; the technique is called chemical shift imaging (CSI) or MR spectroscopic imaging (MRSI).[9] For instance, in PRESS-based CSI, the three overlapping slabs define a large VOI that is further subdivided into smaller elements by means of phase encoding as in conventional MRI.[c]

5.1.2 ^{1}H MRS IN THE SPINAL CORD

5.1.2.1 Introduction

Twenty years passed after the first human in vivo MRS experiment, before localized MRS in the spinal cord was performed. The group that first investigated it was based in the Institute of Neurology in University College London in 1997–2000.[10] It took a further four years for other groups to pick up the challenge.[11–13] Currently there are still only a few groups worldwide that routinely undertake spinal cord MRS, and one of the reasons for this is that it is technically challenging.

A selection of studies that have reported spinal cord MRS methodology are listed in Table 5.1.1 and will be referred to in more detail in the next sections.

---

[c]This "phase encoding" is applied along one, two, or three orthogonal directions for 1D-CSI, 2D-CSI, and 3D-CSI, respectively.

TABLE 5.1.1 Selection of Spinal Cord MRS Papers

Publication	Year	B_0	RF Coil	Sequence	Water Supp.	Cardiac Trigger	TR (s)	TE (ms)	NSA	Voxel Size	Position	Shim Method	Subject Group
Gomez-Anson[10]	2000	1.5 T	Volume	PRESS	CHESS	–	3	30/144	256	$9 \times 60 \times 40$	–	–	Healthy
Cooke[11]	2004	2 T	Surface	PRESS	CHESS	Yes (400 ms)	3	30	256	$9 \times 7 \times 35$	Above C2	B_0 mapping	Healthy
Kendi[12]	2004	1.5 T	Phased array	PRESS	MOIST	–	1.5	35	196	$6 \times 6 \times 50$	C3–C7	Auto	MS
Kim[13]	2004	1.5 T	Flexible surface	STEAM	CHESS	–	2	30	256	–	Spinal tumor mass	–	Spinal mass lesions
Blamire[14]	2007	2 T	Surface	PRESS	CHESS	Yes (400 ms)	3	30	256	$9 \times 7 \times 35$	Center C3	B_0 mapping	MS
Ciccarelli[15]	2007	1.5 T	Saddle	PRESS	CHESS	Yes (150 ms)	3RR	30	192	$6 \times 8 \times 50$	C1–C3	Manual	MS
Edden[16]	2007	3 T	Flexible surface	1D-PRESS CSI	Dual HS pulses	No	2200	144	64	FOV $10 \times 12 \times 90$	Medulla-C3	FASTMAP	Healthy
Henning[17]	2008	3 T	12 Channel spine	PRESS	CHESS	Yes (300 ms)	2	42	512	$6.5 \times 8.5 \times 27$	C2–C3, Thoracic lumbar	B_0 mapping	Healthy + Various pathologies
Holly[18]	2009	1.5 T	–	PRESS	–	Yes	1.5/3	30	256	$10 \times 10 \times 20$	Center C2	Manual	Cervical Spondilotic myelopathy
Ciccarelli[19]	2010	1.5 T	Saddle	PRESS	CHESS	Yes (150 ms)	3RR	30	192	$6 \times 8 \times 50$	C1–C3	Manual	MS
Marliani[20]	2010	3 T	8 Channel spinal	PRESS	CHESS	–	2	35	396	$7 \times 9 \times 35$	C2–C3	Auto non-triggered	MS
Carew[6]	2011	3 T	Volume	PRESS	CHESS	–	2	35	256	$8 \times 5 \times 35$	Above C2	B_0 mapping	ALS at risk
Kachramanoglou[26]	2011	3 T	8 Channel	PRESS	CHESS	–	3	30	~160	–	C1–C3	B_0 mapping	MS and brachial plexus
Elliott[21]	2011	3 T	–	PRESS	–	–	3	30	~220	$10 \times 10 \times 20$	C1–C3	Auto	Whiplash
Hock[22]	2011	3 T	16 Channel	PRESS	VAPOR/None	Yes	>2.5	30	512	$6 \times 9 \times 35$	–	FASTERMAP	Healthy

5.1.2.2 Challenges

The main factors limiting the quality of spinal cord MRS spectra are:

- adequate VOI positioning, avoiding CSF contamination
- motion of cord and surrounding CSF
- resulting challenge of shimming an elongated VOI surrounded by CSF
- low SNR with respect to conventional brain studies due to the small cross-sectional area of the cord; longer acquisition times also incur more subject motion.

5.1.2.3 Main Metabolites Observed in the Spinal Cord

The relatively low SNR achievable in spinal cord MRS in sessions of reasonable duration (e.g., up to 20 min) does not generally allow for the detection of as many metabolites as in the brain where around 15 metabolites can be measured in less than 10 min acquisitions, depending on location and VOI volume. However most publications quantify the most prominent features in spectra from the CNS, which are outlined following:

- NAA, often reported together with NAAG from which it cannot be easily differentiated in vivo; NAA is selectively localized within neurons, and a decrease is commonly used as a marker of neuronal injury; reduced relative NAA concentrations are said to reflect axonal loss and/or metabolic dysfunction.
- total Choline (tCh) (including contribution from free choline, glycerol-phosphoryl-choline [GPC] and phosphorylcholine [PC]). Changes in tCh levels are generally associated with membrane composition with increased signal associated, for example, with cancer, ischemia, and head trauma.
- total Creatine (Cr) (creatine plus phosphocreatine) levels are related to energy metabolism as phosphocreatine behaves as reservoir for the generation of adenosine triphosphate (ATP). Cr is relatively stable across age or disease and is thus often used as reference compound.
- myo-Inositol (mIns) mIns is considered to be a glial marker; its increase can be related to astrocytic activation and proliferation.
- Glutamate (Glu) is the major excitatory neurotransmitter in mammals. Despite is relatively high abundance it is particularly difficult to quantify, since its signal is spread over many low-intensity resonances. It is often quantified together with glutamine (Gln), an important component of metabolism (Glu + Gln = Glx). Few spinal cord MRS studies have reported Glu or Glx levels.[13,17,23]

ppm	Metabolite	Properties
2.01	N-acetylaspartate	Neuro-axonal marker
2.0–2.4	Glutamate/Glutamine	Neurotransmitters
3.03	Creatine/Phosphocreatine	Energy metabolism
3.22	Choline compounds	Cell membrane marker
3.56	Myo-inositol	Glial cell marker

5.1.2.4 Short Summary of Findings from Clinical Applications

Looking again at Table 5.1.1, it is apparent that the main clinical application of spinal cord MRS has been to multiple sclerosis (MS), with a few reports on other pathologies including amyotrophic lateral sclerosis (ALS),[24] cervical spondylotic myelopathy,[18] spinal mass lesions,[13] tumors,[25] whiplash,[21] and brachial plexus avulsion.[26,27] The most commonly and consistently reported finding is that of reduced NAA/Cr concentration ratio in pathological spinal cord compared to healthy subjects. In MS, reduced NAA concentration (concentration is denoted by [])[28] was also observed,[12,14,15,29] together with the NAA/Cho ratio whilst Cho/Cr and mIns/Cr increased.[20] It has also been reported that reduced NAA at the onset of an MS relapse can be followed by a partial recovery over time with greater increase at one month correlated to greater recovery.[29] NAA was also shown to correlate with cerebellar scores of neurological assessment.[14]

mIns was measured to be slightly higher in MS patients than controls, but the difference was not statistically significant; however, it did correlate with EDSS.[29] mIns/Cr was significantly elevated in MS vs. controls in another study,[20] whilst lower mIns/Cr than in controls was found in a case series of five patients with neuromyelitis optica (NMO), potentially reflecting astrocytic damage.[30]

5.1.3 TECHNICAL ISSUES

5.1.3.1 Anatomy/Geometry of the Cord

On axial images at the level of the cervical spinal cord it can be seen that the cord has an oval cross section, with an LR axis of approximately 8–11 mm and an AP axis of 6–9 mm. It is "padded" all around by CSF in a thickness of 2–8 mm.

Typically the minimum VOI volumes used in single-voxel MRS are around 4–8 ml, however, rarely voxels larger than 2–2.5 ml can be achieved from the spinal cord.

As summarized before in Eqn (5.1.2), if the VOI volume is halved, four signal averages are necessary to recover the original SNR, so the VOI needs to be maintained as large as possible, as long as it does not span outside the cord.

The obvious approach to increasing the VOI dimensions for spinal cord is to extend it in the HF direction, however, given the VOI has a cuboidal shape, the maximum usable length depends on the curvature of the cord in the chosen section. In diseases that involve neuronal loss, atrophy of the spinal cord also limits the size of the VOI.

Other considerations affecting voxel positioning include B_0 inhomogeneity (see Chapter 2.2 or Section 5.1.3.7 of this chapter on shimming).

5.1.3.2 Main Field Strength

MR scanners of higher and higher fields are increasingly popular and widespread. The highest B_0 currently used for in vivo studies in humans is 9.4 T, though 11.7 T scanners are currently being built. As described in Chapter 2.4, one benefit of higher field strength is that signal to noise (SNR) increases approximately linearly with field strength. Moreover, higher field strength also offers higher spectral resolution—the capability to resolve two adjacent spectral peaks, thereby making it possible to investigate other metabolites such as GABA which is overlapped by NAA and Cr at 3 T but resolved at 7 T given the larger chemical shift. Similarly, at 7 T the higher field results in the added information from Glu and Gln, which cannot be resolved at 3 T without spectral editing pulse sequences.[31] At the same time, with increased B_0 we also observe increased longitudinal relaxation times T_1, increased magnetic susceptibility differences between tissue/air/bone structures causing increased susceptibility-dependent effects, causing line broadening in MRS as well as chemical shift positioning errors (see following).

The first few spinal cord MRS studies have been conducted at lower clinical field strengths of 1.5 T[10,12,13,18,29] and 2 T,[11,14] whilst since 2007 3 T has been more commonly employed.[16,17,22,24,32,33] Higher field strengths are employed predominantly for brain applications. In addition to the lack of high field studies on the spinal cord there are limited sites with coils that are built for spinal cord purposes. In addition to hardware constraints for spectroscopy at 7 T or higher, field strengths would also need to overcome issues related to chemical shift positioning errors, which would make MRS VOI placement in the spinal cord more challenging.

These chemical shift errors are related to the limited effective bandwidth of the selective excitation and refocusing pulses used for VOI localization and result in signal from different metabolites arising from different spatial locations, much the same as in the fat appearing shifted from the water signal in conventional MRI. For instance the main resonance used for NAA quantification occurs at 2.01 ppm whilst for mIns it appears at 3.56 ppm, a 1.55 ppm difference; this corresponds to 99 Hz at 1.5 T ($\omega_L = 64$ MHz) and twice as much at 3 T. Using for instance a 1 kHz bandwidth refocusing pulse, defining one of the short dimensions of the VOI, say 6 mm, it will result in a spatial shift between NAA and mIns VOIs of 0.6 mm and 1.2 mm (20%) at 1.5 T and 3 T, respectively, and 1.8 mm at 4.7 T. In other words, the greater the field strength, the greater the chance that the signal from one of the metabolites comes at least partially from outside the cord and could include CSF contributions. Whilst using higher bandwidths would drastically reduce this issue, in practice realistic pulse bandwidths are restricted as higher bandwidths are associated with higher tissue heating, especially at higher B_0s (see, for instance, Kinchesh 2005, *JMR*, for issues in carrying out MRS at 4.7 T).[34] In addition to chemical shift–associated problems, magnetic susceptibility effects further exacerbate shimming issues within the cord, and hence even though an increase in SNR is theoretically possible at higher fields, unless MRS acquisition sequences are carefully and cleverly optimized, spectral quality in the spinal cord may suffer.

5.1.3.3 Coil Selection

Similarly to MRI, in spinal cord MRS the choice of RF coil is particularly important; a thorough description of spinal cord coils is given in Chapter 2.1. A few considerations though are worth repeating with particular reference to MRS. The small anatomy and the shape of the surrounding area (i.e., neck) must be considered, as some coils do not have adequate sensitivity for this region. Simple "scout" imaging protocols can give information on the cervical cord area and potential sensitivity drop-offs as distance from the coil increases.

The sensitivity of the coil, the ability to produce accurate flip angles for correct localization, and the filling factor of the coil (the fraction of the coil detection volume filled with sample) all need to be considered to get the highest SNR and hence quicker scans as a result. Following, two types of coil are considered and the advantages and drawbacks of each discussed.

5.1.3.3.1 Surface Coils

Surface coils, which both transmit (Tx) and receive RF signal (Rx), were traditionally favored in MRS protocols due to their high local sensitivity. However the sensitivity falls off rapidly (for a loop, as distance[3]) and is roughly only acceptable within one radius of the coil. This means the anatomically deep cervical spine, which lies approximately 7–8 cm from the surface of the neck, is only within the sensitive region of relatively large surface coils. Flat surface coils are unlikely to offer a good filling factor due to the small width and curvature of the neck when lying in a supine position. This curvature of the neck also leaves a gap between the tissue and the coil, exacerbating shimming issues.

Given the rapid drop off in the B_1 profile of surface coils, when they are used for excitation, adiabatic pulses (pulses that are insensitive to B_1 variations) must be used to give more accurate excitation and inversion profiles over the sensitive region. However, these adiabatic pulses are usually much longer than conventional RF pulses and result in: (1) significantly increased minimum TE, thus reduced SNR and reduced number of metabolites detectable before dephasing due to T_2 relaxation, and (2) increased heating (specific absorption rate, SAR), especially at medium and high magnetic field strengths.

The suitability of a surface coil largely depends on the diameter and shape of the coil available. Some studies have used flexible surface coils, which offer better filling factors and can be volunteer specific in shape.[13,16]

It is advised to compare suitable surface coils against a volume coil in the first instance.

The quality of structural images needed for voxel placement must also be taken into account. These will suffer due to B_1 inhomogeneities and/or signal drop off if these are acquired with a surface coil, resulting in images with spatially variable SNR.

Alternatively to overcome the Tx B_1-inhomogeneity issues whilst keeping the sensitivity of the surface coil, RF coils, which are only active during signal detection (Rx), may provide a solution (see following).

Surface coils have been chosen over volume coils at all field strengths 1.5 T–3 T and provided successful metabolite detection in scan times comparable to volume coils.[11,13,14,16] However, more recently they are used less and less due to the availability of volume coils and modern array coils where the individual elements can be chosen and combined on a subject-to-subject basis.

5.1.3.3.2 Volume and Phased Array Coils

Volume coils generally offer much better spatially uniform inversion and excitation profiles. The main drawback of such coils when used in combined Tx/Rx mode is that signal is received from the entire coil whose sensitive volume is much greater than the VOIs used in MRS. Hence, most of the coil is not sensitive to the region of interest and simply adds noise to the spectrum.

Many modern scanners offer a single body–Tx coil for excitation. Whilst the resulting $\mathbf{B_1}$ is very uniform, the large diameter (typically 50–60 cm) causes the coil to

be very inefficient for a small VOI, and the maximum bandwidth that can be obtained is much lower than if, for instance, a head-only Tx/Rx coil was used.

The issues related to choosing a single surface or volume head coil for both Tx and Rx have effectively been overcome by the widespread use of Rx-only phased array coils. Phased array coils consist of a number of different coils that all receive like small surface coils that are highly sensitive only to the surrounding area. At the same time, given that the coil array spans a larger area, a relatively high and uniform spatial sensitivity is achieved across the whole area covered.

Roughly speaking, if we replaced a cylindrical "volume coil" with smaller coils placed on the same surface, the sensitivity would increase with the number of coils used close to the surface itself; in the middle of the cylinder, the sensitivity would remain approximately the same as for the equivalent volume coil.

In a realistic situation, for single voxel MRS, only a few of the coils would be sensitive to the VOI. The others would only add noise to the spectrum. To overcome this potential drawback, usually the raw spectrum from each coil is weighted according to the received signal from an MRS reference scan of the VOI with no water suppression and appropriately phased.[35] In this manner coils further away from the VOI will be assigned lower weighting than those closer and most sensitive to the VOI. Some MRS sequences have an option to turn on sensitivity weighting, although often this may not be available for MRS, but only for imaging, so this should be checked when selecting the appropriate coil. A number of studies have successfully detected signal from the main metabolites using a phased array coil even without using sensitivity weighting.[12,20,24,32,33]

5.1.3.3.3 Filling Factor and Shimming

An inherently inhomogeneous B_0 field surrounds the cervical cord area.[11] To overcome the adverse effects of this, active shimming and dielectric foams and beads can help to alleviate this similarly to imaging. When employed for spinal cord MRS, rather than giving a more homogenous signal over the area scanned, these methods and materials are likely to result in better-resolved, higher-SNR spectra.

5.1.3.3.4 Combined and Selective Coils

Many systems allow the user to also select a priori the parts of a multiple array coil to be used for MRS data collection, whilst still using the full array of coils when performing structural scans and a separate coil for transmission.[22,32] An example of spectra from the cervical cord is given in Figure 5.1.2 for a 32-channel head coil, and for a 16-channel coil where only the four elements close to the neck were used for signal reception.

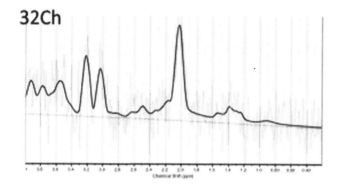

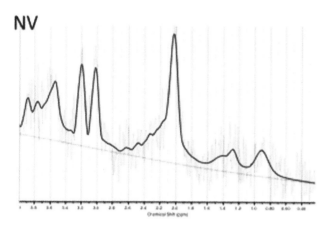

FIGURE 5.1.2 MR spectra from a healthy volunteer with a VOI based in the C1–C3 region. Acquisition parameters were TE = 36 ms, NSA = 192, TR = 3 s. Two receiver coils were tested using the same acquisition sequence: A 32-channel head coil (32-ch, top) and a 16-channel neurovascular coil (NV, bottom). When using the NV coil it is possible to select just the neck elements closest to the VOI; this leads to increased SNR for the cervical spinal cord VOI (volume 1.9 ml). LCModel reported SNR of 3 and 4 for 32-Ch and NV coils, respectively, showing the selectivity of the NV coil boosts the SNR. %SD of tCh, Cr, NAA were 12%, 15%, and 9% for the 32-ch coil and 9%, 9%, and 8% for the NV coil, showing this improvement in SNR is also reflected in lower quantification errors.

5.1.3.4 Subject Positioning and Motion

As seen in Figure 5.1.3, care must be taken to position the VOI so that it does not encompass any surrounding CSF. Typical voxel sizes for single voxel MRS in the cord are between 5 and 9 mm in the left-right (LR) and anterior-posterior (AP) direction and 30–45 mm in the cranio-caudal direction.

Reducing motion is important in all aspects of MRI to reduce blurring and artifacts in imaging. Motion during multiple-acquisition MRS protocols causes the effective VOI to shift and encompass different tissue proportions. In addition, even if the VOI shifted to tissue exactly equivalent to that in the original VOI, there may be phase and frequency variations compared to the initial spectra. When spectra are summed postacquisition, if these frequency and phase shifts are not corrected for, the resulting spectrum will appear broadened and show a reduced SNR.

Given the timescales involved in spinal cord MRS (10–20 mins), potential movement during the scan must be carefully considered and action taken to minimize its occurrence during the scan.

When dealing with such small regions of interest as the cervical spine patient immobilization is all the more important. For example assuming an AP voxel size of 5 mm, just a small 1 mm shift in the AP direction could lead to a potential VOI shift of 20%. The recommendation is thus to leave a small gap between VOI and the edge of the cord so CSF contamination is less likely to occur in the event of small shifts.

Large macroscopic movements can be reduced by a number of immobilization techniques (Figure 5.1.4). Many studies have been reported using no immobilization, however. when looking at metabolites that are spectrally close to each other or very low in SNR, then to ensure no frequency drifts due to motion, immobilization may offer better resultant spectra. The methods discussed here are not exhaustive and are used in a few research labs, but are suggested techniques.

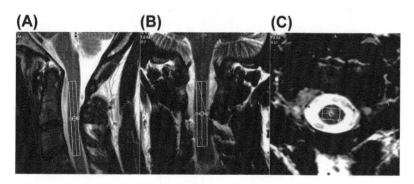

(A)   **(B)**   **(C)**

FIGURE 5.1.3 Sagittal, coronal, and axial views of the voxel placement in the cervical cord for one subject. Of particular importance was the avoidance of CSF inclusion in the voxel in all planes. Note that C1–C5 is straight due to the cervical collar allowing easier placement of long voxels. The box corresponds to the "plan metabolite" (in this case NAA). The position of other chemically shifted voxels (such as water) should also be checked.

FIGURE 5.1.4 Examples of immobilization equipment: (A) Foam pads — these are used to fill the gaps between the head and neck areas and the coil so the volunteers' motion is restricted. (B) The cervical collar — this comes low onto the shoulders and can lead to discomfort. (C) A vacuum bag that can mold around the neck, head, and shoulders providing support as well as helping to reduce patient motion. (D) Left—Axial 3D-FFE image (resolution $0.5 \times 0.5 \times 5$ mm^3) through the C2–C3 intervertebral disc acquired with standard immobilization padding displaying motion artifacts (note the blurred edges at the WM/GM interface within the cord). Right—the same image acquisition protocol after the introduction of the cervical collar, demonstrating the major benefits of the immobilization procedure in reducing considerably the effect of motion, resulting in an increased sharpness of the GM/WM boundaries. *Source: Images courtesy of Dr M Yiannakas, UCL Institute of Neurology, London, UK*

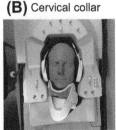 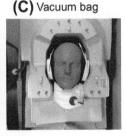

(A) Foam Pads   **(B)** Cervical collar   **(C)** Vacuum bag

(D) Effect of immobilisation on images

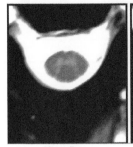 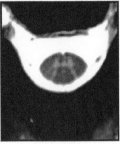

No collar   With collar

5.1.3.4.1 Cervical Collar

An MR compatible rigid collar has been suggested to reduce macroscopic movement. The collar also acts to straighten the cervical cord, making voxel placement much simpler. The effectiveness of the collar is illustrated in Figure 5.1.4 for imaging and Figure 5.1.5 for MRS.

The restriction results in reduced frequency drifts due to reduction in subject involuntary movements, more consistent shimming, and improved water suppression for every acquisition. However the length of time a volunteer can realistically tolerate the collar is limited, and hence this may impose restrictions on the overall MR session time (unless the collar is removed after the MRS acquisition). Another downside of using the cervical collar is that it can add distance between the subject and the coil, thereby reducing the SNR. Hence, you

should choose a model of cervical collar that is relatively thin in the posterior side (also it should be MRI compatible).

Alternatively a more simple way toward straightening the cord is to ask the subject to lie with their chin lowered toward their chest.

5.1.3.4.2 Polystyrene Vacuum Cast

Vacuum cushion immobilizers are filled with polystyrene spheres, which create a mold of the patient's position when negative pressure is generated within the cushion with the use of a pump. These are useful in adapting to different patient shapes and filling gaps between the coil and tissue. They also offer more comfort than the cervical collar as the cast can be set when the patient is in a more natural supine

FIGURE 5.1.5 Example of cervical cord VOI placement without the use of a cervical collar (top row) and with the use of the collar (bottom row). When not using the collar there is substantial subject-to-subject variation in the spinal cord curvature; when the collar is used, the spinal cervical cord appears consistently straight. In addition, with the collar involuntary motion during the scan is reduced.

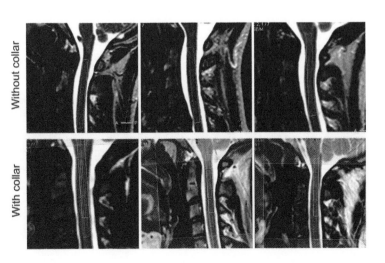

Without collar

With collar

position, supporting their neck and head, rather than the rigid cervical collar, which may not suit the length of the patient's neck. It is also important to design the cushion to suit the spinal cord as "off the shelf" ones are often too big or too thick for using around the neck. This allows for longer scans, but voxel positioning may not be as straightforward when the volunteer is in a more natural position, due to curvature of the cord (VacFix, QADOS, Berkshire, UK).

5.1.3.4.3 Navigator Scans

Given the low concentration of metabolites, many averages are needed to acquire good SNR spectra. These acquisitions can be split into blocks and then summed and averaged at the postprocessing stage to get the resultant spectra. This has a twofold advantage: in the first instance any longitudinal frequency drifts can be corrected for (see Section 5.1.3.8 following), and second, the blocks can be interleaved with navigator scans. These scans allow the voxel position to be checked after each block of FIDs. If patient motion is identified, the voxel position can be updated for the next block of FIDs.[22] This method does require more scanning time for the extra navigator acquisitions but may improve overall spectral quality. It can also be combined with immobilization methods.

Recently EPI volume navigators (vNavs) have been developed for use with spectroscopy. In the brain, this has been shown to both measure and correct head movement and B_0 changes in real time.[36] If such a method could also be developed for spinal cord spectroscopy, it could make a difference to the quality of the spectra where motion is an issue.

5.1.3.4.4 In Bore Optical Tracking Systems

In recent years systems using MR compatible cameras have been introduced to correct for motion in the head. Accurate tracking by the cameras during acquisition yields information that allows prospective motion correction by adjusting RF pulses and gradients.[37] This requires a stable marker and a line of sight from the camera to the marker and the subject. This method could be applied to spinal cord.

5.1.3.4.5 NMR Field Probes

For brain imaging active probes are secured to the head; the position of these can be measured used to correct for motion before the next line of k-space/spectrum is acquired.[38] Pruessmann et al. have shown the use of NMR probes and gradient tones to produce continuous motion correction without the need for extra sequence elements or scan time.[39] Both these methods could also be extended for use in the spinal cord.

TABLE 5.1.2 Average T_1 and T_2 Values for Brain Metabolites at 3 T That Can be Used for Correcting Signal Intensities and Quantifications[5,16,40,41,42]

	NAA	Total Choline	Total Creatine	Myo-Inositol	Water (White Matter)
T_1 (s)	1.48	1.29	1.38	1.03	0.83
T_2 (s)	0.26	0.2	0.15	0.17	0.11

5.1.3.5 Sequence Selection

The sequence chosen for localization in the cord depends largely on the metabolites of interest. The most commonly reported metabolites are mIns, Cr, tCh, and NAA. Each metabolite has unique T_1 and T_2 relaxation times (Table 5.1.2). It is with these metabolites and relaxivities in mind that traditional spectroscopy sequences (STEAM, PRESS, and CSI)[7–9] will be discussed.

5.1.3.5.1 Point Resolved Spectroscopy (PRESS)

PRESS is the ^{1}H MRS sequence of choice in most spinal cord studies published to date, with the exception of two that used STEAM and 1D-PRESS-CSI, respectively.[13,16] Sequence diagrams for PRESS and STEAM are shown in Figure 5.1.6. PRESS offers moderately short TE's ($\sim$ >30 ms), which are capable of capturing the majority of metabolites. In contrast to STEAM the initial excitation pulse is followed by two longer refocusing pulses, hence the minimum effective TE is longer with PRESS than with other sequences. On the other hand, unlike with STEAM localization,[43] all the signal available is refocused. Given the small voxels involved in spinal cord MRS, this is greatly beneficial and can reduce the scan times needed to get adequate SNR.

5.1.3.5.2 Stimulated Echo Acquisition Mode

This sequence is suitable for short T_2, low SNR or highly coupled metabolites, such as mIns, which has six coupled protons, as shorter echo times are possible. This is due to the use of three short 90° pulses for localization during STEAM. During the mixing time TM, defined as the time between the second and third RF pulse, the signal is not influenced by T_2 relaxation, and hence TE is determined by the interval between the first two 90° pulses, which is shorter than the interval between the first 90° pulse and the subsequent 180° pulse that determines TE in PRESS. This leads to less scalar evolution of coupled metabolites, which changes the phase across coupled multiplets. Whilst the signal yield is potentially higher due to shorter TE's, for equivalent TE's STEAM produces 50% less signal yield than PRESS. Given the lower SNR and the impact of small voxels prescribed in the spinal cord ($\sim$2 ml) it can be seen from

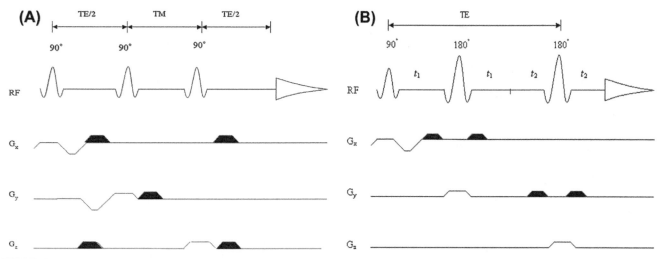

FIGURE 5.1.6   Pulse sequence diagrams for both STEAM (A) and PRESS (B). Both have three slice selective pulses, with crushers to spoil anything outside of these slices, where the three pulses intersect the signal will be unspoilt and detected at time TE. The main difference here is in the second and third pulses: STEAM has two 90° pulses and PRESS has two 180° pulses to refocus the signal in the voxel. STEAM allows shorter TE relative to PRESS as during the time between the 2nd and 3rd pulse (TM) the magnetization decays with T_1 rather than T_2.

Table 5.1.3 that STEAM has been rarely used in the cord. One such study has used STEAM to report ratios of NAA, Cr, tCh, mIns, and Glx in meningiomas in the spinal cord.[13] This study shows low SNR and uses a TE of 30 ms, which can be matched by PRESS on most systems.

5.1.3.5.3 Chemical Shift Imaging

The sequences described previously are for the localization of a single VOI. This offers a well-defined origin of the MRS data that can be prescribed easily within the spinal cord. The voxel shim can be optimized to that area improving spectral resolution and the effectiveness of water suppression. However, with the single-voxel approach the data is limited to only one area of interest. Chemical shift imaging can potentially offer spectroscopic imaging over a large portion of the cord, giving the spatial distribution of metabolites. Figure 5.1.7 shows a CSI matrix covering the cervical spine.

Edden et al. looked at the medulla and cervical cord using water-suppressed proton 1D-CSI. High resolution data from the medulla down to C3 were achieved and NAA, Cr, and tCh successfully quantified.[16] The practicalities of achieving a good shim and water suppression in all voxels in addition to the longer scan time has hindered the publication of further studies. Alternatively some studies have examined more than one voxel of interest and different areas of the cord using serial single voxel MRS.[12,13,17,25] The results of Henning et al.'s study showed that acceptable quality spectra can only be

TABLE 5.1.3   Summary of Published "Absolute Concentrations" in mmol/l from Spinal Cord MRS

Paper	Sequence/TE	Water Supp.	Voxel Size (mm)	Area Placed	TR	n	NAA	Cr	Ch
Blamire[14]	PRESS TE 30 ms	CHESS	$9 \times 7 \times 35$	C3	3	256	12.4	7.1	2.7
Ciccarelli[15]	PRESS TE = 30 ms	CHESS	$6 \times 8 \times 50$	C1–C3	3	192	6.7	3.2	1.2
Edden[16]	PRESS 1D-CSI TE = 144 ms	Dual HS	$10 \times 12 \times 90$	Medulla to C3	2.2	64	11.4[a]	9.1[a]	2.9[a]
Cooke[11]	PRESS TE = 30 ms	CHESS	$9 \times 7 \times 35$	Above C2	3	256	17.3	9.5	2.7
Marliani[33]	PRESS TE = 35 ms	CHESS	$7 \times 9 \times 35$	C2–C3	2	396	6.8	4.8	2.2
Gomez-Anson[10]	PRESS TE = 30/144	Unknown	$9 \times 6 \times 40$	Unknown	3	256	2.93	2.62	1.05

[a] Values in C2.

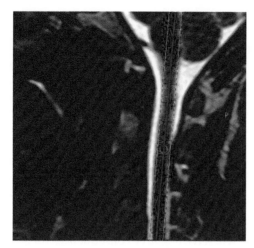

FIGURE 5.1.7 Example of a 1D-CSI matrix covering the cervical spinal cord area. A bar split into 27 voxels is placed along the cord, each voxel in the bar is $6 \times 11 \times 14 \, mm^3$ are placed along the cord. OVS can also be applied to reduce CSF contamination. Each voxel in the matrix gives its own spectrum, and hence regional variations in metabolite concentrations can be assessed from a single acquisition.

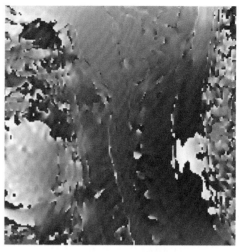

FIGURE 5.1.8 Sagittal view of the phase difference map for a volunteer covering C1–C7. The large phase differences at the discs are areas of high B_0 inhomogeneity.

consistently achieved in the cervical cord due to limited movement, less CSF artifacts, and higher sensitivity of the RX coil, whilst other areas of the cord can be scanned for spectral acquisition but are more challenging.[17]

5.1.3.6 Voxel of Interest Dimensions and Positioning

5.1.3.6.1 Dimensions of Voxel of Interest

Typical sizes in healthy cord to quantify the main metabolites are about 2 ml, which require 196–256 averages at 3 T for achieving the required SNR (Table 5.1.3). It must be noted that in diseased states cord volume often changes, and this will impact the size of the voxel in the AP and RL dimensions and consequently impact on the SNR. With large reductions in voxel size it may be necessary to increase the number of averages to get good quality spectra, though this has obvious implications on scan time.

5.1.3.6.2 VOI Positioning and Chemical Shift Displacement Artifacts

Voxel positioning is imperative to good spectral quality especially in the spinal cord, failure to ensure this will lead to contamination or poorly shimmed spectra, increasing scan times and lowering spectral quality. As mentioned before, the majority of good resolution spectra from the spinal cord have originated from the cervical cord, usually placed between C1 and C3. Good spectra are largely dependent on B_0 homogeneity within the voxel.

B_0 homogeneity within the cord is strictly related to cord anatomy. Cooke 2004 and Edden 2007 demonstrated this with sagittal B_0 maps through the cord, showing periodic variations of B_0 corresponding to interspinal processes.[11] A B_0 map acquired at 3 T prior to localized VOI shimming is displayed in Figure 5.1.8.

Having established this underlying B_0 variation, the Cooke et al. 2004 study systematically tested the optimal voxel placement within the cord: it was found that a $9 \times 7 \times 35$ mm voxel placed just above the C2 vertebral disc gave the best spectra.[11] These dimensions, however, may be optimum for a particular system (in this case a 2 T Bruker) as pulse shapes and the way in which excitation bandwidths and voxel dimensions relate to each other may differ between scanners by different manufacturers. Indeed successful studies have been reported using long voxels up to 50 mm in the FH direction.[19,29] Also larger axial dimensions may not be possible in patient populations with spinal cord atrophy.

Using anatomical landmarks such as vertebral levels to help position the voxel ensures good reproducibility of voxel positioning, both between subjects and longitudinally for a single subject. Cooke et al. 2004[11] showed that better lineshapes are produced when shimming on shorter voxels (comparison of 30 mm, 40 mm and 50 mm voxels) because the VOI spans a smaller number of the B_0 inhomogeneities associated to interspinal processes; however, SNR is affected by voxel size, with lower SNR associated to smaller voxels, so both factors (good shim and sufficient SNR) should be considered when deciding voxel size and scan time as more averages are needed for smaller voxels.

To accurately place the voxel it is advisable to acquire a set of sagittal/coronal/axial images covering the region of interest such that the contrast between

CSF and the cord can easily be seen. Cooke recommends making sure that the VOI of interest is approximately on-resonance before acquiring these scout images, as failure to do so may result in additional positioning errors.

Saturation bands can also be used more effectively in this area by prescribing a large voxel and using saturation bands to suppress signal from parts of the voxel that lie in CSF or areas of high susceptibility (inner volume saturation [IVS]).[17] The dimensions and angulation of the voxel depend on whether inner volume saturation is applied; if not, the voxel must lie wholly within the cord and be planned according to the frequency of the metabolite of interest, e.g., NAA or the center of the spectral range (e.g., between mIns and NAA). It is useful to also visualize the chemical shift of the voxel at the water and lipid frequencies, and, if possible, care should also be taken to avoid contamination of CSF and exterior tissue in these shifted voxels.

The assignment of the dimensions of the voxel must take into account how the dimensions are prescribed; this will vary depending on scanner manufacturer. For example a 5 mm width may correspond to the full width half maximum (FWHM) or the width at 99% of the excited profile. In the FWHM case, the 5 mm will be an underestimate of the effective voxel size and significant magnetization will come from outside the selected area. The latter case (99% of the excitation bandwidth) will result in less signal from the same prescribed voxel dimensions, due to an overestimation of the voxel size. The advantage here is that minimal outer volume contamination will occur, at the expense of lower SNR.

Inner volume saturation together with a bigger prescribed voxel has been shown to produce good spectral quality.[17] Here highly selective polynomial phase response (PPR) pulses are used for outer volume suppression but are offset to cover the chemically shifted voxel from lipid and water, making sure magnetization only from within the assigned voxel within the cord is available to sample.[17] A study using this method showing MRS data from voxels placed in the thoracic region has also been reported.[17,44]

The voxel dimensions may be limited due to spinal cord atrophy or placement of the voxel away from areas of susceptibility.

5.1.3.7 Shimming and Water Suppression

Shimming is important for all MR spectroscopy scans to correct for B_0 inhomogeneities over the selected VOI, caused by the different magnetic susceptibilities of different tissues or tissue–air interfaces.

A spatially homogenous B_0 field not only reduces linewidths therefore resulting in better resolution and higher SNR but also reduces artifacts from spurious echoes and outer volume excitation. Shimming is performed on the water resonance as this is by far the largest resonance, and a good shim on the water peak will translate to all peaks in the spectrum.

A poorly shimmed VOI will result in fast decaying metabolite signals or reduced T_2^*, which will produce artificially broadened resonance peaks. A well-shimmed VOI results in smaller linewidths and higher SNR (see Figure 5.1.9). The ability to consistently get a good shim on the MRS VOI will depend on the shimming routine and the correct placement of the VOI within the spinal cord. Severe degeneration of the cord, for example, resulting in the intrusion of the disk into CSF will have negative consequences for shimming, often introducing significant local magnetic field shifts to the extent that shimming on a voxel in this area cannot converge the water peak to one peak.

Reported methods for shimming a voxel in the spinal cord differ, and this is partly due to the fact that limited options are generally available on each given scanner. Even assignment of the area to shim over is conflicting, with some research groups shimming just over the VOI and others choosing a larger area. Also, shimming performance could depend on software and hardware, therefore on vendor and shim gradients characteristics. However the general consensus is that cardiac triggering should be employed in this phase of the preparation too if possible. Typically reported linewidths for the water resonance are between 8 and 14 Hz. Here we describe widely available shimming techniques that have been published in reports of spinal cord spectroscopy.

5.1.3.7.1 Iterative Shimming

Iterative shimming can usually be performed both on the VOI or on a larger volume. Gradient coils in the X, Y, and Z directions are used to optimize field homogeneity, by iteratively running through different X, Y, and Z combinations. The best shim is found by determination of the largest integral for the time-domain signal—this corresponds to the longest signal with the largest amplitude, which will result in a high intensity, narrow water peak in the frequency domain. The time required for this method is a matter of minutes, and for some vendors it is used for first order shimming only. Also shimming results depend on the size of the area shimmed over, with poorer shims for larger areas covering a greater extent of magnetic field susceptibility changes within the region.

5.1.3.7.2 Projection-Based or FASTMAP Shimming

Automatic fast shimming routines have been implemented utilizing a linear projection scheme and used in both imaging and spectroscopy to achieve excellent shims in less than a minute.[45] This is based on taking

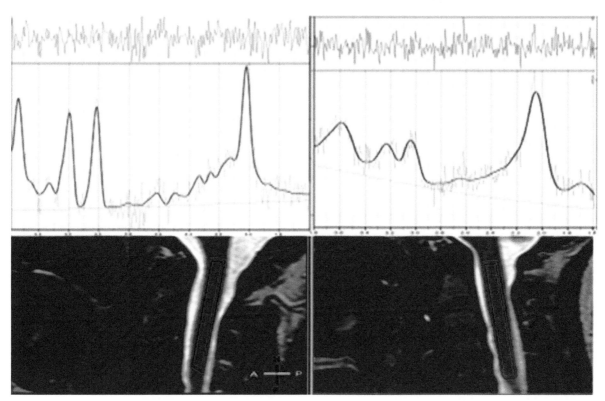

FIGURE 5.1.9   Spectra from two different subjects: one subject with a longer C1–C3 region (A) where the voxel spans across two intervertebral discs, and another with a shorter region (B) where given the shorter cord the voxel spans across three intervertebral discs. The VOI size was 2.13 ml in both cases. In (B) the VOI spans across more regions affected by magnetic susceptibility changes due to bone, i.e., it goes through more regions close to discs. The spectrum on the left (A), which is less affected by magnetic susceptibility changes corresponding to discs, shows good shimming with narrow well-resolved peaks (FWHM 7.8 Hz); to the right (B) the effect of a poor shim can be seen (FWHM 17.6 Hz). The peaks on a poorly shimmed spectrum are broader reducing spectral resolution and SNR (SNR ~3 vs. SNR ~6). Acquisition parameters were PRESS with TE = 30 ms, NSA = 376, TR = 3 s.

measurements along a limited number of linear projections over the volume of interest to characterize the B_0 field in each direction (e.g., in X, Y, Z, XY, XZ etc.). Both first and second order shims can be optimized relatively quickly, even when cardiac triggering is employed. The only drawback is that the scheme assumes a shim volume that can be nicely approximated by a sphere, and hence MRS voxels with roughly equal dimensions perform best. For spinal cord spectroscopy, voxels are elongated cuboids, with FH dimension 5–10 times greater than the orthogonal cross-sectional area, diverging drastically from the assumed sphere, which may cause shim routines such as this to fail or perform suboptimally. Despite this a fast automatic shimming technique by mapping along projections (FASTMAP)[45] has nevertheless been successfully implemented in the cervical cord to give good spectra.[22,32] As with any shim routine, one should keep a careful eye on the resultant water spectrum to ensure that a single narrow peak does result. This method is the fastest method, and no time is lost attempting this routine in the first instance if it is available.

5.1.3.7.3 Shimming Based on B_0 Mapping

B_0 field maps over the VOI, of appropriate spatial resolution, can be calculated using images acquired at two echo times (typically $TE_1 < 0.5$ ms and TE_2 2–5 ms). The phase accumulation between TEs gives an indication of the change in B_0 across the tissue. Considering the B_0 field changes that can be produced by the available first and second order shims, these initial field maps allow calculation of the changes in shim currents needed to achieve the best B_0 homogeneity across the area of interest. (Actual, rather than theoretical, shim performance can also be taken into account if shim calibration data is available.)

This method typically requires a scan for the field-mapping data followed by shim calculations and can show B_0 changes at the voxel edge (in which case a larger voxel maybe selected), and the optimization of higher order shims can be very helpful when focusing on small VOIs. Cardiac-triggered B_0 mapping has also been successfully established. As such it has found popularity in spinal cord imaging despite the slightly longer protocol.[11,14,24,32,44] Typical sagittal B_0 maps have 1 mm in-plane resolution and 2 mm slice thickness. The optimum difference in echo times to remove interference from the B_0-dependent fat signal at 3 T is 2.46 ms. A recent study used B_0 maps as a guide to plan the voxel size to ensure the entire voxel lies in a homogenous area.[24]

5.1.3.7.4 Water Suppression

The signal of water is several orders of magnitude greater than that of metabolites in vivo (up to 50 M vs. ~10 mM), and traditionally the limited dynamic range of the signal receiver did not allow distinguishing resonances from low concentration metabolites on top of the large water signal. While modern analog-to-digital receivers circumvent this problem with large dynamic ranges (16 or 32 bits), the water signal can lead to baseline distortions and the appearance of artificial vibration-induced sidebands that can affect spectral analysis and metabolite quantification. Suppression of the water signal is thus usually carried out for ^{1}H MRS. Several suppression methods exist based on the frequency and T_1 relaxation of water, such as excitation, inversion, chemical shift selective suppression

(CHESS),[46] multiply optimized insensitive suppression train (MOIST; a water suppression module available on Philips scanners), and variable pulse power and optimized relaxation delays (VAPOR).[47] CHESS is the most popular method, however, studies have shown good spectra using both MOIST and VAPOR too. Figure 5.1.10 shows a comparative example of these water suppression methods, and in this case MOIST performed the best in all four healthy volunteers tested. Care should be taken when choosing a method that is sensitive to T_1 as contamination from CSF will introduce overwhelming water signals with T_1s very different to that of white and gray matter in the cord. Water suppression itself is also cardiac triggered; reported delays range from 150 to 400 ms after the diastole, but this may be due to differences in how each scanner defines the start and end of the delay within the sequence. About two-thirds of all spinal cord spectroscopy publications successfully used CHESS for water suppression with cardiac gating.

In a recent paper, Hock et al. presented non-water-suppressed MRS in the spinal cord.[22] This has the advantage of allowing use of the prominent water

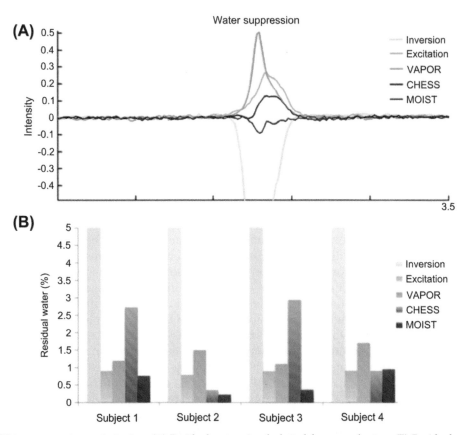

FIGURE 5.1.10   Water suppression optimization. (A) Residual water signal plotted for one volunteer. (B) Residual water heights as a percentage of reference water signal for each of four subjects shown for CHESS, Excitation, Inversion, MOIST, and VAPOR water suppression techniques. Y-axis cut off at 5% to help visualize and compare the more efficient water suppression modules. Acquisition parameters were TE = 30 ms, NSA = 376, TR = 3 s.

peak to correct for frequency drifts and to phase each individual spectrum, improving resolution when a number of averages are added, which may otherwise be difficult due to the low SNR of individual spectra. This resulted in resonances with lower linewidths and better automated fitting.

5.1.3.8 Sequence Parameters for Acquisition

Table 5.1.3 summarizes recent reports on spinal cord MRS to provide a comprehensive account of sequence parameters that have given rise to successful reports of NAA, Cr, tCh, and mIns ratios or their absolute values.

The most popular sequence is short TE (30–35 ms) PRESS using 2 ml volumes with 196–256 averages. Repetition times of 2–3000 ms are commonly used as minimal T_1 saturation occurs,[d] and many averages can be acquired in a short time. However, as the spectra are not fully relaxed, the resulting spectra will be sensitive to pathological T_1 changes.

To cover the chemical shifts of most ^{1}H compounds (approximately 10 ppm), a spectral bandwidth of 2 kHz is more than sufficient at 3 T; 1024 points adequately sample the whole free induction decay. The transmit and receive frequency should be centered on the middle of the spectrum or on the metabolite of interest.

A water reference scan (the exact same sequence with zero amplitude for the water suppression pulses) should also be taken from the same voxel. The transmit frequency should now be set on the water frequency. This spectrum can be used for eddy current correction purposes and internal water referencing for quantification.

5.1.3.8.1 Phase Cycling

Phase cycling is commonly employed in MRS protocols; it is used to suppress unwanted signals generated from spectrometer hardware and coherent noise or tissue outside the VOI. When the phase of the excitation pulse is cycled, the phase of the resulting signal will correspondingly change, and in this way NMR signal can be distinguished from background interference where the phase will not change. The receiver phase is alternated accordingly, hence when FIDs are summed, unwanted background interference is canceled whilst the desired VOI signal is added coherently.

5.1.3.8.2 Saturation Bands

Similarly to MR imaging, saturation bands can be employed when planning the scan to suppress spurious signals from fat and water contaminating the spectrum. As saturation bands are large compared to the size of the VOI prescribed in spinal cord MRS, care should be taken when placing saturation bands close to the voxel, as their profile may encroach into the small VOI, leaving significantly less signal. It is therefore wise to perform calibration experiments to measure the actual spatial profile of the saturation bands used for MRS. If saturation pulses are used to define the voxel, they can also act to reduce chemical shift artifacts and unwanted resonances from fat and water.[17] Saturation bands can also be placed over areas of magnetic susceptibility changes to facilitate convergence of shimming routines.

5.1.3.8.3 Addressing Physiological Motion

Spectral quality is highly susceptible to physiological motion, with motion causing shifts in VOI position resulting in changes in phase, frequency drifts, increased linewidths and effectively reduced SNR and water suppression efficiency. In the spinal cord the two most prominent offenders are the cardiac-induced pulsation of the CSF and blood[48–50] and respiratory motion.[51] A number of studies have shown that good spectra giving quantitative results can be acquired with the help of cardiac triggering that minimizes the effect of any pulsation in the spinal cord. Due to SAR and T_1 saturation effects, the scans are usually triggered at 2–3 times the volunteers' heart rate, which in healthy subjects results in 2–3 s repetition times.

In the study by Cooke et al., it is mentioned that spectra were acquired at different positions within the cardiac cycle and found that a delay of 400 ms after the cardiac electrical systole was found to give the most consistent spectra.[11] However, variable repetition times are likely to result when cardiac triggering is employed. Felblinger et al. investigated the possibility of "retrogating" to overcome this effect in the brain.[52] As the pulsatile motion causes phase dispersion, non-water-suppressed scans can be used to record a phase calibration curve. Using this together with information from the time response of the cardiac cycle it is possible to retrogate the subsequent water-suppressed scans.[52] This has not yet been applied to the spinal cord, although pulsatile motion may be more exacerbated compared to the brain.

Edden et al. reported 1D-PRESS CSI in the cervical cord and showed that good quality spectra can be obtained even without any cardiac triggering.[16] Respiratory gating has also been employed,[11,22] although this affects the C2–C3 level much less than the lumbar and thoracic spine.

---

[d]assuming $T_1 = 1.5$ s, with TR = 2 s or 3 s we get 74% or 86% of M_0, respectively.

5.1.3.8.4 Acquisition in Blocks

Due to the relatively long duration of single voxel spectroscopy scans, especially in the spinal cord, the number of averages may be split into blocks.[11,14,22] This is a method employed routinely in all MRS, not just in the spinal cord. It has the advantage of allowing postacquisition correction for any frequency or phase drifts occurring during the scan.[e] This procedure can also give a surrogate measure of patient or physiological motion and allows spectral quality control as any blocks with motion induced artifacts can be removed. The averaged frequency/phase corrected spectra will produce better resolution spectra than if no correction had been applied.

5.1.3.9 Data Processing and Metabolite Quantification

Very few publications have reported absolute concentrations of metabolites in the spinal cord, with the majority of reports quoting metabolite concentration ratios. A number of reviews exist covering quantification methods in ^1H MRS.[53–59] A brief outline follows.

If the spectral data from the spinal cord is of sufficiently good quality, then the same steps used for any other spectral quantification process should be followed.

There are a number of available spectral preprocessing and analysis packages that are widely used. These have become sophisticated packages, which not only measure simple peak integrations but also use prior knowledge about the spin systems and sequences to provide model spectra with which to fit the data. The most widely used programs are LCModel[57] and jMRUI.[60] LCModel fits the data in the frequency domain using a basis set computed using prior knowledge or a phantom basis set. jMRUI[60] fits the data in the time domain to a superposition of sine waves very often using the AMARES or VARPRO algorithms.[59,61] The practicalities of getting to an absolute measure of metabolites are discussed in the following sections.

5.1.3.9.1 Preprocessing

Basic preprocessing steps such as referencing the spectra (e.g., to NAA at 2.01 ppm) and phasing are usually done automatically when using LCModel but need user input for jMRUI. At long TE, if good water and fat suppression have been applied then the spectral baseline should be relatively flat and phasing the spectrum should result in upright peaks for all metabolites. At short TE, these same peaks will lie on top of a set of broad macromolecule resonances, which ideally should

be taken into consideration when determining the amplitude of each resonance. Some software packages allow frequency correction, but not many perform phase correction of time series of sequential blocks of MRS spectra.

5.1.3.9.2 Apodisation and Zero-Filling

Apodisation (line broadening) simplifies the spectrum making the resonances easier to see whilst smoothing out the noise. Line broadening should be consistent across groups as values used will affect SNR. By definition line broadening reduces spectral resolution so it may not be indicated when trying to resolve slightly overlapping peaks. LCModel does not use line broadening in its analysis, but it is an option in other packages.

Zero filling is also commonly applied, which artificially increases the digital resolution in the spectral domain. It does not add information to the available data, however, it can be useful for visualization purposes. Zero filling to 2048 points is usually sufficient.

5.1.3.9.3 Lineshape and Eddy Current Correction

During an MR experiment, the time-dependent magnetic fields used for signal encoding and detection can cause unwanted "eddy"—currents in conductors within the magnet bore and casing. These currents end up producing time-varying magnetic fields that interfere with the MR experiment and can distort the detected signal.

This gives rise to resonance lineshapes that depart from the theoretical Gaussian or Lorentzian shapes. As most algorithms are designed to deal with Gaussian or Lorentzian shapes (or can use a mixture of the two), strong deviations from these symmetric shapes can make fitting the spectrum difficult and introduce bias. These distortions can be eliminated or at least reduced by the use of a water signal from a non-water-suppressed reference scan that experiences the same time-varying B_0 field experienced by metabolites, giving rise to lineshape distortions. By using this information it is possible to remove the time domain modulations from the metabolite spectra (or equivalently, use the measured distorted lineshape for the fitting), effectively removing the effects of eddy currents on the data.[62,63]

5.1.3.9.4 Baseline Correction

If sufficient water suppression has been applied, then the baseline rolls will most probably be independent of residual water. Fast relaxing macromolecular metabolites such as lipid may still be present/contaminants in

---

[e]Frequency correction is typically done in the frequency domain using one of the highest peaks available. Phase correction is then performed easily in the time domain by measuring and adjusting the phase of the first one or first few FID points.

short TE spectra. LCModel incorporates these fast decaying metabolites in the basis set as prior knowledge. These can also be added in a similar fashion to the prior knowledge used for jMRUI with known resonant frequencies and T_2 relaxation times to estimate linewidths. In addition to this, jMRUI also has a range of functions to correct the baseline during the postprocessing steps, leaving a spectrum with a flat baseline where the remaining metabolites are easily fit. If the origin of the signal is due to outer volume contamination, using fat-specific saturation slabs may eliminate this artifact at data collection point and this specific postprocessing step is not needed. Also if the macromolecule resonances are due to pathology in the voxel, then this will be evident if correct fat suppression outside the volume is used. Using a longer TE (such as TE > 80 ms) reduces the information from short T_2 metabolites and helps to alleviate any macromolecular contamination (at the cost of reduced SNR). This is true at any field strength as macromolecule T_2 is independent of field strength.[64]

DATA PREPROCESSING

- Eddy current correction
- Offset correction
- Apodisation
- Phase correction
- Baseline correction
- Residual water correction

5.1.3.9.5 Relative and Absolute Metabolite Quantification

When MRS data are analyzed the main goal is to fit the FID/spectrum so the result is a set of sine waves/resonances that adequately represent the acquired spectrum. The integral of each resonance will be proportional to the concentration of the metabolite. This data can be used to express metabolite ratios or, if calibrated, can be used to get absolute concentrations for each metabolite.

A word of warning is necessary here. Though "absolute concentrations" in mmol/l are often reported, in many cases several assumptions have been made that may cause the results to be institution- or scanner-dependent estimates of concentrations rather than "absolute" concentrations. This is obvious from Table 5.1.3 where the main metabolite concentrations obtained on healthy subjects by several groups are listed, and they appear to vary substantially between studies.

The steps leading to concentration quantifications are discussed in more detail following.

5.1.3.9.6 Prior Knowledge

5.1.3.9.6.1 jMRUI

After referencing, apodising, phasing, zero-filling, and baseline correction within jMRUI, the data are ready for quantification using one of its in-built algorithms, e.g., AMARES. To help the fitting algorithm the user can enter in prior knowledge to reduce the number of free variables used to fit the data. The simplest starting points are defining the frequency of each resonance and its FWHM linewidth. These two pieces of information provide jMRUI with the approximate frequency of each sinusoidal component and an initial estimate of how fast it is decaying. This information can be derived in two ways: (1) directly from in vivo data (by manually clicking on the individual peaks and defining linewidth graphically on the spectra within JMRUI); (2) using reference information, such as that found in Govindaraju et al. for peak positions, and employing as minimum linewidth that of the water peak FWHM calculated during shimming.[65]

Other more sophisticated information can be entered using knowledge of resonance splittings, relative chemical shifts, and T_2 relaxation times. For example, if a triplet is being fitted then the ratio of amplitudes will be 1:2:1, which can be entered into the prior knowledge. If the metabolite chemical shift is independent of temperature and pH, for example, NAA at 2.01 ppm and tCr at 3 ppm, then the chemical shift can also be added as a hard constraint (i.e., 0.99 ppm apart) or soft constraint (0.96–1.02 ppm shift). Given these additional pieces of information the number of free variables is reduced again, improving the performance of the fitting algorithm. The result of the fitting algorithm will give the amplitude of each peak identified in the prior knowledge step. Users should always check the original and the fitted peaks to see if the linewidth, lineshape, and phase are a good match before using the amplitudes for quantification. An example of the output from a jMRUI fit is shown in Figure 5.1.11.

5.1.3.9.6.2 LCMODEL

Prior knowledge in LCModel is entered in the form of a basis set that can be used for all spectra acquired with the same technique. Basis sets can be simulated or acquired from phantoms of known concentration, and again contain information on the spectral features attributable to each metabolite. Following the formation of a basis set, the analysis of the spectra is fairly automated, taking away any user dependency on the spectral analysis. Referencing, phasing, lineshape estimation, and baseline correction are automatic, as is quantitation and eddy current correction if a non-water-suppressed reference dataset is available. Data are quantified in "institutional units". Using the water

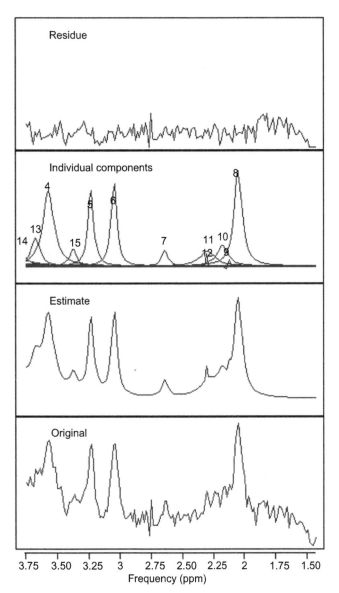

FIGURE 5.1.11   Example of the results window in jMRUI. The original spectrum is shown at the bottom; above this is the estimate spectrum calculated using the AMARES algorithm using user-defined prior knowledge. The individual peaks that have been fitted are shown; here broad peaks and peaks where the phase is distorted can be seen more clearly. The area under each peak is also given, which can be used for quantification. A residual signal is also shown (top), which gives an indication of noise.

reference dataset, the information about water and metabolite relaxation times and the known or assumed concentration of water in tissue, LCModel allows to quantify the data in mmol/l. Alongside each metabolite concentration value, LCModel calculates the %SD (or Cramer Rao Lower Bounds; CRLBs), giving an indication of the goodness of the fit. Values of %SD < 20% have been used by many groups as a measure of acceptable reliability.

5.1.3.9.7 Data Calibration

5.1.3.9.7.1 INTERNAL – RELATIVE TO WATER

As mentioned before, using LCModel absolute quantification of ^{1}H metabolites can also be achieved using the water signal measured at the same location as the metabolites as a reference and making a few assumptions on the NMR visible water concentration in the voxel,[66] and the water and metabolites T_1 and T_2 relaxation times. It is often assumed that spinal cord water concentration is similar to brain water concentration, and potential differences due to pathology are not accounted for (unless these are specifically quantified). By taking the ratio of the areas of the water reference and metabolite resonances, and taking into account how many protons contribute to each signal, an absolute concentration for each metabolite can be determined. This has been the method applied in most quantification in the spinal cord where absolute concentrations are reported.[10,11,14–16,19,33] If further corrections based on T_1 and T_2 are made, these have used T_1 and T_2 values of metabolites as previously measured and reported in the brain.

5.1.3.9.7.2 RELATIVE TO CREATINE

To avoid errors in quantification related to incorrect/unknown relaxation times and pathological changes in water density, many studies have reported metabolites as ratios in particular to Cr to provide semiquantitative measures.[12,13,18,20,22,24,26,32] In healthy tissues and in several pathologies the concentration of Cr remains stationary and reporting values in relation to Cr is considered a reliable way of portraying changes in metabolite values. However, in some cases, e.g., MS, Cr may also change so the metabolite(s) driving the change in metabolic ratios to Cr becomes unclear, making interpretation of the results more difficult.[67] This however remains a popular and widely applied reporting strategy.

5.1.3.9.7.3 EXTERNAL CALIBRATION

Another method for calibrating the data for quantification is to run the same MRS protocol used in vivo on an external phantom. This can be done either while the subject is still in the scanner by placing a small calibration phantom of known concentration next to him or her, or immediately after the scan as long as the exact same protocol is used, including VOI positioning within the coil and coil loading as used in vivo.

The use of small calibration phantoms positioned next to the subject avoids any errors due to loading; it is, however, a different experiment as the voxel cannot be placed at the same position within the coil as the VOI of interest, therefore the measured data may be acquired in a position where the coil sensitivity is different from the coil sensitivity at the in vivo VOI, and the scanner also needs to be reshimmed before this reference data is acquired. While the replacement phantom technique overcomes this issue, careful design of the phantom to make loading similar to the in vivo situation must be undertaken. T_1 and T_2 values of the phantom solution must also be accounted for.

Similarly to the water resonance once the number of protons (N_H), averages (n) are corrected for, the calibration factor can be calculated to get absolute quantification of metabolites from resonance amplitudes (S) using the following equation and correction factors (C):

$$[conc_{met}] = (S_{phan}/S_{met}) * C_{NH} \cdot C_n \cdot C_l \qquad (5.1.3)$$

where [$conc_{met}$] is the concentration of the metabolite, S_{phan} is the peak amplitude of the phantom, and S_{met} of the metabolite in vivo, C_{NH} corrects for any difference in the number of protons, C_n corrects for any difference in the number of averages, and C_l corrects for any differences in loading between the phantom and in vivo experiments.

5.1.4 NON-PROTON MRS OF THE SPINAL CORD

Owing to larger chemical shifts in spectra originating from other nuclei (e.g., ^{31}P and ^{13}C) and the lower sensitivities of other nuclei, multinuclear MRS in the cord is an area just beginning to be explored. The simplest example is that of ^{23}Na. Like ^{31}P and ^{13}C it has a lower gyromagnetic ratio leading to lower sensitivity and a much lower abundance. In addition to this and similarly to other non-^1H MRS the sequence needs to be sensitive to short T_2s as ^{23}Na has T_2s ranging from 0.5 to 20 ms in tissue to 40–50 ms in unbound states. Only one example of sodium MRS has been presented to date in healthy subjects.[68] This study used image selected in vivo spectroscopy (ISIS), which collects an FID rather than an echo, minimizing T_2 dephasing in the time between excitation and acquisition.[69] The lower T_1 relaxation time of sodium means that scan times can be comparable to ^1H MRS of the spinal cord given the lower TRs that can be used allowing to perform more averages in the same scan time. One of the reasons perhaps that ^{23}Na has been pursued before the relatively more common ^{31}P MRS and ^{13}C MRS is the presence of only one peak in the spectrum, which results in no chemical shift displacement. In comparison, ^{31}P and ^{13}C have large chemical shift scales of 60 and 200 ppm, respectively, hence chemical shift displacements into CSF and bone are very likely pitfalls, which may need to be overcome or eliminated with saturation bands giving real quantification on just a fraction of the spectrum.

5.1.5 RECOMMENDED PROTOCOL

5.1.5.1 Suggestions for Cervical Spine MRS Data Acquisition

Below is a summary table of recommendations (with drawbacks of the choice).

Issue	Recommendation and Advantages	Disadvantages
Field strength	Higher fields for more sensitivity	Higher fields give larger linewidths; there are also greater chemical shift displacement effects unless pulses with higher bandwidths can be employed
Coils	Local surface coil reception for greater sensitivity	Need volume coil for homogenous excitation; need array of coils to investigate extended areas

(Continued)

Issue	Recommendation and Advantages	Disadvantages
Patient immobilization	Cervical collar for straighter cord and reduced motion artifacts. Vacuum bag providing immobilization and support	Cervical collar can be uncomfortable for subjects
Sequence selection	PRESS gives twice the signal as STEAM	Minimum echo times are sometimes longer than for STEAM
Echo time	Short, ~30 ms if detection of mIns is required	Macromolecular signals can produce a distorted baseline. TE = 144 ms gives a flatter baseline at the expense of SNR
Voxel positioning	Use software allowing visualization of VOI for both NAA and water	Not available on all MR scanners
Outer volume suppression	Use to avoid contamination from CSF and subcutaneous fat on the neck. Needs prior assessment of effective saturation profile of saturation bands to avoid saturating signal within VOI	Can increase minimum TR. Can affect VOI signal if not properly calibrated
Cardiac triggering	Use for reduction of pulsation artifacts resulting in smaller linewidths	Can make repetition time variable between averages
Shimming	Passive shimming can be effective if available For gradient-based active shimming, use method appropriate for elongated voxel with small cross section ($\sim 6 \times 6$ mm^2), (i.e., if field maps are used they should have appropriate spatial resolution). Always visually assess results from automated shimming procedures and consider manual adjustments	Visual assessment and manual adjustments can be time consuming
Water suppression	Use best method available on system	If postacquisition frequency correction is required, consider partial suppression

5.1.5.2 Future Methodological Improvements

With the emergence of higher field strength magnets and advancements in coil design for the spinal cord, there is scope for the sensitivity to this region to be improved allowing more widespread applications. In addition to this, spinal cord MRS is still in its junior steps; as pitfalls are addressed and overcome, more sophisticated sequences looking at a larger range of metabolites can be applied, such as to provide information on glutamate, GABA, and other more elusive metabolites, as well as more instances of multinuclear applications.

References

1. Lauterbur PC. Image formation by induced local interactions: examples employing nuclear magnetic resonance. *Nature.* 1973; 242:190–191.
2. Mansfield P, Grannell PK. NMR 'diffraction' in solids? *J Phys C Solid State Phys.* 1973;6(22):L422.
3. Bloch F, Hansen WW, Packard M. The nuclear induction experiment. *Phys Rev.* 1946;70:474–485.
4. Purcell EM, Torrey HC, Pound RV. Radiation absorption by nuclear magnetic moments in a solid. *Phys Rev.* 1946;69:37–38.
5. de Graaf RA. *In Vivo NMR Spectroscopy: Principles and Techniques.* 2nd ed. John Wiley & Sons Ltd; 2007.
6. Hore PJ. *Nuclear Magnetic Resonance.* Oxford: Oxford University Press; 1995.
7. Bottomley PA, Smith LS, Edelstein WA, et al. Localized P-31, C-13, and H-1-Nmr spectroscopy studies of the head and body at 1.5-T. *Magn Reson Med.* 1984;1(2):111–112.
8. Frahm J, Merboldt KD, Hanicke W. Localized proton spectroscopy using stimulated echoes. *J Magn Reson.* 1987;72(3):502–508.
9. Brown TR, Kincaid BM, Ugurbil K. NMR chemical-shift imaging in 3 dimensions. *Proc Natl Acad Sci India Sect B.* 1982;79(11): 3523–3526.
10. Gomez-Anson B, MacManus DG, Parker GJM, et al. In vivo ^{1}H-magnetic resonance spectroscopy of the spinal cord in humans. *Neuroradiology.* 2000;42(7):515–517.
11. Cooke FJ, Blamire AM, Manners DN, Styles P, Rajagopalan B. Quantitative proton magnetic resonance spectroscopy of the cervical spinal cord. *Magn Reson Med.* 2004;51(6):1122–1128.
12. Kendi AT, Tan FU, Kendi M, Yilmaz S, Huvaj S, Tellioglu S. MR spectroscopy of cervical spinal cord in patients with multiple sclerosis. *Neuroradiology.* 2004;46(9):764–769.
13. Kim YG, Choi GH, Kim DH, Kim YD, Kang YK, Kim JK. In vivo proton magnetic resonance spectroscopy of human spinal mass lesions. *J Spinal Disord Tech.* 2004;17(5):405–411.
14. Blamire AM, Cader S, Lee M, Palace J, Matthews PM. Axonal damage in the spinal cord of multiple sclerosis patients detected by magnetic resonance spectroscopy. *Magn Reson Med.* 2007;58(5): 880–885.
15. Ciccarelli O, Wheeler-Kingshott C, McLean M, et al. Spinal cord diffusion imaging and spectroscopy to assess the impact of acute lesions in multiple sclerosis. *J Neurol Neurosurg Psychiatr.* 2007; 78(9):1024.
16. Edden RA, Bonekamp D, Smith MA, Dubey P, Barker PB. Proton MR spectroscopic imaging of the medulla and cervical spinal cord. *J Magn Reson Imaging.* 2007;26(4):1101–1105.
17. Henning A, Schar M, Kollias SS, Boesiger P, Dydak U. Quantitative magnetic resonance spectroscopy in the entire human cervical spinal cord and beyond at 3 T. *Magn Reson Med.* 2008;59(6): 1250–1258.

18. Holly LT, Freitas B, McArthur DL, Salamon N. Proton magnetic resonance spectroscopy to evaluate spinal cord axonal injury in cervical spondylotic myelopathy. *J Neurosurg Spine*. 2009;10(3): 194–200.

19. Ciccarelli O, Altmann DR, McLean MA, et al. Spinal cord repair in MS: does mitochondrial metabolism play a role? *Neurology*. 2010; 74(9):721–727.

20. Marliani AF, Clementi V, Riccioli LA, et al. Quantitative cervical spinal cord 3 T proton MR spectroscopy in multiple sclerosis. *Am J Neuroradiol*. 2010;31(1):180–184.

21. Elliott JM, Pedler AR, Cowin G, Sterling M, McMahon K. Spinal cord metabolism and muscle water diffusion in whiplash. *Spinal Cord*. 2012;50(6):474–476.

22. Hock A, MacMillan E, Fuchs A, et al. Non-water suppressed proton MR spectroscopy allows spectral quality improvement in the human cervical spinal cord. In: *Nineteenth ISMRM Proceedings*. Montreal; 2011;406.

23. Solanky BS, Abdel-Aziz K, Yiannakas MC, Berry AM, Ciccarelli O, Wheeler-Kingshott CA. In vivo magnetic resonance spectroscopy detection of combined glutamate-glutamine in healthy upper cervical cord at 3 T. *NMR Biomed*. 2013;26(3):357–366.

24. Carew JD, Nair G, Pineda-Alonso N, Usher S, Hu X, Benatar M. Magnetic resonance spectroscopy of the cervical cord in amyotrophic lateral sclerosis. *Amyotroph Lateral Scler*. 2011;12(3): 185–191.

25. Dydak U, Kollias SS, Schar M, Meier BH, Boesiger P. MR spectroscopy in different regions of spinal cord and in spinal cord tumors. In: *Proceedings of ISMRM Thirteenth Scientific Meeting and Exhibition*. Miami; 2005;813.

26 Kachramanoglou C, De Vita E, Thomas DL, et al. Metabolic changes in the spinal cord after brachial plexus root re-implantation. *Neurorehabil Neural Repair*. 2013;27(2):118–124.

27. Kachramanoglou C, De Vita E, Thomas DL, et al. Metabolic changes in the spinal cord after brachial plexus root re-implantation. *Neurorehabil Neural Repair*. 2013;27(2):118–124.

28. Chokkalingam K, Tsintzas K, Snaar JE, et al. Hyperinsulinaemia during exercise does not suppress hepatic glycogen concentrations in patients with type 1 diabetes: a magnetic resonance spectroscopy study. *Diabetologia*. 2007;50(9):1921–1929.

29. Ciccarelli O, Wheeler-Kingshott CA, McLean MA, et al. Spinal cord spectroscopy and diffusion-based tractography to assess acute disability in multiple sclerosis. *Brain*. 2007;130:2220–2231.

30. Ciccarelli O, Thomas D, De Vita E, et al. Low myo-inositol indicating astrocytic damage in a case series of NMO. *Ann Neurol*. 2013;74(2):301–305.

31. Stephenson MC, Gunner F, Napolitano A, et al. Applications of multi-nuclear magnetic resonance spectroscopy at 7 T. *World J Radiol*. 2011;3(4):105–113.

32. Carew JD, Nair G, Andersen PM, et al. Presymptomatic spinal cord neurometabolic findings in SOD1-positive people at risk for familial ALS. *Neurology*. 2011;77(14):1370–1375.

33. Marliani AF, Clementi V, Albini-Riccioli L, Agati R, Leonardi M. Quantitative proton magnetic resonance spectroscopy of the human cervical spinal cord at 3 Tesla. *Magn Reson Med*. 2007;57(1): 160–163.

34. Kinchesh P, Ordidge RJ. Spin-echo MRS in humans at high field: LASER localisation using FOCI pulses. *J Magn Reson*. 2005;175(1): 30–43.

35. Brown MA. Time-domain combination of MR spectroscopy data acquired using phased-array coils. *Magn Reson Med*. 2004;52(5): 1207–1213.

36. Hess AT, Tisdall MD, Andronesi OC, Meintjes EM, van der Kouwe AJW. Real-time motion and B(0) corrected single voxel spectroscopy using volumetric navigators. *Magn Reson Med*. 2011; 66(2):314–323.

37. Qin L, van Gelderen P, Derbyshire JA, et al. Prospective head-movement correction for high-resolution MRI using an in-bore optical tracking system. *Magn Reson Med*. 2009;62(4):924–934.

38. Ooi MB, Krueger S, Thomas WJ, Swaminathan SV, Brown TR. Prospective real-time correction for arbitrary head motion using active markers. *Magn Reson Med*. 2009;62(4):943–954.

39. Haeberlin M, Kasper L, Brunner DO, Barmet C, Preussmann KP. Continuous motion tracking and correction using NMR probes and gradient tones. In: *Proceedings of Twentieth Annual Meeting of ISMRM*. Melbourne, Australia; 2012:595.

40. Choi C, Patel A, Douglas D, Dimitrov I. Measurement of proton T2 of coupled-spin metabolites in gray and white matter in human brain at 3 T. In: *Proceedings Eighteenth Annual Meeting of ISMRM*. Stockholm, Sweden; 2010:1406.

41. Srinivasan R, Sailasuta N, Hurd R, Nelson S, Pelletier D. Evidence of elevated glutamate in multiple sclerosis using magnetic resonance spectroscopy at 3 T. *Brain*. 2005;128:1016–1025.

42. Wansapura JP, Holland SK, Dunn RS, Ball Jr WS. NMR relaxation times in the human brain at 3.0 Tesla. *J Magn Reson Imaging*. 1999; 9(4):531–538.

43. Moonen CT, von Kienlin M, van Zijl PC, et al. Comparison of single-shot localization methods (STEAM and PRESS) for in vivo proton NMR spectroscopy. *NMR Biomed*. 1989;2(5–6):201–208.

44. Henning A, Schar M, Kollias A, Meier D, Boesiger P, Dydak U. Quantitative magnetic resonance spectroscopy in the entire human cervical spinal cord and beyond at 3T. *Magn Reson Med*. 2008;59(6):1250–1258.

45. Gruetter R. Automatic, localized in vivo adjustment of all first- and second-order shim coils. *Magn Reson Med*. 1993;29(6):804–811.

46. Haase A, Frahm J, Hanicke W, Matthaei D. H-1-NMR chemical-shift selective (Chess) imaging. *Phys Med Biol*. 1985;30(4):341–344.

47. Tkac I, Starcuk Z, Choi IY, Gruetter R. In vivo H-1 NMR spectroscopy of rat brain at 1 ms echo time. *Magn Reson Med*. 1999; 41(4):649–656.

48. Mikulis DJ, Wood ML, Zerdoner OA, Poncelet BP. Oscillatory motion of the normal cervical spinal cord. *Radiology*. 1994;192(1): 117–121.

49. Pattany PM, Khamis IH, Bowen BC, et al. Effects of physiologic human brain motion on proton spectroscopy: quantitative analysis and correction with cardiac gating. *AJNR Am J Neuroradiol*. 2002; 23(2):225–230.

50. Schroth G, Klose U. Cerebrospinal fluid flow. III. Pathological cerebrospinal fluid pulsations. *Neuroradiology*. 1992;35(1):16–24.

51. Schroth G, Klose U. Cerebrospinal fluid flow. II. Physiology of respiration-related pulsations. *Neuroradiology*. 1992;35(1):10–15.

52. Felblinger J, Kreis R, Boesch C. Effects of physiologic motion of the human brain upon quantitative ^{1}H-MRS: analysis and correction by retro-gating. *NMR Biomed*. 1998;11(3):107–114.

53. Cavassila S, Deval S, Huegen C, van Ormondt D, Graveron-Demilly D. Cramer-Rao bounds: an evaluation tool for quantitation. *NMR Biomed*. 2001;14(4):278–283.

54. Helms G. The principles of quantification applied to in vivo proton MR spectroscopy. *Eur J Radiol*. 2008;67(2):218–229.

55. in 't Zandt H, van Der Graaf M, Heerschap A. Common processing of in vivo MR spectra. *NMR Biomed*. 2001;14(4):224–232.

56. Mierisova S, Ala-Korpela M. MR spectroscopy quantitation: a review of frequency domain methods. *NMR Biomed*. 2001;14(4): 247–259.

57. Provencher SW. Automatic quantitation of localized in vivo ^{1}H spectra with LCModel. *NMR Biomed*. 2001;14(4):260–264.

58. Stoyanova R, Brown TR. NMR spectral quantitation by principal component analysis. *NMR Biomed*. 2001;14(4):271–277.

59. Vanhamme L, Sundin T, Hecke PV, Huffel SV. MR spectroscopy quantitation: a review of time-domain methods. *NMR Biomed*. 2001;14(4):233–246.

60. Naressi A, Couturier C, Devos JM, et al. Java-based graphical user interface for the MRUI quantitation package. *Magn Reson Mater Phys Biol Med.* 2001;12(2–3):141–152.

61. van der Veen JW, de Beer R, Luyten PR, van Ormondt D. Accurate quantification of in vivo 31P NMR signals using the variable projection method and prior knowledge. *Magn Reson Med.* 1988; 6(1):92–98.

62. Klose U. In vivo proton spectroscopy in presence of eddy currents. *Magn Reson Med.* 1990;14(1):26–30.

63. Riddle WR, Gibbs SJ, Willcott MR. Removing effects of eddy currents in proton MR-spectroscopy. *Med Phys.* 1992;19(2): 501–509.

64. de Graaf RA, Brown PB, McIntyre S, Nixon TW, Behar KL, Rothman DL. High magnetic field water and metabolite proton T1 and T2 relaxation in rat brain in vivo. *Magn Reson Med.* 2006;56(2): 386–394.

65. Govindaraju V, Young K, Maudsley AA. Proton NMR chemical shifts and coupling constants for brain metabolites. *NMR Biomed.* 2000;13(3):129–153.

66. Ernst T, Kreis R, Ross BD. Absolute quantitation of water and metabolites in the human brain; part I: compartments and water. *J Magn Reson.* 1993;B102:1–8.

67. Vermathen M, Rooney WD, Goodkin DE, Weiner MW. Creatine and myo-Inositol are increased in multiple sclerosis normal appearing white matter. In: *Proceedings of ISMRM Seventh Scientific Meeting and Exhibition.* Philadelphia, USA; 1999:1440.

68. Solanky BS, Riemer F, Golay X, Wheeler-Kingshott CA. Sodium quantification in the spinal cord at 3 T. *Magn Reson Med.* 2013; 69(5):1201–1208.

69. Ordidge RJ, Connelly A, Lohman JA. Image-selected in vivo spectroscopy (ISIS). A new technique for spatially selective NMR spectroscopy. *J Magn Reson.* 1986;66:283–294.

Annex: Anatomy of the Spinal Cord

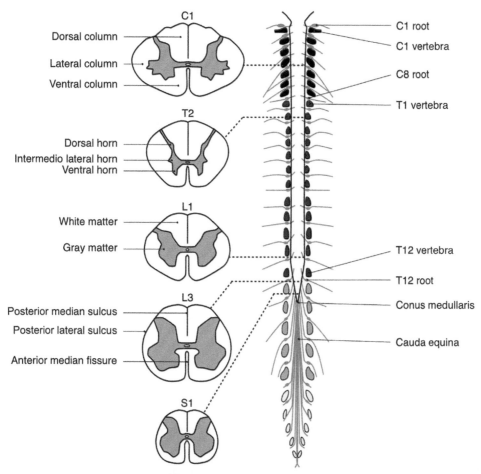

FIGURE A.1 **Schematic view of vertebral levels with spinal root distributions.** Axial slices are shown on the left at various levels. *Source: Figure inspired by (i) Anatomy and physiology of the Spinal Cord. Rossignol S. In: Essentials of Spinal Cord Injury. New York: Thieme Medical Publishers Inc.; 2012. Chapter 1: p.3–17. and by (ii) Netter FH. Nervous system: anatomy and physiology. In: Brass A, Dingle RV, eds. The Ciba Collection of Medical Illustrations, 2 Section II, plates 14 and 17.*

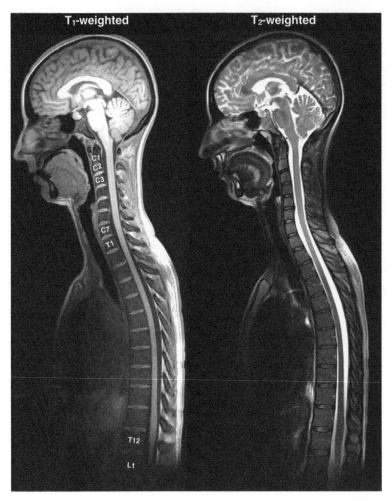

FIGURE A.2 **T$_1$- and T$_2$-weighted MRI of the spinal cord.** Sagittal T$_1$-weighted (MPRAGE) and T$_2$-weighted (3D FSE) MRI of a 27-year-old healthy female. Each image was acquired by stitching two acquisitions together (top and bottom). Resolution is 1 mm isotropic. The spinal cord is well visible on both contrasts. The cerebrospinal fluid is dark on the T1w sequence (due to the inversion recovery pulse) and appears as hypersignal on the T$_2$-weighted sequence. Here the spinal cord is about 40 cm long and terminates at the T12-L1 vertebral level.

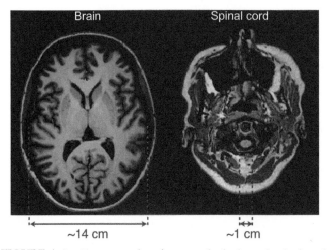

FIGURE A.3 Size comparison between the brain and spinal cord.

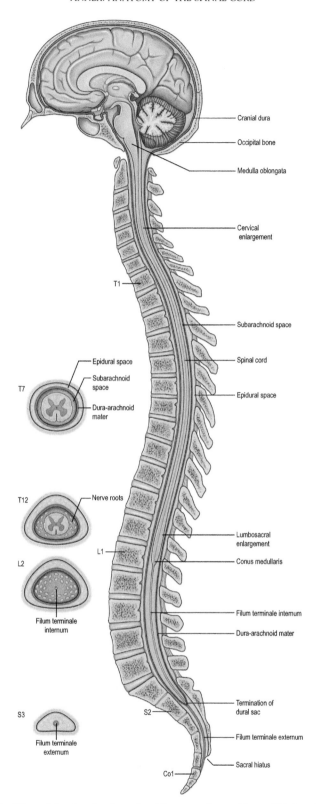

FIGURE A.4 **The epidural and subarachnoid spaces.** *Source: Figure 43.2 from Gray's Anatomy.*

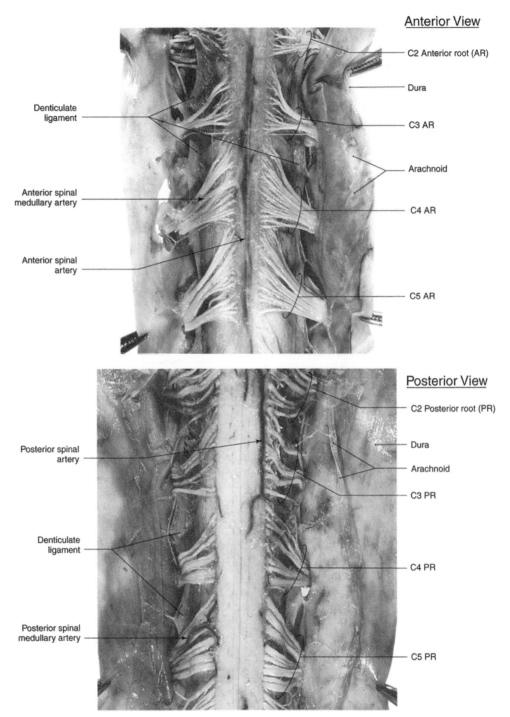

FIGURE A.5 **Ex vivo pictures of the spinal cord showing rootlet distributions.** Anterior (top) and posterior (bottom) views showing the general features of the spinal cord as seen at levels C2–C5. The dura and arachnoid are reflected, and the pia is intimately adherent to the spinal cord and rootlets. Posterior and anterior spinal medullary arteries follow their respective roots. The posterior spinal artery is found medial to the entering posterior rootlets (and the dorsolateral sulcus), whereas the anterior spinal artery is in the anterior median fissure. Radiculopathy results from spinal nerve root damage. The most common causes are intervertebral disc disease/protrusion or spondylolysis, and the main symptoms are pain radiating in a root or dermatomal distribution, and weakness, and hyporeflexia of the muscles served by the affected root. The discs most commonly involved at cervical (C) and lumbar (L) levels are C6–C7 (65–70%), C5–C6 (16–20%), L4–L5 (40–45%), and L5–S1 (35–40%). Thoracic disc problems are rare, well under 1% of all disc protrusions. *Source: Reproduced with permission from Haines, Neuroanatomy: An Atlas of Structures, Sections, and Systems. Figure 2.1.*

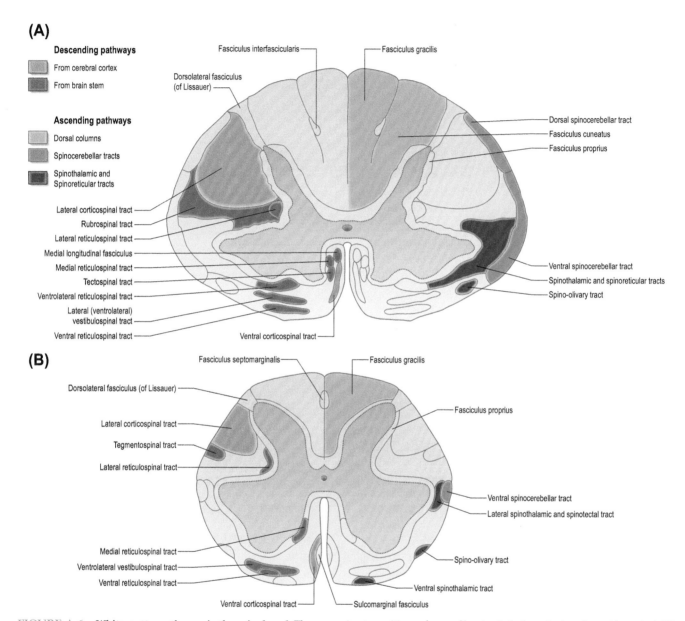

FIGURE A.6 **White matter pathways in the spinal cord.** The approximate positions of nerve fiber tracts in the spinal cord at mid-cervical (A) and lumbar (B) levels. *Source: Figure 18.9 from Gray's anatomy.*

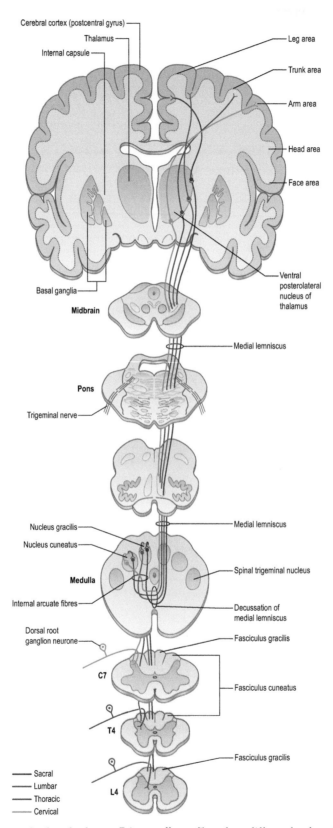

FIGURE A.7 **White matter pathway: the dorsal columns.** Primary afferent fibers from different levels and their associated second- and third-order neurons are depicted in different colors. *Source: Figure 18.10 from Gray's Anatomy.*

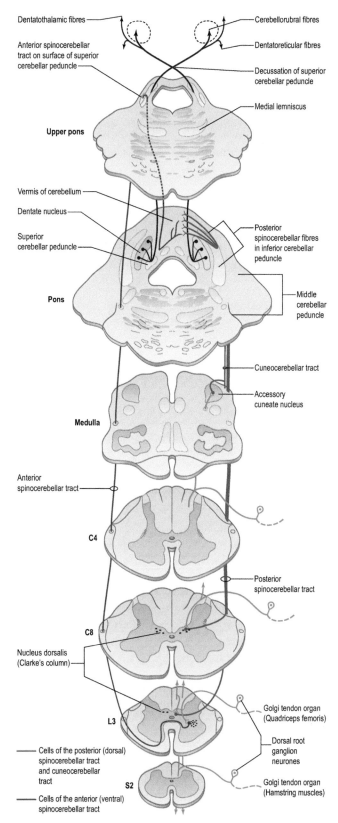

FIGURE A.8 **White matter pathway: the spinocerebellar tracts.** *Source: Figure 18.11 from Gray's Anatomy.*

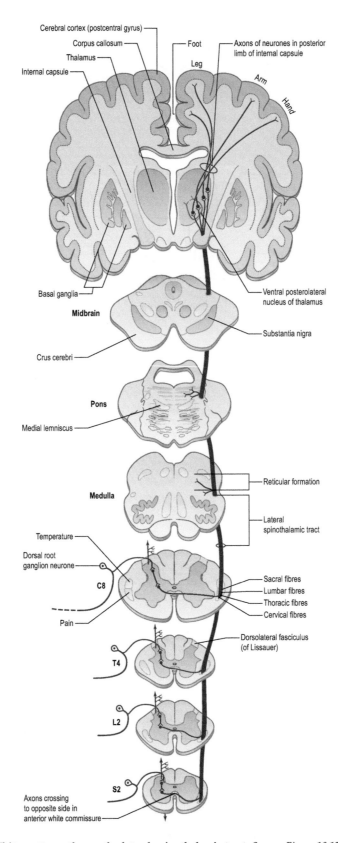

FIGURE A.9   **White matter pathway: the lateral spinothalamic tract.** *Source: Figure 18.12 from Gray's Anatomy.*

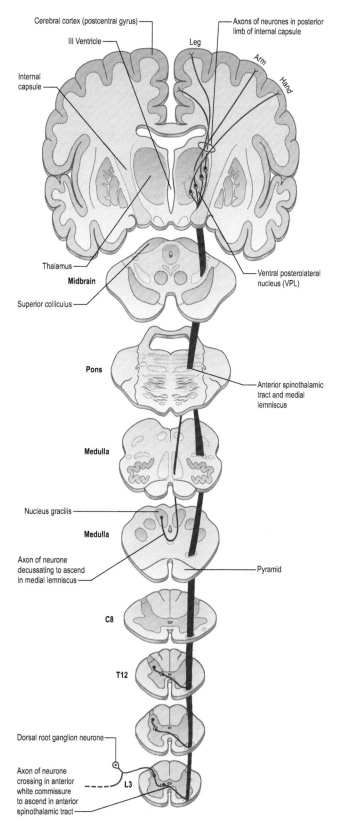

FIGURE A.10   **White matter pathway: the ventral (anterior) spinothalamic tract.** *Source: Figure 18.13 from Gray's Anatomy.*

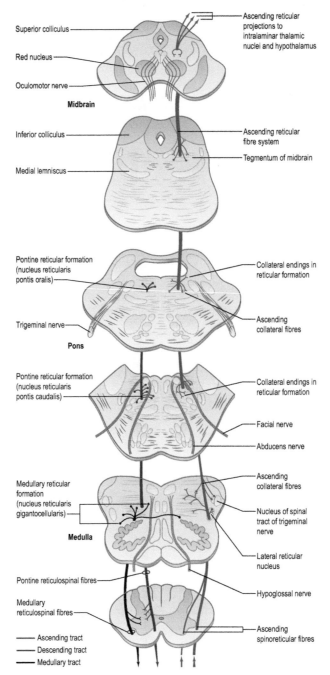

FIGURE A.11 **White matter pathway: the reticular tracts.** *Source: Figure 18.16 from Gray's Anatomy.*

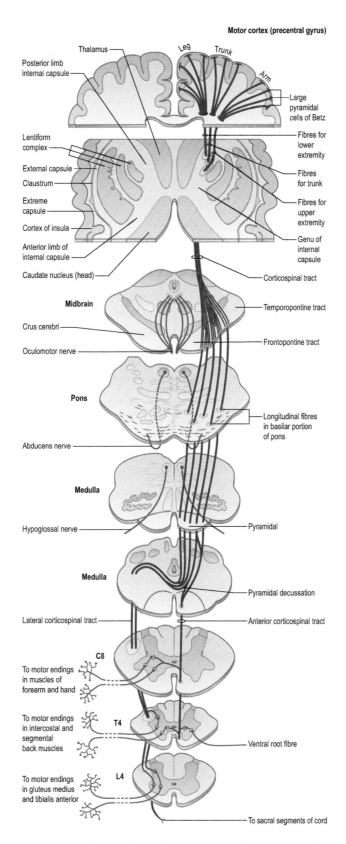

FIGURE A.12   **White matter pathway: the corticospinal tracts.** *Source: Figure 18.17 from Gray's Anatomy.*

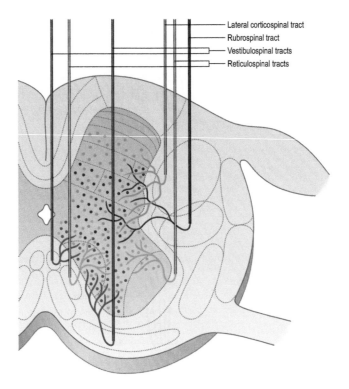

FIGURE A.13   **Spinal terminations of descending white matter pathways.** A simplified scheme of some of the major descending pathways of the spinal cord including their overlapping zones of termination in the gray matter. Within the gray matter the dotted lines show the laminar pattern, while within the white matter they are an approximate guide to the topography of the tracts. *Source: Figure 18.18 from Gray's Anatomy.*

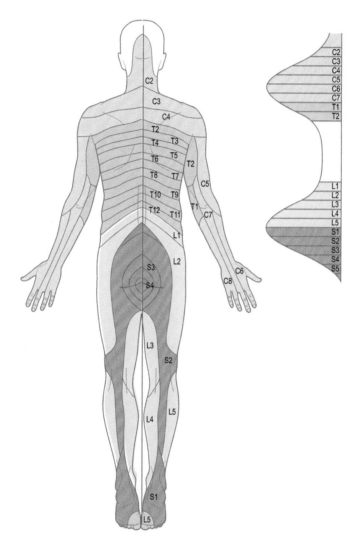

FIGURE A.14 **Dermatomes on the dorsal surface of the body.** The small diagram shows the regular arrangement of dermatomes in the upper and lower limbs of the embryo. *Source: Figure 42.3 from Gray's Anatomy.*

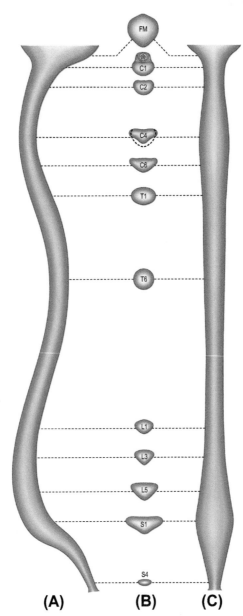

FIGURE A.15   **The vertebral canal.** In section: (A) sagittal; (B) transverse (axial); (C) coronal. FM: foramen magnum. *Source: Figure 42.16 from Gray's Anatomy.*

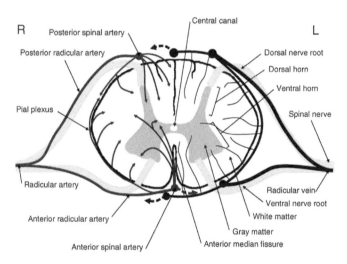

FIGURE A.16 **Vasculature of the human spinal cord.** For clarity reasons, arteries are drawn only on the right side of the cord, veins only on the left. *Source: Reproduced with permission from Giove et al. (2004) Magn Reson Imaging, 22 1505–1516.*

Index

Printed and bound by CPI Group (UK) Ltd, Croydon, CR0 4YY

08/05/2025

01865034-0001